S0-BBH-094

Middle Range Theories

APPLICATION TO NURSING RESEARCH

Middle Range Theories

APPLICATION TO NURSING RESEARCH

2nd Edition

Sandra J. Peterson, PhD, RN

Professor and Department Chair

Bethel University

St. Paul, Minnesota

Timothy S. Bredow, PhD, RN

Professor

Bethel University

St. Paul, Minnesota

Wolters Kluwer | Lippincott Williams & Wilkins
Health

Philadelphia · Baltimore · New York · London
Buenos Aires · Hong Kong · Sydney · Tokyo

Senior Acquisitions Editor: Margaret Zuccarini
Managing Editor: Michelle Clarke
Editorial Assistant: Brandi Spade
Production Project Manager: Cynthia Rudy
Director of Nursing Production: Helen Ewan

Senior Managing Editor/Production: Erika Kors
Design Coordinator: Joan Wendt
Manufacturing Coordinator: Karin Duffield
Production Services/Compositor: Aptara, Inc.

2nd edition

Copyright © 2009 Wolters Kluwer Health | Lippincott Williams & Wilkins.

Copyright © 2004 by Lippincott Williams & Wilkins. All rights reserved. This book is protected by copyright. No part of this book may be reproduced or transmitted in any form or by any means, including as photocopies or scanned-in or other electronic copies, or utilized by any information storage and retrieval system without written permission from the copyright owner, except for brief quotations embodied in critical articles and reviews. Materials appearing in this book prepared by individuals as part of their official duties as U.S. government employees are not covered by the above-mentioned copyright. To request permission, please contact Lippincott Williams & Wilkins at 530 Walnut Street, Philadelphia, PA 19106, via email at permissions@lww.com, or via our website at lww.com (products and services).

9 8 7 6 5 4

Printed in the United States of America

Library of Congress Cataloging-in-Publication Data

Middle range theories : application to nursing research / [edited by] Sandra J. Peterson, Timothy S. Bredow. – 2nd ed.
    p. ; cm.
  Includes bibliographical references and index.
  ISBN-13: 978-0-7817-8562-4 (alk. paper)
  ISBN-10: 0-7817-8562-6 (alk. paper)
  1. Nursing—Philosophy. 2. Nursing–Research. 3. Nursing. I. Peterson, Sandra J. II. Bredow, Timothy S.
  [DNLM: 1. Nursing Theory. 2. Nursing Research. WY 86 M6269 2009]
  RT84.5.M535 2009
  610.7301–dc22

                                                         2007047700

Care has been taken to confirm the accuracy of the information presented and to describe generally accepted practices. However, the authors, editors, and publisher are not responsible for errors or omissions or for any consequences from application of the information in this book and make no warranty, expressed or implied, with respect to the currency, completeness, or accuracy of the contents of the publication. Application of this information in a particular situation remains the professional responsibility of the practitioner; the clinical treatments described and recommended may not be considered absolute and universal recommendations.

The authors, editors, and publisher have exerted every effort to ensure that drug selection and dosage set forth in this text are in accordance with the current recommendations and practice at the time of publication. However, in view of ongoing research, changes in government regulations, and the constant flow of information relating to drug therapy and drug reactions, the reader is urged to check the package insert for each drug for any change in indications and dosage and for added warnings and precautions. This is particularly important when the recommended agent is a new or infrequently employed drug.

Some drugs and medical devices presented in this publication have Food and Drug Administration (FDA) clearance for limited use in restricted research settings. It is the responsibility of the health care provider to ascertain the FDA status of each drug or device planned for use in his or her clinical practice.

LWW.com

DRC0910

My special thanks to my husband, Ray, and my mother,
Margaret Cairns. My fan club of two members
is much appreciated.

Sandra J. Peterson

My appreciation is extended to my wife, Kate Bredow.
She is my life companion, best friend,
confidant, and constructive critic.

Timothy S. Bredow

Contributors

Georgene Gaskill Eakes, RN, MSN, EdD
Retired from School of Nursing
East Carolina University
Greenville, North Carolina

Audrey G. Gift, PhD, RN, FAAN
Professor Emeritus of Nursing
Michigan State University
East Lansing, Michigan

Marion Good, PhD, RN, FAAN
Arline H. and Curtis F. Gavin
Professor of Nursing Excellence
Frances Payne Bolton
School of Nursing
Case Western Reserve University
Cleveland, Ohio

Joan E. Haase, PhD, RN, FAAN
Emily Holmquist Professor,
School of Nursing
Indiana University
Indianapolis, Indiana

Sonya Hardin, PhD, RN, CCRN
Associate Professor, School of Nursing
University of North Carolina at Charlotte
Charlotte, North Carolina

Katherine Kolcaba, PhD, RN
Associate Professor Emeritus
College of Nursing
The University of Akron
Akron, Ohio

Marjorie McCullagh, PhD, RN
Associate Professor
North Dakota State University
Fargo, North Dakota

Mertie Potter, DNP, ARNP, BC
Nurse Consultant/Nurse Practitioner
Concord, New Hampshire

Barbara Resnick, PhD, CRNP, FAAN, FAANP
Sonya Gershowitz Chair in Gerontology
University of Maryland
Baltimore, Maryland

Kristin E. Sandau, PhD, RN
Associate Professor
Bethel University
St. Paul, Minnesota

Marjorie A. Schaffer, PhD, RN
Professor
Bethel University
St. Paul, Minnesota

Ellen D. Schultz, PhD, RN, CHTP
Professor, College of Nursing and
Health Sciences
Metropolitan State University
St. Paul, Minnesota

Danuta Wojnar, RN, PhD
Assistant Professor
College of Nursing
Seattle University
Seattle, Washington

Reviewers

Nagia S. Ali, PhD, RN
Professor, School of Nursing
Ball State University
Muncie, Indiana

Cynthia Arslanian-Engoren,
PhD, MSN, RN, CNS
Assistant Professor, School of Nursing
University of Michigan
Ann Arbor, Michigan

Jo Azzarello, PhD, RN
Assistant Professor, College of Nursing
University of Oklahoma
Oklahoma City, Oklahoma

Dot Baker, RN, MS(N), CS, EdD
Associate Professor
Wilmington College
Georgetown, Delaware

Lynne Bryant, PhD, RN
Assistant Professor, Beth-El College of
Nursing and Health Sciences
University of Colorado, Colorado Springs
Colorado Springs, Colorado

Alexander M. Clark, PhD, BA, RN
Assistant Professor
University of Alberta
Edmonton, Alberta

Judith A. Cohen, PhD, RN
Professor
University of Vermont
Burlington, Vermont

Sarah C. Fogel, PhD, RN
Assistant Professor
Vanderbilt University
Nashville, Tennessee

Linda Holbrook Freeman, RN, DNS
Professor, School of Nursing
University of Louisville
Louisville, Kentucky

Margit B. Gerardi
Clinical Instructor
UTHSCSA (Graduate School), Webster University
San Antonio, Texas

Angela Gillis, PhD, RN
Professor, School of Nursing
St. Francis Xavier University
Antigonish, Nova Scotia

Melanie Kalman, PhD, CNS
Associate Professor
SUNY Upstate Medical University
Syracuse, New York

Vicky P. Kent, PhD, RN, CNE
Clinical Associate Professor
Towson University
Towson, Maryland

Katherine Kolcaba, PhD, RN, C
Associate Professor Emeritus,
College of Nursing
The University of Akron, Akron, Ohio

Joan C. Masters, MA, MBA, RN
Assistant Professor
Bellarmine University
Louisville, Kentucky

Magdalena A. Mateo,
PhD, RN, FAAN
Associate Professor, Nursing
Northeastern University
Boston, Massachusetts

Patricia A. McCarthy, PhD, RN, CNS
Professor, Department of Nursing
Youngstown State University
Youngstown, Ohio

Nancy McGowan, RH, PhD, CEN
Assistant Professor
University of Texas Health Science Center,
San Antonio
San Antonio, Texas

Mitzi Grace Mitchell
Lecturer, School of Nursing
York University
Toronto, Ontario

Lorrie L. Powel, PhD, RN
Associate Professor, School of Nursing
University of Florida
Orlando, Florida

Jane E. Ransom, PhD, MSN, BSN, RN
Associate Professor, College of Nursing
University of Toledo
Toledo, Ohio

Loretta M. Reinhart, PhD, RN
Dean and Professor
Malone College
Canton, Ohio

Katherine Morton Robinson,
PhD, RN, CCNS
Associate Professor, School of Nursing
University of North Florida
Jacksonville, Florida

Beth L. Rogers, PhD, RN, FAAN
Professor, College of Nursing
University of Wisconsin–Milwaukee
Milwaukee, Wisconsin

Phyllis Skorga, PhD, RN, CCM
Professor and Director, College of Nursing
and Health Professions
Arkansas State University
Jonesboro, Arkansas

Ida L. Slusher, RN, DSN
Professor
Eastern Kentucky University
Richmond, Kentucky

Sandra Talley, PhD, APRN, BC, FAAN
Associate Professor and Director of
Psychiatric Mental Health Nursing
Yale University
New Haven, Connecticut

Michele J. Upvall, PhD, RN, FNP
Associate Dean and Director
Carlow University
Pittsburgh, Pennsylvania

Teresa Walsh, PhD, RN
Assistant Professor, College of Nursing
Texas Woman's University
Houston, Texas

Jane H. White, PhD, APRN, BC
Professor of Nursing, Associate Dean for
Research, Director of Graduate Programs
Adelphia University
Garden City, New York

Barbara Wilder, DSN, CRNP
Associate Professor, School of Nursing
Auburn University
Auburn, Alabama

Meg Wilson, PhD, RN
Professor, Department of Nursing
University of Saint Francis
Fort Wayne, Indiana

Diane Young, PhD, CNE, RN
Professor
Allen College
Waterloo, Iowa

Preface

Several authors have expressed the perspective that middle range theories are the preferred direction for knowledge development in the discipline of nursing (Blegen & Tripp-Reimer, 1997; Lenz, 1998; Liehr & Smith, 1999). "Middle range theory will create the disciplinary fabric of the new millennium as nurse theorists spin and twist fibers from the past-present into the future" (Liehr & Smith, 1999, The future: Where does nursing theory go from here?, para. 3). The prediction of the emergence of middle range theory as a major contribution of nurse scholars to the profession of nursing is becoming a reality. With increasing frequency, middle range theories are being both generated and tested through practice-oriented nursing research.

The second edition of *Middle Range Theories: Application to Nursing Research* attempts to meet the same needs as that of the first edition. We hope that this edition serves as a resource for nurse scholars, making middle range theories more accessible for their research and practice. Critical Thinking Exercises have been added to this edition, which serve to expand the focus of the book to include applications to practice.

As the number of middle range theories increases, selecting the ones to include in the book becomes increasingly difficult. As for the previous edition, we reviewed published research, identified the theories most frequently cited, and then attempted to enlist authors who had used the theories in their research or practice. That process resulted in the addition of two middle range theories, Theory of Synergy, promoted by the American Association of Critical Care Nurses, and Theory of Caring, developed by Kristin Swanson.

ORGANIZATION

Part I

Part I is devoted to an overview of the state of nursing's body of knowledge. In this edition there is a brief discussion of epistemology, with a summary of Carper's conceptualization of nurses' ways of knowing. Chapter 1 considers the hierarchy of nursing knowledge and particularly the place of middle range theory within that hierarchy (i.e., paradigm, philosophy, conceptual framework, and theories). For each component of the hierarchy, the chapter includes a description of its nature, a review of its development, a discussion of its contributions to nursing knowledge, consideration of controversies related to its nature or use, and examples of nurse scholars' work. The section devoted to middle range theories includes a table referencing multiple examples of middle range theories. Chapter 2 emphasizes the analysis and evaluation of middle range theories, including issues to consider in the selection of a middle range nursing theory for research purposes. This chapter also describes a brief evaluative process that is used as a feature throughout the rest of the chapters. Using this evaluation process, readers can compare and contrast their conclusions about the theory as presented in the chapter with those of a nurse scholar who has also used this evaluation process.

Parts II to VI

Parts II to VI are devoted to specific middle range theories. The selected theories are labeled by their developers or by nurse scholars as middle range theories and are the ones most frequently cited in published nursing research. Many of the chapters contain unique nursing theories; some are borrowed from related disciplines but are, nonetheless, useful to nursing. All theories in the text, however, have the intrinsic capability to be applied to nursing research and practice and address a wide range of phenomena that allow the researcher to consider a variety of nursing research questions. The theories have been organized by categories to reflect the type of research questions or practice applications that could most likely be considered. The categories are not presented as absolute, but more as a guide to direct users of the book to the theories that might be most relevant to their issue of interest.

- Physiological—Pain: A Balance Between Analgesia and Side Effects; Unpleasant Symptoms; Synergy Model
- Cognitive—Self-Efficacy
- Emotional—Chronic Sorrow
- Social—Social Support, Caring, Interpersonal Relations
- Integrative—Modeling and Role-Modeling, Comfort, Health-Related Quality of Life, Health Promotion, Deliberative Nursing Process, Resilience

SPECIAL FEATURES

Each theory chapter provides the nurse researcher with a variety of tools, updated from the first edition. In addition to those features included in the previous edition, Critical Thinking Exercises have been included at the end of each chapter.

- **Definition of Key Terms:** appears at the beginning of each chapter; provides conceptual definitions to aid students' understanding of the theory
- **Using Middle Range Theories:** provides examples of how the theory has been used in published research
- **Research Application:** provides a sample application of the theory, modeling the research process
- **Analysis of Theory:** appears at the end of each chapter; allows readers to arrive at their own conclusions about the theory and then compare them to a nurse scholar's evaluation, found in Appendix A
- **Critical Thinking Exercises:** engage readers in analysis of the theory and its application to practice
- **Web Resources:** guide readers to valuable web sites to aid them in their research
- **Instruments:** discussed in the chapters, with specific examples found in Appendix B

Many chapters also contain an extensive bibliography that provides additional references for the development of a review of the literature.

We hope this text provides the readers with the background to appreciate the relationship between nursing theory, research, and practice, and the specific content to enable them to make use of this background in their scholarly work. We also hope the book promotes a sense of excitement about and commitment to the development of nursing's body of knowledge.

REFERENCES

Blegen, M. A., & Tripp-Reimer, T. T. (1997). Implications of nursing taxonomies for middle-range theory development. *Advances in Nursing Science, 19*(3), 37(3). Retrieved December 14, 1999, from http://web7.infotrac. galegroup.

Lenz, E. R. (1998). Role of middle range theory for nursing research and practice. Part 1. Nursing research. *Nursing Leadership Forum, 3*(2), 24–33.

Liehr, P., & Smith, M. J. (1999). Middle range theory: Spinning research and practice to create knowledge for the new millennium. *Advances in Nursing Science, 21*(4), 8–91. Retrieved June 11, 2002, from CINAHL/Ovid database.

Acknowledgments

There is a sense of accomplishment that accompanies the completion of a project such as this text. We would have never been able to experience that rather pleasant sensation without the significant involvement of many others. The quality of the scholarship of the chapter authors will be evident to all those who read the text. Their willingness to invest themselves in this project, consistently providing what was needed in a timely fashion, is much appreciated. Those who completed the Analysis of Theory, found in Appendix A of the book, have added what we believe will be a useful resource to readers, enabling them to clarify their understanding of the theories.

The staff at Lippincott Williams & Wilkins was invaluable. Margaret Zuccarini, Senior Acquisitions Editor, continued to see this book as a contribution to the body of nursing literature and helped us launch this project. Michelle Clarke, Managing Editor, guided us through the publication process of this second edition. And finally, we are profoundly grateful for the forbearance of our family and friends (especially husband, Ray Peterson, and wife, Kate Bredow). They helped us have "lives" beyond the scope of completing this book.

Contents

PART V   Middle Range Theories: Social   161

PART VI   Middle Range Theories: Integrative   231

Overview of Theory

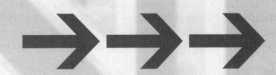

Introduction to the Nature of Nursing Knowledge

■ SANDRA J. PETERSON

DEFINITION OF KEY TERMS

Concept	Symbolic representation of a phenomenon or set of phenomena
Conceptual model	"Set of abstract and general concepts and the propositions" (Fawcett, 1997, pp. 13–14) that represents a phenomenon of interest
Deduction	Reasoning from the general or universal to the particular or specific
Discipline	A field or branch of knowledge that involves research
Domain	Related components or items that reflect the unified subject matter of a discipline
Empiricism	A philosophical theory of knowledge acquisition through experience, observation, and experiment
Ethics	A branch of philosophy concerned with moral principles
Epistemology	A branch of philosophy concerned with the sources of knowledge of truth and the methods used to acquire it
Induction	Reasoning from the individual or particular to the general or universal
Logic	A branch of philosophy concerned with sound reasoning and validity of thought
Logical positivism	Philosophical perspective that espouses logic, objectivity, falseness/truth, observable and operationally defined concepts, and prediction
Metaparadigm	Global concepts specific to a discipline that are philosophically neutral and stable

(Key Terms continued on next page)

DEFINITION OF KEY TERMS continued

Metaphysics	A branch of philosophy concerned with the study of ultimate cause and underlying nature of that which exists
Metatheory	A philosophical theory about theories, concerned with "logical and methodological foundations of a discipline" (Beckstrand, 1986, p. 503). Examines "how theory affects and is affected by research and practice within nursing, and philosophy and politics outside nursing" (McKenna, 1997, p. 92)
Ontology	Examination of the nature of being or reality
Paradigm	A worldview, a common philosophical orientation, that serves to define the nature of a discipline
Phenomenon	A designation of an aspect of reality
Philosophy	(a) A set of beliefs or values; (b) science concerned with the study of reality and the nature of being. Composed of but not limited to aesthetics, epistemology, ethics, logic, and metaphysics
Science	A systematized body of knowledge that has as its main purpose the discovery of "truths about the world" (Jacox, 1974, p. 4), confirmed through empirical investigation
Theory	"Set of interrelated concepts, based on assumption, woven together through a set of propositional statements" (Fitzpatrick, 1997, p. 37) used to provide a perspective on reality

INTRODUCTION

What is knowledge? Attempts to answer that question have been primarily the domain of the branch of philosophy referred to as epistemology. Traditionally knowledge has been defined as a belief that was justified as true with absolute certainty. This definition requires that for knowledge to exist it must be believed; if not believed, something cannot be known. It also must be true; if not true, even if well justified and believed, it cannot be considered knowledge. Finally, there must be sound reasons for the belief; if there are no sound reasons for a belief, it would be more a probable opinion or lucky guess than knowledge. There is not universal agreement about the nature of a sound reason or adequate evidence for a belief.

There are multiple epistemological theories to describe the nature of knowledge and explain its sources, or how something can be known. Examples of epistemological theories include idealism, pragmatism, rationalism, and relativism. The theory of empiricism, most closely associated with natural science, considers knowledge to be a result of human experience. Ideas and theories can then be tested against reality and accepted or rejected on the basis of how well they are congruent with observable facts.

The traditional ideas about the nature of knowledge are being challenged on an ongoing basis. Edmund Gettier in the 1960s proposed several cases in which a person had a sound justification to believe that something was true; it was true, but for reasons other than those believed. The issue then is the nature of the justification of a belief. The two contemporary approaches to consideration of that issue are foundationalism and coherentism. Foundationalism identifies basic beliefs as the justification for a belief. A belief is basic if it is self-evident, providing support for other beliefs. Coherentism rejects the notion of basic beliefs as a form of justification. Instead, this theory of justification claims that it is the interrelationship of a set of beliefs that supports the truth of a belief.

Nurses obviously need knowledge to practice. This discussion of the nature of knowledge is clearly basic but establishes a foundation for consideration of nursing knowledge and the roles that theory and research play in its development.

NURSING KNOWLEDGE

Nurses are fundamentally "knowledge workers" in that they synthesize "a broad array of information and knowledge from a wide variety of sources and bring that synthesis to bear on nursing work" (Porter-O'Grady, 2003, para. 2). The knowledge that nurses need to practice has been conceptualized by Carper (1978) as four distinct patterns: (a) empirics, the science of nursing; (b) aesthetics, the art of nursing; (c) personal knowing, the intra- and interpersonal nature of nursing; and (d) ethics, the moral component of nursing.

Empirical knowing is positivistic science, which means that it is logically determined and based on observable phenomenon. It is knowledge that is systematically organized into general laws and theories that serve to describe, explain, and/or predict the phenomena of interest to nursing (Carper, 1978). The sources of empirical knowledge are research and theory and model development. There is no coherent conceptual structure that is generally accepted as nursing's scientific paradigm, which can lead to the possibility of a confusing and sometimes conflicting knowledge base. For the practicing nurse empirical knowledge must always be interpreted within the context of specific clinical situations.

Aesthetic knowing is a process of "perceiving or grasping the nature of a clinical situation; interpreting this information in order to understand its meaning for those involved, while envisioning desired outcomes in order to respond with appropriate skilled action; and subsequently reflecting on whether the outcomes were effectively achieved" (Johns, 1995, Aesthetics, para. 1). Aesthetic knowing comes from the nurse's ability to grasp and interpret the meaning of a situation. It makes use of the nurse's intuition and empathy. This type of knowing also involves the nurse's skills in imagining a desired and practical outcome in the actual situation and responding based on an interpretation of the whole situation, analyzing the interrelationships of its various aspects. Unfortunately, aesthetic knowing cannot be articulated; it is not transferable to others. It is based solely on the skill of the nurse in a specific situation. This type of knowing has also been criticized for the role of empathy in nursing knowledge acquisition. White (2004) claims that empathy is a psychological phenomenon that has been uncritically adopted by nursing.

Personal knowing is knowledge of the concrete, individual self; it is not knowledge about the self. It involves encountering and actualization of the self in a way that enables the nurse to transcend the notion of other individuals as objects but instead to engage with others in authentic personal relationships. The type of knowing and the nature of these relationships result in an increasing willingness to accept ambiguity, vagueness, and discrepancy in oneself and others. Personal knowing is the basis of the therapeutic use of self in the nurse–patient relationship. Reflection is the primary means by which personal knowing occurs. It involves three interrelated factors:

1. Perceiving the self's feelings and prejudices within the situation
2. Managing the self's feelings and prejudices in order to respond appropriately (to the other)
3. Managing anxiety and sustaining the self (Johns, 1995, The Personal Way of Knowing, para. 2).

Like aesthetic knowing, personal knowing cannot be described; it can only be actualized. In order to escape the problem of self-delusion, there is a need for individual reflection that is informed by the responses of others. But data about self from others can also be problematic in that it can be misperceived. In addition, personal knowing presents the nurse with a dilemma; personal knowledge needs to be integrated or reconciled with the professional responsibility of the nurse to manipulate the environment in order to work toward a desired health outcome (Carper, 1978, p. 19). Personal knowing of all the ways of knowing is the most difficult to teach and to master (White, 2004, p. 253).

Ethical knowing is knowledge of what is right or wrong and the commitment to act on the basis of that knowledge. It involves "judgments of moral value in relation to motives, intentions and traits of character" (Carper, 1978, p. 20) and focuses on obligations, on what ought to be done related to those judgments. Sources of ethical knowledge include nursing's ethical codes and professional standards. It is also important for the nurse to have an understanding of different philosophical positions as to what is considered good and what is identified as an obligation. Consideration of the philosophical positions can also create confusion since ethical theories of what is good and what constitutes an obligation can conflict. For instance, the teleological perceptive considers what is good on the basis of its production of the greatest good for the greatest number (consequentialism), whereas the deontological perspective identifies good not by the consequences of actions, but by the nature of the actions themselves.

Each of the ways of knowing represents a necessary but incomplete representation of the discipline of nursing. There is also an inherent interrelationship between the four patterns. For instance, aesthetic knowing would require empirical knowledge in order to envision what the desired and practical outcomes in a situation might be and what would constitute valid means of helping to bring about that desired outcome. With an acknowledgement of the contributions of all the ways of knowing to the practice of nursing, this book focuses on empirical knowing and on nursing theories, especially those that are considered middle range.

Two claims can be made about the state of empirical knowledge in nursing: (a) it exists in varying degrees of abstraction, and (b) it is characterized by a lack of consistency in the use of its language. Fawcett (2005) recommends what she refers to as a structural "holarchy" of contemporary nursing knowledge to establish the relationships between the various components that comprise nursing's body of knowledge. The components are arranged from most abstract to most concrete in the following order: metaparadigm, philosophy/paradigm, conceptual model, and theories. The types of theories available to nurses also exist on a continuum from most abstract to most concrete, with grand theories identified as most abstract, practice theories as most concrete, and middle range theories in the logical middle.

There are few components in the hierarchy that appear consistently in the literature with a single label. The terms *conceptual models, conceptual frameworks,* and *theories* are sometimes used interchangeably. The terms *grand theory, macro theory,* and *general theory* all refer to the same level of theory development.

This chapter addresses each component of the conceptual hierarchy, with special emphasis on middle range theories. The nature of the component, its development, its contributions to nursing's body of knowledge, and the debates engaged in by nurses in relation to the component are considered.

PHILOSOPHY

In the nursing literature, the term *philosophy* is used in two distinct ways: as a unique discipline and as a set of beliefs of a separate discipline (e.g., nursing). As a discipline, it is often defined by its main branches: metaphysics, epistemology, ethics, logic, and aesthetics. Well into the 19th century, the classical Greek thought persisted that philosophy represented humanity's total knowledge (Silva, 1997). The scientific revolution, ushered in by a knowledge explosion related to new thinking about survival of species, cause of disease, nature of matter and energy, and the workings of the human mind, came with new ways of knowing and forms of inquiry. This revolution also resulted in new ways of thinking about philosophy and science. Philosophy is concerned with the nature of being, the meaning and purpose of life, and the theory and limits of knowledge, whereas science is more concerned with causality (Silva, 1997). Philosophy is considered discursive, noninvestigative, and dependent on common experience, contrasting with science, which is considered investigative and dependent on special experience (Simmons, 1992, pp. 16–17).

For a discipline, philosophies represent its beliefs and values, and its mindset or worldview. "Nursing philosophy is a statement of foundational and universal assumptions, beliefs, and principles about the nature of knowledge and truth (epistemology)" (Reed, 1995, Nursing Philosophy: Metaparadigms for Knowledge Development, para. 1). Like other disciplines, nursing has reflected and is reflecting the modern, postmodern, and some would include neomodern thinking, or worldview of its time.

Development

Philosophies emerge as a reflection on the issues of interest to philosophers, primarily logic, ethics, aesthetics, metaphysics, and epistemology. In the 20th and 21st centuries, these reflections or philosophies have been often characterized as either modern or postmodern perspectives. Although modernism and postmodernism do not represent singular philosophies but, rather, a collection of philosophies (Burbules, n.d., para. 2), each possesses commonly occurring themes that can serve as points of contrast. The most basic comparison between the schools of thinking is in their perspectives on metanarratives, defined as efforts to offer "general and encompassing accounts of truth, value, and reality" (Burbules, n.d., para. 5). In modernism, the metanarratives are a primary concern. In postmodernism, metanarratives are dismissed. This dismissal is not necessarily rejection or denial, but instead doubt and uncertainty about what metanarratives have to offer. These schools of thought also differ in their view of the nature of problems. In modern thinking, problems are to be solved. In postmodern thinking, they are to be deconstructed, requiring a disassembling of the metanarratives that are entangled in values and beliefs that fail to reveal reality or liberate the oppressed (Reed, 1995, Historical Background: Modernism and Postmodernism, para. 3). Reed (1995) also identifies distinctions in epistemology: modernism, concerned with the truth of findings, and postmodernism, concerned with the usefulness of findings. She also suggests a neomodernism perspective, which rejects modernism's logical positivism and postmodernism's radical relativism and lack of coherent vision to focus instead on a plurality of realistic visions of a possible future (Bisk, n.d.). Reed's neomodern perspective for nursing embraces the metanarratives of health and the processes of healing but integrates them with the postmodern assumptions that knowledge is value laden and that context is critical in order to achieve the desired future.

Within these schools of thought—modern, postmodern, and neomodern—a variety of philosophies or philosophical schemes have been used to describe the nature of nursing. Adam (1992) identified the following: (a) Socratic—know self; (b) realism—be self; (c) humanism—give self; (d) rationalism—understand self; (e) naturalism—describe self; (f) pragmatism—prove self; (g) idealism—imagine self; and (h) existentialism—choose self (p. 56).

Another schema, proposed by Lerner (1986), which considered the nature of human development, is useful in categorizing nursing philosophies. Three worldviews of most interest are:

1. Mechanistic, in which the machine is the metaphor for the human being. The whole is equal to the sum of the parts, and the goal is a return to equilibrium.
2. Organistic, in which a biologic organism composed of complex interrelated parts is the basic metaphor. The organism is active in a passive environment. Change is probable, goal directed, and developmental.
3. Developmental–contextual, in which historical events are the metaphor. The individual is immersed in a dynamic context. Change in the person and the environment is ongoing, irreversible, innovative, and developmental. Chaos and conflict are an energy source for change (Reed, 1995).

Uses

Phillips (1992) claims that "without an understanding of philosophy in nursing there can be no science of nursing" (p. 45). The branches of philosophy suggest a set of questions with relevance to nursing. For instance, ethical nursing questions would be concerned with what is good to do and to seek to attain nursing's goals (Kikuchi, 1992). Epistemological questions would focus on the structure, scope, and reliability of nursing's knowledge, and ontological questions would relate to the meaning of nurses' and clients' realities (Silva, Sorrell, & Sorrell, 1995). But these important questions are ones that are best addressed through philosophical inquiry.

The contribution the branches of philosophy make to nursing knowledge is more directly related to research methods than to the nature of the questions generated. Research requires logic in the use of the research process, with a logical progression from problem identification and hypotheses, to methods, and finally to data analyses and conclusions (Silva, 1997). Epistemology leads nurse researchers to consider the nature of not only evidence obtained through research, but also truth and belief. Metaphysics addresses causality, an important issue for nurse researchers. Ethics are of concern to nurse researchers as they consider the ethical implications of research problems, research methods, and dissemination of the research findings.

Philosophy, theory, and research are inextricably linked. "All nursing theory or research derives from or leads to philosophy" (Phillips, 1992, p. 49). Philosophy makes a significant contribution to the development of nursing theories. The conceptual clarification specified by the philosopher of science helps the theorist generate better theories, and the speculation engaged in by the philosopher of science can also suggest the theories of the future (Smart, 1968, p. 17). Analysis of a theory reveals the underlying assumptions and worldview (philosophy). By considering these philosophical statements, nurses can determine the fit between the values and beliefs expressed through the theory and their own. This enables researchers and practitioners to select theories that are philosophically congruent with their own perspectives on nursing. Therefore, philosophy plays a critical role in the formulation of questions important to nursing, the consideration of research methods, and the development of theories and their analysis and use in practice.

Controversy

The controversy about nursing philosophy centers on the belief systems that exist within the discipline of nursing and the relative value of unity or diversity in nursing thought. Roach (1992) argues that philosophical inquiry in nursing is the pursuit of universal, transcendent principles and suggests metaphysics as the basis for nursing's unity. Others refer to this search for a coherent philosophical foundation in nursing as a pursuit of unity in diversity of thought (Newman, 2002; Phillips, 1992). The diversity of perspectives represented in the variety of existing nursing models requires philosophical inquiry as a means of determining underlying philosophical themes and patterns. This search for the unitary nature of phenomena of concern to nursing will lead to the recognition of core beliefs:

- A holistic view of persons (Phillips, 1992; Roach, 1992)
- A commitment to caring as an expression of the human mode of being (Newman, Sime, & Corcoran-Perry, 1996; Roach, 1992)
- A perspective on education that acknowledges the unity of mind–body–spirit and recognition of the universe of knowledge that is necessary to achieve and makes a contribution to human understanding (Roach, 1992)
- A view of humans in relationship, with awareness of ethical–moral bonds (Roach, 1992)

Though diversity may result in confusion and lack of clarity in nursing's theory development and research agenda, others believe that a philosophy that represents the worldview of all nurse scientists would be diluted to the point of becoming meaningless and useless (Landreneau, 2002). Diversity of philosophies may be viewed as a more accurate representation of reality, a perspective consistent with postmodern thinking, and may have the potential of stimulating greater creativity and variety in the development of nursing models and theories.

PARADIGMS AND METAPARADIGM

The terms *paradigm* and *metaparadigm* are frequently found in the nursing literature. Paradigms provide the basic parameters and framework for organizing a discipline's knowledge. Similar to philosophies, they are an abstract means of expressing that knowledge. Paradigms generally are considered to be discipline specific, philosophical, and mutable. The metaparadigm of a discipline is distinguished from a paradigm in that the metaparadigm is global, philosophically neutral, and fairly stable.

Paradigms

Kuhn introduced the term *paradigm* and stimulated interest in its use as a method of defining and analyzing the nature of a discipline. He also acknowledged the existence of multiple and conflicting definitions of the term (Kuhn, 1977, p. 294). Kuhn (1996) included the following as the components of paradigms or, as he later referred to them, disciplinary matrices: (a) symbolic generalizations, the laws accepted by a scientific community and the language used to express them; (b) shared commitments to beliefs in particular models, shared beliefs about and commitment to the prevailing theories of the discipline and the motivation and methods used to create and test them; (c) values, shared values that serve to identify what is significant or meaningful to the scientific community; and (d) exemplars, the specific problems to be solved and the methods used to solve them. Guba (1990) suggested a means of differentiating paradigms. Paradigms can be distinguished by the answers to three questions:

1. *Ontological:* What is the nature of the "knowable"? Or, what is the nature of "reality"?
2. *Epistemological:* What is the nature of the relationship between the knower (the inquirer) and the known (or knowable)?
3. *Methodological:* How should the inquirer go about finding out knowledge (p. 18)?

The components identified by Kuhn and the answers to the questions posed by Guba express the nature of existing paradigms. Before a paradigm is identified, the facts generated by the discipline and the methods used to generate them are disorganized. The discipline is considered to be in a pre-paradigm stage of development.

DEVELOPMENT

Paradigms emerge when they are recognized as a dominant way of thinking about the discipline by its scientific community. Kuhn (1996) refers to the emergence of a new paradigm as a revolution in which the new paradigm replaces an older one. "Scientific revolutions are inaugurated by a growing sense, again often restricted to a narrow subdivision of the scientific community, that an existing paradigm has ceased to function adequately in the exploration of an aspect of nature to which that paradigm itself had previously led the way" (Kuhn, 1996, p. 92).

Shapere (1980) criticized the notion of revolution, noting that scientific advances can be cumulative in that later sciences build on that which was earlier. This is a more evolutionary perspective on paradigm development. Integration has also been proposed as a form of paradigm development. This form of paradigm development describes a pattern in progress that is created "through accommodation, refinement, and collaboration between thoughts, ideas, and individuals" (Meleis, 1997, p. 80). Meleis believes paradigm development in nursing is characterized by this approach.

There are multiple paradigms and systems of classifying the paradigms used to express the worldview of the discipline of nursing. Stevens-Barnum (1998) suggests a paradigm that focuses on nursing action that is composed of intervention, conservation, substitution, sustenance/support, and enhancement. Newman, Sime, and Corcoran-Perry (1991) describe three existing paradigms that provide different perspectives on the phenomena of caring and health, identified as the concepts most central to nursing: particulate–deterministic, interactive–integrative, and unitary–transformative. In the particulate–deterministic paradigm, phenomena exist as separate entities, possess properties that can be measured, and relate to each other in predictable and linear ways. Knowledge is identified in terms of facts and universal laws. The interactive–integrative paradigm, an extension of the particulate–deterministic paradigm, considers context and experience from subjective perspectives as a means of understanding the intrarelated nature of the properties of phenomena and the reciprocal interrelated nature that exists among phenomena. This paradigm is concerned with probabilistic predictability of interactive–integrative phenomena. The unitary–transformative paradigm is quite distinct, emphasizing the unitary and self-organizing nature of phenomena that exist in a larger but also self-organizing field. Knowledge is derived from both the mutuality that exists between phenomena and those who are observing them and focuses on the personal nature of knowledge and pattern recognition.

The classification of nursing paradigms proposed by Parse (1987) is the one most frequently cited in nursing literature. Parse identifies two distinct paradigms that describe the relationship between persons and their environments as they relate to health: totality and simultaneity. In the totality paradigm "man is considered a bio-psycho-socio-spiritual organism whose environment can be manipulated to maintain or promote balance" (Parse, 1987, p. 32) and health is viewed as a dynamic state and process of well-being. The goals of nursing are health promotion, illness prevention, and care and cure of the sick. Research from this paradigmatic perspective would be quantitative. In the simultaneity paradigm man is greater than the sum of parts, a self-initiating being in rhythmical interchanges with environments, living in the "relative Now experiencing what was, is, and will be, all at once" (Parse, 1987, p. 136). Health is the process of becoming, which can be experienced and described only by the individual.

"There is no optimum health; health is simply how one is experiencing personal living" (Parse, 1987, p. 136). The goal of nursing in this paradigm is to illuminate meaning and move beyond the immediate or present to changing patterns of health with the person and family. The nurse is considered a guide and the other is the decision maker. Research conducted from this paradigmatic perspective is qualitative in nature.

There are a number of similarities in the paradigms proposed by Newman et al. and Parse, with the particulate–deterministic paradigm sharing features in common with the totality paradigm, and the unitary–transformative paradigm similar to the simultaneity paradigm. There are a number of other classifications of paradigms identified in the literature to describe actual or preferred perspectives of nursing. Many seem to be a renaming of or very similar to the conceptualizations of previously identified paradigms, particularly Parse's. For instance, Monti and Tingen (1999) suggest empiricism and interpretative; Guiliano, Tyer-Viola, and Lopez (2005) identify received view and perceived view; Weaver and Olson (2006) propose positivism/postpositivism and interpretive; and Pilkington and Mitchell (1999, 2003) refer to natural science and human science. A summary of three of the major paradigms is found in Table 1.1.

Table 1.1 EXAMPLES OF NURSING'S PARADIGMATIC SCHEMES

AUTHOR	CATEGORIZATION OF PERSPECTIVES
Parse (1987)	• *Totality*. Man is a total, summative organism, comprised of bio-psycho-social-spiritual features. The environment is a source of external and internal stimuli to which Man m adapt in order to maintain balance and achieve g • *Simultaneity*. Man is a unitary being in continuous and reciprocal interrelationships with the environment. Health is an unfolding phenomenon.
Newman, Sime, & Corcoran-Perry (1996)	• *Particulate–deterministic*. Phenomena are specific, reducible, measurable entities. Relationships between and within entities are causal and linear. Change, as a result of prior conditions, can be predicted and controlled. • *Interactive–integrative*. Phenomena include experiences and subjective data. Multiple interrelationships that are contextual and reciprocal exist between phenomena. Change is a function of multiple prior conditions and probabilistic relationships. • *Unitary–transformative*. A phenomenon is a unitary, self-organizing field and is identified through pattern recognition and interaction with the larger whole. Change is unidirectional and unpredictable.
Fawcett (1995)	• *Reaction*. Person is viewed as composed of discrete biological, psychological, sociological, and spiritual aspects, who responds in a reactive manner to environmental stimuli. Change occurs when survival is challenged. • *Reciprocal interaction*. Person is holistic, interactive being. Interactions with the environment are reciprocal. Change occurs as a result of multiple factors at varying rates throughout life and can only be estimated, not predicted. • *Simultaneous action*. Person is viewed as a holistic, self-organized field. Person–environment interactions are mutual and rhythmical processes. Change is unpredictable and evolutionary.

Note. These philosophical schemes are also referred to as paradigms.
Fawcett, J. (1995). *Analysis and evaluation of conceptual models of nursing* (3rd ed.). Philadelphia: F. A. Davis Company.

USES

One function of a paradigm is to identify the boundary or limits of the subject matter of concern to a discipline (Kim, 1989). A paradigm also provides a summary of the intellectual and social purposes of the discipline. It provides the "perspective with which essential phenomena of concern are conceptualized" (Kim, 1997, p. 32). A paradigm is considered to represent a worldview, "a coherent and common philosophical orientation" (Sarter, 1988, p. 52).

Therefore paradigms can provide the frames of reference for the construction of nursing theory and the use of nursing and non-nursing theories in nursing research. "The paradigm determines the way in which scientists make sense of the world. Therefore, without it, there is nothing about which to construct theories" (Antognoli-Toland, 1999, p. 39). Multiple theories generally emerge from a single paradigm. Paradigms also are important to nursing researchers. Researchers need to be assured that what is being studied will contribute to the body of nursing knowledge. By providing definitions of the discipline's boundaries, paradigms provide researchers with a nursing context for their research. Paradigms more specifically suggest the types of research questions that need to be addressed and appropriate methods used to answer the questions (Guiliano et al., 2005). Thus, nursing paradigms function as a means for nurse theorists and researchers to determine the congruence of their work in both focus and methods with the discipline of nursing, as expressed through a particular worldview.

CONTROVERSY

The topic of nursing paradigms is much debated by nurse scholars with differing opinions articulated about which paradigm best serves the discipline's needs regarding knowledge development. This debate has not always been viewed as particularly constructive. "The paradigm debates have done more to create divisiveness with theoretical nursing than to clearly define our unique mission and facilitate effective communication among nurses" (Thorne et al., 1998, A Unifying Definition, para. 1). The nursing literature reveals four major positions: (a) emergence of a singular dominant paradigm; (b) integration of the most predominant paradigms (i.e., totality and simultaneity); (c) the coexistence of multiple paradigms; and (d) avoidance of the issue.

Kikuchi and Simmons (1996), arguing from the perspective of the logic of truth, which holds that "two contradictory positions cannot both be true—one must be true and the other false" (p. 8), seem to support the necessity of a single dominant paradigm for the discipline of nursing. It has been argued that a predominant paradigm demonstrates the legitimacy of the science of a discipline. When Parse (1987) labeled and described the totality and simultaneity paradigms, she acknowledged the existence of a dominant paradigm and suggested the emergence of a new and preferred perspective for nursing. She identified the simultaneity paradigm as "an alternative to the traditional predominant worldview in nursing [totality]," one that moves "nursing away from the particulate view of Man" (p. 135). She noted that the simultaneity paradigm was gaining "recognition among scientists" and was "beginning to have an impact on research and practice competitive with the totality paradigm" (p. 135). Her use of the term *competition* initiated a debate over a preferred paradigm for nursing that is ongoing. The case for a single dominant paradigm is articulated by Leddy (2000); citing Kim, she concluded that multiple paradigms, instead of leading to coherence and patterning, actually result in "chaos, fragmentation, and arbitrariness" (p. 229).

Others support the existence of a single dominant paradigm, one that has not yet been identified. "The dialog is not to determine which [existing] paradigm is, finally, to win out. Rather it is to take us to another level at which all of these paradigms will be replaced by yet another paradigm whose outlines we can see now but dimly, if at all" (Guba, 1990, p. 27). Some nurse scholars have suggested new paradigms. For instance, Georges (2003) recommends a paradigm that claims social justice as the central teleology of its scholarship, is critical of dominant practices, and embraces diversity and the contextual nature of phenomena.

A variation on the position that nursing is best served by a single paradigm is the recommendation made by some nurse scholars that a paradigm integrating both the totality and simultaneity paradigms become the dominant perspective of the discipline. Rawnsley (2003) believes that "constructing new paradigms to complement totality and simultaneity is one way of respecting the contributions of colleagues without compromising philosophical integrity" (p. 11). Several nurse scholars have suggested this approach, and Winters and Ballou (2004) identified integration as a trend that values not only the traditional scientific worldview, but also the phenomenological and philosophical worldviews (p. 535). Arguing for "a less extreme and more integrated reference point for nursing's theory and practice," Thorne et al. (1998) proposed a unifying definition of nursing (p. 1257).

> Nursing is the study of human health and illness processes. Nursing practice is facilitating, supporting, and assisting individuals, families, communities, and/or societies to enhance, maintain and recover health and to reduce and ameliorate the effects of illness. Nursing's relational practice and science are directed toward the explicit outcome of health related quality of life within the immediate and larger environmental contexts (Thorne et al., 1998, A Unifying Definition, p. 1265).

Engebretson (1997) proposed an integrative paradigm, derived from the Heterdox Explanatory Paradigms Model for health practice. This model consisted of a horizontal axis with a continuum from logical positivism to metaphysics and a vertical axis with mind–body dualistic types of healing. Rawnsley (2003) conceptualized two paradigms that she believed promoted an inclusive nursing science, the heuristic paradigm and the complementarity paradigm. The focus of the heuristic paradigm is a valuing of the process of discovery, and of the complementarity paradigm a valuing of inclusiveness. Roy is also a proponent of an integrative paradigm, which she refers to as unity in diversity (Guiliano et al., 2005, p. 246). She believes in the existence of universal truths and that knowledge generated from multiple perspectives can and should be unified to serve the needs of nursing practice.

The third position in this debate is that nursing science is best served by a multiparadigm perspective in which the various paradigms are complementary. As noted by Pilkington and Mitchell (2003), other disciplines exist with multiple and distinctively different paradigms (pp. 107–108), and Barrett (1992) claims that uniformity of perspective is neither possible nor desirable (p. 156). Other nurse scholars express similar views. Whitehead (2005) claims "that the *real reality* is that there is not single reality or truth in nursing practice and subsequently no one method [for acquiring knowledge] prevails over the next" (p. 144). Fawcett (2003) also acknowledges the contributions of both the totality and simultaneity paradigms (p. 273). Those who support the multiple paradigm perspective have concluded that the complexity of the knowledge base that nurses need to practice requires paradigmatic plurality.

Though not as common as the other positions, some nurse scholars are suggesting that the paradigm debate be suspended. Thorne, Kirkham, and Henderson (1998) claim that "paradigm discourse inhibits rather than fosters productive knowledge development within the discipline" (p. 124), certainly a serious indictment. They identify the dichotomies in perspectives (old versus new) that become the focus of discussions on paradigms as unhelpful in synergistic knowledge development. Kikuchi (2003) suggests a rejection of worldviews (i.e., paradigms) in favor of a philosophy of moderate realism with its emphasis on probable not absolute truths and on a belief that reality exists independent of the human mind. This approach to nursing knowledge development is viewed as a public enterprise, one in which (a) questions are posed that all scholars can answer; (b) questions are answered in a piecemeal fashion; (c) there is both agreement and disagreement regarding the answers proposed; (d) disagreements are resolved using accepted standards; and (d) scholarly work is cooperative so that the cumulative knowledge can better answer the questions. This avoidance of the paradigm dilemma may be a trend. In 2002, Cody and Mitchell noted that there were decreasing numbers of publications addressing the fundamental philosophical issues of nursing (i.e., ontology and epistemology). By definition, paradigms cannot be discussed without consideration of questions of ontology and epistemology.

The paradigm debate remains unresolved. Without the emergence of a single dominant paradigm, nursing is left with multiple paradigms that are either competing or complementary or the need to develop an integrated paradigm that dialectically combines the perspectives of the multiple paradigms. With this state of paradigm confusion, it would be helpful for nurse theorists to identify the paradigmatic perspective from which the theory is developed and nurse researchers to identify the paradigmatic perspective from which the research questions were posed and the research methods chosen.

Metaparadigm

Metaparadigm is defined as the global concepts specific to a discipline and the global propositions that define and relate the concepts (Fawcett, 2005, p. 4). A metaparadigm transcends all specific philosophical or paradigmatic orientations. There are four requirements for the metaparadigm of any discipline: (a) a domain distinctive from other disciplines; (b) inclusive of all phenomena of interest to the discipline in a parsimonious way; (c) perspective neutral; and (d) international in scope and substance (Fawcett, 1996, p. 94). The metaparadigm is composed of several domains, often referred to as a typology. These domains are a classification system to identify the constructs or phenomena that are the focus of nursing. Several nursing metaparadigms have been suggested. For instance, Kim (2000) suggested a four-domain typology consisting of client, client–nurse, practice, and environment. The client domain is concerned with only those phenomena that pertain to the client. The client–nurse domain focuses on the phenomena that emerge from nurse–client interactions. The practice domain refers to what nurses do as professionals. The environment domain is composed of physical, social, and symbolic components of the client's external world, both past and present. The four-domain typology most frequently cited in nursing literature includes man/person, health, society/environment, and nursing (Fawcett, 1978; Yura & Torres, 1975). The metaparadigm described by Fawcett is also composed of four nonrelational and four relational propositions. The nonrelational propositions provide the definitions of the four domains and the relational propositions describe the linkages between the domains. See Table 1.2 for an overview of these propositions.

DEVELOPMENT

A metaparadigm is not so much constructed as it is identified. This identification process occurs through the analysis of the recurring themes of nursing's theories (Sarter, 1988). This analysis is philosophical in nature and allows for recognition of the "common and coherent philosophical orientation" (p. 52) of the discipline of nursing.

USES

Metaparadigms, or in Kim's (1983) words, typologies, are "boundary-maintaining devices" (p. 19) and as such help delineate nursing's frame of reference. The primary purpose then is to provide a means of focusing on that which is inherently nursing and marginalizing that which is not. This enables nurse practitioners, theorists, and researchers to concentrate their energies on the business of nursing. In addition, the

Table 1.2 FAWCETT'S RELATIONAL AND NONRELATIONAL PROPOSITIONS OF METAPARADIGM

Nonrelational	1. Person refers to individuals, families, communities, and other groups who are involved in nursing.
	2. Environment refers to the person's social network and physical surroundings and to the setting in which nursing is taking place. It also includes all local, regional, national, cultural, social, political, and economic conditions that might have an impact on a person's health.
	3. Health refers to a person's state of well-being at the time of engagement with nursing. It exists on a continuum from high-level wellness to terminal illness.
	4. Nursing refers to the definition of the discipline, the actions taken by nurses on behalf of and/or with the person, and the goals or outcomes of those actions.
Relational	1. Nursing is concerned with the principles and laws that govern life processes, well-being, and optimal functioning of human beings, sick or well.
	2. Nursing is concerned with the patterning of human behavior in the interaction with the environment in normal life events and critical situations.
	3. Nursing is concerned with the nursing actions or processes by which positive changes in health status are effected.
	4. Nursing is concerned with the wholeness or health of human beings, recognizing that they are in continuous interaction with their environment.

Source: Fawcett, J. (2000). *Analysis and evaluation of contemporary nursing knowledge: Nursing models and theories* (3rd ed., pp. 5). Philadelphia: F. A. Davis. Reprinted with permission from F. A. Davis Company, Philadelphia, PA.

metaparadigm is used for the purpose of analysis, a framework for comparing the perspectives of various nursing theorists (Fawcett, 2000; Fitzpatrick & Whall, 1983; Kim, 1983). For instance, Fitzpatrick and Whall noted that Levine defined health as wholeness, whereas Johnson found health to be a moving state of equilibrium.

CONTROVERSY

By definition, a discipline possesses only one metaparadigm. The controversy involves what that metaparadigm should be. Fawcett (2000) critiqued nine other paradigms using the criteria of distinctiveness, inclusiveness, neutrality, and internationality. The paradigms suggested by Newman; Conway; Kim; Meleis; King; Newman et al.; Malloch et al.; Parse; and Leininger/Watson all failed to meet one or more of the stated criteria. Fawcett's most common criticism was failure of the paradigms to meet the criterion of inclusion. For example, Kim (1983) did not address health; King (1984) eliminated environment and nursing; and Newman et al. (1996) failed to include environment. Obviously, nursing is still in search of a commonly shared metaparadigm and requires further philosophical analysis to arrive at this metaparadigm.

The metaparadigm proposed by Fawcett has also received criticism. It was faulted for using outdated language (Fawcett, 2003), being oriented to a particular paradigm (Fawcett, 2003), providing a limited perspective of the domains (Malone, 2005), and reflecting a cultural bias (Kao, Reeder, Hsu, & Cheng, 2006). Leininger criticized use of the term *person* as being too individualistic, and Fawcett now proposes using the term *persons* (Fawcett, 2003, p. 273). Malone (2005) found the conceptualization of the domain environment to be underdeveloped; she believed greater emphasis was needed on the policy environment.

The Western orientation of the metaparadigm is also criticized. In light of the fact that nursing is a global enterprise, this criticism seems warranted. Kao et al. (2006) provided definitions of each of the four domains from the perspective of Chinese philosophies. For instance, the concept of person can be defined in part as a social being engaged in ethical relationships, relationships governed by certain rules (p. 93). Fawcett (1996) believes that the nursing metaparadigm that she proposed is the final conceptualization for the discipline. "Indeed, it is anticipated that modifications in the metaparadigm concepts and propositions will be offered as the discipline of nursing evolves" (p. 95). Recent nursing literature reveals only limited consideration of the discipline's metaparadigm.

CONCEPTUAL MODELS

Conceptual models are a "set of interrelated concepts that symbolically represent and convey a mental image of a phenomen[on]" (Fawcett & Alligood, 2005, p. 228). Adam (1992) claims that they are the cornerstone of nursing's development (p. 61). Conceptual models are considered less abstract and more explicit and specific than philosophies but more abstract and less explicit and specific than theories (Adam, 1992; Alligood & Tomey, 2006; Caper, 1986; Fawcett, 2005). The term *conceptual model* has been used interchangeably, accompanied by some controversy, with conceptual framework, theoretical framework, conceptual system (King, 1997), philosophy (Adam, 1992), disciplinary matrix, paradigm (Fawcett, 2005), theory (Dickhoff & James, 1968; Fitzpatrick & Whall, 2005; Meleis, 1997), and macrotheory (Adam, 1992).

Beginning in the 1960s, conceptual models emerged as nursing attempted to distinguish itself from other disciplines, especially medicine (Kikuchi, 1992; Schlotfeldt, 1992). Since the 1960s, nursing models have been developed, proposed, analyzed, critiqued, and refined. Table 1.3 provides examples of the work of nurse scientists that has been labeled as conceptual models.

Development

Conceptual models are typically developed through the three stages of conceptualization or formulation, model formalization, and validation (Young, Taylor, & Renpenning, 2001, p. 11). The process can be empirical or intuitive, deductive or inductive. Empirically, nurse scholars make observations from practice; intuitively, they develop insights; deductively, they combine ideas from a variety of areas of inquiry, particularly other theories (e.g., general systems) and scientific bases; and inductively, they generalize from specific situations or observations. Conceptual nursing models reflect assumptions, beliefs, and values and, according to Adam (1992), are composed of six units, with commonly occurring philosophical perspectives. The following list summarizes the units and philosophical perspectives with examples from Johnson's Behavioral System Model.

1. Goal of nursing, generally idealistic, pragmatic, and humanistic; for instance, "fostering effective and efficient behavioral functioning" (Johnson, 1990, p. 24)
2. Conceptualizations of the client, usually existential and humanistic, and almost certainly holistic, as evidenced by Johnson's eight behavioral subsystems (Grubbs, 1974)
3. Social role of nurse, often humanistic and idealistic; for example, nursing viewed as a service that makes a unique contribution to the health and well-being of individuals—specifically, nurses acting to "provide a distinctive service to society" (Grubbs, 1974, p. 160) and "to seek the highest possible level of behavioral functioning [for the patient]" (Grubbs, 1974, p. 161)

Table 1.3 CONCEPTUAL MODELS

MODEL	SELECTED SOURCES
Johnson's Behavioral System Model	Johnson, D. E. (1959). The nature and science of nursing. *Nursing Outlook, 7,* 291–294.
	Johnson, D. E. (1980). The behavioral system model for nursing. In J. P. Reihl & C. Roy (Eds.), *Conceptual models for nursing practice* (2nd ed., pp. 207–216). New York: Appleton-Century-Crofts.
	Johnson, D. E. (1990). The behavioral system model for nursing. In M. E. Parker (Ed.), *Nursing theories in practice* (pp. 23–32). New York: National League for Nursing.
King's General Systems Framework	King, I. M. (1968). A conceptual frame of reference for nursing. *Nursing Research, 17,* 27–31.
	King, I. M. (1971). *Toward a theory of nursing: General concepts of human behavior.* New York: Wiley.
	King, I. M. (1981). *A theory for nursing: Systems, concepts, process.* New York: Wiley.
Levine's Conservation Model	Levine, M. E. (1969). The pursuit of wholeness. *American Journal of Nursing, 69,* 93–98.
	Levine, M. E. (1991). The conservation model: A model for health. In K. M. Schaefer & J. B. Pond (Eds.), *The conservation model: A framework for nursing practice* (pp. 1–11). Philadelphia: F. A. Davis.
	Levine, M. E. (1996). The conservation principles: A retrospective. *Nursing Science Quarterly, 9*(1), 38–41.
Neuman's Systems Model	Neuman, B. (1982). *The Neuman systems model: Application to nursing education and practice.* Norwalk, CT: Appleton-Century-Crofts.
	Neuman, B. (1995). *The Neuman systems model* (3rd ed.). Norwalk, CT: Appleton & Lange.
	Neuman, B. (1996). The Neuman system model in research and practice. *Nursing Science Quarterly, 9*(1), 67–70.
Rogers' Science of Human Beings	Rogers, M. E. (1980). Nursing: A science of unitary man. In J. P. Reihl & C. Roy (Eds.), *Conceptual models for nursing practice* (2nd ed., pp. 207–216). New York: Appleton-Century-Crofts.
	Rogers, M. E. (1990). Nursing: A science for unitary, irreducible human beings: Update 1990. In E. A. M. Barrett (Ed.), *Visions of Rogers' science-based nursing* (pp. 5–11). New York: National League for Nursing.
	Rogers, M. E. (1994). The science of unitary human beings: Current perspectives. *Nursing Science Quarterly, 7,* 33–35.
Roper-Logan-Tierney Model for Nursing	Roper, N., Logan, W., & Tierney, A. (1996). *The elements of nursing: A model for nursing based on a model of living* (4th ed.). Edinburgh: Churchill Livingstone.
	Roper, N., Logan, W., & Tierney, A. (1983). A nursing model. *Nursing Mirror, 156*(22), 17–19.
	Roper, N., Logan, W., & Tierney, A. (1997). The Roper-Logan-Tierney model. In P. Hinton-Walker & B. Neuman (Eds.), *Blueprint for use of nursing models.* New York: National League for Nursing.

(table continued on page 18)

Table 1.3 **CONCEPTUAL MODELS** *(continued)*

MODEL	SELECTED SOURCES
Roy's Adaptation Model	Roy, C. (1971). Adaptation: A conceptual framework for nursing. *Nursing Outlook, 18*(3), 42–45.
	Roy, C. (1976). *Introduction to nursing: An adaptation model.* Englewood Cliffs, NJ: Prentice-Hall.
	Roy, C. & Andrews, H. A. (1999). *The Roy adaptation model: The definitive statement.* Norwalk, CT: Appleton & Lange.

4. Source of difficulty, primarily pragmatic, because it identifies the scope of nursing's responsibility; for instance, behavioral disequilibrium and unpredictability, indicating a malfunction in the behavioral system (Grubbs, 1974)
5. Intervention, typically humanistic, idealistic, and pragmatic; for example, restrict (e.g., set limits on dysfunctional behavior), defend (e.g., use isolation techniques), inhibit (e.g., teach new skills), and facilitate (e.g., provide adequate nutrition) (Grubbs, 1974)
6. Desired consequences, also typically humanistic, idealistic, and pragmatic, as evidenced by Johnson's goal of system balance and stability (Grubbs, 1974; Johnson, 1990)

Though Johnson's Behavioral System Model was used as one example of how these components are addressed in a conceptual model, all the conceptual models found in Table 1.3 consider these six components, each from its unique perspective.

Uses

The development of conceptual models is essential to the professional identity of nursing. The conceptual models delineate the goals and scope of nursing and provide frameworks for considering the outcomes of nursing. In general, they can direct a professional discipline's theory development, practice, education, and research.

Conceptual models can give birth to nursing theories. Fawcett (2005, p. 19) claims that "grand theories are derived directly from conceptual models." Because, by definition, conceptual models are considered more abstract and less specific than theories, several can develop from a single conceptual model. For instance, several grand theories were derived from Roger's conceptual model, the Science of Unitary Human Beings. The Theory of Power as Knowing Participation in Change (Barrett, 1986) is one example of a theory with its origins in Roger's conceptual model. The alternate view is that conceptual models are "not necessary, and, perhaps, not even important for theoretical growth (Rodman, 1980, p. 436). For instance, Leininger's Theory of Cultural Care Diversity and Universality was derived from anthropological concepts, research (the first being a study of the Gadsup people in Papua, New Guinea), and her beliefs about nursing. Peplau's Theory of Interpersonal Relations was based on an integration of theories from the field of psychology and the recorded interactions between student nurses and patients.

The relationship between nursing's conceptual models and practice is a reciprocal one. Conceptual models can provide a structure for nursing practice and practice experiences can provide evidence of the credibility of the model (Kahn & Fawcett, 1995). In order for a conceptual model to be considered useful it must demonstrate (a) social utility—content is understandable and the interpersonal and psychomotor skills needed to apply the model can be mastered; (b) social congruence—nursing activities are culturally congruent with the expectations of the patient, community, and members of the health care team; and (c) social significance—the use of the model provides outcomes of social value, particularly as it relates to patients' health status (Kahn & Fawcett, 1995, p. 189). In practice, the models have most often been used as a framework for implementation of the nursing process (Archibald, 2000, Nursing Models, para. 2). Assessment based on a conceptual model tends to be more comprehensive, focused, and specific (Hardy, 1986). Because of their level of abstraction, models tend to be less effective in prescribing specific nursing interventions. Instead, the conceptual models suggest general areas of nursing action. The unique focus of each conceptual model also implies criteria for determining when problems have been solved, thus aiding the process of evaluation.

Many schools of nursing used conceptual models as a framework for their curricula. The use of nursing's conceptual models ensured that the focus of the students' education was on nursing, not medicine. It provided students with a perspective for considering nursing issues and a language for expressing such. Beginning in the 1960s and through the 1990s, schools of nursing have identified the use of specific conceptual models in their curricula, for example, Johnson's Behavioral System Model (Harris, 1986), King's General Systems Framework (Brown & Lee, 1980), Neuman's Systems Model (Kilchenstein & Yakulis, 1984), and Roy's Adaptation Model (Brower & Baker, 1976).

Conceptual models can also guide research. "Research is nursing research only if it examines phenomena of special interest to nursing, that is, phenomena that are indicated by one or the other of the conceptual models for nursing" (Adam, 1992, p. 59). Since conceptual models for nursing represent foci of scientific inquiry, they can identify questions for research. For instance, conceptual models generated the following questions: (a) In Johnson's Behavioral System Model, what are the effects of the stage of cancer on the eight behavioral subsystems? (Derdiarian, 1988); (b) In King's General Systems Framework, what factors interfere with goal attainment? (Kameoda & Sugimori, 1993); and (c) In Neuman's System Model, what effect did experience with the model have on the quality of nursing diagnoses? (Mackenzie & Spence Laschinger, 1995). It is important to note that avenues of questioning suggested by conceptual models are not the same as those of empirical testing, which less abstract theories undergo.

Controversy

There are some controversies about the use and usefulness of conceptual models. Although conceptual models cannot be tested or validated because of their level of abstractness (Adam, 1992; Downs, 1982), they can and should be evaluated. Evaluation of conceptual models has revealed some general limitations. They have been criticized for:

- Their level of abstraction, limiting their usefulness
- Rigidity and inflexibility, which inhibits change
- The subjectivity of perspective, which may not be shared by professional colleagues or clients
- The use of a unique language or jargon, requiring specialized education or resulting in confusing communication
- Potential to be used in inappropriate situations and for incorrect purposes (Adam, 1992; Hardy, 1986; Littlejohn, 2002; Tierney, 1998; Young et al., 2001)

Controversy about the use of conceptual models in relation to theory development is complicated by lack of consistency in labeling the work of nurse scientists. Fawcett's (2005) position is that conceptual models are more abstract and global and less specific than theories. Kramer (1997) identifies conceptual models as a type of theory but claims not all theories are conceptual models. Meleis (1997) concludes that most of the differences between the two are semantic and noted that the nurse scientists themselves referred to their work using a variety of terms. For instance, Rogers called her conceptualization of nursing a science (Science of Unitary Human Beings); Erickson referred to her work as both a theory and a paradigm (Modeling and Role-Modeling: A Theory and Paradigm); and Watson identified her thinking as both philosophy and theory (Watson's Philosophy and Theory of Human Caring). In this book, conceptual models and theories have been treated as distinct entities. Although there is some confusion about the term and some limitations regarding their use, conceptual models have proved valuable for the advancement of nursing research and the development of theories.

THEORY: GENERAL ISSUES

Similar to conceptual models, theories are composed of concepts and propositions. In a theory, the concepts are defined more specifically and the propositions are more narrowly focused. Though theory and paradigm are sometimes used interchangeably, theories differ from both paradigms and philosophies in that they represent what is rather than what should be (Babbie, 1995, pp. 37, 47). A theoretical body of knowledge is considered an essential characteristic of all professions (Johnson, 1974). Therefore, theories serve to further specify the uniqueness or distinctiveness of a profession. "Theories have in fact distinguished nursing from other caring professions by fixing professional boundaries" (Rutty, 1998, Theory, para. 2). The definition of theory by Kerlinger is classic and comprehensive. "Kerlinger (1973) defines theory as follows: A theory is a set of interrelated constructs (concepts, definitions, and propositions) that present a systematic view of phenomena by specifying relations among variables, with the purpose of explaining and predicting phenomena" (King, 1978, p. 11). In addition to explanation and prediction of phenomena, Glaser and Straus (1967) identify other uses of theory. They believe theories by definition should also be able to further advance theory development, guide practice by providing understanding and the possibility of controlling some situations, offer a perspective on behavior, offer a means of interpreting data, and provide an approach or style for the research of a specific area of human behavior. Theories should be inherently useful.

In addition to considering the development, uses, and controversies surrounding nursing theories, it is important to address the classifications of theories. Theories can be classified in a number of ways, such as by their purposes, sources, and levels. The three major levels of nursing are grand, middle range, and practice, with middle range theory of special interest as it grows in importance in nursing research and practice.

Development

The development of a theory involves both content and process. Theories are composed of concepts, and their relationships and are constructed through a variety of processes. The history of theory development in nursing helps provide a context for understanding the ongoing work of nurse scientists in the advancement of nursing's body of knowledge.

COMPONENTS

A variety of terms are used to describe concepts and propositions, the two basic elements of a theory. The terms *concept, construct, descriptor,* and *unit* are often used interchangeably, with concept being the most common. Definitions of the concepts can be considered an aspect of the basic element or concept or as a separate and additional component of a theory. Statements of relationships or propositions refer to the same notion. Also, some scientists include axioms and postulates as other components of a theory, because, though they are relational statements, they are assertions assumed to be true that lay the groundwork for the propositions (Babbie, 1995, p. 48).

Concepts. Concepts are considered the basic building blocks of theory. Kim (2000, p. 15) defines concepts as "a symbolic statement describing a phenomenon or a class of phenomena." In other words, a concept is a mental image of a phenomenon, an idea or construct of an object or action (Walker & Avant, 2005, p. 26). Although there are several more complicated classifications of concepts (or units), basically they can be classified on a continuum of abstractness, which some label primitive, abstract, and concrete (Meleis, 1997) and others global, middle range, and empirical (Moody, 1990). They can also be categorized as property or process concepts (Kim, 2000).

Primitive concepts are those that have a culturally shared meaning (Walker & Avant, 2005, p. 26) or are those that are introduced as new in the theory (Meleis, 1997, p. 252). For instance, in culturally derived concepts, a color is usually primitive because it cannot be defined except by giving examples of another color different from the original color. Grass, leaves, and apples would be examples of green, and sky, bark, and grapefruit would be examples of not green. As an original concept in a new theory, role supplementation in the theory of Role Insufficiency and Role Supplementation would be an example of a theory-specific primitive concept (Meleis, 1997, p. 252). Concrete concepts are those that exist in a spatial–temporal reality. They can be defined in terms of primitive concepts. Grass, leaves, apples, sky, bark, and grapefruit would all be examples of concrete concepts. In nursing, touch used by the nurse would be considered a concrete concept. Abstract concepts can be defined by primitive or concrete concepts but are not limited by time or space. "They refer to general cases" (Kim, 2000, p. 16). Communication could be identified as an abstract concept that would be of interest to nursing. Theories can be composed of both concrete and abstract concepts.

For theories using abstract concepts, operational definitions of those concepts are an important inclusion because the definitions enable the theory to be more easily tested empirically through research. An operational definition "assigns[s] explicit meaning to that [abstract] concept" (Duldt & Giffin, 1985, p. 95). Operational definitions can be (a) experimental, providing specific details necessary to manipulate the concept; (b) measurable, describing the means by which the concept can be measured; (c) administrative, including particular information on how to obtain data about the concept; and (d) evaluative, establishing the criteria for operationalizing the concept and the means of determining the degree to which the criteria are met.

The classification of concepts as property or process is significant because it promotes understanding of the concept as defined by the theorist. Property concepts are those that deal with the state of things, and process concepts are those that relate to the way things happen. Stage of grief would be a property concept, whereas grieving as the means by which an individual deals with loss would be a process concept. A concept can be considered both a property and process concept, such as communication. In general, theories contain both types of concepts. "The classification system of concepts into property and process types is useful in an analytic sense" (Kim, 2000, p. 18). It provides a clearer sense of the nature of the concepts included in the theory and thus a better understanding of the theory itself.

Propositions. Propositions, defined as statements of the relationships between two or more concepts, provide a theory "with the powers of description, explanation or prediction" (Meleis, 1997, p. 252). Propositional statements can be considered either relational or nonrelational. Relational statements can be either correlational or causal. Nonrelational statements include descriptions of the properties and dimensions of the concept in the definition of the term *proposition* (Meleis, 1997).

In propositional statements that are correlational, the assertion is that two or more concepts exist together or are associated. The associations can be positive, negative, or neutral. Orem's Self-care Deficit Nursing Theory provides examples of positive and neutral correlational statements. The nurse affects the movement from the "'present state of affairs' to 'a desirable future state of affairs' by using the 'nursing means' the nurse selects" (Orem, 2001, p. 151) is an example of a positive statement. "Engagement in self-care or dependent-care is affected by persons' valuation of self care measures with respect to life, development, heath, and well-being" (Orem, 2001, p. 146) is an example of a more neutral or direction-less statement.

Causal propositional statements establish cause-and-effect relationships. Examples of causal statements are found in Parse's Man-Living-Health Theory of Nursing. "In a nurse–family process, by synchronizing rhythms, the members uncover the opportunities and limitations created by the decisions made in choosing irreplaceable ways of being together. The choices of new ways of being together mobilizes transcendence" (Parse, 1987, p. 170). Causal statements are more difficult to establish than correlational statements and are therefore more rare.

"Nonrelational statements serve as adjuncts to relational statements"; they are the means by which theorists clarify meanings in the theory (Walker & Avant, 2005, p. 27). They provide assertions of the existence of concepts or definitions of concepts of a theory and thus help explain the nature of the theory. An example of an existence proposition would be Parse's statement that the practice methodology of her theory is composed of three dimensions: illuminating meaning, synchronizing rhythms, and mobilizing transcendence (Parse, 1987, p. 167). Parse also provides definitional propositions, for example, "health is Man's unfolding. It is Man's lived experiences, a non linear entity that cannot be qualified by terms as good, bad, more, or less" (Parse, 1987, p. 160).

The nature of the elements of the theory relates to the purposes for which the theory can be used. Theories with only nonrelational prepositional statements serve to describe, whereas theories with relational prepositional statements have the potential to explain (correlational statements) and predict (causal statements).

PROCESS

Theory development can be accomplished by inductive or deductive processes or by a combination of both. The content of a theory comes from other theories, practice, or research, or a combination of two or more of these sources. Using other theories as a source of generating a theory involves a deductive process, whereas using practice experience or research findings for developing a theory requires an inductive process.

Walker and Avant (1995) describe strategies of theory development that include both inductive and deductive processes. Analysis, synthesis, and derivation are applied to concepts, statements, and theories. Analysis is solely an inductive process, whereas synthesis and derivation can involve both inductive and deductive processes (Walker & Avant, 1995, p. 32). Table 1.4 presents a matrix of the purposes of the nine strategies that Walker and Avant (1995) describe in detail in their book, *Strategies for Theory Construction in Nursing*.

This process of theory construction is modeled in the work of Lenz, Suppe, Gift, Pugh, and Milligan (1995), as they collaborated on the development of the middle range theory of unpleasant symptoms. For instance, the researchers used existing literature for concept analysis, examining attributes, characteristics,

Table 1.4 **MATRIX OF APPROACHES TO THEORY CONSTRUCTION**

	CONCEPT	STATEMENT	THEORY
Analysis	Distinguish between defining and irrelevant attributes of the concept by breaking a concept into simpler elements and considering similarities and differences	Determine how useful, inform-ative, and logically correct the statements are through an orderly examination	Determine the strengths and weaknesses of theory by applying an analytical frame-work
Synthesis	Generate new ideas by examining data for new insights	Develop statements about relationships through obser-vations of phenomena	Construct a theory from empiri-cal evidence
Derivation	Generate new ways of thinking about phenomena by developing a new voca-bulary based on the relation-ships between phenomena	Formulate statements about a poorly understood phenom-enon by clarifying relation-ships between phenomena	Explain and predict phenomena that are poorly understood, for which no methods of study are known, or for which no theory exists

Source: Walker, L. O., & Avant, K. C. (1995). *Strategies for theory construction in nursing* (3rd ed.). Norwalk, CT: Appleton & Lange. Reprinted with permission of Pearson Education, Inc., Upper Saddle River, NJ.

and dimensions of the concept of dyspnea. The literature review also served as a basis of concept deriva-tion, resulting in the identification of pain as an analog of dyspnea. And through synthesis of the literature and the researchers' own experiences, they conceptualized dyspnea as having five components: sensation, perception, distress, response, and reporting.

Walker and Avant (1995) identify other theories as a source of additional theory development. Theo-ries from other disciplines are one source of nursing theory content. Peplau made use of psychoanalytic theory and Johnson made use of systems theory, informed by their clinical practices, psychiatric and pedi-atric nursing, respectively. Nursing theories and conceptual models often give rise to middle range the-ory. For instance, from Orem's Self-care Deficit Theory came the Theory of Dependent-care Deficit, Theory of Self-care, and Theory of Nursing Systems (Alligood & Tomey, 2005, p. 53).

"Some theories are driven by clinical practice situations and are inductively developed" (Meleis, 1997, p. 230). This grounded theory approach uses observations and analysis of similarities and differences of observed phenomena to develop concepts and establish their relationships. The works of Peplau, Orlando, Travelbee, and Wiedenbach have been associated with this approach.

Research is often cited as the most common and acceptable source for theory development, most often leading to the development of a middle range theory. "Theories evolve from replicated and confirmed research findings" (Meleis, 1997, p. 231). This is considered an empirical quantitative approach and involves (a) identifying a phenomenon, listing all its characteristics; (b) measuring these characteristics in a variety of settings; (c) analyzing the results to determine if patterns exist; and (d) formalizing these patterns as theoretical statements (Reynolds, 1971, p. 140). Johnson and Rice's (1974) theory of sensory and distress components of pain was developed using this approach.

Qualitative research is often referred to as theory generating with grounded theory and phenomenol-ogy often used by nurse scientists to develop theories. Fagerhaugh's (1974) theory of pain expression and control is an example of theory developed through qualitative research. Metasynthesis is emerging as an approach for developing theory, especially middle range theory (Annells, 2005; Walsh & Downe, 2005).

This method addresses the criticism that theory development from qualitative research relies on a small number of homogeneous participants (Estabrooks, Field, & Morse, 1994). Metasynthesis involves aggregation of qualitative data, employing four processes—"comprehending, synthesizing, theorizing, and recontextualizing" (Estabrooks et al., p. 505), with greatest emphasis on theorizing and recontextualizing. Kylma's (2005) substantive theory on dynamics of hope in adults living with HIV/AIDS was developed using metasynthesis. McKenna (1997) noted similarities between the quantitative and qualitative approaches: Both use inductive methods, and both generally result in the development of middle range theories.

HISTORY

Nursing theory development can trace its roots to the work of Florence Nightingale (Alligood & Tomey, 2005; Dunphy, 2001; Fitzpatrick & Whall, 2005; Meleis, 1997), with her concern for the relationship between health and environment and the nurse's role in that relationship. Hildegard Peplau is credited with being the first contemporary nurse theorist (McKenna, 1997). Other theorists of the 1950s (Henderson [in Henderson and Harmer], 1955; Orem, 1959; Johnson, 1959; Hall, 1959) (McKenna, 1997, p. 95) were influenced by Peplau's conceptualization of interpersonal relationships in nursing. Others were influenced by their involvement at Columbia University's Teachers' College and the practical-oriented philosophy of John Dewey, who served on its staff. From Teachers' College in the 1950s, Abdellah, King, Wiedenbach, and Rogers emerged as nurse theorists (Meleis, 1997). Not all of the work of these nurse scientists would be considered theory by today's definition. The theoretical work that did take place in the 1950s focused on what nurses did, not why they did it, and the conceptual frameworks developed at this time were more often used as a basis for the development of curricula than as a guide for practice. The 1950s also saw the introduction of the journal *Nursing Research,* which provided a forum for the development of nursing theories and their testing.

In addition to continuing development of individual nursing theories, the 1960s brought a more national and coordinated approach to theory development. Federal financial support became available in 1962 to nurses pursuing doctoral education; the American Nurses Association stated in 1965 that theory development was a significant goal for the profession; and in 1967, Case Western Reserve University sponsored a national nursing symposium, a third of which was devoted to nursing theory. The theorists associated with this decade include "Abdellah et al. (1960), Orlando (1961), Wiedenbach (1964), Levine (1966), Travelbee (1966) and King (1968)" (McKenna, 1997, pp. 95–96). Theorists, particularly Wiedenbach and Orlando, began to consider not only what nurses did, but also what effect it had on patients. Debate, stimulated by the metatheorists, focused on the issue of the types of theories that nursing should develop rather than the content of theories.

Although nursing theorists continued to develop and publish their work, such as Roy (1970), Rogers (1970), Neuman (1972), Riehl (1974), Adam (1975), Patterson and Zderad (1976), Leininger (1978), Watson (1979) and Newman (1979) (McKenna, 1997, p. 97), the questions posed by metatheorists dominated the decade of the 1970s (Meleis, 1997). Efforts were made to determine what is meant by theory, to identify the structural components of theories, and to clarify the methods of analysis and critique of theory. The previously developed theories were criticized for a failure to include explicated propositions and for their lack of empirical testing (McKenna, 1997, p. 97). The development and use of nursing theories were advanced by (a) the adoption by the National League for Nursing of an accreditation criterion requiring a theory base to nursing curricula; (b) the formation of two groups (Nursing Theories Conference Group and Nursing Theory Think Tank) that considered application of theory to practice; and

(c) the publication of *Advances in Nursing Science,* a journal dedicated to the development of nursing science.

Alligood and Tomey (2006) refer to the 1980s as the Theory Era, even though few new nursing theories emerged. "Only three new nursing theories were published in the 1980s: the work of Parse (1981), Fitzpatrick (1982) and Erickson, Tomlin and Swain (1983)" (McKenna, 1997, p. 97). Fawcett's (1984) explication of a metaparadigm for nursing allowed for the comparative content analysis of theories, and her delineation of the levels of abstraction of nursing knowledge helped nurse scientists and practitioners make the distinctions between grand, middle range, and practice theories. Her work also clarified how nursing grand theory can be derived from nursing conceptual models and how middle range theory can be derived from grand theory. The importance of nursing theory to the profession was well established and the shift by the end of this decade was away from theory development toward theory use (Alligood & Tomey, 2006, p. 9). There was both an increased interest in the relationship between theory and practice and an increased emphasis on the relationship between theory and research.

The decade of the 1990s was hallmarked by the development of the middle range and practice theories. These theories are less abstract and therefore more directly applicable to practice and more easily tested empirically by research. Interest in nursing theory was evidenced by the publication of *Nursing Science Quarterly,* edited by Parse, focusing on theory development and testing, and by the increasing number of European-based nursing theory conferences.

Uses

Nurse scientists have worked on the development of nursing theory as part of the process of establishing nursing as a profession with a unique body of knowledge. Nursing theories provide nurses with the language of nursing, a means of communicating the nature of the discipline within and outside the profession. In addition, as a component of nursing knowledge considered less abstract than conceptual frameworks, nursing theories generate more specific research questions and provide greater guidance to nursing practice.

Nursing theories provide nursing-specific identifications, definitions, and interrelationships of concepts. This allows the profession to distinguish itself from the medical and behavioral sciences. For example, in nursing, we speak of unitary human beings, self-care, and the centrality of caring. Through analysis of theories, nursing's metaparadigm emerges, providing us with a common and basic frame of reference for communicating about nursing.

The relationship between nursing theory and research is symbiotic. Research provides for both theory generating and theory testing. Qualitative research seeks to identify and define phenomena of interest to nursing, thus serving as a theory-generating tool. By contrast, quantitative research is a means by which the propositions of theories can be substantiated, thus functioning as a theory-testing tool. Theories then serve as a framework for relating the data generated by research, resulting in a more coherent whole nursing body of knowledge than a collection of isolated facts.

In addition, the greater clarification of concepts and their relationships that nursing theories provide allows researchers to formulate more specific and nursing-relevant research questions. The evidence that is generated through the study of these questions, because of the level of specificity and relevance, in turn is more directly applicable to nursing practice. Parse (1999) challenges nurses "to conduct research to ensure that the practice of nursing serves people in a unique way" (Recommendations, para. 1). It is through nursing theories that the profession identifies its unique service to people. The testing of nursing theories also leads to theory-guided evidence-based practice. "Evidence itself refers to evidence about theories. Similarly, theory determines what counts as evidence" (Fawcett, Watson, Neuman, Walker, & Fitzpatrick, 2001, p. 117). Thus, theory as it guides research has the potential to provide the evidence that makes nursing practice more efficient and more effective.

Controversy

There are two recurring themes in criticisms of nursing theories: the issue of consistency in labeling and the appropriateness of the sources of the theories used by nurses. The lack of definitional clarity between what is labeled a conceptual model and what is considered a theory is further complicated by confusion over identification of the level of the theory, that is, grand, middle range, or practice. Nurse scientists have not consistently classified the level of the developed theory in the work they publish. This issue is further addressed in the discussion of the middle range level of theory development. In addition, there is some disagreement over the appropriate source of theories to be used by nurses, borrowed or unique. The debate focuses on to what degree nurses can use theories from other disciplines and still advance nursing's unique body of knowledge. The discussion of this issue is integrated into the section on classification of theories by source.

Classifications

Theories differ in their purposes, sources, and, most importantly, levels of abstraction and scope. These differences lead to classifications. The basic purposes of theory are description, explanation, prediction, and/or control. The sources of theory in nursing include those developed by nurse scientists (unique) and those that are used in nursing but come from other disciplines (borrowed). The terms *theory of nursing* and *theory in nursing* are often used to distinguish between these two sources.

There are multiple terms used to classify the various levels or scope of nursing theories. The broad-scope theories are referred to as *macro, holistic, molar, general, situation,* and, most commonly, *grand.* Narrow-scope theories are called *middle range, circumscribed,* or *situation/factor.* Theories narrowest in scope are labeled *micro, molecular, atomistic, narrow-range, phenomena, prescriptive, factor, situation-specific,* or *practice* (Babbie, 1995; George, 1995; Parker, 2006; Rinehart, 1978). The most common labels for the levels of nursing theory are grand, middle range, and micro or practice. The level is determined primarily by the theory's degree of abstraction. Examination of the level of abstraction of the "purpose, concept, and definitional components of the theory" (Kramer, 1997, p. 65) allows for the identification of the level of the theory.

PURPOSES

Though theories are designed to describe, explain, predict, and/or control, some nurse scientists claim that only theories that enable nurses to control outcomes are legitimate for a practice discipline (Dickhoff & James, 1968). Descriptive theories are limited to naming and classifying characteristics of the phenomenon of interest, which identify what is happening. Peplau's Theory of Interpersonal Relationships has been labeled a descriptive theory.

Explanatory theories expand the knowledge base by delineating the relationships between characteristics of the phenomenon, clarifying why it is happening. Watson's Theory of Human Caring is considered an explanatory theory. But predictive theories provide the conditions that can result in a preferred outcome, determining how it can intentionally happen. Orlando's Theory of the Deliberative Nursing Process is an example of a predictive theory. Theories whose purpose is to control, often referred to as prescriptive theories, guide action to create an intended result. The three ingredients for this type of theory are content of goal, primary prescription for activity to achieve goal, and list of additional recommendations of activity (Dickhoff & James, 1968, p. 201).

The existence of descriptive and explanatory theories is a necessary precursor to the development of predictive and prescriptive theories. "Predictive theory presupposes the prior existence of more elementary types of theories" (Dickhoff & James, 1968, p. 200). The relationship between the purposes of a theory has been conceptualized in some instances as a hierarchy:

1. Factor-isolating theories (descriptive)
2. Factor-relating theories (descriptive/explanatory)
3. Situation-relating theories (explanatory/predictive)
4. Situation-producing theories (prescriptive) (Dickhoff & James, 1968, pp. 200–201)

SOURCES

The source of theory refers to the discipline from which it developed. The possibilities include theories unique to nursing, theories borrowed from other disciplines, and theories from other disciplines adapted for nursing. A borrowed theory is one in which the knowledge "is developed in the main by other disciplines and is drawn upon by nursing" (Johnson, 1986, p. 112). The distinctions between these three sources are difficult to make since "the man-made, more-or less arbitrary divisions between the sciences are neither firm nor constant" (Johnson, 1986, p. 112).

Given that the differences between the sources of theory may be less than perfectly precise, unique theory can be defined "as that knowledge derived from the observation of phenomena and the asking of questions unlike those which characterized other disciplines" (Johnson, 1986, p. 112). Many argue that nursing's identity as a profession and, ultimately, its ability to improve nursing practice are dependent on the existence of nursing theories unique to the discipline. Wald and Leonard (1964), the most frequently cited proponents of this position, claimed that to become an independent discipline, nursing was required to develop its own theories rather than borrow theories or apply principles from other disciplines. They expressed concern about nursing's reliance on these borrowed theories.

Wald and Leonard's concerns seem validated by Jacobson's (1987) findings. When nurses with advanced degrees were asked to identify "conceptual models of nursing," responses included Selye's stress model, Piaget's theory of cognitive development, the general system's theory, problem solving, and Maslow's hierarchy of needs. All of these examples would be considered borrowed rather than knowledge unique to nursing.

More recent examination of the literature reveals continued reliance on theories from fields other than nursing. Fawcett and Bourbonniere (2001) found that of 90 research studies published in two clinical journals, *Geriatric Nursing* and *Nurse Practitioner,* and two research journals, *Nursing Research* and *Research in Nursing and Health,* only nine (10%) used nursing conceptual models or theories (p. 314). The borrowed theories or models used in these studies came from psychology, sociology, medicine, dentistry, physiology, biology, education, decision sciences, economics, ethics, epidemiology, management sciences, marketing, and communications.

Borrowed theories continue to be used with some frequency as the theoretical foundation of nursing research. Of the 47 research articles published in *Nursing Research* in 2006, only four (8.5%) used existing nursing theories, all in the middle range. The Theory of Unpleasant Symptoms was the only nursing theory tested in more than one study. Borrowed middle range theories were cited in 17 studies (36.2%), with social support, health-related quality of life, and self-efficacy the most commonly identified theories. There were no theories identified in 15 (31.9%) of the studies, and in 11 (23.4%) studies, models were created specifically for the research study from a variety of conceptual models and theories.

In past decades, the practice of borrowing theories seemed to be the result of a belief in the superiority of theories "imported" from other disciplines (Meleis, 1997). This perspective was reinforced by nurses whose advanced degrees were in fields other than nursing. Theories from sociology, psychology, education, ecology, physiology, and others were and still are borrowed. The argument for borrowed theories seems to be that theorists and practitioners should not place boundaries on any knowledge that might be useful to nursing because "knowledge does not innately 'belong' to any field of science" (Johnson, 1986, p. 117). Borrowing theories from other disciplines is sometimes referred to as theory adoption and involves the unchanged use of a theory developed from a field other than nursing. The use of unmodified theories from physiology, for instance, acid–base balance, is an example of a completely borrowed theory. Though the need for adopting borrowed theories does exist, there is concern about their prevalence. The preferred approach for the use of borrowed theories seems to be to adapt them to a distinctively nursing perspective.

Adaptation refers to altering the content or structure of a theory that was initially developed for application to a discipline other than nursing. Borrowing and altering theory is seen as necessary "to acquire a means of explanation and prediction about some phenomena that is currently poorly understood, or for which there is no present means to study it, or for which there is no theory at all" (Walker & Avant, 1995, p. 172). Walker and Avant provide a process called theory derivation, which allows nurses to modify the concepts and structures of a theory from another discipline to create a new theory more relevant to nursing. The steps of the process are not considered strictly linear; they are repeated as necessary until the theory being developed is sufficiently complete. Box 1.1 summarizes the steps in theory derivation.

The debate about the value of borrowed theories continues. Fawcett and Bourbonniere (2001) identify premises necessary for a healthy future for the nursing profession. They claim that "the discipline of nursing can survive only if we celebrate our own heritage and utilize nursing knowledge" (p. 311). This premise and

---

BOX 1.1   Steps in the Process of Theory Derivation

1. Become acquainted with the literature that addresses the phenomenon. Evaluate theory in nursing for its adequacy.
2. Read extensively in related fields. Look for unusual relationships between the knowledge in those fields and the phenomenon of interest to nursing.
3. Choose a parent theory as a source of the derivation. Focus on the theory, or parts of the theory, that best explains or predicts the phenomenon.
4. Select the relevant concepts and/or structures. Eliminate those aspects of the theory that are not useful.
5. Develop, refine, or redefine the concepts, statements, and structures from the parent theory to develop a theory more meaningful for nursing. This requires reflection and creativity.

Source: Walker, L. O., & Avant, K. C. (1995). *Strategies for theory construction in nursing* (3rd ed., pp. 172–173). Norwalk, CT: Appleton & Lange.

the future it suggests is challenged by the ongoing dependence of nurses on perspectives of nursing that are grounded in the knowledge of other disciplines. The solution they suggest is to end nursing's "romance" with borrowed theories. Few would argue that nursing needs to attend to the ongoing development of its unique body of knowledge, perhaps not for the sole purpose of divorcing itself from other disciplines, but for creating a body of knowledge that could be shared across disciplines. Thus, nursing theory could be borrowed.

GRAND THEORY

Grand theories, as the most abstract of the three identified levels, attempt "to create a view of the whole of nursing" (Liehr & Smith, 1999, Juxtaposition with Grand Nursing theory, para. 1). They address the nature, mission, and goals of nursing care (Meleis, 1997) in a general fashion and are created through the observations and/or insights of the theorist. The development of grand theories served to differentiate the discipline of nursing from the medical model, stimulated the expansion of nursing knowledge (McKenna, 1997), and provided a general "structure for the organization of nursing knowledge" (Orem, 2001, p. 139). Orem also claimed that the unstructured nature of grand or general theories allows for a wide range of knowledge available to practitioners and scholars within a nursing-specific frame of reference. McKenna (1997) outlined the benefits of grand theories to include (a) a guide for practice as an alternative to practicing solely by tradition or intuition; (b) a framework for education by suggesting a focus and a structure for curricula; and (c) an aid to the professionalization of nursing by providing a basis of practice.

More than 50 grand theories have been identified (McKenna, 1997, p. 93), although that number may vary based on the label assigned to the work. Because of their level of abstraction, there has been some difficulty in distinguishing between grand theories, philosophies, and conceptual models. Examples of nursing theories that have been designated as grand include Leininger's Theory of Culture Care Diversity and Universality, Newman's Theory of Health as Expanding Consciousness, and Parse's Theory of Human Becoming (Fawcett & Bourbonniere, 2001; Fawcett, 2005; Parker, 2006). Parker (2006) also identifies Orem's Self-care Deficit, Roger's Science of Human Beings, and Roy's Adaptation Model as theories, whereas Fawcett (2005) and Alligood and Tomey (2005) label these nursing scientists' work as conceptual models. Orem (2001) refers to her work as a general theory. Table 1.5 provides sources of information about specific grand theories.

The level of abstraction makes it difficult to test grand theories empirically. In fact, Donnelly (2001), citing the work of Lundh, Soder, and Waerness (1988), claimed that because the theories were abstract and normative "rather than facilitating research development [they] actually made research development in nursing 'more difficult'" (p. 337). This conclusion is supported in part by the findings of Moody et al. (1988) that in nursing practice research published from 1977 to 1986, fewer than 13% of the 720 studies identified were linked to one of the grand theories.

Grand theories seem better able to serve as a basis for the development of the more specific theories of the middle and practice range, which can undergo empirical testing. For instance, the middle range theory "A Theory of Sentient Evolution" was derived from Roger's Science of Unitary Human Beings (Parker, 1989). In addition, grand theories have fulfilled the important functions of distinguishing nursing from other helping professions and providing legitimization to its science. But because of their success in fulfilling these functions, grand theories have become less necessary and the focus of theory development has changed to the middle range theories (Suppe, 1996a).

Table 1.5 EXAMPLES OF GRAND THEORIES WITH SOURCES OF INFORMATION

THEORY	PRIMARY SOURCES OF INFORMATION
King's Theory of Goal Attainment	King, I. M. (1981). *A theory of goal attainment: Systems, concepts, process.* New York: Wiley.
	King, I. M. (1990). Health the goal for nursing. *Nursing Science Quarterly, 3,* 123.
	King, I. M. (1992). King's theory of goal attainment. *Nursing Science Quarterly, 5,* 19.
	King, I. M. (1994). Quality of life and goal attainment. *Nursing Science Quarterly, 7,* 29.
	King, I. M. (1996). The theory of goal attainment in research and practice. *Nursing Science Quarterly, 9,* 61.
	King, I. M. (1997). King's theory of goal attainment in practice. *Nursing Science Quarterly, 10,* 180–185.
Leininger's Theory of Culture Care and Universality	Leininger, M. M. (1970). *Nursing and anthropology: Two worlds blend.* New York: Wiley. Leininger, M. M. (1978). *Transcultural nursing: Concepts, theories, and practices.* New York: Wiley.
	Leininger, M. M. (1985). Transcultural care diversity and universality: A theory of nursing. *Nursing and Health Care, 6,* 208–212.
	Leininger, M. M. (1988). Leininger's theory of nursing: Cultural care diversity and universality. *Nursing Science Quarterly, 1,* 152–160.
	Leininger, M. M. (1991). *Cultural care diversity and universality: A theory of nursing.* New York: National League for Nursing.
	Leininger, M. M. (1995). *Transcultural nursing: Concepts, theories, research, and practice.* Columbus, OH: McGraw Hill College Custom Series.
Newman's Theory of Health as Expanding Consciousness	Newman, M. A. (1986). *Health as expanding consciousness.* St. Louis: Mosby. Newman, M. A. (1990). Newman's theory of health as praxis. *Nursing Science Quarterly, 3,* 37–41.
	Newman, M. A. (1994). *Health as expanding consciousness* (2nd ed.). Boston: Jones & Bartlett.
	Newman, M. A. (1997). Evolution of a theory of health as expanding consciousness. *Nursing Science Quarterly, 10,* 22–25.
Orem's Self-care Deficit Theory	Orem, D. E. (1971). *Nursing: Concepts of practice* (2nd ed.). New York: McGraw Hill. Orem, D. E. (1983). *The self-care deficit theory of nursing.* New York: Wiley.
	Orem, D. E. (1987). *Orem's general theory of nursing.* Philadelphia: W. B. Saunders.
	Orem, D. E., & Taylor, S. G. (1986). *Orem's general theory of nursing.* New York: National League for Nursing.
	Orem, D. E. (2001). *Nursing: Concepts of practice* (6th ed.). New York: McGraw Hill.
Parse's Theory of Human Becoming	Parse, R. R. (1981). *Man-living-health: A theory of nursing.* New York: Wiley. Parse, R. R. (1987). *Nursing science: Major paradigms, theories, and critiques.* Philadelphia: W. B. Saunders.
	Parse, R. R. (1992). Human becoming: Parse's theory of nursing. *Nursing Science Quarterly, 5,* 35–42.
	Parse, R. R. (1994). Quality of life: Sciencing and living the art of human becoming. *Nursing Science Quarterly, 7,* 16–21.
	Parse, R. R. (1996). Reality: A seamless symphony of becoming. *Nursing Science Quarterly, 9,* 181–183.
	Parse, R. R. (1997). The human becoming theory: The was, is, and will be. *Nursing Science Quarterly, 10,* 32–38.
	Parse, R. R. (1998). *The human becoming school of thought.* Thousand Oaks, CA: Sage.

MIDDLE RANGE THEORY

Compared to grand theories, middle range theories are less abstract. Merton (1968), whose work served to promote the development of middle range theories, described them as lying between "the minor but necessary working hypotheses that evolve in abundance during day to day research and the all-inclusive systematic efforts to develop a unified theory . . ." (p. 39). Consistent with Merton's conceptualization, nurse authors have described middle range theories in comparison to grand theories as:

- Narrower in scope (Fawcett, 2005; Liehr & Smith, 1999; McKenna, 1997; Meleis, 1997; Parker, 2006; Walker & Avant, 1995)
- Concerned with less abstract, more specific phenomena (Fawcett, 2005; Meleis, 1997)
- Composed of fewer concepts and propositions (Fawcett, 2005; McKenna, 1997; Walker & Avant, 1995)
- Representative of a limited or partial view of nursing reality (Jacox, 1974; Liehr & Smith, 1999; Young et al., 2001)
- More appropriate for empirical testing (Liehr & Smith, 1999; McKenna, 1997; Meleis, 1997; Parker, 2006; Walker & Avant, 1995)
- More applicable directly to practice for explanation and implementation (McKenna, 1997; Walker & Avant, 1995; Young et al., 2001)

These attributes make middle range theories attractive to nurses who wish to engage in theory-based research and practice.

The appeal of these theories to nurse researchers and practitioners is demonstrated by their proliferation in the past 15 years. Lenz (1996) identified a number of the middle range theories developed in the 1980s and 1990s. Table 1.6 provides a partial listing of theories used by nurses in research and/or practice that have been considered to be middle range. Included in the table are middle range theories in various stages of development and testing. The table also includes one reference for each theory.

Although not included in the table, Peplau's Theory of Interpersonal Relationships, Orlando's Theory of Deliberative Nursing Process, and Watson's Theory of Human Caring (Fawcett, 2005; Fawcett & Bourbonniere, 2001; Jones, 2001) have been labeled middle range theories.

Development of Middle Range Theory

Liehr and Smith (1999) outlined the relationships between the intellectual processes and the sources of content related to the development of middle range theories, which included:

- Inductive theory, building theory through research
- Deductive theory, building from grand nursing theories
- Combining existing nursing and nonnursing theories
- Synthesizing theories from published research findings
- Developing theories from clinical practice guidelines (Approaches for Generating Middle Range Theory, para. 1)

Qualitative research, particularly phenomenological and grounded theory studies, has served as a source of middle range theory development. Ten qualitative studies conducted through the Nursing Consortium for Research on Chronic Sorrow provided a foundation for the development of the middle range

Table 1.6 EXAMPLES OF MIDDLE RANGE THEORIES

THEORY	REFERENCE
Physiological	
Acute Pain Management in Infants and Children	Huth, M. M., & Moore, S. M. (1998). Prescriptive theory of acute pain management in infants and children. *Journal of the Society of Pediatric Nurses, 3*(1), 23–32.
Chronic Pain	Tsai, P., Tak. S., Moore, C., & Palencia, I. (2003). Testing a theory of chronic pain. *Journal of Advanced Nursing, 43*(2), 159–169.
Chronotherapeutic Intervention for Postsurgical Pain	Auvil-Novak, S. E. (1997). A mid-range theory of chronotherapeutic intervention of postsurgical pain. *Nursing Research, 46,* 66–71.
Feeding Efficiency for Bottle-fed Preterm Infants	Hill, A. S. (2002). Toward a theory of feeding efficiency for bottle-fed preterm infants. *The Journal of Theory Construction & Testing, 6*(1), 75–81.
Unpleasant Symptoms	Lenz, E. R., Pugh, L. C., Milligan, R. A., Gift, A. G., & Suppe, F. (1997). The middle range theory of unpleasant symptoms: An update. *Advances in Nursing Science, 19,* 14–27.
Cognitive	
Diabetes Self-care Management	Sousa, V. D., & Zauszniewski, J. A. (2005). Toward a theory of diabetes self-care management. *The Journal of Theory Construction & Testing, 9*(2), 61–67.
Health Belief*	Champion, V. L. (1985). Use of the health belief model in determining frequency of breast self-examination. *Research in Nursing Health, 8,* 373–370.
Learned Response to Chronic Illness	Braden, C. J. (1990). A test of the Self-Help Model: Learned response to chronic illness experience. *Nursing Research, 39,* 42–47.
Life After Liver Transplantation	Chappell, S. M. (2001). Toward a theory of life after a liver transplant. *The Journal of Theory Construction & Testing, 5*(1), 12–14.
Emotional	
Chronic Sorrow	Eakes, G. G., Burke, M. L., & Hainsworth, M. A. (1998). Middle-range theory of chronic sorrow. *Image, 30,* 179–184.
Empathy	Olson, J., & Hanchett, E. (1997). Nurse-expressed empathy, patient outcomes, and development of a middle-range theory. *Image, 29,* 71–76.
Fulfillment	Kylma, J., & Vehvilainen-Julkunen, K. Hope in nursing research: A meta-analysis of the ontological and epistemological foundations of research on hope. *Journal of Advanced Nursing, 25*(2), 364–371.
Grief	Chapman, K. J., & Pepler, C. (1998). Coping, hope anticipatory grief in family members with palliative home care. *Cancer Nursing, 21*(4), 226–234.
Hardiness	Pollack, S. E., & Duffy, M. E. (1990). The health-related hardiness scale: Development and psychometric analysis. *Nursing Research, 39*(4), 218–222.
Hope*	Change, E. C., & DeSimone, S. L. (2001). The influence of hope on appraisals, coping, and dysphoria: A test of hope theory. *Journal of Social & Clinical Psychology, 20*(2), 117–129.
Inner Strength in Women	Dingley, C., Bush, H., & Roux, G. (2001). Inner strength in women recovering from coronary heart disease: A grounded theory. *Journal of Theory Construction and Testing, 5*(2), 45–52.

*Theories used in nursing research that are not nursing-developed theories.

THEORY	REFERENCE
Inner Strength in Women *(continued)*	Roux, G., Dingley, C., & Bush, H. (2002). Inner strength in women: Metasynthesis of qualitative findings in theory development. *Journal of Theory Construction and Testing, 6*(1), 4–15.
Patient Satisfaction	Comley, A. L. (1998). Toward a derived theory of patient satisfaction. *The Journal of Theory Construction & Testing, 2*(2), 44–50.
Peaceful End of Life	Ruland, C. M., & Moore, S. M. (1998). Theory construction based on standards of care: A proposed theory of the peaceful end of life. *Nursing Outlook, 46*(4), 169–175.
Postpartum Depression	Beck, C. T. (1993). The lived experience of postpartum depression: A substantive theory of postpartum depression. *Nursing Research, 42*, 42–48.
Tidal Model	Barker, P., & Buchanan-Barker, P. (2004). *The Tidal Model: A guide for mental health professionals.* London: Brunner-Routledge.
Uncertainty	Mishel, M. H. (1991). Reconceptualization of the uncertainty in illness theory. *Image, 2*, 256–261.
Uncertainty of Illness	Deane, K. A., & Degner, L. F. (1998). Information needs, uncertainty, and anxiety in women who had a breast biopsy with benign outcome. *Cancer Nursing, 21*(2), 117–126.
Social	
Bureaucratic Caring	Ray, M. (1989). The theory of bureaucratic caring for nursing practice in the organizational culture. *Nursing Administrative Quarterly, 13*(2), 31–42.
Caring Through Relation and Dialogue	Sanford, R. C. (2000). Caring through relation and dialogue: A nursing perspective for patient education. *Advances in Nursing Science, 22*(3), 1–15.
Entry into Nursing Home as Status Passage	Chenitz, W. C. (1983, March/April). Entry into a nursing home as status passage: A theory to guide nursing practice. *Geriatric Nursing*, 92–97.
Mastery over Stress	Younger, J. (1991). A theory of mastery: Philosophy of nursing science. *Advances in Nursing Science, 17*(2), 24–28. Younger, J. (1993). The Mastery of Stress Instrument. *Nursing Research, 42*(2), 68–73.
Perceived Family Dynamics of Persons with Chronic Pain	Smith, A. A., & Friedemann, M. (1999). Perceived family dynamics of persons with chronic pain. *Journal of Advanced Nursing, 30*(3), 543–551.
Maternal Role Attainment	Mercer, R. T. (1986). *First time motherhood: Experiences from teens to forties.* New York: Springer.
Negotiating Partnerships	Powell-Cope, G. M. (1994). Family caregivers of people with AIDS: Negotiating partnerships with professional health care providers. *Nursing Research, 43*, 324–330.
Patient Education: Caring Through Relation and Dialogue	Sanford, R. C. (2000). Caring through relation and dialogue: A nursing perspective for patient education. *Advances in Nursing Science, 22*(3), 1–15.
Precarious Ordering: A Theory of Women's Caring	Wuest, J. (2001). Precarious ordering: Toward a formal theory of women's caring. *Health Care for Women International, 22*(1/2), 167–193.

(table continued on page 34)

Table 1.6 **EXAMPLES OF MIDDLE RANGE THEORIES** (continued)

THEORY	REFERENCE
Self-Transcendence	Reed, P. (1991). Toward a nursing theory of self-transcendence: Deductive reformulation using developmental theories. *Advances in Nursing Science, 12,* 64–74.
Integrative	
Caregiver Stress	Tsai, P. (2003). A middle-range theory of caregiver stress. *Nursing Science Quarterly, 16*(2), 137–145.
Experiencing Transitions	Meleis, A. I., Sawyer, L. M., Im, E., Hilfinger Messias, D. K., & Schumacher, K. (2000). Experiencing transitions: An emerging middle-range theory. *Advances in Nursing Science, 23*(1), 12–28.
Healing in Internalized HIV-related Stigma	Gray, D. P. (2004). A theory of healing in internalized HIV-related stigma. *The Journal of Theory Construction & Testing, 8*(2), 48–53.
Illness Constellation	Morse, J. M., & Johnson, H. K. (1991). In *The illness experience: Dimensions of suffering.* Newbury Park, CA: Sage.
Interaction Model of Client Behavior	Cox, C. L. (1982). An interaction model of client behavior: A theoretical prescription for nursing. *Advances in Nursing Science, 5*(1), 41–56.
Self-Care Management for Vulnerable Populations	Dorsey, C. J., & Murdaugh, C. L. (2003). The theory of self-care management for vulnerable populations. *The Journal of Theory Construction & Testing, 7*(2), 43–49.
Successful Aging	Flood, M. (2005). A mid-range nursing theory of successful aging. *The Journal of Theory Construction & Testing, 9*(2), 35–39.

theory of chronic sorrow (Eakes, Burke, & Hainsworth, 1998). The research findings of these and of other studies underwent concept analysis as part of the process of developing this theory.

Several conceptual models and grand theories have served as the foundation for the development of middle range theories. For instance, the middle range theory of home care effectiveness was based on Roy's Adaptation Model (Smith et al., 2002). The work of the theorists resulted in increased specificity of the conceptualization of Roy's interdependence mode. Other examples of middle range theories derived directly and specifically from nursing's major conceptual models and grand theories are found in Table 1.7. Middle range theories have been developed from Johnson's Behavioral System Model, Levine's Conservation Principles, Roger's Science of Unitary Beings, and Roy's Adaptation Model (Alligood & Tomey, 2005).

Theories from nursing have been combined with those from other disciplines to create middle range theories. Mercer used Rubin's work on maternal role attainment (i.e., attachment and role identity during pregnancy and early infancy) and integrated role and developmental theories from the field of psychology to arrive at her Theory of Maternal Role Attainment (Meighan, 2006). She also conducted a number of research studies on the subject, the findings of which were reflected in the theory.

Published research findings have been cited as the most common source for constructing middle range theories of nursing (Lenz, 1998). The development of Online Social Support Theory is an example of this

Table 1.7 **MIDDLE RANGE THEORIES DERIVED FROM CONCEPTUAL MODELS**

CONCEPTUAL MODEL	MIDDLE RANGE THEORY
Johnson's Behavioral System Model	Theory of a Restorative Subsystem Theory of Sustenal Imperatives
Levine's Conservation Principles	Theory of Redundancy Theory of Therapeutic Intention
Rogers' Science of Unitary Human Beings	Theory of Perception of Dissonant Pattern
Roy's Adaptation Model	Theory of the Physiologic Mode Theory of the Self-concept Mode Theory of the Interdependence Mode Theory of the Role Function Mode

Source: Alligood, M. R., & Tomey, A. M. (2002). *Nursing theory: Utilization & application* (pp. 46–54). St. Louis: Mosby. With permission from Elsevier Science.

approach (LaCoursiere, 2001). Synthesized research findings from various patient populations (e.g., patients diagnosed with cancer or cardiovascular illness) that reflected the perspectives of those involved with the use of on-line social support (i.e., patient, caregiver, and nurse) served as a foundation for LaCoursiere's theory.

Clinical practice and clinical practice guidelines are sources of middle range theory development. Peplau is credited with introducing the use of clinical data in the development of her theory, the Theory of Interpersonal Relations. She based her understanding of the stages of the nurse–patient relationship on the observations of interactions between student nurses and psychiatric patients. The guidelines established by the Agency for Health Care Policy and Research for the management of acute pain were used by Good and Moore in the development of the theory of a balance between analgesia and side effects in the management of pain.

It is important to note that most of the nurses involved in the development of middle range theories used more than one approach. As part of arriving at the creation of the middle range theory, often findings from previous research studies were reviewed and analyzed, conceptual models and theories were considered, and additional research was conducted that targeted the phenomenon of most interest.

Uses of Middle Range Theory

Middle range theory has been found to be useful in both research and practice. "Theory can serve a heuristic function to stimulate and provide the rationale for studies, as well as help guide the selection of research questions and variables" (Lenz, 1998, p. 26). Middle range theories also can assist practice by facilitating understanding of client's behavior, suggesting interventions, and providing possible explanations for the degree of effectiveness of the interventions.

Reviews of published studies reveal a fairly extensive use of middle range theory in nursing research, most often middle range theories from other disciplines (Lenz, 1998). This is particularly evident when comparing how frequently middle range theories and grand theories of nursing are cited in the nursing research literature. Of 173 studies included in *Nursing Research* from January 1994 through June 1997, only 79 (45.7%) identified any theory. Of the 79 studies that identified a theory, 25 were nursing theories and 54 were middle range theories borrowed from other disciplines, most frequently from psychology.

Nursing's middle range theories accounted for most of the nursing theories used in the studies, 22 of the 25 (Lenz, 1998, p. 27).

Though middle range theory has great potential for guiding nursing practice, the nursing literature suggests that the potential has not been fully realized. Many authors note a gap between theory and practice. And when applications of theory to practice are included in the literature, it is more likely to be a grand rather than a middle range theory (Lenz, 1998). An informal survey of 10 clinical nurse specialists and five staff nurses, conducted by Lenz, revealed few who were able to identify theories they were using in their practice. She attributes this to several factors: (a) the busyness of practicing nurses that does not allow time for consideration of the theoretical bases for their actions; (b) educational programs that do not help students learn the connections between theory and practice; (c) clinical environments that do not value theory-based practice; and (d) the lack of availability and usability of information on middle range theories. Nurse theorists need to address the last factor by producing literature describing their theories in understandable terms, identifying the theories' implications for practice, and placing that information in practice-oriented journals.

Controversy Surrounding Middle Range Theory

The identification of middle range theories is not unambiguous. For instance, Chenitz, primary author of Entry into a Nursing Home as Status Passage, labeled it practice theory, whereas others considered it middle range theory (Liehr & Smith, 1999, Analysis of the Middle Range Theory Foundation, para. 2). "The question about what constitutes theory at the middle range is not a black and white issue for which a precise and clear definition can be offered. Middle range theory holds to a given level of abstraction. It is not too broad nor too narrow, but somewhere in the middle" (Leihr & Smith, 1999, Analysis of the Middle Range Theory Foundation, para. 3). To reduce confusion, nurse theorists are encouraged to clearly identify their work as middle range and provide a name that represents its conceptual components (Liehr & Smith, 1999; Sanford, 2000).

The imprecision of what constitutes a middle range theory is only one of several criticisms of middle range theory. In addition to lack of definitional clarity, middle range theory has been criticized for distinguishing itself from grand theories by its ability to be tested, using a logical positivistic idea of testability. Suppe (1996b) suggests an alternative approach to considering the testability of middle range theory. He rejects the widely accepted notion of theories as a set of propositions and proposes the idea that theories are "state-transitions systems modeling the behaviors of real world systems within the theory's scope" (Suppe, 1996b, p. 10). By this conceptualization of theories, operational concepts become descriptors; the values of these concepts become state specifications; and the propositions become specifications of state-transition relations (Suppe, 1996b, p. 11). The purpose of testing using this understanding of the nature of theories is delineating the scope of the middle range theory rather than subjecting a hypothesis to statistical analysis or qualitative data to coding. The basic research question is for what systems does the theory work and for what systems does it not, a question of scope. This type of research question is well suited to the testing of middle range theories.

Since Merton (1968) first promoted the notion of middle range theories, they have been criticized as being intellectually unambitious. Critics argue that their scope and suggested methods of inquiry are too limited. Merton countered that middle range theory was addressing just the questions that the discipline of sociology was asking, and that middle range theories can undergo the same systematic empirical testing that both more and less abstract theories can (pp. 63–64).

Another criticism of middle range theories is that their increasing numbers can lead to fragmentation of nursing's knowledge base into unrelated and distinct theories. This claim could be as legitimately made about either grand or micro theories. Merton acknowledged that risk and proposed consolidating theories to create groups of like theories at the middle range (Whall, 1996). Nurse scientists have addressed this issue. The identification of a metaparadigm is an attempt to create some conceptual cohesion for nursing's knowledge base. In addition, there has been an intentional effort to relate middle range theories to nursing's conceptual models, grand theories, and taxonomies. For instance, the middle range theory of Therapeutic Intention is clearly linked to Levine's Conservation Principles. Nurse scientists have proposed anchoring middle range theories to nursing's taxonomies of (a) diagnoses, North American Nursing Diagnosis Association (NANDA); (b) interventions, Nursing Interventions Classification (NIC); and (c) outcomes, Nursing Outcomes Classification (NOC) (Blegan & Tripp-Reimer, 1997) and have identified a structure to accomplish that linkage (Tripp-Reimer, Woodworth, McCloskey, & Bulechek, 1996). Others consider these taxonomies as types of middle range theories rather than frameworks for categorizing the theories because they consist of concepts, definitions of concepts, propositional statements, and assumptions (Whall, 1996). As taxonomies, these middle range theories could not be considered unrelated and fragmented aspects of nursing's knowledge base. Nurse scientists continue to recommend persistence in efforts to "create an association between the proposed theory and a disciplinary perspective in nursing" (Liehr & Smith, 1999, p. 90).

Nurse researchers have been denounced for making use of middle range theories from disciplines other than nursing. This was certainly true of nursing research published from the mid-1970s to the mid-1980s. During this period, more than half of the studies made use of theories or models from disciplines other than nursing (Moody et al., 1988). The increasing number of nursing middle range theories is reversing that trend. Liehr and Smith (1999) found 22 middle range nursing theories published in the decade from 1988 to 1999 through a CINAHL search. These theories met a number of criteria, including identification by the author that the theory was of the middle range. The criticism that nurse researchers use middle range theories from disciplines other than nursing is also being addressed by a call to continue to develop theories in the midlevel of scope and abstractness. "Situating middle range theory at the forefront for practice and research is critical to epistemologic and ontologic growth in nursing" (Sanford, 2000, Recommendation 5, para. 1).

PRACTICE THEORY/MICRO THEORY/SITUATION-SPECIFIC THEORY

The literature includes a confusing variety of terms to refer to the level of theory that is considered less abstract, more specific, and narrower in scope than middle range theory. *Practice theory* seems to be the most commonly used term (Jones, 2001; McKenna, 1997; Walker & Avant, 1995). Suppe (1996b), Kramer (1997), and Parker (2006) referred to both practice and micro theory, and Suppe discussed some of the distinctions between the two terms. The term *micro theory* was also used by Kim (2000), Duldt and Giffin (1985), and Chinn and Kramer (1999, 2004), and by George (1995) and Young et al. (2001), who both cited Chinn and Kramer. The most recently introduced term is *situation-specific theory* (Im & Meleis, 1999; Meleis & Im, 2001).

Practice theory can trace its origins to the work of metatheorists Dickhoff and James (1968). Their position is that because nursing is a profession, its theory must have an action orientation that can shape reality to create a desired goal. "The major contention here is that theory exists finally for the sake of practice" (p. 199).

Several authors have provided a list of the components of a practice theory. As stated earlier, Dickhoff and James referred to this goal-oriented theory as "situation-producing" and identified its essential elements as: "1) goal-content specified as aim for activity; 2) prescriptions for activity to realize the goal-content; and 3) a survey list to serve as a supplement to present prescription and preparation for future prescription for activity toward the goal-content" (p. 201). Jones (2001, p. 376) interprets these elements to include the use of nursing diagnosis and outcomes classification systems as components of practice theory. Walker and Avant (1995) and Kramer (1997) referred to these three components in their definitions of practice theory and both suggested additional considerations. Walker and Avant claim that without a basis in situation-relating (predictive) theories, it would require a liberal definition of theory to identify practice or situation-producing theory as theory. They suggest that it would be more legitimate to refer to practice theory as nursing practices (pp. 12–13). Kramer identifies a similar issue, the importance of connecting practice theory to the more encompassing knowledge structures of nursing as identified by metatheory. To the traditional understanding of practice theory she adds theory about nursing practice (e.g., administrative and educational theories). This is not a commonly occurring use.

Like other levels of theory, practice theories as situation producing are derived from middle range theories, practice experiences, and empirical testing. Middle range theories are the source of the prescriptions that are directed at the specified goal (McKenna, 1997; Parker, 2006; Walker & Avant, 1995) and if not specifically derived from these middle range theories, at the very least, practice theories should identify how the concepts from both levels of theory are interrelated. Practice theory also develops from the clinical experiences of nurses that have been subjected to the process of reflection. Reflection on practice leads to insights that can serve as a foundation for developing theory. It provides a real-world basis for the creation of practice theory. Research is also an important source of practice theories. Walker and Avant (1995) note the contributions of the Conduct and Utilization of Research in Nursing project in the formulation of practice theories. This project, initiated in 1975, identified a need for change in practice and summarized the relevant research to arrive at research-based principles for nursing interventions. There were 10 practice theories or protocols that were considered during the project. Examples of the protocols that were developed include (a) lactose-free diet; (b) sensation information: distress; (c) intravenous cannula-change regiment; and (d) prevention of decubiti by means of small shifts of body weight (Haller, Reynolds, & Horsley, 1979, p. 47).

Micro theory, a term sometimes identified as interchangeable with practice theory, is included in the writings of Kim (2000), Suppe (1996b), and Chinn and Kramer (2005). Kim's (1983) definition of micro theory as a set of "theoretical statements, usually hypotheses, that deal with narrowly defined phenomena" (p. 13) suggests a research-based theory. Suppe (1996b) also identifies hypothesis testing as a primary feature of micro theories and claims that this fact provides the primary distinction between micro theory and middle range theory, both of which could be considered practice theories (pp. 12–13). According to Suppe, the term *micro theory* is found with increasing frequency in the literature to refer to theories that are too limited in scope to be considered middle range. He provided a hypothetical example of a micro theory of pain management for a hospitalized patient with acute postamputation pain, who was treated with patient-controlled anesthesia (PCA) with morphine, with possible Valium potentiation, focusing on pain intensity and addiction outcomes (Suppe, 1996b, p. 12). Kim (1983) provided examples of what she labeled as micro theories (i.e., maternal attachment, pressure sores, wound healing, and positioning). Other examples of this level of theory development found in the literature include alcoholism recovery in lesbian women (Hall, 1990), quality of care (Nielson, 1992), milieu therapy for short-stay units (LeCuyer, 1992), caring for patients with chronic skin disease (Kirkevold, 1993), therapeutic touch (Green, 1998), exercise as self-care (Ulbrich, 1999), and ecological view of protection (Shearer, 2002).

Im and Meleis (1999) use the term *situation specific* to refer to that level of nursing theory that focuses on specific nursing phenomena with direct application to nursing practice. There are a number of features that distinguish situation-specific theories from either grand or middle range theories. They exhibit "(1) a lower level of abstraction, (2) reflection of specific nursing phenomenon, (3) context, (4) readily accessible connection to nursing research and practice, (5) reflection of diversities in nursing phenomena, and (6) limitation of generalization" (Properties of Situation-Specific Theories, para. 1). A somewhat unique quality of situation-specific theories is their emphasis on sociopolitical, cultural, and historical contexts, demonstrated by the theory of menopausal transition of Korean immigrant women described by Im and Meleis.

In addition to the debate on the term to use in referring to this level of theory, the controversies about practice theory center on whether it is a theory, and if so, whether it is needed. Walker (1986) suggests that, based on a definition of practice theory as sets of principles or directives, the terms *policy, procedure,* or *principles of practice* might be more appropriate. Her conclusion is based on an understanding of theory as a "systematic description and explanation" (p. 28). Walker's position seems consistent with the increasingly popular phenomena of research utilization and evidence-based practice. Beckstrand's (1986) contention is that practice theory is unnecessary. She claims that "all the theoretical knowledge relevant to practice can be discovered within existing systems of knowledge such as metatheory, philosophy, science, and ethics." Collins and Fielder (1986) respond to Beckstrand's conclusion by emphasizing the unique issues that nursing theories must address. They assert that Beckstrand's position does not consider the nurse's responsibility for caring for the client as a "particular" individual. Nursing still has a need for "a nursing theory that will set out the kinds of nursing practice and the particular set of moral ideals that nursing practice seeks to bring about" (Collins & Fielder, 1986, p. 510). The increasing number of practice theories or their semantic equivalent identified in the literature in the 1990s seems to be supporting, if not a need, at least an interest in this level of theory development.

SUMMARY

The development of nursing knowledge is an ongoing process, though debates continue on the direction that this development should take. For instance, there are differences of opinion on whether diversity or unity of paradigms and philosophies is preferred. The language of nursing science is not firmly established or used consistently; there still is not consensus on the use of some of the terms that refer to the components of the structural hierarchy of nursing knowledge. One term used fairly consistently in the literature is *middle range theory,* and it is the development of this level of theory verified by research and useful for practice that is the focus of the efforts of many nurse scientists.

CRITICAL THINKING EXERCISES

1. In the debate on nursing paradigms, which of the currently proposed considerations—emergence of a single paradigm, coexistence of complementary paradigms, or creation of an integrated paradigm from the two most prominent paradigms—seems to best serve the advancement of nursing knowledge? What would be the implications of the chosen perspective on paradigms for the development of nursing knowledge?

2. Make a case for the ongoing development and use of nursing grand theories. Conversely, make a case for the obsolescence of nursing grand theories for today's practice and research.

3. Identify a research topic or develop a research question. Refer to the table *Examples of Middle Range Theories*. Which middle range theory might be applicable to the research topic or question? If none seems appropriate, why might that be?

WEB RESOURCES

Philosophy

1. **http://www.ksl.stanford.edu/kst/what-is-an-ontology.html** provides expanded definitions of ontology and links to several on-line articles.
2. **http://www.formalontology.it/index.htm** traces historical development and lists relevant readings.

Theory

There are several Internet sites that provide links to the home pages of individual nursing theorists. These home pages often include biographical information and bibliographies of the theorists' publications, and sometimes provide descriptions of the theories, reviews of their published work, and the E-mail addresses of the theorists.

The links to theorists include but are not limited to:

Faye Abdellah
Anne Boykin and
  Savina Schoenhofer
Helen Erickson, Evelyn
  Tomlin, and Mary
  Ann Swain
Joyce Fitzpatrick
Lydia Hall
Virginia Henderson
Dorothy Johnson
Ionnis Kalofissudi
Imogene King

Kathy Kolcaba
Madeleine Leininger
Myra Levine
Alaf Meleis
Ramona Mercer
Betty Neuman
Margaret Newman
Florence Nightingale
Ida Jean Orlando
Josephine Paterson and
  Loretta Zderad
Nola Pender

Hildegard Peplau
Joan Riehl-Sisca
Martha Rogers
Sister Callista Roy
Nancy Roper, Winifred
  Logan, and Alison
  Tierney

Cornelia Ruland
Jean Watson
Ernestine Wiedenbach

The following Internet sites provide links to the theorists and to other nursing theory pages:

1. **http://www.sandiego.edu/academics/nursing/theory/** organizes its links to the web pages of the nurse scientists by categorizing them as general theories, middle range theories, and models. In addition to links to middle range theories, the site provides a description of this level of theory development. Other features included are discussion forums and lists of resources (books and videos).
2. **http://www.healthsci.clayton.edu/eichelberger/nursing.htm** includes a list of theory books, links to electronic resources, and advice for searching on-line for information on nursing theories, in addition to the links to specific theorists.
3. **http://www.enursescribe.com/nurse_theorists.htm** classifies the nurse theorists as models: adaptation, anthropological, energy fields, humanist, self-care, and systems. There are also sections devoted to the early nurse theorists, middle range theories, and book reviews.

4. **http://www.nursingtheory.net** organizes content as models, midrange, grand, and other theories.

These sites can also be located through a web search on "nursing theory."

Another source of information on nursing theorists, though not an Internet site, is the video series *The Nurse Theorists: Portraits in Excellence.* The individual videos provide biographical information and description of the theory, with an interview of the theorists conducted by

Jacqueline Fawcett. The following theorists are included in this series: Johnson, King, Levine, Neuman, Orem, Rogers, Roy, Leininger, Newman, Orlando, Parse, Peplau, Watson, Rubin, Henderson, and Nightingale. This resource is available from Fuld Institute for Technology in Nursing Education (FITNE) at their address, 5 Depot Street, Athens, OH 45701; their telephone numbers, 1-800-691-8480 or 740-592-2511; or on-line at http://fitne.net.

REFERENCES

Adam, E. (1992). Contemporary conceptualization of nursing: Philosophy or science? In J. F. Kikuchi & H. Simmons (Eds.), *Philosophic inquiry in nursing* (pp. 55–63). London: Sage.

Alligood, M. R., & Tomey, A. M. (2006). *Nursing theory: Utilization & application* (3rd ed.). St. Louis: Mosby.

Annells, M. (2005). Guest editorial: A qualitative quandary: Alternative representations and meta-synthesis. *Journal of Clinical Nursing, 14*(5), 535–536.

Antognoli-Toland, P. L. (1999). Kuhn and Reigel: The nature of scientific revolutions and theory construction. *The Journal of Theory Construction & Testing, 3*(2), 38–41.

Archibald, G. (2000). A postmodern nursing model. *Nursing Standard, 14*(34), 40–42.

Babbie, E. (1995). *The practice of social research* (7th ed.). Belmont, CA: Wadsworth.

Barrett, E. (1986). Investigation of the principle of helicy: The relationship of human filed motion and power. In V. Mailinski (Ed.), *Explorations on Martha Rogers' science of unitary human beings* (pp. 173–184). Norwalk, CT: Appleton-Century-Crofts.

Barrett, E. A. M. (1992). Diversity reigns. *Nursing Science Quarterly, 5*(4), 155–157.

Beckstrand, J. (1986). A critique of several conceptions of practice theory in nursing. In L. H. Nicholl (Ed.), *Perspectives on nursing theory* (pp. 494–504). Boston: Little, Brown and Company.

Bisk, T. (n.d.). Utopianism come to age: From postmodernism to neo-modernism. Retrieved August 16, 2006, from http://www.wfs.org/bisk.htm.

Blegan, M. A., & Tripp-Reimer, T. (1997). Implications of nursing taxonomies for middle-range theory development. *Advances in Nursing Science, 19*(3), *37*(13). Retrieved December 14, 1999, from Health Reference Center–Academic database.

Brower, H. T. F., & Baker, B. J. (1976). Using the adaptation model in a practitioner curriculum. *Nursing Outlook, 24*, 686–689.

Brown, S. T., & Lee, B. T. (1980). Imogene King's conceptual framework: A proposed model for continuing nursing education. *Journal of Advanced Nursing, 5*, 467–473.

Burbules, N. C. (n.d.). Postmodern doubt and philosophy of education. Retrieved June 6, 2002, from University of Illinois at Urbana-Champaign Web site: http://www.ed.uiuc.edu/EPS/PES-Yearbook/95_docs/burbules.html.

Caper, C. F. (1986). Some basic facts about models, nursing conceptualizations, and nursing theories. *The Journal of Continuing Education in Nursing, 16*(5), 149–154.

Carper, B. A. (1978). Fundamental patterns of knowing in nursing. *Advances in Nursing Science, 1*(1), 13–23.

Chinn, P., & Kramer, M. (1995). *Theory and nursing: A systematic approach* (4th ed.). St Louis: Mosby Year-Book.

Chinn, P. L., & Kramer, M. K. (1999). *Theory and nursing: Integrated nursing knowledge* (5th ed.). St. Louis: Mosby.

Chinn, P. L., & Kramer, M. K. (2004). *Theory and nursing: Integrated nursing knowledge* (6th ed.). St. Louis: Mosby.

Cody, W. C., & Mitchell, G. J. (2002). Nursing knowledge and human science revisited: Practical and political considerations. *Nursing Science Quarterly, 15*(1), 4–13.

Collins, R. C., & Fielder, J. H. (1986). Beckstrand's concept of practice theory: A critique. In L. H. Nicholl (Ed.), *Perspectives on nursing theory* (pp. 505–511). Boston: Little, Brown and Company.

Derdiarian, A. K. (1988). Sensitivity of the Derdiarian behavioral system model instrument to age, sit, and stage of cancer: A preliminary validation study. *Scholarly Inquiry for Nursing Practice, 2*, 103–121.

Dickhoff, J., & James, P. (1968). A theory of theories: A position paper. *Nursing Research, 17*(3), 197–203.

Donnelly, E. (2001). An assessment of nursing theories as guides to scientific inquiry. In N. L. Chaska (Ed.), *The nursing profession: Tomorrow and beyond* (pp. 331–344). Thousand Oaks, CA: Sage.

Downs, F. S. (1982). A theoretical question. *Nursing Research, 3,* 259.

Duldt, B. W., & Giffin, K. (1985). *Theoretical perspectives for nursing.* Boston: Little, Brown and Company.

Dunphy, L. H. (2001). Florence Nightingale care actualized: A legacy for nursing. In M. E Parker (Ed.), *Nursing theories and nursing practice* (pp. 31–53). Philadelphia: F.A. Davis.

Eakes, G. G., Burke, M. L., & Hainsworth, M. A. (1998). Middle-range theory of chronic sorrow. *Image, 30*(2), 179–184.

Engebretson, J. (1997). A multiparadigm approach to nursing. *Advances in Nursing Science, 20*(1), 21–33. Retrieved June 3, 2002, from CINAHL/OVID database.

Estabrooks, C. A., Field, P. A., & Morse, J. M. (1994) Aggregating qualitative findings: An approach to theory development. *Qualitative Health Research, 4*(4), 503–511.

Fagerhaugh, S. Y. (1974). Pain expression and control on a burn care unit. *Nursing Outlook, 22,* 645–650.

Fawcett, J. (1978). The "what" of theory development. In D. E. Johnson & I. M. King (Eds.), *Theory development: What, why, how?* (pp. 17–33). New York: National League of Nursing.

Fawcett, J. (1984). *Analysis and evaluation of conceptual models of nursing.* Philadelphia: F. A. Davis Company.

Fawcett, J. (1996). On the requirements for a metaparadigm: An invitation to dialogue. *Nursing Science Quarterly, 9*(3), 94–97.

Fawcett, J. (1997). The structural hierarchy of nursing knowledge: Components and their definitions. In I. M. King & J. Fawcett (Eds.), *The language of nursing theory and metatheory* (pp. 11–17). Indianapolis, IN: Sigma Theta Tau.

Fawcett, J., Watson, J., Neuman, B., Walker, P. H., Fitzpatrick J. J. (2001). On nursing theories and evidence. *Journal of Nursing Scholarship, 33*(2), 115–119.

Fawcett, J. (2003). Critiquing contemporary nursing knowledge: A dialogue. *Nursing Science Quarterly, 16*(3), 273–276.

Fawcett, J. (2005). *Contemporary nursing knowledge: Analysis and evaluation of nursing models and theories* (2nd ed.). Philadelphia: F.A. Davis Company.

Fawcett, J., & Alligood, M. R. (2005). Influences on advancement of nursing knowledge. *Nursing Science Quarterly, 18*(3), 227–232.

Fawcett, J., & Bourbonniere, M. G. (2001). Utilization of nursing knowledge and the future of the discipline. In N. L. Chaska (Ed.), *The nursing profession: Tomorrow and beyond* (pp. 311–320). Thousand Oaks, CA: Sage.

Fitzpatrick, J. J. (1997). Nursing theory and metatheory. In I. M. King and J. Fawcett (Eds.), *The language of nursing theory and metatheory,* (pp. 37–39). Indianapolis, IN: Sigma Theta Tau.

Fitzpatrick, J., & Whall, A. (2005). *Conceptual models of nursing: Analysis and application* (4th ed.). Bowie, MD: Robert J. Brady.

George, J. B. (1995). *Nursing theories: The base for professional nursing practice* (4th ed.). Norwalk, CT: Appleton & Lange.

Georges, J. M. An emerging discourse: Toward epistemic diversity in nursing. *Advances in Nursing Science, 26*(1), 44–52.

Green, C. A. (1998). Critically exploring the use of Rogers' nursing theory of unitary beings as a framework to underpin therapeutic touch practice. *European Nurse, 3*(3), 158–169.

Grubbs, J. (1974). An interpretation of the Johnson behavioral system model for nursing practice. In J. P. Riehl & C. Roy, *Conceptual models for nursing practice* (pp. 160–206). New York: Appleton-Century-Crofts.

Glaser, B. G., & Straus, A. L. (1967). *The discovery of grounded theory: Strategies for qualitative research.* Chicago: Aldine.

Guiliano, K. K., Tyer-Viola, L., & Lopez, R. P. (2005). Unity of knowledge in the advancement of nursing knowledge. *Nursing Science Quarterly, 18*(3), 242–248.

Guba, E. G. (1990). *The paradigm dialog.* Newbury Park, CA: Sage.

Hall, J. M. (1990). Alcoholism recovery of lesbian women: A theory in development. *Scholarly Inquiry for Nursing Practice, 4*(2), 109–122.

Haller, K. B., Reynolds, M. A., & Horsley, J. A. (1979). Developing research-based innovation protocols: Process, criteria, and issues. *Research in Nursing and Health, 2,* 45–51.

Hardy, L. K. (1986). Janforum: Identifying the place of theoretical frameworks in an evolving discipline. *Journal of Advanced Nursing, 11,* 103–107.

Harris, R. B. (1986). Introduction of a conceptual model into a fundamental baccalaureate course. *Journal of Nursing Education, 25,* 66–69.

Im, E. O., & Meleis, A. (1999). Situation-specific theories: Philosophical roots, properties, and approach. *Advances in Nursing Science, 22*(2), 11–24. Retrieved June 3, 2002, from CINAHL/OVID database.

Jacobson, S. F. (1987). Studying and using conceptual models of nursing. *Image: Journal of Nursing Scholarship, 19*(2), 78–82.

Jacox, A. (1974). Theory construction in nursing: An overview. *Nursing Research, 23*(1), 4–13.

Johns, J. (1995). Framing learning through reflection within Carper's fundamental way of knowing in nursing. *Journal of Advanced Nursing, 22*(2), 226–234. Retrieved August 26, 2005 from ovid.

Johnson, D. E. (1974). Development of theory: A requisite for nursing as a primary health profession. *Nursing Research, 23*(5), 372–377.

Johnson, D. E. (1986). Theory in nursing: Borrowed and unique. In L. H. Nicholl (Ed.), *Perspectives on nursing theory* (pp. 112–117). Boston: Little, Brown and Company.

Johnson, D. E. (1990). The behavioral system model for nursing. In M. E. Parker (Ed.), *Nursing theories in practice* (pp. 23–32). New York: National League for Nursing.

Johnson, J. E., & Rice, V. H. (1974). Sensory and distress components of pain. *Nursing Research, 23*, 203–209.

Jones, D. A. (2001). Linking nursing language and knowledge development. In N. L. Chaska (Ed.), *The nursing profession: Tomorrow and beyond* (pp. 373–386). Thousand Oaks, CA: Sage.

Kahn, S., & Fawcett, J. (1995). Critiquing the dialogue: A response to Draper's critique of Fawcett's "Conceptual models and nursing practice: The reciprocal relationship." *Journal of Advanced Nursing, 22*(1), 188–192.

Kameoda, T., & Sugimori, M. (1993, June). Application of King's goal attainment theory in Japanese clinical setting. Paper presented at the meeting of Sigma Theta Tau International's Sixth International Nursing Research Congress, Madrid, Spain.

Kao, H. S., Reeder, F. M., Hsu, M., & Cheng, S. (2006). A Chinese view of the western metaparadigm. *Journal of Holistic Nursing, 24*(2), 92–101.

Kikuchi, J. F. (1992). Nursing questions that science cannot answer. In J. F. Kikuchi & H. Simmons (Eds.), *Philosophic inquiry in nursing* (pp. 26–37). Newbury Park, CA: Sage.

Kikuchi, J. F. (2003). Nursing knowledge and the problem of worldviews. *Research & theory for Nursing Practice, 17*, 7–17.

Kikuchi, J. F., & Simmons, H. (1996). The whole truth and progress in nursing knowledge development. In J. F. Kikuchi, H. Simmons, & D. Romyn (Eds.), *Truth in nursing inquiry* (pp. 5–18). Newbury Park, CA: Sage.

Kilchenstein, L., & Yakulis, I. (1984). The birth of a curriculum: Utilization of the Neuman health care system model in an integrated baccalaureate program. *Journal of Nursing Education, 23*, 126–127.

Kim, H. S. (1983). *The nature of theoretical thinking in nursing.* Norwalk, CT: Appleton-Century-Crofts.

Kim, H. S. (1989). Theoretical thinking in nursing: Problems and perspectives. *Recent Advances in Nursing, 24*, 106–122.

Kim, H. S. (1997). Terminology in structuring and developing nursing knowledge. In I. M. King & J. Fawcett (Eds.), *The language of nursing theory and metatheory* (pp. 27–35). Indianapolis, IN: Sigma Theta Tau.

Kim, H. S. (2000). *The nature of theoretical thinking in nursing* (2nd ed.). New York: Springer.

King, I. M. (1978). The "why" of theory development. In National League for Nursing, *Theory development: What, why, how?* (pp. 11–16). New York: National League for Nursing.

King, I. M. (1984). Philosophy of nursing education: A national survey. *Western Journal of Nursing Research, 6,* 387–406.

King, I. M. (1997). Knowledge development for nursing: A process. In I. M. King & J. Fawcett (Eds.), *The language of nursing theory and metatheory* (pp. 19–25). Indianapolis, IN: Sigma Theta Tau.

Kirkevold, M. (1993). Toward a practice theory of caring for patients with chronic skin disease. *Scholarly Inquiry for Nursing Practice, 7*(1), 37–57.

Kramer, M. K. (1997). Terminology in theory: Definitions and comments. In I. M. King & J. Fawcett (Eds.), *The language of nursing theory and metatheory* (pp. 61–71). Indianapolis, IN: Sigma Theta Tau.

Kuhn, T. S. (1977). *The essential tension.* Chicago: Chicago University Press.

Kuhn, T. S. (1996). *The structure of scientific revolutions* (3rd ed.). Chicago: Chicago University Press.

Kylma, J. (2005). Dynamics of hope in adults living with HIV/AIDS: A substantive theory. *Journal of Advanced Nursing, 52*(6), 620–630.

LaCoursiere, S. P. (2001). A theory of online social support. *Advances in Nursing Science, 24*(1), 60–77.

Landreneau, K. J. (2002). Response to: "The nature of philosophy of science, theory and knowledge relating to nursing and professionalism." *Journal of Advanced Nursing, 38*(3), 283–285. Retrieved November 6, 2002, from CINAHL/OVID database.

LeCuyer, E. A. (1992). Milieu therapy for short stay units: A transformed practice theory. *Archives of Psychiatric Nursing, 6*(2), 108–116.

Leddy, S. K. (2000). Toward a complementary perspective on worldviews. *Nursing Science Quarterly, 13*(3), 225–233.

Lenz, E. R. (1996). Role of middle range theory for research and practice. Paper presented at the Proceedings of the Sixth Rosemary Ellis Scholars' Retreat, Frances Payne Bolton School of Nursing, Case Western Reserve University, Cleveland, OH.

Lenz, E. R. (1998). Role of middle range theory for nursing research and practice. Part 1. Nursing research. *Nursing Leadership Forum, 3*(1), 24–33.

Lenz, E. R., Suppe, F., Gift, A. G., Pugh, L. C., & Milligan, R. A. (1995). Collaborative development of middle-range theories: Toward a theory of unpleasant symptoms. *Advances in Nursing Science, 17*(3), 1–13.

Lerner, R. M. (1986). *Concepts and theories of human development* (2nd ed.). New York: Random House.

Liehr, P., & Smith, M. J. (1999). Middle range theory: Spinning research and practice to create knowledge for the new millennium. *Advances in Nursing Science, 21*(4), 81–91. Retrieved June 11, 2002, from CINAHL/OVID database.

Littlejohn, C. (2002). Are nursing models to blame for low morale? *Nursing Standard, 16*(17), 39–41.

Mackenzie, S., & Spence Laschinger, H. (1995). Correlates of nursing diagnoses in public health nursing. *Journal of Advanced Nursing, 21*(4), 772–777.

Malone, R. E. (2005). Assessing the policy environment. *Policy, Politics, & Nursing Practice, 6*(2), 135–143.

McKenna, H. (1997). Nursing theories and models. London: Routledge.

Meighan, M. (2006). Mercer's becoming a mother theory in nursing practice. In M. R. Alligood & A. M. Tomey (Eds.), *Nursing theory: Utilization & application* (3rd ed., pp. 399–411). St. Louis: Mosby.

Meleis, A. I. (1997). *Theoretical nursing: Development and progress* (3rd ed.). Philadelphia: Lippincott-Raven.

Meleis, A. I., & Im, E. (2001). From fragmentation to integration in the discipline of nursing: Situation-specific theories. In N. L. Chaska (Ed.), *The nursing profession: Tomorrow and beyond* (pp. 881–891). Thousand Oaks, CA: Sage.

Merton, R. K. (1968). *On social theory and social structure.* New York: Free Press.

Monti, E. J., & Tingen, M. S. (1999). Multiple paradigms in nursing. *Advances in Nursing Science, 21*(4), 64–80.

Moody, L. E. (1990). *Advancing nursing science through research* (Vol. 1). Newbury Park, CA: Sage.

Moody, L. E., Wilson, N. E., Smyth, K., Schwartz, R., Tittle, M., & Van Cott, M. L. (1988). Analysis of a decade of nursing practice research: 1977–1986. *Nursing Research, 37*(6), 374–379.

Newman, M. (2002). The pattern that connects. *Advances in Nursing Science, 24*(3), 1–7.

Newman, M. A., Sime, A. M., Corcoran-Perry, S. A. (1991). The focus of the discipline of nursing. *Advances in Nursing Science, 14*(1), 1–6.

Newman, M. A., Sime, A. M., & Corcoran-Perry, S. A. (1996). The focus of the discipline of nursing. In J. W. Kenney (Ed.), *Philosophical and theoretical perspectives for advanced nursing practice* (pp. 297–301). Boston: Jones and Bartlett.

Nielson, P. A. (1992). Quality of care: Discovering a modified practice theory. *Journal of Nursing Care Quality, 6*(2), 63–76.

Orem, D. E. (2001). *Nursing: Concepts of practice* (6th ed.). St. Louis: Mosby.

Parker, K. P. (1989). The theory of sentience evolution: A practice-level theory of sleeping, waking, and beyond waking patterns based on the science of unitary human beings. *Rogerian Nursing Science News, 2*(1), 4–6.

Parker, M. E. (2006). *Nursing theories and nursing practice* (2nd ed.). Philadelphia: F.A. Davis.

Parse, R. R. (1987). *Nursing science: Major paradigms, theories, and critiques.* Philadelphia: W. B. Saunders.

Parse, R. R. (1999). Nursing science: the transformation of practice. *Journal of Advanced Nursing, 30*(6),

1383–1387. Retrieved November 6, 2002, from CINAHL/OVID database.

Phillips, J. R. (1992). The aim of philosophical inquiry in nursing: Unity or diversity of thought? In J. F. Kikuchi & H. Simmons (Eds.), *Philosophic inquiry in nursing.* Newbury Park, CA: Sage.

Pilkington, F. B., & Mitchell, G. J. (1999). A dialogue on the comparability of research paradigms—and other theoretical things. *Nursing Science Quarterly, 12*(4), 283–289.

Pilkington, F. B., & Mitchell, G. J. (2003). Mistakes across paradigms. *Nursing Science Quarterly, 16*(2), 102–108.

Porter-O'Grady, T. (2003). Nurses as knowledge workers. *Creative Nursing, 9*(2). Retrieved August 22, 2005 from Academic Search Premier.

Rawnsley, M. M. (2003). Dimensions of scholarship and the advancement of nursing science: Articulating a vision. *Nursing Science Quarterly, 16*(1), 5–15.

Reed, P. G. (1995). A treatise on nursing knowledge development for the 21st century: Beyond postmodernism. *Advances in Nursing Science, 17*(3), 70–84. Retrieved June 3, 2002, from CINAHL/OVID database.

Reynolds, P. D. (1971). *A primer for theory construction.* Indianapolis, IN: Bobbs-Merrill.

Rinehart, J. M. (1978). The "how" of theory development in nursing. In National League for Nursing, *Theory development: What, why, how?* (pp. 67–74). New York: National League for Nursing.

Roach, M. S. (1992). The aim of philosophical inquiry in nursing: Unity or diversity of thought. In J. F. Kikuchi & H. Simmons (Eds.), *Philosophic inquiry in nursing* (pp. 38–44). Newbury Park, CA: Sage.

Rodman, H. (1980). Are conceptual frameworks necessary for theory building? The case of family sociology. *The Sociology Quarterly, 21,* 429–441.

Rutty, J. E. (1998). The nature of philosophy of science, theory and knowledge relating to nursing and professionalism. *Journal of Advanced Nursing, 28*(2), 243–250. Retrieved July 16, 2002, from CINAHL/OVID database.

Sanford, R. C. (2000). Caring through relation and dialogue: A nursing perspective for patient education. *Advances in Nursing Science, 22*(3), 1–15. Retrieved April 15, 2002, from CINAHL/OVID database.

Sarter, B. (1988). Philosophical sources of nursing theory. *Nursing Science Quarterly, 1*(2), 52–59.

Schlotfeldt, R. M. (1992). Answering nursing's philosophical questions: Whose responsibility is it? In J. F. Kikuchi and H. Simmons (Eds.), *Philosophic inquiry in nursing* (pp. 97–104). Newbury Park, CA: Sage.

Shapere, D. (1980). The structure of scientific revolutions. In G. Gutting (Ed.), *Paradigms & revolutions* (pp. 27–38). Notre Dame, IN: University of Notre Dame Press.

Shearer, J. E. (2002). The concept of protection: A dimensional analysis and critique of a theory of protection. *Advances in Nursing Science, 25*(1), 65–78.

Silva, M. C. (1997). Philosophy, science, theory, interrelationships and implications for nursing research. *Image: Journal of Nursing Scholarship, 29*(3), 210–213. Retrieved June 7, 2002, from CINAHL/OVID database.

Silva M. C., Sorrell, J. M., & Sorrell, C. D. (1995). From Carper's ways of knowing to ways of being: An ontological philosophical shift. *Advances in Nursing Science, 18*(1), 1–13.

Simmons, H. (1992). Philosophic and scientific inquiry: The interface. In J. F. Kikuchi & H. Simmons (Eds.), *Philosophic inquiry in nursing* (pp. 9–25). Newbury Park, CA: Sage.

Smart, J. J. C. (1968). *Between science and philosophy.* New York: Random House.

Smith, C. E., Pace, K., Kochinda, C., Kleinbeck, S., Koehler, J., & Popkess-Vawter, S. (2002). Caregiver effectiveness model evolution to a midrange theory of home care: A process for critique and replication. *Advances in Nursing Science, 25*(1), 50–64.

Stevens-Barnum, B. J. (1998). *Nursing theory: Analysis, application, evaluation* (5th ed.). Philadelphia: Lippincott Williams & Wilkins.

Suppe, F. (1996a, May). Middle-range theory: Nursing theory and knowledge development. Paper presented at the Proceedings of the Sixth Rosemary Ellis Scholars' Retreat, Frances Payne Bolton School of Nursing, Case Western Reserve University, Cleveland, OH.

Suppe, F. (1996b, July). *Middle-range theories: Historical and contemporary perspectives.* (Available from Institute for Advanced Study, Indiana University, Poplars 335, Bloomington, IN 47405).

Thorne, S., Canam, C., Dahinten, S., Hall, W., Henderson, A., & Kirkham, S. R. (1998). Nursing's metaparadigm concepts: Disimpacting the debates. *Journal of Advanced Nursing, 27*(6), 1257–1268.

Thorne, S. E., Kirkham, S. R., & Henderson, A. (1998). Ideological implications of paradigm discourse. *Nursing Inquiry, 6*(2), 123–131.

Tierney, A. J. (1998). Nursing models: Extant or extinct? *Journal of Advanced Nursing, 28*(1), 77–85. Retrieved June 3, 2002, from CINAHL/OVID database.

Tripp-Reimer, T., Woodworth, G., McCloskey, J. C., & Bulechek, G. (1996). The dimensional structure of nursing interventions. *Nursing Research, 45*(1), 10–17.

Ulbrich, S. L. (1999). Nursing practice theory of exercise as self-care. *Image, 31*(1), 65–70. Retrieved August 1, 2002, from CINAHL/OVID database.

Wald, F. S., & Leonard, R. C. (1964). Towards development of nursing practice theory. *Nursing Research, 13,* 309–313.

Walker, L. O. (1986). *Toward a clearer understanding of the concept of nursing theory.* In L. H. Nicholl (Ed.), *Perspectives on nursing theory* (pp. 29–39). Boston: Little, Brown and Company.

Walker, L. O., & Avant, K. C. (1995). *Strategies for theory construction in nursing* (3rd ed.). Norwalk, CT: Appleton & Lange.

Walker, L. O., & Avant, K. C. (2005). *Strategies for theory construction in nursing* (4th ed.). Upper Saddle River, NJ: Pearson/Prentice Hall.

Walsh, D., & Downe, S. (2005). Meta-synthesis method for qualitative research: A literature review. *Journal of Advanced Nursing, 50*(2), 204–211.

Weaver, K., & Olson, J. K. (2006). Understanding paradigms used for nursing research. *Journal of Advanced Nursing, 53*(4), 459–468.

Whall, A. L. (1996, May). Overview of middle-range theory. Paper presented at the Proceedings of the Sixth Rosemary Ellis Scholars' Retreat, Frances Payne Bolton School of Nursing, Case Western Reserve University, Cleveland, OH.

White, J. (2004). Patterns of knowing: Review, critique, and update. In P .G. Reed, N. C. Shearer, and L. H. Nicoll (Eds.), *Perspectives in nursing theory* (6th ed., pp. 247–258). Philadelphia: Lippincott Williams & Wilkins.

Whitehead, D. (2005). Guest editorial: Empirical or tacit knowledge as a basis for theory development. *Journal of Clinical Nursing, 14*(2), 143–144.

Winters, J., and Ballou, K. A. (2004). The idea of nursing science. *Journal of Advanced Nursing, 45*(5), 533–535.

Young, A., Taylor, S. G., & Renpenning, K. (2001). *Connections: Nursing research, theory, and practice.* St. Louis: Mosby.

Yura, H., & Torres, G. (1975). Today's conceptual frameworks within baccalaureate nursing programs. In National League for Nursing, *Faculty-curriculum development part III: Conceptual frameworks—its meaning and functioning* (pp. 17–30). New York: National League for Nursing.

Analysis, Evaluation, and Selection of a Middle Range Nursing Theory

■ TIMOTHY S. BREDOW

DEFINITION OF KEY TERMS

Adequacy	Determines how completely the theory addresses the topics it claims to address. Establishes if there are holes or gaps that need to be filled in by other work or further refinement of the theory. Addresses if the theory accounts for the subject matter under consideration
Clarity	Addresses if the theory clearly states the main components to be considered. Determines if it is easily understood by the reader
Complexity	Reviews how many concepts are involved as key components in the theory. Decides how complicated the description of the theory is, and if it can be understood without lengthy descriptions and explanations: considers the number of variables being addressed, and exists on a continuum from parsimony–limited number of variables to complex–extensive number of variables
Consistency	Addresses whether the theory maintains the definitions of the key concepts throughout the explanation of the theory. Determines if it has congruent use of terms, interpretations, principles, and methods throughout
Discrimination	Addresses whether the hypothesis generated by the theory led to research results that could not be arrived at using some other nursing theory. Determines how unique the theory is to the area of nursing that it addresses. Decides if it has precise and clear boundaries and definitive parameters of the subject matter

(Key Terms continued on next page)

DEFINITION OF KEY TERMS continued

External criticism
Considers the fit between the theory and criteria external to the theory, such as the social environment and the prevailing views on the nursing metaparadigm. Criticism here is dependent on individual preference. It depends on reasonableness and perceptions of the evaluator

Internal criticism
Deals with the criteria concerning the inner workings (internal dimensions) of the theory and how the theory's components fit with each other

Logical development
Resolves the questions, Does the theory logically follow a line of thought of previous work that has been shown to be true or does it launch out into unproven territory with its assumptions and premises? Do the conclusions proceed in a logical fashion? Are the arguments well supported?

Nursing metaparadigm
Global concepts that identify the phenomena of nursing, including person, environment, health, and nursing (Fawcett, 1995)

Pragmatic
Determines if the theory can be operationalized in real-life settings

Reality convergence
Determines if the theory's underlying assumptions ring true. Decides if the theory's assumptions represent the real world, and if it represents the real world of nursing. Does the theory reflect the real world as understood by the reader?

Scope
Determines how broad or narrow the range of phenomena is that this theory covers. Does it stay in a narrow range of scope to keep it a middle range theory? (Narrower implies more applicable to practice; wider implies more global and all-encompassing.)

Significance
Will the result of the research that is conducted because of the hypotheses generated by the theory have any impact on the way nurses carry out nursing interventions in the real world, or does it merely describe what nurses do? Does the theory address essential, not irrelevant, issues to the discipline?

Theory analysis
Systematic examination of exactly what was written by the theory author(s)

Theory evaluation
The identification of component parts of a theory and the judgment of them against a set of predetermined criteria

Utility
Determines if the theory can be used to generate hypotheses that are researchable by nurses

INTRODUCTION

Middle range nursing theories can help nurses and graduate nursing students alike meet and accomplish their goals of carrying out sound nursing research. When nursing theories are analyzed and evaluated in a thorough, systematic fashion, it is easier to determine which middle range nursing theory will provide the proper guidance and direction for the research under consideration. This chapter should help graduate student nurses and research nurses deal with the problem of how to analyze, evaluate, and choose a middle range nursing theory for their assignments, and apply it to their research interests.

Theory analysis is the systematic examination of what was personally written over time by the theory author(s) about the theory. When performing a middle range theory analysis, the component parts are identified and the relationships of these components to each other and to the whole theory are examined. This analysis can provide the nurse researcher a thorough understanding about the theory. Theory evaluation is the identification of the theory's same components and judging them against a set of predetermined criteria. The criteria used for judging theories are not standardized within the field of nursing, but, rather, have evolved over time and are different depending on who is presenting the evaluation. Nonetheless, a thorough evaluation of a middle range theory will help the nurse researcher determine the robustness of the theory and the goodness of fit for application to a particular research project.

Over the years, nursing theorists have emerged with different theoretical positions and theories proposing how various nursing concepts and the nursing metaparadigm are uniquely linked. Most of these theorists have constructed theories of nursing that could be termed grand theories, while later theorists have constructed middle range nursing theories. There are now more than 50 different grand nursing theories (McKenna, 1997) and several dozen middle range nursing theories for nursing researchers to choose from.

HISTORICAL BACKGROUND

Historically, nursing theorists worked hard to explain the nature of nursing, carving out a differentiated scientific field to call their own. At the same time, nursing researchers wanted nursing theory to be constructed to aid the generation of testable research hypotheses and also have the ability to affect the practice of nursing. As nursing theory developed and progressed through different stages of maturity, so did the evaluation process of what constitutes sound nursing theory.

In the past, nurses had Nightingale's environmental model, the medical model, and borrowed theories to use as a basis for nursing research. Through the 1960s, '70s, and '80s, several different grand nursing theories and some middle range theories were developed for nurses to use as a basis for their research. In the 1990s and beyond, many more middle range theories have emerged, allowing nurses to move away from using Nightingale, the medical model, borrowed theories, and grand nursing theories. When compared to grand theories, middle range theories contain fewer concepts, with relationships that are adaptable and concrete enough to be tested. Middle range theories have a particular substantive focus and consider only a limited aspect of reality. For example, Orem's Self-care Deficit grand nursing theory would consider patients who are unable to carry out the activities of daily living and provide nursing care necessary to aid them back to a level of living where they were able to provide self-care. The middle range theory of unpleasant symptoms would use this same situation and consider the actual unpleasant symptom that was causing the problem for the patient. It would address the patient's symptom as a consideration for a multidimensional approach to health care symptom management. Kolcaba states "that for these reasons middle range theories are particularly cogent as nursing science addresses the challenges of the 21st century" (2001, p. 86). The use of many different middle range nursing theories for research purposes became a relatively new and exciting possibility for nurses during the 1990s. Now, researchers are expanding the knowledge base of nursing by enhancement of nursing's frameworks and theories (Parse, 2001). Because of this evolutionary process of theory building, nurses need to understand the historical roots for the analysis and evaluation of grand and middle range nursing theory. Additionally, understanding the process of analysis and evaluation provides insight to the evaluator about the strengths and weaknesses of the individual theory itself, as well as its possible use and application to nursing research and practice.

Meleis (1997, p. 245) states that "nurses have always evaluated theories." She provides the reasons why evaluation of theory is an essential component of nursing research:

1. To decide which theory is more appropriate to use as a framework for research
2. To identify effective theories for guiding a research project
3. To compare and contrast different explanations of the same phenomenon
4. To identify epistemological approaches of a discipline through attention to the sociocultural context of the theorist and the theory
5. To assess the ontological beliefs and schools of thought in a discipline
6. To define research priorities (Meleis, 1997)

THEORY ANALYSIS

Theory Analysis by Early Authors

The analysis of nursing theory has evolved over time as nurses have proposed increasingly sophisticated methods for reviewing and analyzing nursing theory. Three "early approaches" to theory analysis by Duffy and Muhlenkamp, Hardy, and Chinn and Jacobs will be discussed followed by a discussion of "recent approaches" by Barnum, Meleis, and Fawcett.

In 1974, Duffy and Muhlenkamp wrote that nursing theory should be examined using four distinct questions. They suggested looking at the origin of the problem, the methods used in the pursuit of knowledge, the subject matter, and the kind of outcomes of testing generated by this theory.

These four questions when used alone to examine a nursing theory provided a fairly good evaluation of the theory; however, additional evaluation questions were proposed when the theory was used for research. Their additional questions for analyzing a nursing theory for nursing research included:

- Does it generate a testable hypothesis, and is it complete in terms of subject matter and perspective?
- Are the biases or values underlying the theory made explicit?
- Are the relationships among the propositions made explicit, and is it parsimonious?

With all of these questions in hand, a nurse could do what was thought, at the time, to be a thorough and complete assessment of any particular nursing theory to be used for nursing research.

During the same period of time, Hardy (1974) developed another way to analyze nursing theories. Her analysis method contained some unique criteria when compared to Duffy and Muhlenkamp's and included more criteria related to the process and outcome of theory evaluation. Her evaluation criteria identified the need for the theory to have adequacy, meaning, logic, and pragmatism. She wanted the theory to provide empirical evidence, have the ability to be generalized, contribute to further understanding, and be able to predict outcomes.

These two positions within the same historical time period contain some unique as well as overlapping criteria for the analysis and evaluation of nursing theory.

In the 1980s, Chinn and Jacobs (1983) proposed a combination of the previous two positions and recommended five brief criteria for evaluating nursing theories. They stated that a theory could be evaluated by asking if it had clarity, simplicity, generality, empirical applicability, and consequences. Clarity was further expanded to include semantic clarity, semantic consistency, structural clarity, and structural consistency. Apparently they felt that semantics and clarity were becoming issues in the nursing community, and they were attempting to address these particular issues.

Recent Approaches to Theory Analysis

In addition to consideration of criteria for evaluation of theories, nursing theorists have proposed steps for the analysis process of nursing theories. Barnum, Meleis, and Fawcett all present several steps for the analysis of a nursing theory.

Recognizing the underlying assumptions of a theoretical work is an analyst's first task in understanding the theory (Barnum, 1998; Meleis, 1997). These assumptions may not be stated but may be inferred by the reader on the basis of other statements made about the given nursing theory in other publications and writings. However, recognizing underlying assumptions may not be possible for some middle range theories, because many of these middle range theories are not constructed by any one particular nursing author but are the work of multiple authors. It then becomes difficult to understand all of the different assumptions from the variety of publications written by them. Additionally, not all middle range theories are named after some nursing author or even have a particular author's name attached to the theory. For example, most of the middle range theories contained in this text do not have a theorist name attached to them, yet they have proved useful in the furthering of nursing understanding. Additionally, there are middle range theories such as Quality of Life or Reasoned Action that are borrowed from other disciplines unrelated to nursing but are used by nurses to describe and build the understanding of nursing. Nonetheless, there are some middle range theories that do have information available about the underlying assumptions, and for them, it is important to understand and relate these assumptions to the research problem.

Barnum (1990, p. 22) asserts that analysis of a theory demands that the analyst "dig beneath the surface for a deeper insight into a thesis in all its meaning and implications." This "reading between the lines" work may be difficult for some nurses because they may not be comfortable with criticism at this level. Meleis (1997) would like to see reviews of theorists; their education, experience, and professional network; and the sociocultural context of their theories. Because theory development in nursing did not take place in a vacuum, Meleis (1997) feels that it is important to carefully consider the paradigmatic origins of the theory through careful analysis of the references and citations cited by the author. In addition, she wants the analysis to include a thorough review of the assumptions, concepts, propositions, and hypothesis that the author employed, and she wants the theory to be examined for beginnings. Analysis of beginnings looks at where the theory started. Did it begin in the mind of the theorist as an attempt to explain what ought to be, or did it arise out of experience and explain what is? Fawcett (1995) suggests that analysis needs to include a thorough review of all the author's original works and presentations. However, for some middle range theories, because they are relatively new to the field of nursing, there may not be enough published work produced by a particular author or group of authors for the analyst to read and grasp this level of understanding about the theory's meaning and implications.

Barnum believes that the analyst should determine who or what performs an activity within the theory, as well as to determine whom or what is the recipient of the activity. A third area that should be evaluated in each theory is in what context the activity is performed and what the end point of the activity is. Two additional concepts that need to be addressed include the procedures that guide the activity and the energy source of the activity. Other concepts Barnum considered essential for theory analysis include nursing acts, the patient, and health (1998). Also included for good theory analysis are the relationship of nursing acts to the patient, the relationship of nursing acts to health, and the relationship of the patient to health. These concepts from Barnum are closely associated with the nursing metaparadigm that includes the concepts of nursing, person, health, and environment.

Barnum presents several devices for theory analysis. These devices use common nursing concepts to define nursing theory elements and their interrelationships. They also include determination of the level of theory development, descriptive or explanatory, and the need to discriminate nursing acts from non-nursing acts. Barnum (1990) adds that every nursing theory is based upon one or more dominant principles. These dominant principles contain an idea that is essential for stating or explaining a theory. It is important to identify and to consider the nature of each key principle. A principle is a fundamental or basic concept with an explanatory function. It explains the basis upon which the theory rests. The theorist's interpretation of reality if it is given should be analyzed by asking, "What is reality like?" Many of these considerations were geared toward the analysis of grand theories and have to be adapted for use when considering middle range theories. For example, if a middle range theory has been formulated over time by several authors, then it will be difficult, if not impossible, to determine the theorist's interpretation of reality.

Meleis includes internal dimensions as a criterion of her method of theory analysis. Internal dimensions include assumptions and concepts upon which the theory is built. She includes several units of analysis as part of this inquiry. Her units of analysis include content, context, and methods, and are similar to the units of analysis contained in Barnum's list. Other items unique to Meleis include the rationale, the system of relations, beginnings, scope, goals, and abstractness. Examining the rationale of a theory's construction provides clarification of how the elements of the theory are united. Meleis wants the analyst to discover the theory's system of relations. This is accomplished by asking the question, "Do relations explain elements or do the elements explain relations?" (Meleis, 1997, p. 258). The scope of a theory determines how broad or narrow the range of phenomena is that the theory covers. Middle range theories keep their scope narrow, helping to make the theory more applicable to research and practice. The scope of a theory also deals with the breadth of the explanations it attempts to accomplish. The scope is narrower, more specific, and more concrete for middle range theories than it is for grand theories (Fawcett, 1999).

The goals of a theory also need to be examined. Does the theory attempt to describe, explain, predict, or prescribe? Each theory must attempt to accomplish at least one of these goals. Middle range theories can be classified as falling into three distinct categories. These categories are descriptive, explanatory, and predictive (Fawcett, 2000). These three categories are closely aligned with the definition given by Meleis (1997) for a grand theory that includes describing, explaining, and predicting different phenomena.

Abstractness is another point that Meleis says is necessary to examine when analyzing a theory. Analyzing abstractness is an attempt to determine the width of the gaps between the theories, propositions, concepts, and reality. In middle range theories, this gap should be small, or nonexistent, since middle range theories deal with what is and not with what ought to be.

Fawcett (2000) has several recommendations for theory analysis that are similar to Meleis's and Barnum's. She has two additional components to consider. They are theory context and theory content.

Theory context is the environment in which the theory's nursing action takes place. It tells about the nature of the nurses' world and may describe the nature of the client environment. Theory context is also concerned with which nursing metaparadigm concepts are addressed by the theory (Fawcett, 2000). In middle range theories, the focus of the theory may be purposefully limited to just one of the nursing metaparadigm concepts, such as in Pain Theory.

Theory content identifies the theory elements that are the subject matter of the theory. The content is stated through the concepts and propositions (Fawcett, 2000). Middle range theories should have their content well defined and their concepts clearly stated in the description of the theory.

A theory's process refers to the activities that either the nurse or the client has to perform to implement the theory. This should be a strength of middle range theories as they give clear direction to some process or activity carried out in application of the theory in research or practice.

THEORY EVALUATION

Barnum's Theory Evaluation Recommendations

Barnum (1990, p. 20) states that "a thorough criticism (both analysis and evaluation) of a theory requires that attention be given to both aspects of internal and external criticism." Internal criticism refers to the internal construction of how the components of the theory fit together, while external criticism considers the theory and its relationship to people, nursing, and health. Internal criticism requires the reviewer to answer the following questions:

- Given the theorist's underlying assumptions, does the theory logically follow?
- Is the theory consistent with and logical in light of the underlying assumptions?

For external criticism, the reviewer would ask the following questions:

- Do the theory's underlying assumptions ring true?
- Do the assumptions represent the "real world" out there, especially the real world of nursing?

Barnum's criteria for evaluating theories include both internal and external criticism based on specific criteria. Her criteria for judging theories for internal criticism include clarity, consistency, adequacy, logical development, and level of theory development. Her criteria for judging theories using external criticism include reality convergence, utility, significance, discrimination, scope of theory, and complexity (Barnum, 1998).

Internal criticism is first evaluated by deciding the clarity of the theory. Two questions should be answered to determine clarity:

- Does the theory clearly state the main components to be considered?
- Is it easily understood by the reader?

Next on Barnum's list is consistency. Two more questions help to determine if the theory is consistent:

- Does the description of the theory continue to maintain the definitions of the key concepts throughout the explanation of the theory?
- Does it have congruent use of terms, interpretations, principles, and methods?

The next criterion is adequacy. Three questions help to determine if the theory is adequate:

- How completely does the theory speak to the topics it claims to address?
- Are there holes or gaps that need to be filled in by other work or further refinement of the theory?
- Does it account for the subject matter under consideration?

Her fourth criterion is logical development. The quality of this criterion is determined by asking three questions:

- Does the theory logically follow a line of thought of previous work that has been shown to be true or does it launch out into unproven territory with its assumptions and premises?
- Do the conclusions proceed in a logical fashion?
- Are the arguments well supported?

The final criterion for evaluating the internal portion of the theory is the level of the theory development, which can be determined by asking the following questions:

- Is it in early development, just at the stage of naming its elements, or has it been around a long time and is able to explain or even predict outcomes?
- How often have different nurse researchers conducted independent research studies applying the theory to different situations and reported the findings in the literature?

Barnum (1998, p. 178) states that "external criticism evaluates a nursing theory as it relates to the real world of man, of nursing and of health." She recommends that the following criteria should be considered: reality convergence, utility, significance, and capacity for discrimination. In addition, two other criteria may be included: scope and complexity (Barnum, 1998).

Reality convergence deals with how well the theory builds upon the premises from which it is derived and then relates that to reality. Some nursing theorists build on past work and remain within the framework of traditional thinking. Other nurse theorists deconstruct the past and develop a new framework to build upon. These theorists are termed *deconstructionists*. Deconstructionists start with a different set of presuppositions than the historical nursing leaders did, and the resulting nursing theories may not represent the same worldview of nursing as described in the past. At this point, the person doing the evaluation may choose to disagree as to whether a particular theory achieves reality convergence, based primarily on the differences between the beliefs and values that he or she holds to be true and those proposed by the theory. This part of theory evaluation may have more applicability to grand theories than middle range theories, but is an important point to consider as new and different middle range theories are developed in the future.

Utility simply requires that the theory be useful to the nurse researcher employing it. It should suggest subject material that could be investigated and lend itself to methods of inquiry. Middle range theories generally lend themselves to a greater ease of usefulness by nurse researchers than grand nursing theories. This is because they tend to be very narrow in scope and focused on specific concepts, like health promotion, pain, and quality of life.

The significance of a nursing theory depends upon the extent to which it addresses the phenomena of nursing and lends itself to further research.

Discrimination is the capacity to differentiate nursing from other health-related disciplines through the use of well-defined boundaries. The boundaries need to be clear and precise so that judgments can be made about any given action performed by a nurse.

Barnum includes the scope of a theory as a necessary criterion for external criticism. Important questions to consider here are, Does it have a narrow range of scope to help identify it as a middle range theory, and does that narrow focus make it easier to use in a research setting?

Complexity is the final criterion in Barnum's list. Complexity is at the opposite pole from the criterion of parsimony. The level of complexity is determined by the number of variables. Middle range nursing theories are less complex than grand nursing theories because they deal with fewer variables, resulting in a fewer number of relationships between the concepts.

Meleis's Theory Evaluation Recommendations

Meleis (1997) provides a complex model for theory evaluation. It includes several integral parts: theory description, theory support, theory analysis, and theory critique. She proposes that this complete model represents the necessary elements needed to thoroughly evaluate a theory. Meleis begins the description of her model by listing two criteria that help describe the theory. These two criteria are structural and functional components. Within the criterion of structural components, there are separate units of analysis to consider. The first is assumptions. Assumptions are "givens" in the theory and are based on the theorist's values. They are not subject to testing but lead to the set of propositions that are to be tested. In nursing theories, there are many assumptions made about the concepts included in the nursing metaparadigm and, additionally, to the concepts of human behavior, life, death, and illness. Again, it must be stated that it will not be possible to find the assumptions of all middle range theories.

Another part of Meleis's theory description includes functional components. A functional assessment of a theory carefully considers the anticipated consequences of the theory and its purposes. The units of analysis of the functional components are the theory's focus, that is, the client, nursing, health, nurse–patient interactions, the environment, nursing problems, and nursing therapeutics (p. 251).

Meleis offers several questions to ask when considering the functional components of a nursing theory (p. 254). They include the following:

1. Who does the theory act upon?
2. What definitions does the theory offer for the elements of the nursing metaparadigm?
3. Does the theory offer a clear idea of what the sources of nursing problems are?
4. Does the theory provide interventions for nurses?
5. Are there guidelines for intervention modalities?
6. Does it provide guidelines for the role of the nurse?
7. Are the consequences of the nurse's actions articulated?

Meleis feels that these criteria are consistent with the ones offered by Barnum.

Another major area of theory evaluation for Meleis is theory support. She includes theory testing in this area. Theory testing consists of four separate tests: tests of utility, tests of nonnursing propositions, tests of concepts, and tests of propositions.

A final area of evaluation in the model is what Meleis calls theory critique. Theory critique is made up of several criteria. Many of her criteria are similar to ones developed by Barnum, but some are unique to Meleis. The duplicated criteria similar to Barnum's are clarity, consistency, simplicity/complexity, and usefulness. Some unique criteria are tautology/teleology and diagrams.

Tautology considers evaluating the needless repetition of an idea in separate parts of the theory. Overuse of repetition can confuse a reader and make the theory explanation unclear.

Teleology is assessed by considering the extent to which causes and consequences are kept separate in the theory. Meleis (1997) says teleology occurs when the theorist defines concepts by consequences and then introduces totally new concepts, rather than getting to the definitions of the original concepts. As this process continues, there is never a clear definition of the theory's concepts, and the theory remains unclear.

Diagrams are useful to visually see the interrelationship of the concepts to each other before doing research. They can be especially useful for reviewing the strength of statistical correlations between the theories concepts.

Fawcett's Theory Evaluation Recommendations

Fawcett (2000) made the following recommendations to be used for the evaluation of nursing theories. Her criteria include significance, internal consistency, parsimony, testability, empirical adequacy, and pragmatic adequacy. She also recommends that the evaluation of a theory requires judgments to be made about the extent to which a theory satisfies the criteria.

Significance may be determined by asking the following questions: Are the metaparadigm concepts and propositions addressed by the theory explicit? In middle range theories, all aspects of the metaparadigm for nursing are not always covered, and that should not detract from its use by nursing researchers. Are the philosophical claims on which the theory is based explicit? Here again, some middle range theories will be devoid of philosophical claims. Is the conceptual model from which the theory was derived explicit? Are the authors of antecedent knowledge from nursing and adjunctive disciplines acknowledged, and are bibliographical citations given? (Fawcett, 2000, p. 504).

Fawcett's second criterion of internal consistency requires that all the elements of the theory are congruent. These elements may include conceptual model and theory concepts and propositions. Additionally, Fawcett suggests that semantic clarity and consistency are required for internal consistency to be maintained. She proposes that the following questions be asked when evaluating the internal consistency of a theory: Are the content and the context of the theory congruent? Do the concepts reflect semantic clarity and consistency? Do the theory propositions reflect structural consistency? (Fawcett, 2000).

Parsimony is concerned with whether the theory is stated clearly and concisely. This criterion is met when the statements clarify rather than obscure the topic of interest. This is as important in middle range theory as it is in grand theory. Even though the scope of the theory may be narrow in a middle range theory, it is still important to be clear and concise in the explanations of the concepts.

The goal of theory development in nursing is the empirical testing of interventions that are specified in the form of middle range theories (Fawcett, 2000). The concepts of a middle range theory should be observable and the propositions measurable. Fawcett (2000, p. 506) suggests that the following questions should be asked when evaluating the testability of a middle range theory: Does the research methodology reflect the middle range theory? Are the middle range theory concepts observable through instruments that are appropriate empirical indicators of those concepts? Do the data analysis techniques permit measurement of the middle range theory propositions?

Empirical adequacy is the fifth step that Fawcett says is necessary in the evaluation of nursing theories. This step requires that assertions made by the theory are congruent with empirical evidence found through studies done using the theory as a basis for research. It usually takes more than one research study to establish empirical adequacy. The end result of using empirical adequacy is to establish the level of confidence in the theory from the best studies yielding empirical results. The question to be considered here is, are the middle range theory's assertions harmonious with the research studies' empirical results?

The final and sixth step in Fawcett's framework for evaluation of nursing theories is the criterion of pragmatic adequacy. This criterion evaluates the extent of how well the middle range theory is utilized in clinical practice. The criterion also requires that nurses fully understand the full content of the theory. Additionally, the theory should help move resulting nursing action toward favorable client outcomes. Ask the following questions when evaluating a theory for pragmatic adequacy:

- Do nurses need special education and skill training to apply the theory in clinical practice?
- Is it possible to derive clinical protocols from the theory?
- How often has the theory been used as the basis of nursing research?
- Do favorable outcomes result from using the theory as a basis for nursing actions? (Fawcett, 2000)

Kolcaba's Theory Evaluation Recommendations

A recent contribution to this discussion of theory evaluation comes from Kolcaba. According to Kolcaba (2001), there are several criteria that determine a good middle range theory. Her criteria involve evaluation and do not mention steps for theory analysis. They include questions concerning the theory's concepts and propositions, and whether or not they are specific to nursing. She also wants to determine if the theory has components that are readily operationalized and can be applied to many situations. She asserts that a middle range theory's propositions can range from causal to associative, depending on their application. The assumptions provided fit the middle range theory. The theory should be relevant for the potential users. The middle range theory should be oriented to outcomes that are important for patients and not merely describe what nurses do. Finally, Kolcaba thinks that middle range theory should describe nursing-sensitive phenomena that are readily associated with the deliberate actions of nurses.

An interesting review process of the Synergy Middle Range Theory (see Chapter 5, Synergy Model) took place during its development. A committee of experts in the analysis of theoretical and conceptual frameworks was assembled to review this theory in order to identify its strengths and weaknesses, and to obtain recommendations regarding the refinement of the model (Sechrist, 2005). This review committee was made up of the following nurse leaders: Barbara Stevens Barnum, RN, PhD; Marion Broome, RN, PhD; Rose Constantino, RN, PhD; Jacqueline Fawcett, RN, PhD; Edna Menke, RN, PhD; Carolyn Murdaugh, RN, PhD; Patrica Moritz, RN, PhD; Bonnie Rogers, DPH, COHN-S; and Marilyn Frank-Stromborg, EdD, JD, ANP. This esteemed committee developed a review instrument that was organized into six criteria. These criteria included the headings of clarity, consistency, adequacy, utility, significance, and summary. When compared to the recommended criteria listed in this chapter, the expert review committee decided to evaluate the synergy theory on fewer criteria. Their evaluation left out "logical development" and "determining the level of theory development" in the appraisal of internal theory analysis. When determining which criteria to include for the external middle range theory analysis, they chose to reduce the list to just three criteria, leaving out complexity, discrimination, reality convergence, pragmatic, and scope. They did add one new criterion, which may act as a "catch all" for the criteria left out, which they called the summary. In a PowerPoint presentation that was posted on the world wide web, Fawcett has suggested an even smaller set of criteria to evaluate middle range theories. Her list is short and includes just four total criteria: significance, internal consistency, and two new criteria, parsimony and testability (Fawcett, 2005).

It is evident that there are several distinct differences between the analysis and evaluation process for grand theories and middle range theories. At the same time, there are several similarities. Many of the principles applied to the analysis and evaluation of grand theories can be readily applied to middle range theories and, with some minor modification, can be used to determine the adequacy of a middle range theory. With this in mind, the next section will address the selection of a middle range theory for use in nursing research.

SELECTING A THEORY FOR NURSING RESEARCH

Before starting to write a proposal, Fawcett (1999) suggests that each investigator become familiar with the research topic and the conceptual model that will guide the study. She reiterates that this is done by an immersion into the literature and a thorough study of the research topic. Additionally, a comprehensive literature search should be done several months before making a proposal of the study. This much time must be given to allow the proper amount of time for reading and thinking about both the content of the proposed study and the conceptual model to provide the basis for the study. It is during this time that the most appropriate middle range theory can be decided upon for use in the research.

As nurse researchers shift away from using grand nursing theories and begin to consider using middle range theories, the philosophical underpinnings of the theory itself become of decreased importance. The emphasis shifts from the philosophical basis of the nursing theory to how the middle range theory is applied in research and practice. Thus, time previously spent with the philosophy and background of the theorist can now be devoted to ensuring the proper fit between the research questions to be studied and the middle range theory. Each nurse researcher should ask the following questions about the middle range theory proposed for use in his or her research:

- Does the theory seem to fit the research that you wish to do?
- Is it readily operationalized?
- What has been the primary application for this theory in the past?
- Where has the theory in question been applied and used before?
- How well has the theory performed at describing, predicting, and/or explaining the phenomena that it relates to?
- Does the theory relate to and address the research hypothesis in its description and explanation?
- Does the hypothesis flow from the research problem?
- Does the theory address the primary and secondary research questions?
- Are the theory's assumptions congruent with the assumptions that are made for this research?
- Is it oriented to outcomes that are critical to patients and does not describe what nurses perform?
- Are tools available to test relationships of the theory or do they need to be developed?

The nurse researcher should consider several different middle range theories as possibilities for use. A thorough analysis and evaluation of these theories in question should be done before selecting one. Subsequently, the nurse researcher should become familiar with all aspects of the theory, using the questions provided in the discussion above. It is essential to have a sound understanding and be in total agreement with the theory selected before beginning the study. This is accomplished by becoming immersed in the literature about the middle range theory in question and arriving at a thorough and complete understanding of the theory before using it. The nurse researcher should try to understand the middle range theory by identifying all the major concepts. The definitions of these concepts, in turn, should be studied for this particular theory, to make sure the meanings have not been changed slightly over time as they are described in the literature.

Additionally, the major concepts should be examined to determine how they relate to each other. Next, the researcher needs to decide if he or she can accept the premises, rationale, and presuppositions that the nursing theory is based upon before adopting it for use (McKenna, 1997). Finally, it is necessary to determine what means of measurement have been used with previous studies employing this theory. It will be important to know if new measurement tools will need to be obtained or if similar tools can be employed for the study at hand.

It is evident that to decide upon and use a middle range theory effectively in nursing research, the potential nurse researcher must do a thorough analysis and evaluation of the middle range nursing theory. The following analysis exercise will provide the guidance for conducting an evaluation of a middle range theory before selecting it for use in a research study.

MIDDLE RANGE THEORY EVALUATION PROCESS

This evaluation process, to be applied at the end of each subsequent chapter as an intellectual educational exercise, is a synthesis of the works of the authors reviewed in this chapter. After careful review of the theory presented in each chapter, taking into consideration the examples given where the middle range theory is applied in practice and the case study provided, the reader should be able to carry out this theory evaluation, taking into account the following criteria listed here with their definitions. Answer the questions posed for each criterion. Summarize the findings in a concluding paragraph for both internal and external criticism. Finally, make a judgment as to whether this theory could be adapted for use in research. Start the process by evaluating internal criticism.

Internal Criticism

Adequacy: How completely does the theory address the topics it claims to address? Are there holes or gaps that need to be filled in by other work or further refinement of the theory? Does it account for the subject matter under consideration?

Clarity: Does the theory clearly state the main components to be considered? Is it easily understood by the reader?

Consistency: Does the description of the theory address whether the theory maintains the definitions of the key concepts throughout the explanation of the theory? Does it have congruent use of terms, interpretations, principles, and methods?

Logical development: Does the theory logically follow a line of thought of previous work that has been shown to be true, or does it launch out into unproven territory with its assumptions and premises? Do the conclusions proceed in a logical fashion? Are the arguments well supported?

Level of theory development: Is it consistent with the conceptualization of middle range theory?

External Criticism

Complexity: How many concepts are involved as key components in the theory? How complicated is the description of the theory? Can it be understood without lengthy descriptions and explanations? (considers the number of variables being addressed, exists on a continuum from parsimony–limited number of variables to complex–extensive number of variables).

Discrimination: Is this theory able to produce hypotheses that will lead to research results that could not be arrived at using some other nursing theory? How unique is this theory to the area of nursing that it addresses? Does it have precise and clear boundaries and definitive parameters of the subject matter?

Reality convergence: Do the theory's underlying assumptions ring true? Do these assumptions represent the real world? Do they represent the real world of nursing? Does the theory reflect the real world as understood by the reader?

Pragmatic: Can the theory be operationalized in real-life settings?

Scope: How broad or narrow is the range of phenomena that this theory covers? Does it stay in a narrow range of scope to keep it a middle range theory? (Narrower implies more applicable to practice; wider implies more global and all-encompassing.)

Significance: Will the result of the research that is conducted because of the hypothesis generated by the theory have any impact on the way nurses carry out nursing interventions in the real world, or does it merely describe what nurses do? Does the theory address issues essential, not irrelevant, to the discipline?

Utility: Is the theory able to be used to generate hypotheses that are researchable by nurses?

After completing the evaluation based on the criteria listed above, compare and contrast responses to the ones done by contributors for each chapter listed in Appendix A at the end of the text.

CRITICAL THINKING EXERCISES

1. Recently groups of nurses and nurse theorists alike have migrated to an abbreviated process for middle range theory analysis. What information about the theory is not available from this abbreviated review?
2. Do you think that the shorter method of analysis results in a "good enough" analysis of any one middle range theory? Why or why not?
3. If you were going to use a particular middle range theory for your own research study, would you be satisfied with the abbreviated method of analysis before you begin the project?

WEB RESOURCES

The Hardin Library for the Health Sciences Electronic Resources home page has full-text journals, subject-specific web resources, governmental and statistical resources, medical databases, and more. You can access it at **http://www.lib.uiowa.edu/hardin/md/ nurs.html.**

Advice for searching nursing theory references can be found at **http://www.wwnurse.com/ topsites/topsites.cgi?ID=364.**

REFERENCES

Barnum, B. (1990). *Nursing theory, analysis application, evaluation* (3rd ed.). Glenview, IL: Scott, Foresman, Little Brown.

Barnum, B. (1998). *Nursing theory: Analysis, application and evaluation* (5th ed.). Philadelphia: Lippincott Williams & Wilkins.

Chinn, P., & Jacobs, M. (1983). *Theory and nursing: A systematic approach.* St. Louis: Mosby.

Duffy, M., & Muhlenkamp, A. (1974). A framework for theory analysis. *Nursing Outlook, 22*(9), 570–574.

Fawcett, J. (1995). *Analysis and evaluation of conceptual models of nursing* (3rd ed.). Philadelphia: F.A. Davis.

Fawcett, J. (1999). *The relationship of theory and research* (3rd ed.). Philadelphia: F.A. Davis.

Fawcett, J. (2000). *Analysis and evaluation of contemporary nursing knowledge: Nursing models and theories.* Philadelphia: F.A. Davis.

Fawcett, J. (2005). Evaluating conceptual-theoretical-empirical structures for science of unitary human beings-based research. Retrieved July 2005 from http://medweb.uwcm. ac.uk/martha/Repository/Fawcett2005.ppt#398,1.

Hardy, M. (1974). Theories: Components, development, evaluation. *Nursing Research, 23*(2), 100–107.

Kolcaba, K. (2001). Evolution of the middle range theory of comfort for outcomes research. *Nursing Outlook 49*(2), 86–92.

McKenna, H. (1997). *Nursing theories and models.* London: Routledge.

Meleis, A. (1997). *Theoretical nursing: Development & progress* (3rd ed.). Philadelphia: Lippincott-Raven.

Parse, R. (2001). Rosemary Rizzo Parse the human becoming school of thought. In M. Parker (Ed.), *Nursing theories and nursing practice.* Philadelphia: F.A. Davis.

Sechrist K., Berlin, L., & Biel, M. (2000). The synergy model: Overview of theoretical review process. *Critical Care Nurse, 20*(1), 85–86.

BIBLIOGRAPHY

Alligood, M. R., & Marriner-Tomey, A. M. (2002). *Nursing theory: Utilization & application* (2nd ed.). St. Louis: Mosby.

Barns, B. (1999). *Nursing theories' conceptual and philosophical foundations.* New York: Springer Publishing Company.

Chinn, P., & Kramer, M. (1995). *Theory and nursing: A systematic approach* (4th ed.). St. Louis: Mosby.

Chinn, P., & Kramer, M. (1999). *Theory and nursing: Integrated knowledge development* (5th ed.). St. Louis: Mosby.

Dubin, R. (1978). *Theory building.* New York: The Free Press.

Fawcett, J. (1993). *Analysis and evaluation of nursing theories.* Philadelphia: F.A. Davis.

Fawcett, J. (1994). Analysis and evaluation of nursing theories. In V. Malinski & E. Barrett (Eds.), (1994). *Martha E. Rogers: Her life and her work.* Philadelphia: F.A. Davis.

Fawcett, J. (1995). *Analysis and evaluation of conceptual models of nursing* (3rd ed.). Philadelphia: F.A. Davis.

Fawcett, J. (1999). *The relationship of theory and research* (3rd ed.). Philadelphia: F.A. Davis.

Fawcett, J. (2000). *Analysis and evaluation of contemporary nursing knowledge: Nursing models and theories.* Philadelphia: F.A. Davis.

George, J. (1995). *Nursing theories: The base for professional nursing practice* (4th ed.). Norwalk, CT: Appleton & Lange.

Gift, A. (1997). *Clarifying concepts in nursing research.* New York: Springer Publishing Company.

Greenwood, J. (Ed.). (2000). *Nursing theory in Australia: Development and application.* Sydney: Harper Collins.

Huck, S., & Cormier, W. (1996). *Reading statistics & research.* New York: Harper Collins College Publishers.

Kim, H., Kollak, I., & Parker, M. (Eds.). (1990). *Nursing theories in practice.* New York: National League for Nursing, Publ. #15-2350.

McKenna, H. (1997). *Nursing models and theories.* London: Routledge.

McQuiston, C., & Webb, A. (Eds.). (1995). *Foundations of nursing theory.* Thousand Oaks, CA: Sage Publications.

Meleis, A. I. (1997). *Theoretical nursing: Development and progress* (3rd ed.). Philadelphia: Lippincott-Raven.

Nicoll, L. H. (1992). *Perspectives on nursing theory.* Philadelphia: J. B. Lippincott.

Nolan, M., & Grant, G. (1992). Middle range theory building and the nursing theory-practice gap: A respite case study. *Journal of Advanced Nursing, 17,* 217–223.

Parker, M. (Ed.). (1990). *Nursing theories in practice.* New York: National League for Nursing.

Parker, M. (Ed.). (1993). *Patterns of nursing theories in practice.* New York: National League for Nursing, Publ. #15-2548.

Parker, M. E. (2000). *Nursing theories and nursing practice.* Philadelphia: F.A. Davis.

Tomey, A. M., & Alligood, M. R. (Eds.). (2002). *Nursing theorists and their work* (5th ed.). St. Louis: Mosby.

Walker, L. O., & Avant, K. C. (1997). *Strategies for theory construction in nursing.* New York: Appleton-Century-Crofts.

Wesley, R. L. (1995). *Nursing theories and models* (2nd ed.). Springhouse, PA: Springhouse.

Whall, A. (1996). The structure of nursing knowledge: Analysis and evaluation of practice, middle range and grand theory. In J. Fitzpatrick & A. Whall (Eds.), *Conceptual models of nursing: Analysis and application* (3rd ed.). Norwalk, CT: Appleton & Lange.

Winstead-Fry, P. (Ed.). (1986). *Case studies in nursing theory.* New York: National League for Nursing.

Young A., Taylor, S. G., & Renpenning, K. (2001). *Connections: Nursing research, theory and practice.* St. Louis: Mosby.

Middle Range Theories: Physiological

Pain: A Balance Between Analgesia and Side Effects

■ MARION GOOD

DEFINITION OF KEY TERMS

Analgesia	Pain relief
Balance between analgesia and side effects	Patient satisfaction with relief of pain and relief or absence of side effects
Identification of lack of pain or side effect relief	Pain intensity greater than the mutual goal; side effects of opioids reported by the patient or observed by the nurse
Intervention, reassessment, and reintervention	Immediate intervention for pain and side effects; reassessment when peak effect is expected, and reintervention if pain and side effects are still unacceptable
Mutual goal setting	Mutually agreed upon, safe, realistic goals for relief
Nonpharmacological adjuvant	Complementary nursing therapies for pain relief (relaxation, music, imagery, massage, and cold)
Pain	An unpleasant sensory and affective experience associated with tissue damage
Patient teaching	Patient instruction encouraging attitudes, expectations, and action in reporting pain; obtaining medication, preventing pain during activity, and use of complementary therapies
Pharmacological adjuvant	Analgesic given as a supplement
Potent pain medication	Opioid analgesic or local anesthetic given systemically or by epidural for acute pain
Regular assessment of pain and side effects	Report of pain and side effects every 2 hours until under control, and then every 4 hours
Side effects	Unpleasant sensory and affective experiences associated with adverse effects of pain medication

INTRODUCTION

Pain is the most common reason that people seek health care, and although pain is known to be a part of life, it is compelling in its unpleasantness and is sometimes overwhelming in its effect. Patients who are in pain endure considerable suffering and are at risk for long-term adverse effects that include slower wound healing, down-regulation of the immune system, and metastasis of tumor cells (Page, 1996). There are many different types of pain: acute pain of injury, surgery, labor, and sickle cell crisis; chronic pain of musculoskeletal or gastrointestinal disorders; procedural pain of lumbar puncture, venipuncture, and chest tube removal; cancer pain from the enlarging tumor, its metastases, or its treatment; and pain in infants, in the critically ill, and at the end of life. Health care professionals today have a duty and an obligation to identify the source, to treat the cause, and to relieve the pain. Theories have been developed to explain and manage pain, and researchers have an obligation to test interventions for relief.

To study pain, researchers experimentally induce it in animals and humans using noxious stimuli such as heat, cold, constriction, and sharpness. In animal research, surgically exposed pain pathways provide information about the transmission of noxious impulses to the thalamus, sensory cortex, and limbic system. However, in animals, the affective component of pain is difficult to discern. When conducting human laboratory studies of induced pain, researchers do not measure pain invasively, but they can obtain a report of the affective component of pain. However, experimentally induced pain in human beings does not have the holistic physical and emotional impact over time that clinical pain does. The pain of illness and surgery can limit life functions and arouse existential fears. The emotional impact is more intense and interacts with the sensory pain. Therefore, clinical studies are needed.

HISTORICAL BACKGROUND

To those who experience pain, there is no mystery as to how it feels. Health professionals may or may not have experienced similar pain themselves. However, they must believe their patients. Only the person in pain can tell them what the pain is like, and describe it in terms of intensity, quality, duration, and trajectory. These will vary depending on the type of pain and the person experiencing it.

Theories of Pain Mechanism

The earliest pain theory was illustrated by Descartes in his 17th-century drawing of a child whose foot was too close to a fire. Pain transmission was drawn as a direct cord ascending from the foot, up through the back to the brain. Descartes described it as similar to pulling a rope to ring a bell (Melzack & Wall, 1962, 1965). Years later, in 1895, von Frey published evidence of a specificity theory proposing that there are nerve fibers specific to pain, which, if stimulated, invariably allow impulses to travel to the pain centers in the brain, resulting in the experience of pain. The specificity theory was followed by pattern theories proposing that stimulus intensity, temporal–spatial transmission patterns, central summation, and input control were critical to pain. However, physiological evidence did not fully support these early theories, and they focused only on sensory pain without accounting for the complex and highly developed central nervous system in humans. Evidence of affective pain was dramatically demonstrated by Beecher (1959). She described extensively wounded American soldiers who reported no pain, probably because they were so elated to be alive and to be going home. These descriptions showed that pain was more complex than simply the transmission of impulses along nerve pathways. Pain had a psychological component that could attenuate the transmission of impulses. The diverse early theories were in need of a unifying perspective (Melzack & Wall, 1965).

GATE CONTROL THEORY

A major watershed or turning point in pain theory was the paradigm shift initiated by the gate control theory that Melzack and Wall published in 1965. Melzack was a psychologist who was searching for a more comprehensive understanding of pain, one that included the brain. He linked with Wall, a neurophysiologist who had described lamina II in the dorsal horn of the spinal cord, where nociceptive impulses were modified by neural input from other areas of the central nervous system (CNS). Together they created the gate control theory, which unified several sensory pain theories and added the affective, motivational, and central control elements. Touch, attention, and emotion were then theoretically capable of increasing or decreasing pain by descending mechanisms from the brain to the dorsal horn.

ENDOGENOUS ANALGESIC THEORIES

Discoveries of endogenous opiates in the periaqueductal gray area of the brain, opioid receptors in the CNS, and later catecholamines, serotonin, and neuropeptide receptors all produced new theories that some scientists viewed as refuting the gate control theory. Others viewed them as explanatory mechanisms for descending control of noxious impulse transmission. Today, descending control is known to occur through neurons, neurotransmitters, and opioid receptors, and also indirectly through the sympathetic nervous system. The gate is no longer localized solely in lamina II of the dorsal horn, but the "gate" has been broadened to refer to repeated modulation, filtering, and abstraction of input in many areas of the CNS via numerous mechanisms (Melzack, 1982). At the close of the 20th century, Melzack presented his new neuromatrix theory of pain that encompassed existing knowledge about the complexity of pain in humans (Melzack, 1996).

The gate control, endogenous opiate, and neuromatrix theories, however, only describe and explain the *mechanisms* of pain. They propose the way pain occurs and is modulated. They offer valuable insight into therapies that health professionals can use for pain, but are only suggestive of therapeutic modalities. They do not specify effective interventions and therefore are not the prescriptive theories needed by nurses for providing and testing interventions (Dickhoff & James, 1968).

Shift to Theories of Pain Relief

A second watershed in pain theory was a paradigm shift from theories of the mechanisms of pain to theories of relief. These included prescriptive and explanatory theories of opioids and of nonopioids such as local anesthetics and nonsteroidal anti-inflammatory drugs (NSAIDs). Health professionals have known this prescriptive theory for years. Even ancient peoples used opium for pain during disease and surgery. Opioids, whether taken orally or injected into blood vessels, muscles, or epidural space, provide potent relief for moderate to severe pain. However, the amount of relief varies among individuals. The explanatory theory (mechanism) for effects was later found to be that opioids attach to mu and kappa opioid receptors in the CNS.

NSAIDs, including aspirin, ibuprofen, acetaminophen, cyclooxygenase-2 (COX-2) inhibitors, and ketorolac, have different mechanisms from centrally acting opioids. Acting at the site of the tissue injury, NSAIDs decrease the release of inflammatory substances that sensitize the nerve fibers to respond to the painful stimuli. NSAIDs do not bind to opioid receptors and do not produce the same side effects as opioids. Therefore, when they are used as adjuvants, they can be opioid sparing, but some could also interfere with blood clotting. Ketorolac is an intravenous NSAID that is often used to add a second mechanism of relief to that of opioids after surgery.

In the discipline of nursing, there are middle range descriptive theories of pain from the perspective of both patients and expert nurses. Qualitative themes obtained from patients have characterized chronic pain as dominating and seemingly endless (Mahon, 1994); it results in vulnerable feelings and thoughts of suicide and death (Morse, Bottorff, & Hutchinson, 1995). Expert nurses have also differentiated between acute and chronic pain (Simon, Baumann, & Nolan, 1995), and know that anxiety and pain have an effect on each other and that self-care accelerates postoperative recovery.

Broad descriptive theories include pain as one of several major concepts. The theory of unpleasant symptoms generalizes across symptoms of pain, dyspnea, nausea, and fatigue, based on the commonalities of these symptoms (Lenz, Pugh, Milligan, Gift, & Suppe, 1997). Other nursing theories are focused on nurse and patient facilitators and barriers to relief (Greipp, 1992), analgesic delivery according to pain diurnal rhythms (Auvil-Novak, 1997), and nurse education for pain management (Dalton & Blau, 1996).

Development of Integrated Prescriptive Approach

A third paradigm shift was the notion that pain alleviation by nurses requires an *integrated* prescriptive approach, proposed in Good and Moore's theory of a balance between analgesia and side effects (Good, 1998; Good & Moore, 1996). This theory prescribes patient teaching, nonpharmacological methods, and expert nursing care in addition to analgesic medication. Do patients need analgesics alone? What can provide additional relief? What patient teaching and what nursing actions produce effective relief? Integrated prescriptive pain theories specify the actions that nurses must take to deliver both pharmacological and nonpharmacological therapies that are effective for relief. There is an integrative pain alleviation theory for adults (Good & Moore, 1996) and also one for children that adds prescriptions for assessment of developmental level, coping strategies, and cultural background (Huth & Moore, 1998).

Acute Pain Management Guidelines

The theory of a balance between analgesia and side effects was originally developed from the acute pain management guidelines published in 1992 by the Agency for Health Care Policy and Research (AHCPR) (Acute Pain Management Guideline Panel, 1992). Cochaired by a nurse, Ada K. Jacox, RN, PhD, FAAN, and an anesthesiologist, Daniel B. Carr, MD, the guidelines were an early interdisciplinary publication to address the inadequate treatment of acute pain following surgery and trauma. However, practice guidelines for acute pain have been revised with the ongoing progress of knowledge, technology, and practice. Today there are many acute pain guidelines—from other countries, pain management organizations, and individual health care agencies. Some current guidelines are written by experts in multiple disciplines, and some by experts in one. An example of current multidisciplinary acute pain guidelines are those published by the American Pain Society Quality of Care Task Force (2005). Single disciplinary examples are the American Society of Anesthesiologists Task Force on Pain Management (2004) and the Research Translation & Dissemination Core, the Gerontological Nursing Interventions Research Center at the University of Iowa (2006).

The American Society of Anesthesiologists Task Force on Acute Pain Management was particularly clear in reporting what the therapies body of scientific literature *supported or suggested,* and also noted when the literature was *equivocal, insufficient, inadequate, or silent,* making recommendations based on their expert opinion. Some of their recommendations were specific to their specialty, such as recommending pharmaceutical agents, routes, and systems for management of pain, and leadership of a dedicated acute pain service. However, other recommendations were about important interactions with the

---

BOX 3.1 • Nonpharmacological Adjuvants

RELAXATION

Jaw relaxation (Good et al., 1999)
Autogenic phrases (Green, Green, & Norris, 1979)
Progressive muscle relaxation (Snyder, Pestka, & Bly, 2002)
Systematic relaxation (Roykulcharoen & Good 2004)
Slow rhythmic breathing

GUIDED IMAGERY

Self-efficacy imagery (Tusek, Church, Strong, Grass, & Fazeo, 1997)

Pleasant imagery (Locsin, 1988; Huth, Broome, & Good, 2004; Lewandowski, 2004)
Hypnosis (Olness, 1981)

MUSIC

Sedative music (Good et al., 1999, Siedlecki & Good, 2006)
Favorite music
Tempos (fast or slow)
Instruments

---

health care team. For example, they recommended that anesthesiologists with responsibility for perioperative analgesia should be *available* for consultation with involved nurses, surgeons, and other physicians *at all times* and should assist in evaluating any patient problems with pain relief 24 hours a day. This recommendation supports the first assumption of the theory between analgesia and side effects that "the nurse and physician collaborate to effectively manage acute pain," found in Box 3.1. The Anesthesiologists Task Force also recommended institutional policies and procedures for education and training for health care providers and interdisciplinary patient and family education for use of opioids and patient-controlled analgesia (PCA), and also for nonpharmacological modalities. Finally, they made recommendations for special populations of pediatric, geriatric, and critically ill patients.

The guidelines published by the American Pain Society (APS) were aimed at institutional quality improvement (QI) programs for the treatment of both acute and cancer pain. They were formed by an interdisciplinary committee of nurses and physicians from several specialties, plus a psychologist and a statistician. After searching the literature and arriving at consensus on a draft, the committee circulated them to APS membership for comments and then carried out formal implementation studies at three medical centers. Their recommendations for QI included introducing "red flags" to raise clinician awareness of unrelieved pain; locating analgesic information at places where orders are written; promising responsive analgesic care to patients; urging patients to report pain; and implementing institutional policies for modern analgesic technologies and monitoring the implementation of these measures.

These acute pain guidelines were created for various purposes by committees of experts, who systematically reviewed the research literature and arrived at consensus of their professional opinions. All of these, plus the Joint Commission (formerly the Joint Commission on Accreditation of Healthcare Organizations), recommend evidence-based acute pain management principles that include analgesics plus complementary therapies, assessment, reassessment, and follow-up; and patient participation, similar to the midrange nursing theory of a balance between analgesia and side effects proposed by Good and Moore in 1996. These principles have stood tests of time and interdisciplinary convergence of recommendations, yet are focused on the role of the individual nurse.

DEFINITION OF THEORY CONCEPTS

The major concepts of the theory A Balance Between Analgesia and Side Effects are found in Table 3.1, along with theoretical definitions and examples of operational definitions that can be used in research. In addition, Figure 3.1 is a graphic representation of the theory. Acute pain is conceptualized as a multidimensional phenomenon occurring after surgery or trauma that includes sensory and affective dimensions. Pain in alert adults is what the person reports. The sensory component of pain following damage to body tissues is the localized physical perception of hurt. It is ordinarily termed "sensation of pain" (Good et al., 2001). The affective component of pain is the unpleasant emotion associated with the sensation and has been named "distress of pain" (Good et al., 2001), "anxiety" (Good, 1995), or "unpleasantness" (Price, McGrath, Rafii, & Buckingham, 1983). The sensory and affective components of pain affect each other (Casey & Melzack, 1967; Johnson & Rice, 1974), and can be measured in terms of intensity magnitude (Good et al., 2001).

The concept of *potent pain medication* refers to the major method used for relief. This may be opioids delivered by patient-controlled analgesia or by subcutaneous, intramuscular, or intravenous injection. However, opioid analgesics have side effects of nausea, vomiting, drowsiness, urinary retention, and respiratory depression. In addition, dependence can occur. To avoid these side effects, patients often take less analgesic than is needed for adequate relief (Acute Pain Management Guideline Panel, 1992). Epidural analgesia can be achieved with the use of opioids, local anesthetics, or both; these are injected into the epidural space of

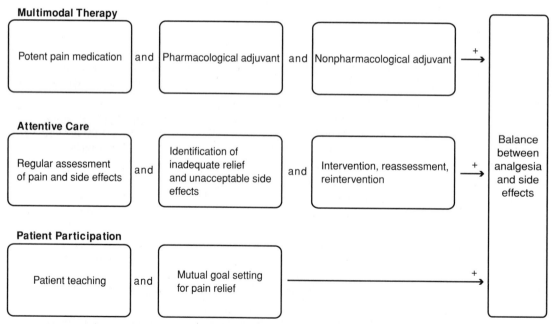

■ **Figure 3.1**   The middle range theory of a balance between analgesia and side effects prescribes nursing actions to encourage patient participation in using multimodal therapy with attentive care. Adapted from Good, M. (1998). A middle range theory of acute pain management: Use in research. *Nursing Outlook, 46*(3), 120–124, with permission from Elsevier.

Table 3.1 CONCEPTS WITH THEORETICAL AND OPERATIONAL DEFINITIONS

CONCEPTS	THEORETICAL DEFINITIONS	OPERATIONAL DEFINITIONS (EXAMPLES)
Outcomes		
Balance between analgesia and side effects	Patient satisfaction with relief of pain and relief or absence of side effects	Patient report of safe and satisfying pain relief with few or no side effects
Pain	An unpleasant sensory and affective experience associated with tissue injury following surgery or trauma	Pain intensity on a visual analog scale
Side effects	Unpleasant sensory and affective experiences associated with pain medication	Opioid Side Effects Scale (Good et al., 2001–2005)
Proposition 1		
Potent pain medication	Opioid analgesic or local anesthetic given systemically or by epidural for acute pain	Drug, dose, frequency, route, and method of administration
Pharmacological adjuvant	Analgesic given as a supplement	Drug, dose, frequency, route, and method of administration
Nonpharmacological adjuvant	Complementary nursing therapies: relaxation, music, imagery, massage, or cold for pain relief	Technique, dose, frequency given, and mastery of use
Proposition 2		
Regular assessment of pain and side effects	Report of pain and side effects every 2 hours until under control, and then every 4 hours	Pain rating scale Patient report or nurse observation of side effects of opioids
Identification of inadequate relief of pain and side effects	Pain/side effect intensity greater than mutual goal	Number and intensity of side effects that are unacceptable to patient/nurse
Intervention, reassessment, and reintervention	Immediate intervention for pain and side effects; reassessment when peak effect is expected, and reintervention if pain and side effects are still unacceptable	Nurse documentation
Proposition 3		
Patient teaching	Patient instruction, encouraging attitudes, expectations, and action in reporting pain, obtaining medication, preventing pain during activity, and using complementary therapies	Documentation of nurse instruction, or patient use of audio/videotape
Mutual goal setting	Mutually agreed upon, safe, realistic goals for relief	Nurse discussions with patient daily, including documentation

the spinal cord. Side effects of epidural analgesia include lower extremity numbness. Other techniques may include postincisional infiltration with local anesthetics, intra-articular analgesia, and peripheral nerve blocks (American Society of Anesthesiologists Task Force on Pain Management, 2004). As these methods often provide insufficient analgesia and uncomfortable side effects, adjuvants are often recommended.

Pharmacological adjuvants may be given because their unrelated mechanism of action increases relief, yet can "spare" the use and the side effects of strong analgesics. The American Society of Anesthesiologists Task Force on Pain Management reports that the literature suggests that two routes of administration may be more effective, and it recommends several combinations (2004), such as (a) epidural opioid analgesia combined with oral or systemic analgesics, or (b) intravenous opioids combined with oral NSAIDs such as ibuprofen, with COX-2 inhibitors (COXIBs) such as celecoxib, or with acetaminophen.

Nonpharmacological adjuvants to analgesic medication can include relaxation techniques, music, hypnosis, guided imagery with self-efficacy messages, or guided imagery with pleasant image messages (Box 3-1). Music can be soft, soothing, sedative instrumental music (Good et al., 2000), and can be combined with relaxation or guided imagery. Nonpharmacological adjuvants have been studied during emergency treatment, following surgery and trauma, during labor, and during painful procedures. Nonpharmacological music interventions have also been found to be effective in cancer, arthritis, and other types of chronic pain.

Regular pain and side effect assessment are actions nurses take to identify patient symptoms. The theory then prescribes that nurses treat these symptoms, rather than simply record them. *Identification of inadequate pain relief and side effects* requires the nurse to believe the patient's report and to know what intensity is less than adequate relief, considering unit norms and the wide variation in patient responses to pain and analgesics. In hospitals, nurses can request and use rescue orders and dose ranges (e.g., 1–2 mg) when the usual dose is insufficient. The nurse can also encourage the use of nonpharmacological interventions. All interventions should be followed by *reassessment* when the greatest effect is expected, and then *reintervention* if pain is still not relieved.

Patient teaching and *mutual goal setting* will assist patients in their important role in managing their own pain. It is proposed that nurses teach patients effective attitudes and accurate expectations of pain and also to report pain, obtain medication, and use adjuvants. It is proposed that nurses initiate dialogue for mutual goal setting of realistic pain relief goals that are acceptable to their patients.

When testing a middle range theory, more specific concepts and testable hypotheses can be deducted from the more general concepts and propositions (Good, 1998). A balance between analgesia and side effects is the general outcome. To deduct more specific concepts, the researcher would think of components of the concept and state their relationships to the general concept. For example, the concept of side effects is a subset of the balance between analgesia and side effects. Less sensation and distress of pain can be deducted from analgesia and studied individually (Good, 1998). Any part of the theory can be examined in research: one concept, new relationships between concepts, part of a proposition, all of a proposition, or the whole theory. In addition, the application to nursing practice or education can be studied.

DESCRIPTION OF THE THEORY OF PAIN: A BALANCE BETWEEN ANALGESIA AND SIDE EFFECTS

The theory of a balance between analgesia and side effects is the first integrative prescriptive middle range pain management theory. It provides a broader and more parsimonious overview than detailed pain management guidelines. Its general principles of acute pain management are a framework for research and a guide for nursing practice. The theorists expect practitioners to use the overall principles, along with the

---

BOX 3.2   Assumptions of the Theory of a Balance Between Analgesia and Side Effects

1. The nurse and physician collaborate to effectively manage acute pain.
2. Systemic opioid analgesics or epidural opioids or anesthetic agents are indicated.
3. Medication for side effects is given as needed.

4. Patients are adults with ability to learn, set goals, and communicate symptoms.
5. Nurses have current knowledge of pain management.

---

detailed knowledge contained in the adult acute pain guidelines and any current empirical evidence. These principles for practice are called "propositions" when theorizing or testing them in research. This terminology is a matter of function: principles for practice and theoretical propositions for research. With the idea that the purpose of theory is research and the purpose of research is theory, but the purpose of both is practice, this theory with its principles/propositions is organized to stimulate additional research and to organize the teaching and communicating of pain management information to nurses. Further, the theory presents a new perspective: that the best pain management practice is an integrated one that combines analgesic medications with nonpharmacological adjuvants, careful nursing care, and patient participation. The goal of the theory is to achieve a more holistic relief outcome than analgesia alone (i.e., to balance greater pain relief with fewer side effects of opioids by using the principles).

The scope for the theory is fairly narrow, encompassing acute postoperative pain or trauma in hospitalized adults. The assumptions of the theory are presented in Box 3.2. They are fairly narrow so that prescriptions can be specific. The theorists meant the theory to be tested and used clinically in adults having moderate to severe acute pain after surgery or trauma. The theory has limits; it does not address the treatment of pain in children, elders, or those with special kinds of acute pain. However, middle range theories have been or can be developed for these phenomena as well.

Propositions

The theory has three prescriptive propositions that can be summarized as follows: In acute pain, patient participation, multimodal interventions, and attentive care are needed for a balance between analgesia and side effects.

The first proposition is about multimodal intervention. It proposes that nurses use potent pain medication plus pharmacological and nonpharmacological adjuvants to achieve a balance between analgesia and side effects. The effect on pain has empirical support published by the Acute Pain Management Guideline Panel (1992) and Good and colleagues (Good et al., 1999; Good, Anderson, Stanton-Hicks, Grass, & Makii, 2002; Good, Anderson, Ahn, Cong, & Stanton-Hicks, 2005).

The second proposition is about attentive care. It proposes that nurses assess, intervene, reassess, and reintervene to achieve a balance between analgesia and side effects. The effect on pain is supported by 30 years of research showing that pain is inadequately treated and by findings that regular assessment alone does not produce relief (Good, Auvil-Novak, & Group, 1994). Intervention, reassessment after a strategic interval, and reintervention by increasing the dose of analgesic and/or adding an adjuvant are needed and should continue until a satisfactory balance is attained (Good & Moore, 1996).

The third proposition is about patient participation. It proposes that patient teaching and goal setting contribute to a balance between analgesia and side effects (see Figure 3.1). This proposition is supported by meta-analyses for patient teaching (Devine, 1992; Devine & Cook, 1986; Shuldham, 1999) and expert opinion for goal setting (Acute Pain Management Guideline Panel, 1992). Patient teaching is a key concept to consider when trying to improve outcomes. Patient teaching should include ways to obtain medication, report pain, and use a nonpharmacological adjuvant.

APPLICATIONS OF THE THEORY

The theory is useful for clinical intervention research with experimental designs, called randomized controlled trials (RCTs), and is useful in alert adult populations in which acute pain is incompletely controlled by medication alone and side effects may prevent increasing analgesic medication. The theory has been adopted by postsurgical nursing units as the basis for their postoperative pain management program, and has been used many times to teach graduate nursing students the usefulness and composition of a focused, concrete nursing theory. It can also be used to teach acute pain management to undergraduate students, using the three principles with current practice guidelines that add the details.

Research Support for the Theory

The first proposition of the theory was partially but directly tested in two studies of abdominal surgical patients. Both studies compared nonpharmacological adjuvants to potent analgesics. Pharmacological adjuvants were not tested, as that was not standard medical practice in the five hospitals we used. Both studies were funded by the National Institute of Nursing Research (NINR). This level of funding for a program of nursing research demonstrates national interest and support for studying nonpharmacological adjuvants for pain management. In the first study, relaxation, music, and the combination of both provided up to 31% more relief than PCA alone following major abdominal surgery. When subgroups of gynecological and intestinal surgical patients were examined from this database, the percent relief compared to opioids alone was even greater (Good et al., 1999; Good et al., 2002; Good et al., 2005).

In the second study, both the first and third propositions were partially tested. The combination of relaxation and music was compared to a short patient-teaching tape that was specific to pain management, plus a third tape that combined them. Pharmacological adjuvants and goal setting were not tested. The patient-teaching tape was intended to lower pain even more than relaxation and music and usual opioids. It taught patients to let go of fears of opioid dependency, to use their PCA system, and to tell their nurse about their pain, until relief was obtained. Postoperative abdominal surgery patients were encouraged to use the tapes as much as possible during the first 2 days. Pain and side effects were measured four times a day. In addition, there were five cross-sectional pre- and posttests in which pain was measured before and after 20 minutes of listening to the tape (or lying in bed for controls) (Good, Anderson, Wotman & Albert, 2001–2005).

The second study demonstrated once again and in a more diverse sample that relaxation and music, in addition to pharmacological interventions, reduced pain during the first 2 postoperative days, giving patients more options and up to 24% more relief. However, preliminary results indicate that the patient-teaching method used did not reduce pain and neither intervention reduced side effects of analgesics (manuscript in preparation). Further study of subpopulations from this database is in progress.

The nonpharmacological adjuvant concept of the theory has been extended to other populations. Music has reduced chronic pain and pain of arthritis and labor, and guided imagery has reduced chronic pain (Lewandowski, 2004; McCaffrey & Freeman, 2003; Phumdoung & Good, 2003; Siedlecki & Good, 2006).

Although these three studies were conceptualized in another theory, the results also support the effectiveness of nondrug adjuvants. Also, massage has reduced back pain after surgery, but not incision pain (Chin, 1999).

In addition, reviews have aggregated the results of many studies of relaxation, music, and guided imagery for acute postoperative pain. Authors of a Cochrane Review of music for pain report heterogeneity in the 14 postoperative studies with 510 participants exposed to music and 493 controls. They found that there was a 0.5-unit (0–10 scale) lower pain intensity in those who listened to adjuvant music. Only four music-for-pain studies reported the proportion of participants in each group who achieved at least 50% pain relief. Based on the four studies, the number of patients needed to treat (NNT) was five in order to have one patient who received 50% relief that they would not have had if they had not listened to music. The authors recommended that future studies report proportions in each group (Cepeda, Carr, Lau, & Alvarez, 2006). However, the correct method of determining the clinical effect of a nonpharmacological adjuvant to a potent drug that is already providing considerable relief is still being established. One issue is that 35% relief is meaningful in people with moderate pain, such as that treated with analgesics (Cepeda, Africano, Polo, Alcala, & Carr, 2003). Another issue is that people with pain less than 3 on a 0 to 10 scale may not need this adjuvant. Perhaps investigators should select only patients with pain levels of 3 or greater out of 10 and report proportions of those in each group with 35% to 50% or greater relief.

Reviews of randomized trials for relaxation revealed findings that support part of the first proposition. A recent review reported support for jaw relaxation and systematic relaxation for relief of pain after surgery (Kwekkeboom & Gretarsdottir, 2006). An earlier review found weaker evidence to support use of relaxation. Only three of seven RCTs demonstrated significantly less pain sensation and/or pain distress in those who had relaxation (Sears & Carroll, 1998). Another review noted that more, 9 of 11, RCTs found significantly less pain sensation and/or pain distress (Good, 1996). These acute pain reviews build on an interdisciplinary Technology Assessment Panel at the National Institutes of Health (NIH) that reported strong evidence for the use of relaxation techniques in reducing chronic pain (NIH Technology Assessment Panel, 1996).

The use of massage and the use of cold therapy have initial support for the effect of nonpharmacological interventions in the first proposition. Five early studies found that massage reduced postoperative pain (Forchuk et al., 2004; Kshettry, Carole, Henly, Sendelbach, & Kummer, 2006; Piotrowski et al., 2003; Taylor et al., 2003; Wang & Keck, 2004), and no ineffective massage studies were found. Although the use of cold therapy is the oldest analgesic still being used clinically, its postoperative testing seems limited to sports and orthopedic surgeries and trauma where prevention of edema-related pain is present. Findings are mixed; some reported an apparent effect of cold on pain (Cohn, Draeger, & Jackson, 1989; Scheffler, Sheitel, & Lipton, 1992; Webb, Williams, Ivory, Day, & Williamson, 1998) and others did not (Edwards, Rimmer, & Keene, 1996; Whitelaw, DeMuth, Demos, Schepsis, & Jacques, 1995). Principles, techniques, and nursing care involved in cryotherapy are reviewed by McDowell, McFarland, and Nalli (1994). Using Middle Range Theories 3.1 summarizes earlier findings supporting the theory's propositions.

Suggestions for Additional Research

The nonpharmacological adjuvant can continue to be tested. The whole-body systematic relaxation technique should be retested. Studies are needed to compare sedative music to music with faster tempos and to compare the effects of various musical instruments and various cultural preferences. New methods of patient teaching for patient integration of pharmacological and nonpharmacological interventions after surgery are needed. An effective patient teaching intervention for PCA use is needed. The second proposition to provide attentive care and intervene until pain is relieved may be incorporated into practice better today than 10 years ago, when the theory was first published. However, nurses in hospitals in which

3.1 USING MIDDLE RANGE THEORIES

The theory of a balance between analgesia and side effects was first tested in a large random-ized clinical trial sponsored by the National Institute of Nursing Research from 1994 to 1998. The researchers wanted to test the effects of jaw relaxation, soft music, and the combination of relaxation and music on postoperative pain in abdominal surgical patients who were receiv-ing patient-controlled analgesia (PCA). Patients were recruited from the preadmission testing departments of five hospitals in northeast Ohio, and were tested at ambulation and rest on postoperative days 1 and 2. Patients marked the sensation and distress of pain visual analog scales before and after listening to the tapes during 15 minutes of rest, and at four times during ambulation each day. Patients in the control group did not receive a tape but were asked to rest in bed during the test and to ambulate according to hospital practice during the test at ambulation. All patients were told they could use PCA as much as they desired. The researchers found that the three nonpharmacological interventions as a group resulted in sig-nificantly less pain (10%–31%) than the control group, and that the three interventions were not different from one another in their effect. Jaw relaxation and music, used separately, reduced pain at most data points, with mixed findings at the after-ambulation point, probably due to increased pain and loss of mental focus on relaxation while getting back into bed (Good et al., 1999).

Based on these findings, the researchers reported support for the part of the theory that they tested: In addition to strong medication, the three nonpharmacological interventions reduced pain. Side effects and pharmacological adjuvants were not studied nor was the balance itself. The concept of pain was deducted from the concept of the balance between analgesia and side effects.

attentive care needs improvement may want to provide inservice education and measure the results in knowledge and practice.

Research Application 3.1 demonstrates the integration of gate control mechanisms in a study of pain after abdominal surgery.

INSTRUMENTS USED IN EMPIRICAL TESTING

In an effort to capture and study the experience of pain, researchers have created so many pain scales that it is sometimes difficult to compare scores across studies, making synthesis of the literature difficult. For example, a five-point scale cannot be equated to an eight-point scale.

Different scales, however, are needed to measure the experience of each type of pain (e.g., acute, chronic, cancer, labor, and pediatric pain) and each component of pain (e.g., sensory and affective pain). Nurses, who are sensitive to these differences, have been instrumental in creating new instruments to measure pain. Within pain types, nurses must consider some sort of standardization across studies so that they can be compared.

Some scales contain both numeric intensity measures and descriptors such as "mild," "moderate," and "severe" to guide responses of subjects. Examples of these combinations are the 0–10 Numeric Pain Intensity Scale and the 0–10 Numeric Pain Distress Scale (Acute Pain Management Guideline Panel,

3.1 RESEARCH APPLICATION

A nurse researcher conducted a study in which the research question was, What is the effect of relaxation and music, patient teaching for pain management, and the combination of both on postoperative pain, side effects of opioids, stress, and secretory immunoglobulin A? Using a randomized clinical trial (RCT), the researcher reviewed the surgery schedule each day to identify males and females scheduled for major abdominal surgery who meet the criterion for age (18–75 years) and are expecting to receive general anesthesia and patient-controlled analgesia (PCA).

The researcher arrived at the hospital at 6:00 AM and introduced herself to Mr. Green, who had been admitted to the surgical waiting area for a 7:30 AM colectomy for cancer, but had not yet received any premedication that would compromise his ability to give consent.

After obtaining written informed consent, the nurse conducted a brief interview and taught Mr. Green to use the Sensation and Distress of Pain Visual Analog Scales (Good et al., 2001). The researcher used a computerized minimization program to randomly assign Mr. Green to one of four groups, while balancing the groups on potentially confounding variables such as age, sex, race, type of surgery, chronic pain, smoking, alcohol use, and time of surgery. The groups were (a) relaxation and music; (b) patient teaching for pain management; (c) the combination of the two; and (d) the control group, which received the usual care. Mr. Green's assignment was the combination of relaxation, music, and patient teaching. He then listened to the 9-minute teaching tape giving him instruction in using the jaw relaxation technique and offering him a choice among six types of sedative instrumental music (Gaston, 1951). He listened to 20 seconds of each type of music: synthesizer, harp, piano, orchestra, jazz, and inspirational. Mr. Green chose the inspirational music.

After surgery, Mr. Green was taken to his postoperative room, and the nurse researcher went to the bedside to conduct the first pretest–posttest. She asked him to rate the intensity of his sensation and distress of pain on the dual visual analog scales, and then she obtained pulse and respirations. She gave him the tape and recorder, and played his assigned tape for 20 minutes. The tape reviewed his role in pain management, guided him in the use of a relaxation technique, and played soft inspirational music for 20 minutes. The researcher asked him to rate his pain again for the posttest and recorded his pulse and respirations. She showed Mr. Green and his wife and daughter how to use the tape recorder and encouraged him to use it as much as possible for the rest of the day and evening, and even during the night. The idea was to get pain under control early in the postoperative period and keep it controlled.

For the next two days at 8 AM, 12 noon, 4 PM, and 8 PM, a research nurse or graduate student came to the bedside to ask about pain and side effects of opioids. In addition, at 10 AM and 2 PM each day, the research nurse conducted 20-minute pre- and posttests. On day 2, she also collected pretest and posttest saliva specimens. The patient's chart was reviewed at each visit for medications and other factors that could confound the outcome. At 8 AM on the third day, the research nurse conducted a structured interview, asking about demographics and information on contextual variables that might confound the outcome. Mr. Green was thanked for participating in the study and for his contribution to nursing knowledge about pain management. A $20 gift certificate was mailed to subjects who completed the study.

The data recorded on the questionnaire was coded and entered into an SPSS statistical program file by graduate student assistants who were learning to become researchers. The principal investigator and the project manager analyzed the data to determine whether or not the interventions reduced pain, side effects of opioids, and stress and/or improved immunity. The findings were written in a manuscript and sent to a peer-reviewed research journal for publication.

Table 3.2 INSTRUMENTS TO MEASURE PAIN

CATEGORY	ABBREVIATION	NAME OF SCALE AND CITATION
Pain	VAS	Visual Analog Scale [a]
Sensory pain	-	VAS Sensation of Pain Scale [b]
Sensory pain	-	Numeric Pain Intensity Scale [c]
Sensory pain	-	Descriptive Pain Intensity Scale [d]
Affective pain	-	VAS Distress of Pain Scale [e]
Affective pain	-	Numeric Pain Distress Scale [f]
Affective pain	-	Descriptive Pain Distress Scale [g]
Affective pain	-	VAS Unpleasantness Scale [h]
Affective pain	-	VAS Anxiety of Pain Scale [i]
Affective pain	MPQ	McGill Pain Questionnaire [j]
Total pain	MPQ-PRI	Pain Rating Index (PRI)
Sensory pain	PRI-sensory	Sensory subscale
Affective pain	PRI-affective	Affective subscale
Pain intensity	MPQ-NWC	Number of Words Chosen
Pain intensity	MPQ-PPI	Present Pain Index
Pain intensity	MPQ-VAS	Visual Analog Scale
Total, sensory, & affective pain	MPQ-SF	McGill Pain Questionnaire–Short Form [k]
Chronic pain	UAB	University of Alabama–Birmingham Pain Behavior Scale [l]
Chronic pain	WHYMPI	West Haven–Yale Multidimensional Pain Inventory [m]
Cancer pain	BPI	Brief Pain Inventory [n]
Cancer pain, relief, mood	MPAC	Memorial Pain Assessment Card [o]
24-hour time-intensity	-	Keele's Pain Chart [p]
Labor pain	-	Behavioral Index for Assessment of Labor Pain [q]
Children's pain	-	Poker Chip Scale [r]
Children's pain	-	Word-Graphic Rating Scale [s]
Children's pain	-	Oucher Scale [t]
Children's pain	-	Wong-Baker Faces Scale [u]
Young children's pain	FLACC	Faces, legs, activity, cry, consolability [v]

- = no abbreviation.
   [a,b,e] Good et al., 2001; [b-g, r, s] Acute Pain Management Guidelines, 1992; [h] Price et al.,1983; [i] McCormack, del Horne & Sheather, 1988; [j, k] Melzack, 1975; [l] Richards, Nepomuceni, Riles, & Suer, 1982; [m] Kerns, Turk, & Rudy, 1985; [n] Daut, Cleeland, & Flanery, 1983; [o] Fishman et al., 1986; [p] Keele, 1948; [q] Bonnel & Boureau, 1985; [t] Beyer, Denyes, & Villarruel, 1992; [u] Wong & Baker, 1988; [v] Merkel, Voepel-Lewis, Shayevitz, & Malviya, 1997.

1992). Visual analog scales (VASs) have a 100-mm horizontal line with no numbers and only descriptive anchors at each end (Good et al., 2001).

The Word–Graphic Rating Scale for adolescents and children is a horizontal line with five verbal descriptors under the line, but no numbers or upright lines. This scale may produce more evenly distributed scores than numerical scales, but the presence of the words may still serve as a clustering factor, even when patients are told to mark anywhere along the line (Good et al., 2001). Patients notice the numbers and verbal descriptors and tend to make their mark near them.

Another solution may be to administer the widely used and sensitive VAS as a "gold standard," followed by a brief descriptor scale (e.g., none, mild, moderate, or severe) and a scale that researchers think is most specific to the health condition. This would provide specificity as well as sensitivity to the type of pain experienced, but could also be used to standardize all three measures of pain in various populations and increase communication and synthesis across studies. Cepeda et al. (2003) have used a similar method to determine the amount of relief that is meaningful to postoperative patients. The McGill Pain Questionnaire contains three measures, including a descriptive scale, a VAS, and a numerical–description rating scale; it could be used for standardization in this manner. Table 3.2 lists instruments and indicates the type of pain measured by each. Other instruments can be found in McDowell and Newell (1996).

SUMMARY

Pain is a universal human experience that has been known since the first human experienced illness, trauma, or labor. Although pain has been studied descriptively for more than a century, it has only recently been studied from a prescriptive nursing perspective. The middle range prescriptive pain management theory of a balance between analgesia and side effects reflects the nursing mission to intervene effectively and holistically to relieve pain and suffering and to prevent their long-term effects. There is increasing empirical support and nurse researchers can continue to test and to provide support and creative extensions of the theory. Practicing nurses are using the evidence-based principles for effective relief of acute pain in their patients.

CRITICAL THINKING EXERCISES

1. Compare two scenarios or scripts for nurses and patients engaging in mutual goal setting for pain management after a specific surgical procedure. With peers, analyze each for advantages and disadvantages to the patient and to those who provide care.

2. Analyze the trajectory of patients undergoing a specific surgical procedure and the places they receive nursing care, from the surgeon's office and the decision for surgery, through the pre- and postoperative hospitalization, to recovery at home. Plan the most effective times, amounts of information, and ways nurses can introduce and reinforce the elements of patient teaching for pain management. *The elements are to encourage attitudes,* *expectations, and action in reporting pain, obtaining medication, preventing pain during activity, and using complementary therapies.* Describe ways this nursing care, delivered in several places, could be streamlined and coordinated with the surgeon's patient teaching.

3. Envision yourself as a leader who is introducing this nursing theory as the basis of postoperative pain management on your unit. Create introductory scripts with arguments for its usefulness to be delivered to the nursing and medical staff. Describe how you would begin to demonstrate its usefulness. Explain your method of presenting its current evidence base. Give the main points of a clinically useable protocol for your unit

WEB RESOURCES

1. National Institute of Nursing Research (NINR): **http://www.ninr.nih.gov**
2. National Center for Complementary and Alternative Medicine: **http://nccam.nih.gov**
3. Sigma Theta Tau International Nursing Society: **http://www.nursingsociety.org**; Virginia Henderson International Nursing Library; keyword, "pain" or **http://www.nursinglibrary.org/portal/main.aspx**
4. The American Pain Society (APS) is the leading U.S. organization committed to pain management. The mission is to advance pain-related research, education, treatment, and professional practice. It is a multidisciplinary society of basic and clinical scientists, clinicians, and others: **http://www.ampainsoc.org**
5. The American Pain Society publishes the following:
   a. *Journal of Pain:* **http://www.ampainsoc.org/pub/journal**
   b. *APS Bulletin:* **http://www.ampainsoc.org/pub/bulletin**
   c. Professional guidelines for pain of arthritis, sickle cell disease, cancer, and fibromyalgia: **http://www.ampainsoc.org/pub/cp_guidelines.htm**
   d. Patient guidelines for pain of arthritis, sickle cell disease, cancer, and fibromyalgia: **http://www.ampainsoc.org/pub/persons_with_pain.htm**
6. The International Association for the Study of Pain (IASP) is the largest multidisciplinary international organization in the field of pain and is dedicated to furthering research and improving patient care. Currently, the IASP has more than 6,900 individual members from 106 countries. **http://www.iasp-pain.org**
7. *PAIN* is the official publication of the IASP. It publishes original research on the nature, mechanisms, and treatment of pain of multidisciplinary interest: **http://www.elsevier.com/locate/pain**
8. The American Society for Pain Management Nursing (ASPMN) is an organization of professional nurses dedicated to promoting and providing optimal care of patients with pain through education, standards, advocacy, and research. ASPMN National Office, PO Box 15473, Lenexa, KS 66285-5473; toll free: (888) 34ASPMN or (913) 752-4975; fax: (913) 599-5340; E-mail: **aspmn@goamp.com; http://www.aspmn.org/Organization/position_papers.htm**
9. *Pain Management Nursing* (PMN) is a peer-reviewed journal with a focus on the realm of pain management as it applies to nursing. It is the official journal of the American Society for Pain Management Nursing. Original and review articles from experts in the field offer key insights in the areas of clinical practice, advocacy, education, administration, and research. Additional features include practice guidelines and pharmacology updates. *Pain Management Nursing* is indexed in CINAHL and MEDLINE: **http://www.us.elsevier health.com/product.jsp?isbn=15249042**
10. The *European Journal of Pain* is a multidisciplinary international journal. It aims to become a global forum on major aspects of pain and pain management: **http://www.us.elsevierhealth.com/product.jsp?isbn=10903801**
11. Alternative therapies: **http://www.holisticonline.com/hol_alt-therapies.htm**
12. Mind–body therapy: **http://www.holisticonline.com/hol_mindcontrol.htm**
13. The Cancer Pain & Symptom Management Nursing Research Group (CPSMNRG) is an innovative group of researchers focused on the generation and dissemination of knowledge related to the pain and other symptoms in persons with cancer and those at the end of life: **http://www.tneel.uic.edu/**
14. Clinical Practice Guidelines Online are now archived and can be accessed through an electronic full-text retrieval system called HSTAT (Health Services Technology Assessment Text) at the National Library of Medicine: **http://hstat.nlm.nih.gov/**

REFERENCES

Acute Pain Management Guideline Panel. (1992). *Acute pain management: Operative or medical procedures and trauma. Clinical practice guideline.* Rockville, MD: Agency for Health Care Policy and Research, Public Health Service, U.S. Department of Health and Human Services. (Vol. AHCPR No. 92-0032). Retrieved on January 16, 2007, from http://www.ncbi.nlm.nih.gov/books/bv.fcgi?rid=hstat6.chapter.8991.

American Pain Society Quality of Care Task Force. (2005). American Pain Society recommendations for improving the quality of acute and cancer pain management. *Archives of Internal Medicine, 165,* 1574–1580.

American Society of Anesthesiologists Task Force on Acute Pain Management. (2004). Practice guidelines for acute pain management in the perioperative setting: An updated Report by the American Society of Anesthesiologists Task Force on Acute Pain Management. *Anesthesiology, 100,* 1573–1581.

Auvil-Novak, S. E. (1997). A middle-range theory of chronotherapeutic intervention for postsurgical pain. *Nursing Research, 46*(2), 66–71.

Beecher, H. K. (1959). *Measurement of subjective responses: Quantitative effects of drugs.* New York: Oxford University Press.

Beyer, J. E., Denyes, M. J., & Villarruel, A. M. (1992). The creation, validation, and continuing development of the Oucher: A measure of pain intensity in children. *Journal of Pediatric Nursing, 7*(5), 335–346.

Bonnel, A. M., & Boureau, F. (1985). Labor pain assessment: Validity of a behavioral index. *Pain, 22*(1), 81.

Casey, K. L., & Melzack, R. (1967). Neural mechanisms of pain: A conceptual model. In E. L. Way (Ed.), *New concepts in pain and its clinical management* (pp. 13–31). Philadelphia: F. A. Davis.

Cepeda, M. S., Africano, J. M., Polo, R., Alcala, R., & Carr, D. B. (2003). What decline in pain intensity is meaningful to patients with acute pain? *Pain, 105*(1–2), 151–157.

Cepeda, M. S., Carr, D. B., Lau, J., & Alvarez, H. (2006). Music for pain relief. *Cochrane Database Systematic Review,* (2), CD004843.

Chin, C-C. (1999). *Effects of back massage on surgical stress responses and postoperative pain.* Unpublished doctoral dissertation. Case Western Reserve University, Cleveland.

Cohn, B. T., Draeger, R. I., & Jackson, D. W. (1989). The effects of cold therapy in the postoperative management of pain in patients undergoing anterior cruciate ligament reconstruction. *American Journal of Sports Medicine, 17*(3), 344–349.

Dalton, J. A., & Blau, W. (1996). Changing the practice of pain management: An examination of the theoretical basis of change. *Pain Forum, 5*(4), 266–272.

Daut, R. L., Cleeland, C. S., & Flanery, R. C. (1983). Development of the Wisconsin brief pain questionnaire to assess pain in cancer and other diseases. *Pain, 17,* 197–210.

Devine, E. C. (1992). Effects of psychoeducational care for adult surgical patients: A meta-analysis of 191 studies. *Patient Education and Counseling, 19,* 129–142.

Devine, E. C., & Cook, T. D. (1986). Clinical and cost saving effects of psychoeducational interventions with surgical patients: A meta analysis. *Research in Nursing and Health, 9,* 89–105.

Dickhoff, J., & James, P. (1968). A theory of theories: A position paper. *Nursing Research, 17*(3), 197–203.

Edwards, D. J., Rimmer, M., & Keene, G. C. (1996). The use of cold therapy in the postoperative management of patients undergoing arthroscopic anterior cruciate ligament reconstruction. *American Journal of Sports Medicine, 24*(2), 193–195.

Fishman, B., Pasternak, S., Wallenstein, S. L., Houde, R.W., Holland, J. C., & Foley, K. M. (1987). The Memorial Pain Assessment Card: A valid instrument for the evaluation of cancer pain. *Cancer, 60*(5), 1151–1158.

Forchuk, C., Baruth, P., Prendergast, M., Holliday, R., Bareham, R., Brimner, S., et al. (2004). Postoperative arm massage: a support for women with lymph node dissection. *Cancer Nursing, 27*(1), 25–33.

Gaston, E. T. (1951). Dynamic music factors in mood changes. *Music Educators Journal, 37,* 42–44.

Good, M. (1995). A comparison of the effects of jaw relaxation and music on postoperative pain. *Nursing Research, 44*(1), 52–57.

Good, M. (1996). Effects of relaxation and music on postoperative pain: A review. *Journal of Advanced Nursing, 24,* 905–914.

Good, M. (1998). A middle range theory of acute pain management; use in research. *Nursing Outlook, 46*(3), 120–124.

Good, M., Anderson, G. C., Ahn, S., Cong, X., & Stanton-Hicks, M. (2005). Relaxation and music reduce pain following intestinal surgery. *Research in Nursing and Health, 28*(3), 240–251.

Good, M., Anderson, G., Stanton-Hicks, M., Grass, J., & Makii, M. (2002). Relaxation and music reduce pain following gynecological surgery. *Pain Management Nursing, 3*(2), 61–70.

Good, M., Anderson, G. C., Wotman, S., & Albert, J. (2001–2005). Supplementing relaxation and music for postoperative pain. National Institute of Nursing Research. (National Institutes of Health, Bethesda, MD, Grant number R013933).

Good, M., Auvil-Novak, S., & Group, M. (1994). Pain and its management: One year after the guidelines. Paper presented at the AHSR & FSHR Annual Conference, June 12–14. Health Services Research, San Diego, CA.

Good, M., & Moore, S. M. (1996). Clinical practice guidelines as a new source of middle-range theory: Focus on acute pain. *Nursing Outlook, 44*(2), 74–79.

Good, M., Picot, B., Salem, S., Chin, C., Picot, S., & Lane, D. (2000). Cultural responses to music for pain relief. *Journal of Holistic Nursing, 18*(3), 245–260.

Good, M., Stanton-Hicks, M., Grass, J. M., Anderson, G. C., Choi, C. C., Schoolmeesters, L., et al. (1999). Relief of postoperative pain with jaw relaxation, music, and their combination. *Pain, 81*(1–2), 163–172.

Good, M., Stiller, C., Zauszniewski, J., Stanton-Hicks, M., Grass, J., & Anderson, G. C. (2001). Sensation and distress of pain scales: Reliability, validity and sensitivity. *Journal of Nursing Measurement, 9*(3), 219–238.

Green, E. E., Green, A. M., & Norris, P. A. (1979). Preliminary observation on a new-drug method for control of hypertension. *Journal of the South Carolina Medical Association, 75*(11), 575–582.

Greipp, M. E. (1992). Undermedication for pain: An ethical model. *Advances in Nursing Science, 15*(1), 44–53.

Huth, M. M., Broome, M. E., & Good, M. (2004). Imagery reduces children's post-operative pain. *Pain, 110*(1–2), 439–448.

Huth, M. M., & Moore, S. M. (1998). Prescriptive theory of acute pain management in infants and children. *Journal of the Society of Pediatric Nursing, 3*(1), 23–32.

Johnson, J. E., & Rice, V. H. (1974). Sensory and distress components of pain: Implications for the study of clinical pain. *Nursing Research, 23*, 203–209.

Keele, K. D. (1948, July 3). The pain chart. *Lancet, 2*, 6–8.

Kerns, R. D., Turk, D. C., & Rudy, T. E. (1985). The West Haven–Yale Multidimensional Pain Inventory (WHYMPI). *Pain, 23*(4), 345.

Kshettry, V. R., Carole, L. F., Henly, S. J., Sendelbach, S., & Kummer, B. (2006). Complementary alternative medical therapies for heart surgery patients: Feasibility, safety, and impact. *Annuals of Thoracic Surgery, 81*(1), 201–205.

Kwekkeboom, K. L., & Gretarsdottir, E. (2006). Systematic review of relaxation interventions for pain. *Journal of Nursing Scholarship, 38*(3), 269–277.

Lenz, E. R., Pugh, L. C., Milligan, R. A., Gift, A., & Suppe, F. (1997). The middle-range theory of unpleasant symptoms: An update. *Advances in Nursing Science, 19*(3), 14–27.

Lewandowski, W. A. (2004). Patterning of pain and power with guided imagery. *Nursing Science Quarterly, 17*(3), 233–241.

Locsin, R. (1988). Effects of preferred music and guided imagery music on the pain of selected postoperative patients. *ANPHI Papers, 23*(1), 2–4.

Mahon, S. M. (1994). Concept analysis of pain: Implications related to nursing diagnoses. *Nursing Diagnosis, 5*(1), 14–25.

McCaffrey, R., & Freeman, E. (2003). Effect of music on chronic osteoarthritis pain in older people. *Journal of Advanced Nursing, 44*(5), 517–524.

McCormak, H. M., del Horne, D. J., & Sheather, S. (1988). Clinical applications of visual analogue scales: A critical review. *Psychological Medicine, 18,* 1007–1009.

McDowell, J. H., McFarland, E. G., & Nalli, B. J. (1994). Use of cryotherapy for orthopaedic patients. *Orthopedic Nursing, 13*(5), 21–30.

McDowell, I., & Newell, C. (1996). *Measuring health: A guide to rating scales and questionnaires* (2nd ed.). New York: Oxford University Press.

Melzack, R. (1975). The McGill Pain Questionnaire: Major properties and scoring methods. *Pain, 1,* 277–299.

Melzack, R. (1982). Recent concepts of pain. *Journal of Medicine, 13,* 147–160.

Melzack, R. (1996). Gate control theory. *Pain Forum, 5*(2), 128–138.

Melzack, R., & Wall, P. D. (1962). On the nature of cutaneous sensory mechanisms. *Brain, 85,* 331.

Melzack, R., & Wall, P. D. (1965). Pain mechanisms: A new theory. *Science, 150*(3699), 971–979.

Merkel, S. I., Voepel-Lewis, T., Shayevitz, J. R., & Malviya, S. (1997). The FLACC: A behavioral scale for scoring postoperative pain in young children. *Pediatric Nursing, 23*(3), 293–297.

Morse, J. M., Bottorff, J. L., & Hutchinson, S. (1995). The paradox of comfort. *Nursing Research, 44*(1), 14–19.

National Institutes of Health (NIH) Technology Assessment Panel. (1996). Integration of behavioral and relaxation approaches into the treatment of chronic pain and insomnia. *JAMA, 276*(4), 313–318.

Olness, K. (1981). Self-hypnosis as adjunct therapy in childhood cancer: Clinical experience with 25 patients. *American Journal of Pediatric Hematology Oncology, 3,* 313–321.

Page, G. G. (1996). The medical necessity of adequate pain management. *Pain Forum, 5*(4), 227–233.

Phumdoung, S., & Good, M. (2003). Music reduces sensation and distress of labor pain. *Pain Management Nursing, 4*(2), 54–61.

Piotrowski, M. M., Paterson, C., Mitchinson, A., Kim, H. M., Kirsh, M., & Hinshaw, D. B. (2003). Massage as adjuvant therapy in the management of acute postoperative pain: A preliminary study in men. *Journal of the American College of Surgeons, 197*(6), 1037–1046.

Price, D. D., McGrath, P. A., Rafii, A. & Buckinham, B. (1983). The validation of visual analogue scales as ration scale measures for chronic and experimental pain. *Pain, 17*(1), 45–56.

The Research Translation & Dissemination Core, the Gerontological Nursing Interventions Research Center at the University of Iowa. (2006). *Acute pain management in the elderly.* Retrieved October 23, 2007 from http://www.nursing.uiowa.edu/products_services/evidence_ased.htm.

Richards, J. S., Nepomuceno, C., Riles, M., & Suer, Z. (1982). Assessing pain behavior: The UAB pain behavior scale. *Pain, 14*(4), 393.

Roykulcharoen, V., & Good, M. (2004). Systematic relaxation relieves postoperative pain in Thailand. *Journal of Advanced Nursing, 48*(2), 1–9.

Scheffler, N. M., Sheitel, P. L., & Lipton, M. N. (1992). Use of Cryo/Cuff for the control of postoperative pain and edema. *Journal of Foot Surgery, 31*(2), 141–148.

Sears, K., & Carroll, D. (1998). Relaxation techniques for acute pain management: A systematic review. *Journal of Advanced Nursing, 27,* 466–475.

Shuldham, C. (1999). A review of the impact of pre-operative education on recovery from surgery. *International Journal of Nursing Studies, 36*(2), 171–177.

Siedlecki, S., & Good, M. (2006). Effect of music on power, pain, depression and disability. *Journal of Advanced Nursing, 54*(5), 553–562.

Simon, J. M., Baumann, M. A., & Nolan, L. (1995). Differential diagnostic validation: Acute and chronic pain. *Nursing Diagnosis, 6*(2), 73–79.

Snyder, M., Pestka, E., & Bly, C. (2002). Progressive muscle relaxation. In M. Snyder & R. Lindquist (Eds.), *Complementary/alternative therapies in nursing* (4th ed., pp. 310–319). New York: Springer.

Taylor, A. G., Galper, D. I., Taylor, P., Rice, L. W., Andersen, W., Irvin, W., et al. (2003). Effects of adjunctive Swedish massage and vibration therapy on short-term postoperative outcomes: a randomized, controlled trial. *Journal of Alternative and Complementary Medicine, 9*(1), 77–89.

Tusek, D. L., Church, J. M., Strong, S. A., Grass, J. A., & Fazio, V. W. (1997). Guided imagery: A significant advance in the care of patients undergoing elective colorectal surgery. *Diseases of the Colon and Rectum, 40*(2), 172–178.

Wang, H. L. & Keck, J. F. (2004). Foot and hand massage as an intervention for postoperative pain. *Pain Management Nursing, 5*(2), 59–65.

Webb, J. M., Williams, D., Ivory, J. P., Day, S., & Williamson, D. M. (1998). The use of cold compression dressings after total knee replacement: a randomized controlled trial. *Orthopedics, 21*(1), 59–61.

Whitelaw, G. P., DeMuth, K. A., Demos, H. A., Schepsis, A., & Jacques, E. (1995). The use of the Cryo/Cuff versus ice and elastic wrap in the postoperative care of knee arthroscopy patients. *American Journal of Knee Surgery, 8*(1), 28–30; discussion 30–31.

Wong, D. L., & Baker, C. M. (1988). Pain in children: Comparison of assessment scales. *Pediatric Nursing, 14*(1), 9–17.

This chapter was supported in part by the National Institute of Nursing Research, NIH, Grant Number R01 NR3933 (1994–2005), to M. Good, PhD, Principal Investigator, and by the General Clinical Research Center, Case Western Reserve University.

Unpleasant Symptoms

■ AUDREY GIFT

DEFINITION OF KEY TERMS

Performance
Performance is the outcome or effect of the symptom experience. It includes functional and cognitive activities. Functional performance includes activities of daily living (ADLs), social interaction, and role performance. Quality of life is a part of performance.

Physiological factors
Physiological factors are the normal or abnormal functioning of bodily systems. They may include indicators of disease severity, comorbidities, nutritional balance, or hydration.

Psychological factors
Psychological factors include the mental state or mood, affective reaction to illness, and the degree of uncertainty and knowledge about the symptoms and their possible meaning.

Situational factors
Situational factors include aspects of the social and physical environment that surround the person and may influence the experience and reporting of symptoms. They also include environmental factors, such as heat, humidity, noise, light, and air quality. They may include socioeconomical factors, marital status, social support, and lifestyle behaviors, such as exercise and diet.

Unpleasant symptoms
Symptoms are the perceived indicators of change in normal functioning as experienced by patients. They are the subjective indicators of threats to health.

INTRODUCTION

The Theory of Unpleasant Symptoms (TOUS) is a middle range nursing theory that was developed and intended for application and use by nurses. The original concept paper appeared in 1995 and was revised in 1997. The theory uniquely allows for the presence of multiple symptoms that interact and/or are multiplicative. It implies that management of one symptom will contribute to the management of other symptoms.

HISTORICAL BACKGROUND

The TOUS originated when Drs. Linda Pugh and Audrey Gift were writing a chapter for the Nursing Clinics of North America. The chapter was to be titled "Dyspnea and Fatigue," Gift writing the dyspnea section and Pugh the fatigue section. They began meeting to develop a common outline for the two sections of the chapter but soon realized that they were similar in their thinking about the two symptoms. Each had hypothesized antecedent or influencing factors that would impact their symptom as occurring in the context of environmental or situational factors that would influence the reporting of the symptom. Additionally, each had hypothesized the symptom as influencing performance. Also, they were both familiar enough with the pain literature to know that similar models had been proposed for pain.

In addition to noting similar models for the symptoms, they realized that similar interventions, such as the use of progressive muscle relaxation, had been proposed and tested for both the symptoms of dyspnea and fatigue. These management techniques were similar to those proposed for the management of pain. They imagined that if a nurse had one model that helped her or him to understand all symptoms and how to manage them, it would advance nursing practice. They decided to call that model the Theory of Unpleasant Symptoms.

After completing the "Dyspnea and Fatigue" chapter, Drs. Gift and Pugh began to work on developing the TOUS. However, they were not able to successfully describe their model in a manner acceptable for publication. After having the manuscript rejected by two journals, they decided they needed collaborators more experienced at writing about theory. They contacted Dr. Elizabeth Lenz, who was an expert on theory development and had done research related to pain in the cardiac patient, and asked her to collaborate on the development of the TOUS. Because the focus of the manuscript was changed to further develop the model, requiring extensive revision of the manuscript, it was agreed that Dr. Lenz would be first author. Since Dr. Pugh had developed many of her ideas about fatigue in her collaboration with Dr. Milligan, she was invited to collaborate on the development of the TOUS. Dr. Lenz took the lead to call the collaborators together to further develop the model. She also contacted Dr. Suppe, a philosopher with much experience related to nursing science. The authors began meeting regularly to develop the model, assign writing tasks, and discuss each other's work. The collaboration became a source of idea development for the authors, and the meetings continued after the manuscript was accepted for publication (Lenz, Suppe, Gift, Pugh, & Milligan, 1995).

It was in the later meetings that work began on the revision of the model. The desire was to make the model less linear and reflect the dynamic clinical situation the authors had observed. The collaborators reviewed the symptom literature once again and began to redesign the model. The work accelerated when there was a call for theory revision manuscripts, and the collaborators decided to publish their update. The second article was published 2 years after the first article (Lenz, Pugh, Milligan, Gift, & Suppe, 1997). Thus, the TOUS originated from clinical observations, a review of the symptom research literature, and a sharing among investigators. Refining the theory and communicating those ideas to the nursing community required the collaboration of those with an in-depth understanding of a clinical population who regularly experienced symptoms, those who knew the research literature related to at least one symptom, and those with expertise in theory development and skill in writing theoretical articles.

SYMPTOM MODELS

While some use symptoms simply as a means to identify and characterize the underlying disease, most symptom models established in the nursing literature conceptualize theories more holistically and include physiological, psychological, cognitive, and/or social aspects. Symptoms rarely present alone in patients but rather occur together; however, not all models include this co-occurrence of symptoms. Most symptom theories within the nursing literature focus on the symptom experience, but some focus more on symptom management.

Nociceptive Model of Dyspnea

An example of a symptom theory that is focused on the symptom experience is the nociceptive model of dyspnea (Steele & Shaver, 1992). This theory is characterized as an ecological model of dyspnea because it provides a psychosocial framework for guiding nursing science, allowing for the interactive effects of multiple individual and environmental influences. It includes multiple feedback loops, with internal and external variables, and biobehavioral outcomes that reflect multiple dependencies. Environmental factors that affect symptoms include living conditions, economic status, air quality, work and family demands, and perceived social support. Individual factors include disease severity, duration of disease, trajectory of disease process, vulnerability, and resilience, as well as the nature of the symptom experience. Biobehavioral outcomes include individual adaptations, life management strategies, and tolerance for the symptom.

Symptom Interpretation Model

Another model of the symptom experience is the Symptom Interpretation Model (SIM), which focuses on cognition from an intrapersonal perspective (Teel, Meek, McNamara, & Watson, 1997). It includes conceptual identification, use of knowledge structures, and reasoning. An individual's knowledge of a symptom and the meaning attached are critical to understanding outcomes relative to the symptom. Three major constructs of the model are input, interpretation, and outcome. Input includes the recognition of a disturbance in the human system. It must be of sufficient magnitude and impact to stimulate an awareness of something being different. The repetition of the stimulus affects the threshold at which the stimulus is brought to awareness to initiate interpretation and cognitive appraisal. Awareness is shaped by personal history, current context, and individual factors.

Interpretation, the second construct in the SIM model, is the naming of the sensation and attaching meaning to the symptom by activating stored information and reasoning about the symptom. Three elements of appraisal are critical to symptom recognition and discrimination. They consist of conceptual identification, knowledge structures, and reasoning. Conceptual identification is a judgment about the similarity between a disturbance and established knowledge structures. Knowledge structures include definitions, exemplars, prototypes, and mental models that are needed for symptom interpretation. Reasoning is the third component of interpretation. It involves a comparative process in which similarity is determined between an input and knowledge structure. Comparisons are made to worst symptom experiences (exemplars) and typical symptom patterns (prototype), leading to the interpretation of symptoms.

Outcome, the third major construct in the SIM model, involves having the individual make decisions about the sensation and doing something or nothing about it. Consequences of these outcome actions and behaviors are fed back into the interpretation of the symptom, modifying knowledge and affecting future symptom interpretations. Over time, the individual recognizes patterns that inform future responses. The outcome component of the SIM is whether or not an individual is going to take action and what action is taken. The meaning attached to the sensation influences the outcome. The SIM explains the process the patient goes through in interpreting symptoms and deciding management strategies. It also points to potential patient education topics, such as focusing on the meaning of symptoms in specific situations.

Model of Chronic Dyspnea

The first known model to examine changes in perception and behavior that occur when a symptom is experienced continuously over time is the Model of Chronic Dyspnea (McCarley, 1999). In this model, dyspnea is seen from a longitudinal perspective as waxing and waning over time, occasionally increasing greatly, only to eventually return to baseline, but with the baseline (usual dyspnea) slowly increasing over time. The model has three components: physiological antecedents, dyspnea, and the consequences of dyspnea. The physiological antecedents are conceptualized as being of lesser importance in chronic dyspnea than in acute dyspnea. The main focus of this model is the ever-present dyspnea, which is depicted as having a gradually increasing baseline interspersed with episodes of acute dyspnea. Acute episodes are precipitated by physical, environmental, or psychoemotional factors. The consequences of chronic dyspnea include reduced activities, fatigue, depression, and social isolation. Reduced activity results in physical deconditioning, leading to dyspnea at a lower level of activity. There is also the constant threat of a bout of acute dyspnea. This threat contributes further to the decrease in physical activities and the downward spiral of physical deconditioning.

Symptom Management Model

The most comprehensive symptom model that focuses on symptom management is the Symptom Management Model (SMM) proposed by the faculty at the University of California at San Francisco, School of Nursing, Symptom Management Faculty Group (1994). This model views the patient's symptom experience, the symptom management strategies, and the symptom outcomes as interrelated. The patient's symptom experience is seen as an interaction of symptom perception, symptom evaluation, and the response to symptoms. Symptoms are managed by the patient, family, health care provider, and/or the health care system. The outcomes of symptom management include functional status, emotional status, self-care ability, financial status, quality of life, mortality, morbidity and comorbidity, and health service use. The advantage of this model is that it identifies ways in which the health care provider can intervene to assist the patient in the management of symptoms. It suggests a multidimensional approach to symptom management.

The Theory of Unpleasant Symptoms

Most models of symptoms focus on one symptom and specifically on the intensity of the symptom, not the quality, distress, or duration. The TOUS was the first to portray multiple symptoms occurring together and relating to each other in a multiplicative manner. Symptoms occurring together are depicted as catalyzing each other. Thus, this theory uniquely allows for the presence of multiple symptoms and implies that management of one symptom will contribute to the management of other symptoms. Current literature refers to these co-occurring symptoms as symptom clusters (Dodd et al., 2001).

DESCRIPTION OF THE THEORY OF UNPLEASANT SYMPTOMS

The TOUS focuses on the symptom experience, with multiple symptoms occurring together, rather than one symptom in isolation. The symptoms are seen as multiplicative, rather than additive. Symptoms have antecedent factors such as physiological factors, psychological factors, and environmental factors. These antecedents are interactive and reciprocal (Figure 4.1).

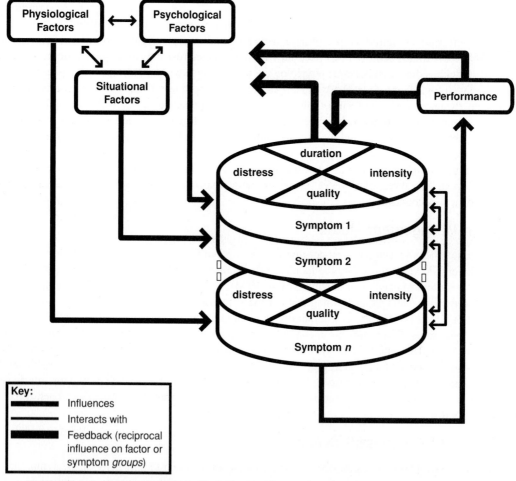

■ **Figure 4.1**   Theory of unpleasant symptoms. From Lenz, E. R., Pugh, L. C., Milligan, R. A., Gift, A., & Suppe, F. (1997). The middle-range Theory of Unpleasant Symptoms: An update. *Advances in Nursing Science, 19*(3), 14–27. Copyright 1997 by Lippincott Williams & Wilkins.

4.1 USING MIDDLE RANGE THEORIES

The TOUS was used to examine the relationship between the symptoms of dyspnea, fatigue, and sleep difficulty and the everyday functional performance of patients with COPD. Antecedents that were measured included age, sex, race, oxygen use, and medications. The researcher explored the influence of dyspnea, fatigue, and sleep difficulty on functional status and found that dyspnea was most important in explaining functional status, with the other symptoms adding very little additional information. The antecedents of age and oxygen use along with the symptom of dyspnea predicted 44% of the variance in functional performance in patients with COPD.

Reishtein, J. (2005). Relationship between symptoms and functional performance in COPD. *Research in Nursing & Health, 28*(1) 39–47.

Symptoms can be considered alone or in combination. Symptoms have the dimensions of intensity (severity), timing (frequency, duration, and relationship to events), distress (the person's reaction to the sensation), and quality (descriptors used to characterize the symptom, location of the symptom, or response to intervention). The quality dimension may be especially difficult, depending on the culture and language of the patient and the number of symptoms experienced at the same time.

The antecedent factors are categorized as physiological, psychological, or situational. Physiological antecedents are commonly what characterize the severity of the disease, such as comorbidities, abnormal blood studies, or other pathological findings. Stages of disease may also be a physiological antecedent factor. Psychological factors affecting the symptom experience may include the person's mood, level of depression, affective reaction to disease, degree of uncertainty regarding the symptoms, and meaning ascribed to the symptoms. Situational factors refer to the social and physical environment that may affect patients' symptom experience and their reporting of that experience, including social support, marital status, and resources.

In the TOUS, symptoms affect performance. Performance includes functional (physical activity, ADLs, and social and role performance) and cognitive performance (ability to concentrate, problem solve, and/or think). Cognitive functioning is also seen as a consequence of symptoms. Those who experience more symptoms are likely to have impaired cognitive functioning.

In the updated version of the theory (Lenz et al., 1997), symptoms are seen as occurring together and interacting with each other, as are antecedent factors. See Figure 4.1 for a model of the TOUS. An interaction and reciprocal relationship between the antecedent factors and symptoms is also hypothesized. While symptoms are seen as influencing performance, performance is, likewise, seen as affecting symptoms. See Using Middle Range Theories 4.1 and 4.2 for examples of the theory's use.

MODELS THAT EXPAND OR MODIFY THE THEORY OF UNPLEASANT SYMPTOMS

Armstrong Model of Symptom Experience

Armstrong (2003) proposed a symptom model that builds on the TOUS but focuses more on the meaning or perception of the symptom as well as the expression. Multiple co-occurring symptoms can interact and

4.2 USING MIDDLE RANGE THEORIES

A study was undertaken, using the TOUS as the conceptual model, to examine a cluster of symptoms consisting of fatigue, weakness, weight loss, appetite loss, nausea, vomiting, and altered taste that were present at the time of diagnosis as well as 3 and 6 months later in a sample of patients with lung cancer. The physiological factor of stage of cancer was the most predictive of the number of cluster symptoms reported. The mean symptom severity and number of symptoms at diagnosis were correlated with later ratings but decreased in severity over time. Symptom severity, age, and stage of cancer were predictive of those who died within the 19 months after diagnosis. Thus, aspects of the TOUS were supported and indicate the importance of symptoms as a predictor of patient prognosis.

Gift, A. G., Stommel, M., Jablonski, A., & Given, W. (2003). A cluster of symptoms over time in patients with lung cancer. *Nursing Research, 52*(6), 393–400.

affect the patient's perception of the symptom as a new event and his perception of his ability to deal with the situation. Armstrong also extends the TOUS to include the meaning of the symptom(s) to the patient, or rather the existential meaning, the patient's sense of vulnerability and mortality. Existential meaning can also be positive, such as the sense that a treatment is working or that the patient's illness has brought the family together. The antecedents have been reorganized as demographic, disease, and individual characteristics. Symptoms are characterized as having the frequency, intensity, and distress dimensions from the TOUS, but also a symptom meaning dimension. This model also expands the consequences of the symptom experience beyond physical, social, and role performance or cognitive functioning to include emotional consequences. This model is appropriate to use when symptom meaning is the focus of investigation and/or when examining the emotional consequences of the symptom experience (Armstrong, 2003).

Symptom Experience in Time Model

This model combines the TOUS with the SMM and a time model to examine the symptom flow and develop the Symptom Experience in Time (SET) Model (Henley, Kallas, Klatt, & Swenson, 2003). In this model symptoms are seen as being initiated by a precipitating event that leads to the onset of symptoms. The influencing factors of the TOUS are broadened to include nursing metaparadigm concepts such as person, health, and environment that mediate or moderate the symptom. The symptom experience has an onset, an experience, a cognitive evaluation, and an emotional response. The symptom dimensions of timing, intensity, distress, and quality are retained from the TOUS. The cognitive evaluation determines if the symptoms are serious, unpleasant, and/or inexplicable. They are also evaluated as either enduring or treatable. If treatable, symptom management can take the form of self-care or help seeking. The outcomes of these strategies can be changes in the symptom itself as well as changes in person, health, and/or environment.

Time, a factor determining the patterning of a symptom experience, may serve as input to the symptom experience, or as output from the symptom management process, and may be a component of an intervention. Time is discussed as having a pattern that differs for perceived time, biological/social and clock/calendar time. Transcendence is the qualitative repositioning in time and is beyond time. The value of this model is the study of changes in symptoms over time (Henley et al., 2003).

Assessment of Symptoms

The distress associated with a symptom relates to both the symptom itself and the individual's interpretation. This may result in over- or underreporting of a symptom. Appropriate symptom assessment depends on the symptom involved, the underlying disease or other cause of the symptom, the stage of the illness, and the patient's prognosis. The medical history is an important part of the assessment, including physical and emotional conditions or symptoms, medications, and previous and current family/living situation, including caregiver needs. Symptoms should be characterized by assessing their rate of onset (sudden or gradual), the factors precipitating or alleviating them, the frequency, the intensity, the duration, the quality, and the distress felt by the patient as a result of the symptom (Meek et al., 1999).

A careful physical examination focusing on possible underlying causes of the symptoms should be performed. Signs supporting progression of the underlying condition should be sought. Is the patient anxious or agitated? Is he or she anemic or cyanotic? Particular attention needs to be paid to signs associated with clinical syndromes. Physical exams, laboratory tests, and interventional procedures need to be undertaken, noting the stage of the illness and treatment being prescribed.

Diagnostic tests helpful in determining the etiology of the symptom are advised. Since many symptoms are contextual and related to movement or exercise, it is important to assess these parameters as well.

INSTRUMENTS USED IN EMPIRICAL TESTING

Symptom measures can either focus on one symptom or include multiple symptoms that are commonly seen in a specific disease entity. Some symptom measures focus only on physical symptoms, while others include both physical and emotional symptoms. Symptom measures may focus only on presence or absence, intensity or frequency, rather than all the dimensions described in the TOUS.

Single Symptom Assessment

Several individual symptoms have been studied over time by a variety of nurses and other health care providers. As a result of this interest, investigators have developed tools for assessing and measuring these particular individual symptoms. Some of these single-symptom assessment scales will be discussed next.

VISUAL ANALOGUE SCALE

Single-symptom measures can be focused only on the intensity of the symptom or on multiple symptom dimensions. A valid symptom measure that focuses on intensity is a visual analogue scale (VAS). This scale was first introduced for the measurement of feelings (Aitken, 1969). It has been validated as a measure of pain, dyspnea, fatigue, and other symptoms. It consists of a 100-mm line (placed either horizontally or vertically) with anchors indicating the low and high end of the scale. The patient is asked to mark the intensity of the symptom on the continuum. Scoring the measure involves measuring the distance (in millimeters) from the lowest end of the line to the patient's mark.

The VAS validated as a measure of dyspnea (VADS) consists of a 100-mm vertical VAS with anchors of "shortness of breath as bad as can be" at the top and "no shortness of breath" at the bottom. Concurrent validity of this scale has been established with chronic obstructive pulmonary disease (COPD) patients, using both a horizontal VAS and a measure of airway obstruction (Gift,

On a scale from 0 to 10, indicate how much shortness of breath you have had in the past week, where 0 = no shortness of breath and 10 = shortness of breath as the worst possible. Circle the number.

0   1   2   3   4   5   6   7   8   9   10

No shortness of breath   Worst possible

■ **Figure 4.2**   Numeric rating scale. From Gift, A. G., & Narsavage, G. (1998). Validation of the numeric rating scale as a measure of dyspnea. *American Journal of Critical Care, 7*(3), 200–204. Copyright 1998 by the American Association of Critical Care Nurses. Used with permission.

Plaut, & Jacox, 1986). Construct validity was established, using the contrasted-groups approach between those expected to have dyspnea and those not expected to have dyspnea. Differences between the two groups were significant for both COPD and asthmatic patients (Gift, 1989). Drawbacks of the VADS are (a) the scale is limited in discerning the different dimensions of dyspnea (Mancini & Body, 1999) and (b) the comparison of ratings between individuals may be problematic because the anchors may be discerned as qualitatively different for each individual (Mahler & Jones, 1997) (Figure 4.2).

NUMERIC RATING SCALE

The Numeric Rating Scale (NRS) has patients rate the intensity of their pain or shortness of breath by choosing a number on a scale from 0, the lowest intensity of the symptom, to 10, the highest intensity of the symptom. The NRS can be administered either in the written or verbal form and is extremely easy to administer and score. This scale has been used clinically as a measure of pain or dyspnea and is a valid measure of these symptoms (Gift & Narsavage, 1998). Cleeland et al. (2000) described an Interactive Voice Response system that uses telephone voiced questions with the patient responding using the phone keypad to indicate his or her symptom severity from a numeric rating scale (Figure 4.3).

McGILL PAIN QUESTIONNAIRE

The McGill Pain Questionnaire (MPQ) was developed by Melzack (1975) at McGill University, with a focus on pain description. The MPQ permits measurement of the sensory, affective, and evaluative dimensions of pain and provides information on the relative intensity of each, as well as several measures of the patient's evaluation of the overall intensity of the pain (Melzack, 1983). The words used to describe pain are classified in three quality categories: (a) sensory (including temporal, spatial, pressure, thermal, and other properties); (b) affective (including tension, fear, and autonomic properties of the pain experience); and (c) evaluative (words describing overall intensity).

These are followed by four miscellaneous items. In addition, patients are asked to rate their present pain intensity (PPI) based on a 0-to-5 scale. Repeated administrations of the questionnaire to cancer patients have established the reliability of the MPQ. The consistency index (average of the individuals' repeated scores) was high, ranging from 66% to 80%. Factor analytical techniques have been used to demonstrate that the affective and evaluative categories are distinctly different from each other.

How much shortness of breath have you had in the last week?
Please indicate by marking the height on the column.

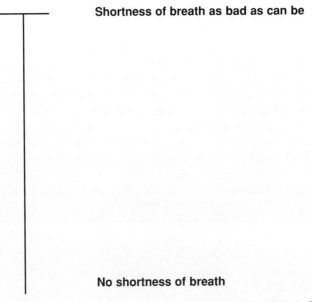

Shortness of breath as bad as can be

No shortness of breath

■ **Figure 4.3** Visual Analogue Dyspnea Scale. From Gift, A. G. (l989). Validation of a vertical visual analogue scale as a measure of clinical dyspnea. *Rehabilitation Nursing, I4*(6), 323–325. Copyright 1989 by the Association of Rehabilitation Nurses.

THE BRIEF FATIGUE INVENTORY

The Brief Fatigue Inventory (BFI) measures the frequency and severity from cancer-related fatigue (CRF) and the amount that fatigue interferes with aspects of the patient's life (Mendoza et al., 1999). Appropriate psychometric properties were found using data on adult patients ($n = 305$) consisting of inpatients and outpatients with varying types of cancer (including persons with lung cancer) and control subjects ($n = 290$) (Mendoza et al., 1999). Through factor reduction, the BFI achieved a high internal consistency level of 0.96. Concurrent validity was established with two previously validated measures, the profile of mood state (POMS)-Fatigue ($r = 0.84$, $P < .001$) and the Fatigue subscale of the functional assessment of cancer therapy (FACT) ($r = -0.88$, $P < .001$). Furthermore, the BFI is sensitive in detecting severe from nonsevere chronic renal failure (CRF) at a cut score of 7 with a range of 7 to 10. Stability of the BFI to detect severity of CRF has been demonstrated (Hwang, Chang, Cogswell, & Kasimis, 2002).

Multiple Symptom Assessment

In addition to single-symptom inventories, several tools have been developed to assess multiple symptoms with just one assessment (see Using Middle Range Theories 4.3 for an example of assessment of clients with multiple symptoms). Two of these multiple-symptom inventory tools will be discussed next.

4.3   USING MIDDLE RANGE THEORIES

The number of Korean women diagnosed with breast cancer has increased rapidly, making it currently the most common type of cancer in Korean women. Treatment for this disease produces multiple symptoms that interfere with the patient's activities and social functioning. Researchers examined the relationships between the situational factor of social support, the psychological factor of mood disturbance, and symptoms. They found that while mood disturbance was positively correlated with symptom experience, this relationship was moderated by social support. Women with a higher level of mood disturbance were at greater risk for experiencing symptoms when the level of social support was low. Thus, the nurse is advised to be especially attentive to evaluate the patient's social support along with mood disturbance when planning interventions to reduce symptoms, especially in Korean women with breast cancer.

Lee, E. H., Chung, B. Y., Park, H. B., & Chun, K. H. (2004). Relationships of mood disturbance and social support to symptom experience in Korean women with breast cancer. *Journal of Pain and Symptom Management, 27*(5), 425–433.

MEMORIAL SYMPTOM ASSESSMENT SCALE

The Memorial Symptom Assessment Scale is one of the most comprehensive symptom scales and one that includes three of the four symptom dimensions included in the TOUS. It includes 24 symptoms, both physical and psychological, and asks the subject to indicate the presence or absence of each of the symptoms. In addition, for all symptoms indicated as occurring, the subject is asked the frequency, intensity, and distress the symptom causes her. Additionally, eight longer-lasting symptoms that commonly occur in the cancer patient are listed, and the subject is requested to indicate how severe the symptom was and how much she was distressed by the symptom. This scale was developed and tested on 246 patients with a variety of cancers. A factor analysis found three factors that were labeled as psychological, high-prevalence physical, and low-prevalence physical. High correlations with the clinical status and quality-of-life measures further supported the validity of the scale. Reliability was established using Cronbach's alpha (Portenoy et al., 1994).

The scale has recently been demonstrated to be of value in assessing symptoms in other patient populations such as patients with congestive heart failure (Zambroski, Moser, Bhat, & Ziegler, 2005). Others have developed a shortened version with only 19 symptoms for the comprehensive assessment of symptoms in patients with COPD (Jablonski, Gift, & Cook, 2006).

SYMPTOM DISTRESS SCALE

The Symptom Distress Scale (SDS) is another example of a measure that includes multiple symptoms. In this scale, patients are asked to rate each symptom on a five-point response format, ranging from 1 (normal or no distress) to 5 (extensive distress). Evidence for validity and alpha reliability (0.82 for the total scale) has been reported (McCorkle & Young, 1978). This is one of the most frequently used measures, often with advanced disease and palliative care.

4.1 RESEARCH APPLICATION

A nurse researcher is interested in reducing pain postoperatively in hip-replacement patients. The researcher decides to use the TOUS to structure the preoperative teaching class. The class has components related to all aspects of the model, such as physiological factors that can be controlled to reduce pain postoperatively, psychological factors, and social or environmental factors that will help patients manage their pain postoperatively. Patients are taught to characterize their pain according to the intensity, frequency, distress, and quality of the sensation, and to record the sensation, so they can note the changes that occur after medication and over time as they recover. They are taught to note other symptoms that may accompany the pain. In addition, patients are told what to expect related to their performance after surgery, and how to gradually increase what they do as the pain is relieved. The effectiveness of this preoperative teaching is assessed by having patients rate their pain using a visual analogue pain scale during the postoperative period and comparing it to pain ratings in those not exposed to the teaching.

Activity Symptom Assessment

This category of measures refers to instruments requiring some activity or report of activity to indicate the intensity of the symptom. These scales focus on the result or impact of symptoms, rather than the symptom itself. Such measures are often referred to as functional scales because they require the patient's report of activities. The symptom of dyspnea has been measured with such a scale. The scales' emphasis on physical activity makes them inappropriate for use in those who are in critical care or at the end stage of disease. They are often used in a rehabilitation setting where the goal is to increase activity. Thus, they measure the consequences of a symptom rather than the symptom itself.

Selection of Instruments

The use of a particular symptom measurement instrument in a research study is dependent upon the needs of the researcher for assessment to adequately answer the research question study. Research Application 4.1 provides an example of how the TOUS may be used, and how symptoms can be assessed using a single-symptom assessment measure.

SUMMARY

Having symptoms as the focus of nursing care, rather than simply being an indication of the underlying "cause" of another problem, is new to the nursing literature. The use of middle range theories to guide the management of symptoms is even newer. They serve the useful purpose of guiding the practitioner to focus on more than the sensation and its intensity but, rather, to have a more comprehensive approach, including the context in which the symptom occurs. The situational aspects that contribute

ANALYSIS OF THEORY

Using the criteria presented in Chapter 2, critique the TOUS. Compare your conclusions about the theory with those found in Appendix A. An experienced nurse has completed the analysis found in Appendix A.

Internal Criticism
1. Clarity
2. Consistency
3. Adequacy

4. Logical development
5. Level of theory development

External Criticism
1. Reality convergence
2. Utility
3. Significance
4. Discrimination
5. Scope of theory
6. Complexity

to the symptom experience need further study. We know that there are environmental, social, and cultural factors that play a part in the interpretation of symptoms, but more detail is needed to guide the clinician in planning nursing care. Although the symptom models advocate the assessment of multiple symptoms rather than only one, such as pain, few clinical settings implement that assessment in their routine patient care.

The effects of symptoms on patient performance are just beginning to be identified. Symptoms affect all aspects of performance, not just the physical aspects. Because proper management of symptoms can be expected to affect patients physically, psychologically, and socially, it is important for nurses to develop their science in this area.

CRITICAL THINKING EXERCISES

1. Using the Theory of Unpleasant Symptoms as your guide, what would you look for in an assessment tool for patient symptoms?
   a. Do you monitor all symptom dimensions, such as how distressing the symptom is, or do you only ask about symptom severity/intensity?
   b. Do you monitor only one symptom or multiple symptoms?
2. In your patient assessment, how might you include the antecedents to symptoms?
3. How would you use the Theory of Unpleasant Symptoms to plan a comprehensive intervention to alleviate symptoms?

   a. What interventions might you plan that would target the antecedents?
   b. What might you do to intervene regarding symptom distress?
4. What outcome might you use to assess the effectiveness of your interventions?
   a. Would you use an outcome measure that focuses on the physical, role, and/or cognitive performance outcome of symptoms? If so, what measure(s) would that be, specifically?
   b. If you were to have symptom alleviation as your outcome measure, which specific measurement tool would you use?

WEB RESOURCES

1. American Academy of Pain Management: **http://www.aapainmanage.org/**
2. American Pain Society: **http://www.ampainsoc. org/**
3. American Thoracic Society Consensus Statement on Dyspnea: **http://www.olivija.com/dyspnea/**
4. Center to Improve Care of the Dying: **http://www.gwu.edu/~cicd/toolkit/physical.htm**
5. Hospice and Palliative Nurses Association: **http://www.hpna.org/**
6. NIH Research Workshop: Symptoms in Terminal Illness: **http://www.nih.gov/ninr/wnew/ symptoms_in_terminal_illness.html**
7. Research Center for Symptom Management at the University of California at San Francisco, School of Nursing: **http://nurseweb.ucsf.edu/ www/rcsm.htm**
8. Theory of Unpleasant Symptoms journal article: *Advances in Nursing Science, 19,* 14. Retrieved March 1, 1997, from the Library of Medicine: **http://www.ncbi.nlm.nih.gov/entrez/query.fcgi ?cmd=Retrieve&db=PubMed&list_uids=9055 027&dopt=Abstract**

REFERENCES

Aitken, R. C. B. (1969). Measurement of feelings using visual analogue scales. *Proceedings of Research Social Medicine, 62,* 989–993.

Armstrong, T. S. (2003). Symptoms experience: A concept analysis. *Oncology Nursing Forum, 30*(4), 601–605.

Cleeland, C. S., Mendoza, T., Wang, X. S., Chou, C., Harle, M. T., Morrissey, M. (2000). Assessing symptom distress in cancer patients. *Cancer, 89*(7), 1634–1645.

Dodd, M., Janson, S., Facione, N., Faucett, J., Froelicher, E. S., Humphreys, J., et al. (2001). Advancing the science of symptom management. *Journal of Advanced Nursing, 33*(5), 668–676.

Dodd, M., Miaskowski, C., & Paul, S. (2001). Symptom clusters and their effect on the functional status of patients with cancer. *Oncology Nursing Forum, 28*(3), 465–470.

Gift, A. G. (1989). Validation of a vertical visual analogue scale as a measure of clinical dyspnea. *Rehabilitation Nursing, 14*(6), 323–325.

Gift, A. G., & Narsavage, G. (1998). Validity of the numeric rating scale as a measure of dyspnea. *American Journal of Critical Care, 7*(3), 200–204.

Gift, A. G., Plaut, S. M., & Jacox, A. K. (1986). Psychologic and physiologic factors related to dyspnea in subjects with chronic obstructive pulmonary disease. *Heart & Lung, 15,* 595–602.

Gift, A. G., Stommel, M., Jablonski, A., & Given, W. (2003). A cluster of symptoms over time in patients with lung cancer. *Nursing Research, 52*(6), 393–400.

Henley, S. J., Kallas, K. D., Klatt, C. M., & Swenson, K. K. (2003). The notion of time in symptom experiences. *Nursing Research, 52*(6), 410–417.

Hwang, S. S., Chang, V. T., Cogswell, J., & Kasimis, B. S. (2002). Clinical relevance of fatigue levels in cancer patients at a Veterans Administration Medical Center. *Cancer, 94*(4), 2481–2489.

Jablonski, A., Gift, A. G., & Cook, K. E. (2007). Symptom assessment of patients with chronic obstructive pulmonary disease. *Western Journal of Nursing Research, 29,* 845–863.

Lee, E. H., Chung, B. Y., Park, H. B., & Chun, K. H. (2004). Relationships of mood disturbance and social support to symptom experience in Korean women with breast cancer. *Journal of Pain and Symptom Management, 27*(5), 425–433.

Lenz, E., Pugh, L. C., Milligan, R. A., Gift, A., & Suppe, F. (1997). The middle range theory of unpleasant symptoms: An update. *Advances in Nursing Science, 19*(3), 14–27.

Lenz, E., Suppe, F., Gift, A. G., Pugh, L. C., & Milligan, R. A. (1995). Collaborative development of middle-range nursing theories: Toward a theory of unpleasant symptoms. *Advances in Nursing Science, 17*(3), 1–13.

Mahler, D. A., & Jones, P. W. (1997). Measurement of dyspnea and quality of life in advanced lung disease. *Clinical Chest Medicine, 18*(3), 457–469.

Mancini, I., & Body, J. J. (1999). Assessment of dyspnea in advanced cancer patients. *Supportive Care in Cancer, 7*(4), 229–232.

McCarley, C. (1999). A model of chronic dyspnea. *Image: Journal of Nursing Scholarship, 31*(3), 231–236.

McCorkle, R., & Young, K. (1978). Development of a symptom distress scale. *Cancer Nursing, 1,* 373–378.

Meek, P. M., Schwartzstein, R. M., Adams, M. M., Altose, M. D., Breslin, E. H., Carrieri-Kohlman, V., et al. (1999). Dyspnea: Mechanisms, assessment, and management: A consensus statement. *American Journal of Respiratory and Critical Care Medicine, 159,* 321–340.

Melzack, R. (1975). The McGill Pain Questionnaire: Major properties and scoring methods. *Pain, 1,* 277–299.

Melzack, R. (1983). The McGill Pain Questionnaire. In Melzack, R. (Ed.), *Pain measurement and assessment* (pp. 41–47). New York: Raven Press.

Mendoza, T. R., Wang, X. S., Cleeland, C. S., Morrissey, M., Johnson, B.A., Wendt, J. K., et al. (1999). The rapid assessment of fatigue severity in cancer patients: Use of the Brief Fatigue Inventory. *Cancer, 85*(5), 1186–1196.

Portenoy, R. K., Thaler, H. T., Kornblith, A. B., Lepore, J. M., Friedlander-Klar, H., Kiyasu, E. (1994). The Memorial Symptoms Assessment Scale: An instrument for the evaluation of symptom prevalence, characteristics and distress. *European Journal of Cancer, 30A*(9), 1326–1336.

Reishtein, J. (2005). Relationship between symptoms and functional performance in COPD. *Research in Nursing & Health, 28*(1) 39–47.

Steele, B., & Shaver, J. (1992). The dyspnea experience: Nociceptive properties and a model for research and practice. *Advances in Nursing Science, 15*(1), 64–76.

Teel, C. S., Meek, P., McNamara, A. M., & Watson, L. (1997). Perspectives unifying symptom interpretation. *Image: Journal of Nursing Scholarship, 29*(2), 175–181.

University of California at San Francisco, School of Nursing, Symptom Management Faculty Group. (1994). A model for symptom management. *Image: Journal of Nursing Scholarship, 26*(4), 272–276.

Zambroski, C. H., Moser, D. K., Bhat, G., & Ziegler, S. (2005). Impact of symptom prevalence and symptom burden on quality of life in patients with heart failure. *European Journal of Cardiovascular Nursing, 4*(3), 198–206.

BIBLIOGRAPHY

Aaronson, L. S., Teel, C. S., Cassmeyer, V., Neuberger, G. B., Pallikkathayil, L. Pierce, J. et al. (1999). Defining and measuring fatigue. *Image, 31*(1), 45–50.

Acheson, A., & MacCormack, D. (1997). Dyspnea and the cancer patient—an overview. *Canadian Oncology Nursing Journal, 7*(4), 209–213.

Algase, D. L., Newton, S. E., & Higgins, P. A. (2001). Nursing theory across curricula: A status report from Midwest nursing schools. *Journal of Professional Nursing, 17*(5), 248–255.

Armstrong, T. S., Cohen, M. Z., Eriksen, L., & Cleeland, C. (2005). Content validity of self-report measurement instruments: An illustration from the development of the brain tumor module of the M.D. Anderson Symptom Inventory. *Oncology Nursing Forum, 32*(3), 669–676.

Armstrong, T. S., Cohen, M. Z., Eriksen, L., & Hickey, J. V. (2004). Symptom clusters in oncology patients and implications for symptom research in people with primary brain tumors. *Journal of Nursing Scholarship, 36*(3), 197–206.

Blegen, M. A., & Tripp-Reimer, T. (1997). Implications of nursing taxonomies for middle-range theory development. *Advanced Nursing Science, 19*(3), 37–49.

Bredin, M., Corner, J., Krishnasamy, M., Plant, H., Bailey, C., & A'Hern, R. (1999). Multicentre randomized controlled trial of nursing intervention for breathlessness in patients with lung cancer. *British Medical Journal, 318,* 901–904.

Carrieri-Kohlman, V., Gormley, J. M., Douglas, M. K., Paul, S. M., & Stulbarg, M. S. (1996). Differentiation between dyspnea and its affective components. *Western Journal of Nursing Research, 18,* 626–642.

Cella, D., Passik, S., Jacobsen, P., & Breitbart, W. (1998). Progress toward guidelines for the management of fatigue. *Oncology, 12*(11A), 369–377.

Cody, W. K. (1999). Middle-range theories: Do they foster the development of nursing science? *Nursing Science Quarterly, 12*(1), 9–14.

Cooley, M. E. (2000). Symptoms in adults with lung cancer: A systematic research review. *Journal of Pain and Symptom Management, 19*(2), 137–153.

Corwin, E. J., Brownstead, J., Barton, N., Heckard, S., & Morin, K. (2005). The impact of fatigue on the development of postpartum depression. *Journal of Obstetric Gynecologic and Neonatal Nursing, 34*(5), 577–586.

Dabbs, A. D., Dew, M. A., Stilley, C. S., Manzetti, J., Zullo, T., McCurry, K. R., et al. (2003). Psychosocial vulnerability, physical symptoms and physical impairment after lung and heart-lung transplantation. *Journal of Heart and Lung Transplantation, 22*(11), 1268–1275.

Dabbs, A. D., Hoffman, L. A., Swigart, V., Happ, M. B., Iacono, A. T., & Dauber, J. H. (2004). Using conceptual triangulation to develop an integrated model of the symptom experience of acute rejection after lung transplantation. *Advances in Nursing Science, 27*(2), 138–149.

Deets, C. (1998). Nursing—A maturing discipline? *Journal of Professional Nursing, 14*(2), 65.

Drevdahl, D. (1999). Sailing beyond: Nursing theory and the person. *Advanced Nursing Science, 21*(4), 1–13.

Ducharme, F., Ricard, N., Duquette, A., Levesque, L., & Lachance, L. (1998). Empirical testing of a longitudinal model derived from the Roy adaptation model. *Nursing Science Quarterly, 11*(4), 149–159.

Dudley-Brown, S. L. (1997). The evaluation of nursing theory: A method for our madness. *International Journal of Nursing Studies, 34*(1), 76–83.

Eakin, E., Prewitt, L. M., Ries, A., & Kaplan, R. (1994). Validation of the UCSD Shortness of Breath questionnaire. *Journal of Cardiopulmonary Rehabilitation, 14,* 322–323.

Eakin, E., Sassi-Dambron, D. E., Ries, A., & Kaplan, R. (1995). Reliability and validity of dyspnea measures in patients with obstructive lung disease. *International Journal of Behavioral Medicine, 2*(2), 118–134.

Gift, A. G., Jablonski, A., Stommel, M., & Given, C. W. (2004). Symptom clusters in elderly patients with lung cancer. *Oncology Nursing Forum, 31*(2), 203–210.

Gift, A. G., Moore, T., & Soeken, K. (1992). Relaxation to reduce dyspnea and anxiety in COPD patients. *Nursing Research, 41*, 242–246.

Given, C. W., Stommel, M., Given, B., Osuch, J., Kurtz, M. E., & Kurtz, J. C. (1993). The influence of cancer patients' symptoms and functional status on patients' depression and family caregivers' reaction and depression. *Health Psychology, 12*, 277–285.

Good, M. (1998). A middle-range theory of acute pain management: Use in research. *Nursing Outlook, 46*(3), 120–124.

Hann, D., Jacobson, P., Azzarillo, M., & Martin, S. (1998). Measurement of fatigue in cancer patients: Development and validation of the fatigue symptom inventory. *Quality of Life Research, 7*, 301–311.

Higgins, P. A. (1998). Patient perception of fatigue while undergoing long-term mechanical ventilation: Incidence and associated factors. *Heart & Lung, 27*(3), 177–183.

Higgins, P. A., & Moore, S. M. (2000). Levels of theoretical thinking in nursing. *Nursing Outlook, 48*, 179–183.

Hopp, J. P., & Duffy, S. A. (2000). Racial variations in end-of-life care. *Journal of the American Geriatrics Society, 48*, 658–663.

Hupcey, J. A., Morse, J. M., Lenz, E., & Tason, M. C. (1996). Wilsonian methods of concept analysis: A critique. *Scholarly Inquiry for Nursing Practice, 10*, 185–210.

Hutchinson, S. A., & Wilson, H. S. (1998). The Theory of Unpleasant Symptoms and Alzheimer's disease. *Scholarly Inquiry for Nursing Practice: An International Journal, 12*(2), 143–158.

Kim, H. J., McGuire, D. B., Tulman, L., & Barsevick, A. M. (2005). Symptom clusters: Concept analysis and clinical implications for cancer nursing. *Cancer Nursing, 28*(4), 270–282.

Liehr, P., & Smith, M. J. (1999). Middle range theory: Spinning research and practice to create knowledge for the new millennium. *Advance Nursing Science, 21*(4), 81–91.

Mahler, D. A., Harver, A., Lentine, T., Scott, J. A., Beck, K., & Schwartzstein, R. M. (1996). Descriptors of breathlessness in cardiorespiratory diseases. *American Journal of Respiratory and Critical Care Medicine, 154*, 1357–1363.

Mahler, D. A., & Wells, C. K. (1988). Evaluation of clinical methods for rating dyspnea. *Chest, 93*(3), 580–586.

McCann, K., & Boore, J. (2000). Fatigue in persons with renal failure who require maintenance haemodialysis. *Journal of Advanced Nursing, 32*(5), 1132–1142.

Meek, P. M., Lareau, S. C., & Anderson, D. (2001). Memory for symptoms in COPD patients: How accurate are their reports? *European Respiratory Journal, 18*, 1–8.

Morse, J. M., Hupcey, J., Mitcham, C., & Lenz, E. (1996). Concept analysis in nursing research: A critical appraisal. *Scholarly Inquiry for Nursing Practice, 10*, 257–281.

Morse, J. M., Hutchinson, S. A., & Penrod, J. (1998). From theory to practice: The development of assessment guides from qualitatively derived theory. *Qualitative Health Research, 8*(3), 329–340.

Morse, J. M., Mitcham, C., Hupcey, J. E., & Tason, M. C. (1996). Criteria for concept evaluation. *Journal of Advanced Nursing, 24*, 385–390.

Nield, M. (2000). Dyspnea self-management in African Americans with chronic lung disease. *Heart & Lung, 29*, 50–55.

Parker, K. P., Kimble, L. P., Dunbar, D. B., & Clark, P. C. (2005). Symptom interactions as mechanisms underlying symptom pairs and clusters. *Journal of Nursing Scholarship, 37*(3), 209–215.

Parshall, M. B., Welsh, J. D., Brockopp, D. Y., Heiser, R. M., Schooler, M. P., & Cassidy, K. B. (2001). Dyspnea duration, distress, and intensity in emergency department visits for heart failure. *Heart & Lung, 30*(1), 47–56.

Piper, B., Dibble, S., Dodd, M., Weiss, M., Slaughter, R., & Paul, S. (1998). The Revised Piper Fatigue Scale: Psychometric evaluation in women with breast cancer. *Oncology Nursing Forum, 25*(4), 677–684.

Pugh, L. C., & Milligan, R. A. (1998). Nursing intervention to increase the duration of breastfeeding. *Applied Nursing Research, 11*(4), 190–194.

Redeker, N. S., Lev, E. L., & Ruggiero, J. (2000). Insomnia, fatigue, anxiety, depression and quality of life of cancer patients undergoing chemotherapy. *Scholarly Inquiry for Nursing Practice, 14*(4), 275–290.

Ruland, C. M., & Moore, S. M. (1998). Theory construction based on standards of care: A proposed theory of the peaceful end of life. *Nursing Outlook, 46*(4), 169–175.

Sarna, L., & Brecht, M. (1997). Dimensions of symptom distress in women with advanced lung cancer: A factor analysis. *Heart & Lung, 26*(1), 23–30.

Schneider, R. (1998). Reliability and validity of the Multidimensional Fatigue Inventory (MFI-20) and the Rhoten Fatigue Scale among rural cancer outpatients. *Cancer Nursing, 21*, 370–373.

Schwartz, A. (1998). The Schwartz Cancer Fatigue Scale: Testing reliability and validity. *Oncology Nursing Forum, 25*(4), 711–717.

Shih, F. J., & Chu, S. H. (1999). Comparisons of American-Chinese and Taiwanese patients' perceptions of dyspnea and helpful nursing actions during the intensive care unit transition from cardiac surgery. *Heart & Lung, 28*(1), 41–54.

Smith, C. E., Pace, K., Kochinda, C., Kleinbeck, S. V. M., Koehler, J., Popkess-Vawter, S. (2002). Caregiving effectiveness model evolution to a midrange theory of home care: A process for critique and replication. *Advances in Nursing Science, 25*(1), 50–64.

Smith, M. C. (1999). Caring and the science of unitary human beings. *Advanced Nursing Science, 21*(4), 14–28.

Vainio, A., Aurinen, A., & Members of the Symptom Prevalence Group. (1996). Prevalence of symptoms among patients with advanced cancer: An international collaborative study. *Journal of Pain and Symptom Management, 12*(1), 3–10.

Wolfe, J., Grier, H. E., Klar, N., Levin, S. B., Ellenbogen, J. M., Salem-Schatz, S., et al. (2000). Symptoms and suffering at the end of life in children with cancer. *The New England Journal of Medicine, 342*(5), 326–333.

Yeh, C. H. (2002). Life experience of Taiwanese adolescents with cancer. *Scandinavian Journal of Caring Sciences, 16*(3), 232–239.

Zeppetella, G. (1998). The palliation of dyspnea in terminal disease. *The American Journal of Hospice and Palliative Care, 15*(6), 322–330.

Zhou, Q., O'Brien, B., & Soeken, K. (2001). Rhodes Index of Nausea and Vomiting—Form 2 in pregnant women. *Nursing Research, 50*(4), 251–257.

The AACN Synergy Model

■ SONYA R. HARDIN

DEFINITION OF KEY TERMS

Health care system	The health care system acts as a facilitator or conduit to support patient needs and the power to nurture the professional practice environment of the nurse.
Nurse competencies	The eight competencies of nursing practice as defined by the model are clinical judgment, caring practices, advocacy/moral agency, response to diversity, clinical inquiry, facilitator of learning, collaboration, and systems thinking.
Patient characteristics	Eight patient characteristics have been identified that span a continuum of health to illness: vulnerability, resiliency, stability, complexity, predictability, resource availability, participation in care, and participation in decision making
Optimal patient outcomes	Patient outcomes include patient satisfaction with care, levels of trust, patient behavior and knowledge, patient functional change, and quality of life.

INTRODUCTION

The American Association of Critical Care Nurses (AACN) has established a vision to create a health care system that is driven by the needs of patients and families where nurses can make optimal contributions in the delivery of care. This vision involved the development of a model that explicates the practice that nurses contribute at the bedside. The model developed was the AACN Synergy Model. The goal of this model was to clearly articulate the competencies brought to patient care by nurses in meeting the needs of patients and families.

HISTORICAL BACKGROUND

During the early 1990s, the AACN Certification Corporation strategically set forth a direction to identify model that described practice. The model was to help articulate the practice that nursing conducted and to move beyond nursing as a set of tasks. The AACN knew that nurses impacted patient outcomes but needed to articulate a framework by which others could come to understand the discipline's unique contributions. In 1993, the AACN Certification Corporation, the certifying body of the AACN, brought together nurses from across the United States into a think tank to draft a document that identified the concepts of nursing practice, most specifically certified practice. The underlying assumption was that certified critical care nurses brought a unique set of skills to the bedside. Members of the think tank included experts in the field of critical care: Martha A. Q. Curley, Mairead Hickey, Pat Hooper, Bonnie Niebuhr, Wanda Johanson, Sarah Sanford, and Gayle Whitman. Consensus of the think tank was that certified practice was more than the sum of its parts, the parts being critical care tasks. The foundation of critical care nursing was in nurses meeting the needs of patients and families while influencing optimal patient outcomes. Historically, certified practice has been based on hours worked in the critical care unit, continuing education, and successful accomplishment of a list of critical tasks (e.g., insertion of a pacemaker, hemodynamic monitoring, ventilator care, intra-aortic balloon pump therapy). Certified practice included a multiple-choice-question exam along with verification of practice in the clinical setting. Movement away from this paradigm of certified practice to one that was more holistic seemed to be the goal.

The think tank identified 13 patient needs: compensation, resiliency, margin of error, predictability, complexity, vulnerability, physiological stability, risk of death, independence, self-determination, involvement in care decisions, engagement, and resource availability. Nine nurse characteristics were identified: engagement, skilled clinical practice, agency, caring practices, system management, teamwork, diversity responsiveness, experiential learning, and innovator–evaluator. The nurse characteristics were based upon the needs of the patient. Matching the nurse characteristics to the needs of the patient would promote optimal patient outcomes. The think tank concluded that a synergetic effect should exist between the patient/family and nurse.

Then in 1995, the AACN Certification Board identified a group of "subject matter" experts from across the United States: Martha A. Q. Curley, Duanne Foster-Smith, Deborah Gloskey, Janet Fraser Hale, Teresa Halloran, Sonya R. Hardin, Mairead Hickey, Pat Hooper, Vickie Keough, Patricia Moloney-Harmon, Kathleen Shurpin, and Daphne Stannard. The experts met over the course of 2 years to refine the conceptual model and devise a survey tool for a study of critical care practice. Professional Examination Services (PES), a nonprofit corporation, which provides consultation on certification exam development, conducted the study of practice using the survey developed by the experts.

Once the results from the study of practice were received and reviewed by the expert panel, recommendation to change the certification process was submitted to the AACN Certification Board of Directors. The Study of Practice served as the basis for the certification exam and ultimately the deletion of requiring the certified nurse to complete skills off of a task list. The findings from the study also supported revision to the model, resulting in eight nurse characteristics and eight patient characteristics.

In February of 2002, the Practice Analysis Task Force expanded the assumption to the model to include the following:

- The nurse creates the environment for the care of the patient. The context/environment of care also affects what the nurse can do.
- There is an interrelatedness between impact areas. The nature of the interrelatedness may change as the function of experience, situation, or setting changes.
- The nurse may work to optimize outcomes for patients, families, health care providers, and the health care system/organization.
- Nurses bring their background to each situation, including various levels of education/knowledge and skills/experience (Practice Analysis Task Force, 2003).

These assumptions underlie the conceptual framework and establish the context for understanding the AACN Synergy Model. These assumptions also support the purpose of nursing as meeting the needs of patients and families while overseeing their safe passage through the health care system. The AACN Synergy Model is a conceptual framework for designing practice and developing the competencies required to care for acute and critically ill patients. Even though the AACN Synergy Model is used as a blueprint for certified practice, the model has far-reaching implications for research, education, and the practice of nursing and other health care professions. The model has been used to develop nursing curriculums and for conducting research focused on the interrelationship of competencies and patient outcomes. According to the AACN Synergy Model, when patient characteristics and nurse competencies match, patient outcomes are optimized.

In March 1996, the AACN Certification Corporation appointed an Outcome Think Tank for the purpose of articulating optimal outcomes. Members of this think tank included Patricia Benner, Melissa Biel, Martha A. Q. Curley, Wanda Johanson, Marion Johnson, Marguerite Kinney, Benton Lutz, Patricia Moloney-Harmon, Alvin Tarlov, and Cheri White. Outcomes are considered patient conditions measured along a continuum (Curley, 1998). Six major quality indicators were identified by the task force:

1. Patient and family satisfaction
2. Rate of adverse incidents
3. Complication rate
4. Adherence to the discharge plan
5. Mortality rate
6. The patient's length of stay (Hardin, 2004)

The Synergy Model was found to be congruent with outcomes derived from the patient, nurse, and health care system (Hardin & Hussey, 2003). Outcomes derived from the eight patient characteristics include functional changes, behavioral changes, trust, satisfaction, comfort, and quality of life. Outcomes derived from the eight nursing competencies include physiological changes, the presence or absence of complications, and the extent treatment objectives were obtained (Curley, 1998). Outcome data derived from the health care system include readmission rates, length of stay, and cost utilization per case.

From 2001 to 2003, the AACN Certification Corporation focused efforts on devising a study of practice. A Practice Analysis Task Force was appointed, consisting of the following members: Patricia Atkins, Deborah Becker, Deborah Bingaman, Nancy Blake, Jo Ellen Craighead, Beth Diehl-Svrjeck, Sonya R. Hardin, Melissa Hutchinson, Linda Jackson, Roberta Kaplow, Marthe Moseley, Marlene Roman, Daphne Stannard, Karen Thomason, and Darla Ura. The Professional Examination Service (PES) facilitated the task force in developing a survey based on the Synergy Model and the levels of practice in acute and critical care nursing. The nurse characteristics were further delineated and expanded through the development of descriptive behaviors for entry-level, competent, and expert critical care nurses as well as descriptors for the nurse practitioner (NP) and clinical nurse specialist (CNS). PES conducted focus panels, critical incident interviews, and subject matter expert interviews. Using the data, the Practice Analysis Task Force further revised the survey before use with entry-level critical care nurses, critical care registered nurses (CCRNs) and advanced-practice critical care nurses (i.e., CNS and NP) (Hardin, 2004). Findings clearly indicated a significant difference in level of nurse characteristics between clinical nurse specialist and nurse practitioner (Becker et al., 2006).

DESCRIPTION OF THE THEORY OF SYNERGY MODEL

Assumption of the Model

The Synergy Model is based on five assumptions:

"1) Patients are biological. Social and spiritual entities who present at a particular developmental stage. The whole patient (body, mind, and spirit) must be considered. 2) The patient, family, and community all contribute to providing a context for the nurse-patient relationship. 3) Patients can be described by a number of characteristics. All characteristics are connected and contribute to each other. Characteristics cannot be looked at in isolation. 4) Nurses can be described on a number of dimensions. The interrelated dimensions paint a profile of the nurse. 5) A goal of nursing is to restore a patient to an optimal level of wellness as defined by the patient. Death can be an acceptable outcome in which the goal of nursing care is to move a patient toward a peaceful death" (AACN, 2000, p. 55).

Definition of Theoretical Concepts

There are a total of 16 concepts in this model: eight patient concepts and eight nursing concept (Tables 5.1 and 5.2). The concepts (characteristics) are descriptors that describe the patient and nursing. The eight concepts used to understand patients are resiliency, vulnerability, stability, complexity, resource availability, participation in care, participation in decision making, and predictability. The eight concepts (characteristics) used to describe the practice of nursing are clinical judgment, advocacy, caring practices, collaboration, systems thinking, response to diversity, clinical inquiry, and facilitator of learning. The patient and nurse characteristics are leveled from 1 to 5 and are presented in Tables 5.1 and 5.2.

Patient characteristic levels are based on a five-point Likert scale, ranging from 1 (the worst patient state) to 5 (the best patient state). Nurse characteristic levels are based on a five-point Likert scale with 1 being novice and 5 being expert. Descriptions of levels 1, 3, and 5 have been described by the AACN. Levels 2 and 4 have not been specifically identified in the literature by the AACN. However, the use of the five levels with levels 1, 3, and 5 as benchmarks has been useful to nursing organizations as they

Table 5.1 PATIENT CHARACTERISTICS AND LEVELS

CHARACTERISTIC	DEFINITION	LEVEL
Stability	Maintain a steady-state equilibrium	**Level 1—Minimally stable:** labile; unstable; unresponsive to therapies; high risk of death **Level 3—Moderately stable:** able to maintain steady state for limited period of time; some responsiveness to therapies **Level 5—Highly stable:** constant; responsive to therapies; low risk of death
Complexity	Entanglement of two or more systems (e.g., body, family, therapies)	**Level 1—Highly complex:** intricate; complex patient/family dynamics; ambiguous/vague; atypical presentation **Level 3—Moderately complex:** moderately involved patient/family dynamics **Level 5—Minimally complex:** straightforward; routine patient/family dynamics; simple/clear cut; typical presentation
Predictability	Allows one to expect a certain course of events	**Level 1—Not predictable:** uncertain; uncommon patient population/illness; unusual or unexpected course; does not follow critical pathway, or no critical pathway developed **Level 3—Moderately predictable:** wavering; occasionally noted patient population/illness **Level 5—Highly predictable:** certain; common patient population/illness; usual and expected course; follows critical pathway
Resiliency	The capacity to return to a restorative level of functioning	**Level 1—Minimally resilient:** unable to mount a response; failure of compensatory/coping mechanisms; minimal reserves; brittle **Level 3—Moderately resilient:** able to mount a moderate response; able to initiate some degree of compensation; moderate reserves **Level 5—Highly resilient:** able to mount and maintain a response; intact compensatory/coping mechanisms; strong reserves; endurance
Vulnerability	Susceptibility to actual or potential stressors	**Level 1—Highly vulnerable:** susceptible; unprotected, fragile **Level 3—Moderately vulnerable:** somewhat susceptible; somewhat protected **Level 5—Minimally vulnerable:** safe; out of the woods; protected, not fragile
Participation in decision making	Extent to which patient/family engages in decision making	**Level 1—No participation:** no capacity for decision making; requires surrogacy **Level 3—Moderate level of participation:** limited capacity; seeks input/advice from others in decision making **Level 5—Full participation:** full capacity; makes decision for self

(table continued on page 104)

Table 5.1 PATIENT CHARACTERISTICS AND LEVELS (continued)

CHARACTERISTIC	DEFINITION	LEVEL
Participation in care	Extent to which patient/family engages in aspects of care	**Level 1—No participation:** patient and family unable or unwilling to participate in care **Level 3—Moderate level of participation:** patient and family need assistance in care **Level 5—Full participation:** patient and family fully able to participate in care
Resource availability	Extent of resources the patient/family/community bring to the situation	**Level 1—Few resources:** necessary knowledge and skills not available; financial support and personal/psychological supportive resources minimal **Level 3—Moderate resources:** limited knowledge and skills available; limited financial support and personal/psychological and supportive resources **Level 5—Many resources:** extensive knowledge and skills available and accessible; strong financial, personal, and supportive resources

Source: Adapted from AACN Certification Corporation web site. The AACN Synergy Model for Patient Care (2000). Retrieved September 27, 2007 from http://www.certcorp.org/certcorp/certcorp.nsf/edcfc72ba47aaa708825666b0064bdcf/ 08482aa8ec2a5b638825666b00654be7?OpenDocument.

develop clinical ladders. Further work has been completed on the nurse characteristics for the advanced-practice role (Becker et al., 2006). Activities of advanced-practice nurses organized by the eight nurse characteristics emerged through a study of practice conducted by the AACN Certification Corporation. While some of these activities overlap with the expert nurse, the study identified four nurse characteristics considered most critical by clinical nurse specialists (clinical judgment, caring practices, facilitator of learning, and clinical inquiry) and two activities most critical by nurse practitioners (clinical judgment and advocacy/moral agency) (Becker et al., 2006).

PATIENT CHARACTERISTICS

Each patient brings a unique set of characteristics to the health care situation. Among many characteristics that are present, eight are consistently seen in acute and critically ill patients. These eight characteristics are consistently assessed by nurses in variable levels given each patient situation. They should be assessed in the patient as well as other patterns that are unique to the given circumstances of the patient. *Resiliency* is the patient's capacity to return to a restorative level of functioning using compensatory coping mechanisms. The level of resiliency is often dependent upon the patient's ability to rebound after an insult. This ability can be influenced by many factors including age, comorbidities, nutritional status, and compensatory mechanisms that are intact. *Vulnerability* is the level of susceptibility to actual or potential stressors that may adversely affect patient outcomes. Vulnerability can be impacted by the patient's physiological/genetic make-up or health behaviors exhibited by the patient, such as risk factors. *Stability* refers to the patient's ability to maintain a steady state of equilibrium. Response to therapies and nursing interventions can impact the stability of the patient. *Complexity* is the

Table 5.2 **NURSE CHARACTERISTICS AND LEVELS**

CHARACTERISTIC	DEFINITION	LEVEL
Clinical judgment	Clinical reasoning	**Level 1:** collects basic-level data; follows algorithms, decision trees, and protocols with all populations and is uncomfortable deviating from them **Level 3:** collects and interprets complex patient data; makes clinical judgments based on an immediate grasp of the whole picture for common or routine patient populations **Level 5:** synthesizes and interprets multiple, sometimes conflicting, sources of data; makes judgment based on an immediate grasp of the whole picture; helps patient and family see the "big picture"; recognizes and responds to the dynamic situation
Advocacy	Working on another's behalf	**Level 1:** works on behalf of patient; self-assesses personal values; is aware of ethical conflicts/issues that may surface in clinical setting; makes ethical/moral decisions based on rules **Level 3:** considers patient values and incorporates in care, even when differing from personal values; supports colleagues in ethical and clinical issues; moral decision making can deviate from rules **Level 5:** advocates ethical conflict and issues from patient/family perspective; suspends rules; empowers the patient and family to speak for/represent themselves
Caring practices	Activities that create a compassionate, supportive, and therapeutic environment for patients and staff	**Level 1:** focuses on the customary needs of the patient; has no anticipation of future needs; bases care on standards and protocols **Level 3:** responds to subtle patient and family changes; engages with the patient as a unique patient in a compassionate manner; recognizes and tailors caring practices to the individuality of patient **Level 5:** has astute awareness and anticipates patient and family changes and needs; is fully engaged with and senses how to stand alongside the patient, family, and community; orchestrates the process that ensures the patient's/family's comfort and concerns surrounding issues of death and dying

(table continued on page 106)

Table 5.2 NURSE CHARACTERISTICS AND LEVELS (continued)

CHARACTERISTIC	DEFINITION	LEVEL
Collaboration	Working with others in a way that promotes each person's contributions toward achieving optimal outcomes	**Level 1:** willing to be taught, coached, and/or mentored; participates in team meetings and discussions regarding patient care and/or practice issues **Level 3:** seeks opportunities to be taught, coached, and/or mentored; elicits others' advice and perspectives; initiates and participates in team meetings and discussions regarding patient care; recognizes and suggests various team members' participation **Level 5:** seeks opportunities to teach, coach, and mentor and to be taught, coached, and mentored; facilitates active involvement and complementary contributions of others in team meetings and discussions regarding patient care and/or practice issues; involves/recruits diverse resources when appropriate to optimize patient outcomes
Response to diversity	Sensitivity to recognize, appreciate, and incorporate differences into the provision of care	**Level 1:** assesses cultural diversity; provides care based on own belief system; learns the culture of the health care environment **Level 3:** inquires about cultural differences and considers their impact on care; accommodates personal and professional differences in the plan of care; helps patient/family understand the culture of the health care system **Level 5:** responds to, anticipates, and integrates cultural differences into patient/family care; appreciates and incorporates differences, including alternative therapies; tailors health care culture, to the extent possible, to meet the diverse needs and strengths of the patient/family
Clinical inquiry	Ongoing process of questioning and evaluating practice and providing informed practice	**Level 1:** follows standards and guidelines; implements clinical changes and research-based practices developed by others; recognizes the need for further learning to improve patient care; recognizes obvious changing patient situation; needs and seeks help to identify patient problem **Level 3:** questions appropriateness of policies and guidelines; questions current practice; seeks advice, resources, or information to improve patient care; begins to compare and contrast possible alternatives **Level 5:** improves, deviates from, or individualizes standards and guidelines for particular patient situations or populations; questions and/or evaluates current practice based on patients' responses, review of the literature, research, and education/learning

CHARACTERISTIC	DEFINITION	LEVEL
Facilitator of learning	Ability to facilitate learning for patients/ families, nursing staff, other members of the health care team, and community	**Level 1:** follows planned educational programs; sees patient/family education as a separate task from delivery of care; provides data without seeking to assess patient's readiness or understanding; has limited knowledge of the totality of the educational needs **Level 3:** adapts planned educational programs; begins to recognize and integrate different ways of teaching into delivery of care; incorporates patient's understanding into practice **Level 5:** creatively modifies or develops patient/family education programs; integrates patient/family education throughout delivery of care; evaluates patient's understanding by observing behavior changes; sets patient-driven goals for education
Systems thinking	Knowledge and tools that enhance the nurse's ability to manage whatever environmental and system resources exist for the patient/family and staff	**Level 1:** uses a limited array of strategies; does not recognize negotiation as an alternative; sees patient and family within the isolated environment of the unit; sees self as key resource **Level 3:** develops strategies based on needs and strengths of patient/family; is able to make connections within components; sees opportunity to negotiate but may not have strategies; recognizes how to obtain resources beyond self **Level 5:** develops, integrates, and applies a variety of strategies; has a global or holistic outlook; knows when and how to negotiate and navigate through the system; anticipates needs of patients and families as they move through the health care system; uses untapped and alternative resources as necessary

Source: Adapted from AACN Certification Corporation web site. The AACN Synergy Model for Patient Care (2000). Retrieved September 27, 2007 from http://www.certcorp.org/certcorp/certcorp.nsf/edcfc72ba47aaa708825666b0064bdcf/ 08482aa8ec2a5b638825666b00654be7?OpenDocument.

intricate entanglement of two or more systems. Systems refer to either physiological or psychological states of the body or family dynamics or environmental interactions with the patient. The more systems involved, the more complex are the patterns displayed by the patient. *Resource availability* is influenced by the extent that resources are brought to the context by the patient, family, and community. The resources can present as pharmaceutical, technical, fiscal, personal, psychological, social, or supportive in nature. A greater potential for a positive outcome exists when a patient has more resources. *Participation in care* is the participation by a patient and family who is engaged in the delivery of care. Patient and family participation can be influenced by health status, educational background, health literacy, resource availability, and cultural background. *Participation in decision making* is the level of engagement of the patient and family in comprehending the information provided by health care providers and acting upon this information to execute informed decisions. Patient and family engagement in clinical decisions can be impacted by the knowledge level of the patient, his or her capacity to make decisions given the insult, cultural background (i.e., beliefs and values), and the level of inner strength during a crisis (AACN Certification Corporation, 2002).

NURSE CHARACTERISTICS

The nurse characteristics can be considered competencies that are essential for providing care to the acute and critically ill. The nursing competencies were confirmed through a study of practice in 1997 conducted by the AACN Certification Corporation. PES mailed the patient characteristics, along with the varying levels of patient acuity, and asked nurses to rate each profile for the intensity of criticality of the patient given the level of the characteristic. All eight competencies reflect an integration of knowledge, skills, and experience of the nurse. The competencies include clinical judgment, advocacy, caring practices, systems thinking, facilitation of learning, collaboration, response to diversity, and clinical inquiry. *Clinical judgment* is the clinical reasoning that is used by a health care provider in the delivery of care. It consists of critical thinking and nursing skills that are acquired through a process of integrating formal and experiential knowledge. The integration of knowledge and experience brings about the clinical decisions made during the course of care for patients, groups, and communities. *Advocacy* is working on another's behalf when the other is not capable of advocating for herself. The nurse serves as a moral agent in identifying and helping to resolve ethical dilemmas within the clinical setting. *Caring practices* are the constellation of nursing interventions that are unique to the needs of the patient and family. Caring behaviors include compassion, vigilance, engagement, and responsiveness to the patient and family. *Collaboration* is the nurse working with others to promote optimal outcomes. The patient, family, and members of various health care disciplines collaborate by working toward promoting the needs and requests of patients. *Systems thinking* is the tools and knowledge that the nurse uses to recognize the interconnected nature within and across the health care system. The ability to understand how one decision can impact the whole is integral to systems thinking. The nurse uses a global perspective in analyzing problems, making decisions, and negotiating for the patient and family internally and externally to the health care system. *Response to diversity* is the sensitivity to recognize, appreciate, and incorporate differences into the provision of care. Nurses need to recognize the individuality of each patient while observing for patterns that respond to nursing interventions. Nurses should be open to the patient's spiritual beliefs, ethnicity, family configuration, lifestyle values, and use of alternative and complementary therapies. *Clinical inquiry* is the ongoing process of questioning and evaluating practice, providing informed practice, and innovating through research and experiential learning. Clinical inquiry evolves as the nurse moves from novice to expert. At the expert level, the nurse enhances, deviates, and/or individualizes standards and guidelines to meet the needs of patients, families, groups, and communities. *Facilitator of learning* is understood as the nurse facilitating learning among patients, families, communities, and staff through tailored educational programs. The educational level of the audience should be considered in the design of the plan to educate. Creative methods should be developed to ensure patient and family comprehension and to make informed decisions. Each nurse and patient characteristic is understood on a continuum from 1 to 5. The level of each patient characteristic is critical in identifying the competency required of the nurse (AACN Certification Corporation, 2002).

Research

The PES has undertaken a number of studies to validate the Synergy Model. Recently results of the 2001–2003 study of practice were reported, concluding that acute and critical care clinical nurse specialists were more experienced than nurse practitioners in clinical judgment and clinical inquiry. While the sample of 261 subjects, both CNSs and NPs, rated the nurse characteristic of clinical judgment as the highest, CNSs identified clinical inquiry as second. NPs identified advocacy and moral agency as second. Table 5.3 displays the differences between NPs and CNSs on the characteristic of clinical judgment. This study indicates that based on the Synergy Model, a difference in practice between CNSs and NPs exists (Becker et al., 2006).

Evidence-based practice is based upon clinical inquiry of scientists in the field or developed protocols through clinical evidence. The integration of research findings into practice or the translation of findings into practice is a skill set within the characteristic of clinical inquiry (Titler, 2004). The tools that have evolved from evidence-based practice and hence clinical inquiry have supported the decision making of nurses. Through evidence-based practice, interventions and outcomes can be identified.

Table 5.3 **NURSE PRACTITIONER (NP) AND CLINICAL NURSE SPECIALIST (CNS) DIFFERENCES IN CLINICAL JUDGMENT**

CNS	NP
Synthesizes, interprets, makes decisions and recommendations, and evaluates responses on the basis of complex, sometimes conflicting sources of data	Orders appropriate diagnostic studies and interprets findings to manage patients' care in collaboration with physicians and other members of the health care team as necessary
Identifies and prioritizes clinical problems on the basis of education, research, and experiential knowledge	Prescribes medications, therapeutics, and monitoring modalities in collaboration with physicians and other members of the health care team as necessary
Facilitates development of clinical judgment in health care team members (e.g., nursing staff, medical staff, and other health care providers) through serving as a role model, teaching, coaching, and/or mentoring	Elicits comprehensive history and performs physical examinations on the basis of each patient's initial signs and symptoms
	Develops a list of differential diagnoses on the basis of findings obtained from each patient's initial signs and symptoms
	Synthesizes, interprets, makes decisions and recommendations, and evaluates responses on the basis of complex, sometimes conflicting sources of data
	Initiates appropriate referrals and performs consultations

Source: Adapted from Becker, D., Kaplow, R., Muenzen, P., Hartigan, C., PES, & AACN. (2006). Activities performed by acute and critical care advanced practice nurses: American Association Of Critical-Care Nurses study of practice. *American Journal of Critical Care, 15*(2), 130–148.

The Synergy Model is useful in identifying optimal patient outcomes given evidence-based nursing interventions (Kaplow & Hardin, 2007). Optimal outcomes can be measured through the use of numerous instruments. For example, as the nurse begins managing the transition of the patient from one setting to another, the outcome of transition without complications is established. The nurse can use numerous research-developed risk-screening instruments to improve postdischarge problems. Or, if the nurse is managing an organ donor, pathways have been developed by the United Network for Organ Sharing to guide the decisions and actions in managing donors. Such pathways have been researched and/or reached through clinical consensus (Kaplow & Hardin, 2007).

Research has been conducted using the Synergy Model to link nursing care to diagnosis-related groups (DRGs) and nurse intensity at Children's Hospital in Boston (Doble, Curley, Hession-Laba, Marino, & Shaw, 2000). However, further research with the model needs to be conducted to further validate the model within other practice settings and patient populations.

Nursing Education

Using the Synergy Model to facilitate the learning of patients, families, communities, and staff has been discussed in the literature (Hardin, 2004; Kaplow, 2002; Zungolo, 2004). Teaching can be enhanced by using the patient and nurse competencies to design care. The patient should be analyzed through identifying data points associated with each of the patient characteristics. Nursing interventions from each of the eight nursing competencies should be chosen to address the patient characteristics. Developing courses or curriculums can be accomplished with the Synergy Model as a framework. An example of the model being used has been described as the framework for the Duquesne University School of Nursing (Zungolo, 2004). In this school, each nurse characteristic has been used as a thread in the undergraduate curriculum across 4 years of study. The nurse characteristic of caring practices is to be demonstrated in freshman year as care of self and caring processes; sophomore year as initiating caring practices; junior year as integrating caring into one's practice; and senior year as displaying a caring attitude in all aspects of one's practice. The graduate curriculum is guided by the three spheres of influence along with the Synergy Model. Table 5.4 displays the three spheres of influence (Moloney-Harmon, 1999) for the clinical nurse specialist and the content in a graduate curriculum.

The Synergy Model has been used to revise and update critical care graduate programs such as the one provided by Marymount University in Arlington, VA, to prepare clinical nurse specialists (Cox & Galante, 2003). The eight nurse competencies became the framework for the courses with the instructor preparing a lecture on each competency and then a seminar focused on specific content areas that could be discussed in relationship to the content. For example, during week 6, the instructor provided a lecture on collabo-

Table 5.4 SYNERGY MODEL IN GRADUATE EDUCATION

NURSE–PATIENT SPHERE	NURSE–NURSE SPHERE	NURSE–SYSTEM SPHERE
Establish and maintain outstanding relationships with patients	Establish ways to maximize use of personnel and enhance patient safety	Analyze the political, economic, and financial realities of the health care industry

Source: Adapted from Zungolo, E. H. (2004). The synergy model in educational practice: A guide to curriculum development. *Excellence in Nursing Knowledge*. Retrieved October 3, 2006, from http://www.nursingknowledge.org/Portal/main.aspx?pageid=3507&ContentID=56394.

ration and then had content in the seminar on hypovolemic shock, acute inflammatory diseases, and dys-rhythmias. The clinical component of the course ensured integration and application of the Synergy Model as students were expected to learn the role of the critical care clinical specialist and to apply the eight nursing characteristics. The students used the nurse characteristics in a journal for reflecting on the experiential knowing of working in the role of a CNS (Cox & Galante, 2003).

Nursing Practice

The Synergy Model is a model of practice. Practice is driven by the characteristics and needs of the patient. Nurses respond to the needs of the patient through nurse characteristics. When the patient and nurse characteristics are matched to facilitate optimal outcomes, synergy occurs (Pacini, 2004). The eight nursing competencies represent nursing practice. However, the core of nursing is *clinical judgment,* which is grounded in the nursing process of assessment, planning, intervention, and evaluation. Making decisions to act or not act is intervention. These decisions come about through the integration of knowledge and critical thinking skills such as distinguishing relevant data from the irrelevant, recognizing patterns and relationships, determining desired outcomes, and continuously evaluating.

Advocacy is doing for the patient that which he cannot do so for himself in that he lacks the knowledge or ability due to alteration in physiological systems. Nurses advocate through their pursuit of supporting the patient's right to self-determination and autonomy, and being a "protective shield" when the client is unable to advocate for himself (Hanks, 2005, p. 76). Advocacy has been described as a semipermeable sphere that allows the client to self-advocate if he is emotionally and physically able or to be advocated for by the nurse when unable (Hank, 2005).

The characteristic of *caring practices* includes interventions of spiritual support for end of life (Levey, Danis, Nelson, & Solomon, 2003), promotion of a "healing environment" (Rex Smith, 2006, pp. 44–45), and the use of listening and therapeutic communication skills. Nurses intervene by providing an unconditional positive regard and nonjudgmental stance toward the patient, and creatively using self to engage in healing practices (Hardin & Kaplow, 2005).

Given the increasing complexity required in the care of patients, *collaboration* is a critical nurse characteristic. Individuals collaborating together are successful when (a) there is a compelling, shared drive or goals; (b) individuals with unique competencies will contribute to successful outcomes; (c) members operate within a formal structure, with defined roles that facilitate collective/collaborative work; and (d) there is mutual respect, tolerance, and trust. Individuals must be willing to take on different roles within a group and be honest and open with their ideas and concerns. There are times when an individual should be a follower and times when he or she should be a leader.

Systems thinking is used to address the most challenging patient and organizational problems in health care. This nurse characteristic allows one to understand reality through the relationships among the system's parts, rather than the parts themselves. Long-term ramifications from a decision and a more accurate picture of reality, so that you can work with a system's natural forces, allow achievement of results desired.

Response to diversity is a characteristic that requires the nurse to approach each situation with an open mind and the ability to use respect when faced with requests or practices that are not understood. Providing culture-specific care is a stance that promotes healing. Nurses must first examine their own biases and values while providing sensitive care to others. To understand another, the nurse must seek knowledge about his or her culture. Assessing the needs of the patient and family requires the skill of obtaining relevant cultural data to promote optimal patient outcomes (Campinha-Bacote, 2002).

Questioning to uncover best practices or innovative strategies to meet the needs of patients and families is a form of *clinical inquiry*. "Clinical inquiry is the ongoing process of questioning and evaluating practice, providing informed practice based on available data, and innovating through research and experiential learning" (Curley, 1998, p. 66). Nurses must remain knowledgeable of the new scientific information for applying the best research evidence while respecting the patient and family's values (Titler, 2004).

Facilitator of learning is a characteristic that uses "teaching moments" throughout the time care is provided. Strategies to improve outcomes or to ensure informed decision making require the nurse to educate patients and families. Besides patients and families, nurses must continually work with new nurses that arrive on the unit as orientees. Psychomotor, critical-thinking, and clinical decision-making skills are role modeled, taught, and facilitated (Kaplow, 2002). Whether the nurse is working with a new orientee or patients and families, taking the lead in providing the knowledge and skills for the delivery of care is an aspect of this competency.

An extension of the model has been proposed by Alspach (2006) to have preceptor characteristics and nurse characteristics to bring about a competent provider through a synergistic mentored experience. Expanding the assumptions of the model by substituting the nurse as the preceptor and the patient as the preceptee was proposed. Further development of this form of thinking may require a different definition of the characteristic of facilitator of learning, which was initially intended to encompass the nurse as facilitating learning with the patient and family, nursing staff and colleagues, and the community.

The use of the model in practice has been articulated with victims of intimate partner violence (IPV) (Cox, 2003). These individuals are typically highly vulnerable and display a maladaptive resiliency, variable stability depending on the degree of physical and psychological injury, and low levels of resource availability. In providing care to victims of IPV, the nurse must possess a moderate to high level of all nurse characteristics. Advocacy and caring characteristics are needed at a high level to enhance prevention and to screen for IPV in a safe environment. At a minimum, moderate levels of clinical inquiry, response to diversity, systems thinking, collaboration, facilitator of learning, and clinical judgment are needed to facilitate the best possible level of wellness (Cox, 2003).

USE OF THE THEORY IN A SYSTEM

Clarian Health Partner is the first hospital system in the United States to integrate the AACN Synergy Model for Patient Care in an organization. Nurses hired into the system are as an Associate Partner, Partner, or Senior Partner. These three levels correlate with the three levels of the nurse characteristics and differentiated practice principles (Kerfoot, 2004). In this organization, the model is used to simplify the needs of the patient. From the orientation of the nurse, to the clinical ladder, to job descriptions and documents, the model provides the framework for this organization. The integration of this model into an organization is an exemplary example of advancing accountability and professionalism in the workplace (Kaplow & Hardin, 2007).

The model has been used as a framework to explicate outcomes in tobacco-dependent patients requiring surgery. Matching a patient's level of vulnerability with a nurse's level of inquiry promotes best practices for tobacco-dependent patients. The majority of smokers are less educated and unemployed with limited resources, requiring nurses with a high level of facilitator of learning (Graham-Garcia, George-Gay, Heater, Butts, & Heath, 2006). Smokers are highly vulnerable and require a high

ANALYSIS OF THEORY

Using the criteria presented in Chapter 2, critique the Synergy Model. Compare your conclusions about the theory with those found in Appendix A. An experienced nurse has completed the analysis found in Appendix A.

Internal Criticism
1. Clarity
2. Consistency
3. Adequacy

4. Logical development
5. Level of theory development

External Criticism
1. Reality convergence
2. Utility
3. Significance
4. Discrimination
5. Scope of theory
6. Complexity

level of clinical inquiry and advocacy by the nurse as evidence-based approaches are required to implement clinical guidelines. Clinical guidelines suggest that all smokers receive a comprehensive tobacco use history, including previous smoking cessation attempts. The Synergy Model provides a framework for the nurse to assess, advise, and determine readiness for smoking cessation (Graham-Garcia et al., 2006).

SUMMARY

The Synergy Model resonates with clinicians because it describes a practice where nurses achieve optimal patient outcomes with patients and families. The mutuality and reciprocal nature of the relationship between nurses and patients are very unique. This uniqueness emerges due to the intimacy from being the primary caregiver and overseer of care across the continuum of care. The nurse is the one constant in the trajectory of disease that has the ability to detect subtle changes due to the intense length of care over time. The use of the Synergy Model enhances the nurse's understanding of the contribution that is brought to the patient and family through the discipline of nursing.

CRITICAL THINKING EXERCISES

1. In today's health care environment, how is it possible to attempt to match patient characteristics to specific nurse competencies in order to optimize patient outcomes?
   • How is this accomplished in the acute care setting?
2. Would it be possible to apply the Synergy Model to other care practice settings where patients are less acutely ill?

• Think of different nursing care practice arenas. What practice areas are most conducive to using the Synergy Model to advance nursing practice and nursing research?
• What could you do as a nursing leader to make your area of practice better equipped to optimize patient outcomes?

WEB RESOURCES

AACN Certification Corporation web site:
**http://www.certcorp.org/certcorp/certcorp.nsf/
edcfc72ba47aaa708825666b0064bdcf/08482aa
8ec2a5b638825666b00654be7?OpenDocument**
AACN Bibliography of the Synergy Model:
**http://www.aacn.org/certcorp/certcorp.nsf/vw
doc/SynBibList?opendocument**
Excellence in Nursing Knowledge, a Sigma
Theta Tau online publication: **http://www.
nursingknowledge.org/Portal/main.aspx?
pageid=3508&ContentID=55889**

REFERENCES

AACN (2000). Assumptions Guiding the AACN Synergy Model for Patient Care. Retrieved September 27, 2007 from http://www.certcorp.org/certcorp/certcorp.nsf/vwdoc/SynModel?opendocument#Assumptions%20Gu

AACN Certification Corporation (2002). The AACN Synergy Model for Patient Care. Retrieved September 27, 2007 from http://www.certcorp.org/certcorp/certcorp.nsf/vwdoc/SynModel?opendocument#Assumptions%20Gu

AACN Practice Analysis Task Force (2003). History of AACN Certification Corporation. Retrieved September 27, 2007 from http://www.certcorp.org/certcorp/certcorp.nsf/vwdoc/AboutUs

Alspach, G. (2006). Extending the Synergy Model to Preceptorship: A Preliminary Proposal. *Critical Care Nurse, 26*(2) 10–13.

Becker, D., Kaplow, R., Muenzen, P., Hartigan, C., PES, & AACN. (2006). Activities performed by acute and critical care advanced practice nurses: American Association of Critical-Care Nurses study of practice. *American Journal of Critical Care, 15*(2), 130–148.

Campinha-Bacote, J. (2002). Readings & resources in transcultural health care and mental health. *Monograph of the Clinical, Administrative, Research & Educational Consultation in Transcultural Health Care* (13th ed.). Cincinnati, Ohio: Transcultural C.A.R.E. Associates.

Cox, E. (2003). Synergy in practice: Caring for victims of intimate partner violence. *Critical Care Nurse Quarterly, 26*(4), 323–330.

Cox, C. W., & Galante, C. M. (2003). An MSN curriculum in preparation of CCNSs: A model for consideration. *Critical Care Nurse, 23*(6), 74–80.

Curley, M. (1998). Patient-nurse synergy: Optimizing patients' outcomes. *American Journal of Critical Care, 7*(1), 64–72.

Doble, R. K., Curley, M. A. Q., Hession-Laba, E., Marino, B., & Shaw, S. (2000). Using the Synergy Model to link nursing care to diagnosis related groups. *Critical Care Nurse, 20*(3), 86–92.

Graham-Garcia, J., George-Gay, B., Heater, D., Butts, A., & Heath, J. (2006). Application of the Synergy Model with the surgical care of smokers. *Critical Care Clinics in North America, 18*(1), 29–38.

Hanks, R. G. (2005). Sphere of Nursing Advocacy model. *Nursing Forum, 40*(3), 75–78.

Hardin, S. R. (2004). Using the Synergy Model with undergraduate students. *Excellence in Nursing Knowledge.* Retrieved October 3, 2006, from http://www.nursingknowledge.org/Portal/main.aspx?pageid=3507&ContentID=56388.

Hardin, S., & Hussey, L. (2003). AACN synergy model for patient care case study of a CHF patient. *Critical Care Nurse, 23*(1), 73–76.

Hardin, S. R., & Kaplow, R. (2005). *Synergy for clinical excellence: The AACN Synergy Model for Patient Care.* Sudbury, MA: Jones and Bartlett Publisher.

Kaplow, R. (2002). Applying the Synergy Model to nursing education—The Synergy Model in Practice. *Critical Care Nurse, 22*(3), 77–81.

Kaplow, R., & Hardin, S. (2007). *Critical care nursing: Synergy for optimal outcomes.* Sudbury, MA: Jones & Bartlett Publishers.

Kerfoot, K. (2004). Synergy from the vantage point of a chief nursing officer. *Excellence in Nursing Knowledge.* Retrieved October 3, 2006, from http://www.nursingknowledge.org/Portal/main.aspx?pageid=3507&ContentID=56442.

Levy, M., Danis, M., Nelson, J. & Solomon, M. Z. (2003). Quality indicators for end-of-life in the intensive care unit. *Critical Care Medicine.* 31, 2255–2262.

Moloney-Harmon, P. (1999). Contemporary practice of the clinical nurse specialist. *Critical Care Nurse, 19*(2), 101–104.

Pacini, C. M. (2005). Synergy: a framework for leadership development and transformation. *Critical Care Nursing Clinics of North America, 17*(2): 113–9, ix.

Rex Smith, A. (2006). Using the synergy model to provide spiritual care in critical care settings. *Critical Care Nurse, 26*(4), 41–47.

Titler, M. G. (2004). Understanding synergy: The model from the perspective of a nurse scientist. *Excellence in Nursing Knowledge.* Retrieved October 3, 2006, from http://www.nursingknowledge.org/Portal/main.aspx?pageid=3507&ContentID=56400.

Zungolo, E. H. (2004). The synergy model in educational practice: A guide to curriculum development. *Excellence in Nursing Knowledge.* Retrieved October 3, 2006, from http://www.nursingknowledge.org/Portal/main.aspx?pageid=3507&ContentID=56394.

Middle Range
Theories: Cognitive

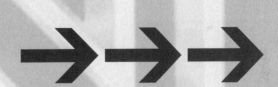

Self-Efficacy

■ BARBARA RESNICK

DEFINITION OF KEY TERMS

Mastery experience	The most influential source of self-efficacy information is the interpreted result of one's previous performance, or mastery experience. Individuals engage in tasks and activities, interpret the results of their actions, use the interpretations to develop beliefs about their capability to engage in subsequent tasks or activities, and act in concert with the beliefs created.
Outcome expectations	The belief that if a specific behavior is completed, there will be a certain outcome. Bandura postulates that because the outcomes an individual expects are the result of the judgments of what he or she can accomplish, outcome expectations are unlikely to contribute to predictions of behavior.
Self-efficacy	People's judgments of their capabilities to organize and execute courses of action required to attain designated types of performances. Self-efficacy beliefs provide the foundation for human motivation, well-being, and personal accomplishment.
Social persuasions	Individuals also create and develop self-efficacy beliefs as a result of the social persuasions they receive from others. These persuasions can involve exposure to verbal judgments of others.
Somatic and emotional states	Somatic and emotional states, such as anxiety, stress, arousal, and mood, also provide information about efficacy beliefs. People can gauge their degree of confidence by the emotional state they experience as they contemplate an action.
Vicarious experience	In addition to interpreting the results of their actions, people form their self-efficacy beliefs through the vicarious experience of observing others perform tasks. This source of information is weaker than mastery experience in helping to create self-efficacy beliefs, but when people are uncertain about their own abilities or when they have limited prior experience, they are more likely to be influenced by observation reactions.

INTRODUCTION

The links between health and lifestyle behavior (i.e., smoking, physical activity, weight, and diet) are now well supported. The challenge remains, however, on how to best help individuals change behavior so as to promote health and well-being. Understanding the determinants of health behaviors and the mechanisms linking health and behavioral processes is an essential step in designing interventions to support health-promoting behaviors and eliminate those that can impair health.

Theories are judged by their explanatory and predictive power. The value of psychological theory must also be judged by the ability of the theory to change people's lives for the better. Self-efficacy theory provides a body of knowledge for social applications to varied health-related activities. The broad scope and variety of applications attests to the explanatory and operative generality of this theory.

Individuals can exercise influence over what they do. Most human behavior, however, is determined by many interacting factors. Individuals are contributors to rather than the sole determiners of what happens to them. The power to make things happen should be distinguished from the mechanics of how things are made to happen. Based on their understanding of what is within the power of humans to do and beliefs about their own capabilities, people try to generate courses of action to suit given purposes. Since control is central in human lives, many theories have been proposed. Individuals' level of motivation, affective states, and actions are based more on what they believe than on what is objectively true. Therefore, it is the individuals' belief in their causative capabilities that is the major focus of behavior.

Many previous theories developed to understand behavior were focused on an inborn drive for control (i.e., self-determination or mastery). Theories that contend that striving for personal control is an expression of an innate drive tend to ignore the importance of the development of human efficacy. The fact that all individuals try to bring at least some influence to bear on some of the things that affect them does not necessarily mean that this is solely driven by an innate motivator. Understanding of whether the individual controls behavior by an inborn drive or is pulled by an anticipated benefit is central to understanding behavior change. Most human behavior, however, is determined by many interacting factors. The theory of self-efficacy, derived from social cognitive theory, has proven to be a useful guide in understanding behavior and facilitating behavior change.

HISTORICAL OR DEVELOPMENT BACKGROUND

The theory of self-efficacy was derived from social cognitive theory. Social cognitive theory favors a conception of interaction based on triadic reciprocity. In this model of reciprocal determinism, behavior, cognitive, and other personal factors and environmental influences all operate interactively as determinants of each other. In this triadic reciprocal determinism, there is mutual action between causal factors. Reciprocity does not, however, mean symmetry in the strength of bidirectional influences. Nor is there a specific pattern of influences. There are times when environmental factors may be the driving force in behavior, and other times when the individual's behavior and its intrinsic feedback are the central factors in determining behavior. Generally, however, when situational constraints are weak, personal factors serve as the predominant influence in the regulatory system.

The theory of self-efficacy is based on the belief that what people think, believe, and feel affects how they behave. The natural and extrinsic effects of their actions, in turn, partly determine their thought patterns and affective reactions and behavior. Freedom of choice is central to the theory. Freedom is considered as the exercise of self-influence. This is achieved through reflective thought, generative use of the knowledge and skills at one's command, and other tools of self-influence, which choice and execution of action require.

The initial work in the development of the theory of self-efficacy was done to test the assumption that psychological procedures could result in behavior change by altering an individual's level and strength of self-efficacy expectations. Treatment of snake phobias was the area of study, and it was demonstrated that certain interventions such as performance of a behavior and observing others perform a behavior strengthen self-efficacy expectations to perform that behavior. In the early studies, Bandura manipulated variables and observed outcomes. The interventions resulted in increased self-efficacy expectations, and positive behavioral changes occurred.

Initial Theory Development and Research

The early research using the theory of self-efficacy was done to test the assumption that psychological procedures could result in behavioral change by altering an individual's level and strength of self-efficacy. In the initial study (Bandura, Adams, & Beyer, 1977), 33 subjects with snake phobias were randomly assigned to different treatment conditions: (a) enactive attainment, which included actually touching the snakes; (b) role modeling, or seeing others touch the snakes; and (c) the control group. Results suggested that self-efficacy was predictive of subsequent behavior, and enactive attainment resulted in stronger and more generalized (to another snake) self-efficacy expectations.

Expansion of the early research included three additional studies (Bandura, Reese, & Adams, 1982): (a) 10 subjects with snake phobias, (b) 14 subjects with spider phobias, and (c) 12 subjects with spider phobias. Similar to the initial self-efficacy study, enactive attainment and role modeling were effective interventions for strengthening self-efficacy expectations and impacting behavior. The study of 12 subjects with spider phobias also considered the physiological arousal component of self-efficacy. Pulse and blood pressure were measured as indicators of fear arousal when interacting with spiders. After interventions to strengthen self-efficacy expectations (enactive attainment and role modeling), heart rate decreased and blood pressure stabilized.

This early self-efficacy research was in an ideal controlled setting in that the individuals with snake phobias were unlikely to seek out opportunities to interact with snakes when away from the laboratory setting. Therefore, there was controlled input of efficacy information. While this ideal situation is not possible in the clinical setting, the theory of self-efficacy has been used to study and predict health behavior change and management in a variety of settings.

It should be recognized that at the core of this theory is the assumption that people can exercise influence over what they do. Based on reflective thought, generative use of the knowledge, and skills to perform a specific behavior, as well as other tools of self-influence, a person will decide how to behave (Bandura, 1995). It has also been suggested that in order to determine one's self-efficacy, the individual must have the opportunity for self-evaluation, or the comparison of individual output to some sort of evaluative criterion (White, Kjelgaard, & Harkins, 1995). It is this comparison process that provides the individual with a sense of how likely it is that he or she can achieve a given level of performance.

EXPANDED DEFINITIONS OF THEORETICAL CONCEPTS

Human Agency

The role of intentionality in self-efficacy theory is essential and is described as personal agency. Personal or human agency refers to acts done intentionally. Actions intended to serve a certain purpose can cause quite different things to happen. Effects are not the characteristics of the individual's actions; they are the consequences of those actions. The power to originate actions for given purposes is the key feature of personal agency.

Human agency operates largely on the basis of control beliefs. That is, in daily life individuals formulate solutions to tasks at hand. They act on their thoughts and later analyze how well their thoughts served them in managing events. The individual reflects on his or her experiences in executing courses of action as well as on the consequences of those actions. In social cognitive theory human agency operates within an interdependent causal structure involving triadic reciprocal causation. In this model of causality, internal personal factors in the form of cognitive affective and biological events, behavior, and environmental influences all operate as interacting determinants that influence each other bidirectionally. The relative influence of each of these factors will vary for different activities and under different circumstances.

Self-Efficacy and Outcome Expectations

Bandura (1977, 1986) suggests that outcome expectations are based largely on the individual's self-efficacy expectations. The types of outcomes people anticipate generally depend on their judgments of how well they will be able to perform the behavior. Individuals who consider themselves to be highly efficacious will expect favorable outcomes. Expected outcomes are highly dependent on self-efficacy judgments; therefore, Bandura postulated that expected outcomes may not add much on their own to the prediction of behavior.

Bandura differentiated between two components of self-efficacy theory: judgments of personal efficacy or self-efficacy, and outcome expectancy. Self-efficacy is a comprehensive summary or judgment of perceived capability for performing a specific task. Self-efficacy is a dynamic construct as the efficacy judgment changes over time as new information and experiences are acquired. Self-efficacy beliefs also involve a mobilization component. That is, self-efficacy reflects a process that involves the construction and orchestration of adaptive performance to fit changing circumstances. Individuals who have the same skills may perform differently based on their utilization of the skills, combination of skills, and sequencing of the skills. Outcome and self-efficacy expectations were differentiated because individuals can believe that a certain behavior will result in a specific outcome; however, they may not believe that they are capable of performing the behavior required for the outcome to occur. For example, Mrs. White may believe that rehabilitation will result in her being able to go home independently; however, she may not believe she is capable of ambulating across the room. Therefore, Mrs. White may not participate in the rehabilitation program or be willing to practice ambulation.

Bandura (1986) does state, however, that there are instances when outcome expectations can be dissociated from self-efficacy expectations. This occurs when either no action will result in a specific outcome or the outcome is loosely linked to the level or quality of the performance. For example, if Mrs. White knows that *even if* she regains functional independence by participating in rehabilitation she will still be discharged to a skilled nursing facility rather than back home, her behavior is likely to be influenced by her outcome expectations (discharge to the skilled nursing facility). In this situation no matter what Mrs. White's performance is the outcome is the same; thus, outcome expectancy may influence her behavior independent of her self-efficacy beliefs.

Expected outcomes are also partially separable from self-efficacy judgments when extrinsic outcomes are fixed. For example, when a nurse provides care to six patients during an 8-hour shift, the nurse receives a certain salary. When the same nurse cares for 10 patients during that shift, the same salary is received. This could negatively impact performance. It is also possible for an individual to believe he or she is capable of performing a specific behavior, but not believe that the outcome of performing that behavior is worthwhile. For example, an older adult in rehabilitation may believe that he is capable of performing the exercises and activities involved in the rehabilitation process, but he may not believe that performing the exercises will result in improved functional ability. Some older adults believe that resting rather than exercising will lead to recovery. In this situation outcome expectations may have a direct impact on performance.

Generally, self-efficacy expectations are more strongly related to performance when compared to outcome expectations (Jenkins, 1985; Neff & King, 1995; Rovniak, Anderson, Winett, & Stephens, 2002). Conversely, other researchers demonstrated the important impact of outcome expectations with regard to predicting behavior (Damush, Stump, Saporito, & Clark, 2001; Grembowski et al., 1993; Jette et al., 1998; Resnick, Palmer, Jenkins, & Spellbring, 2000; Resnick & Spellbring, 2000). Which one is more important in any given situation may depend on the features of the situation, such as the cost of performing the activity, and the perceived certainty of its benefit or outcome. Whether or not the outcomes anticipated associated with a given activity have been achieved seems to also have an influence on behavior (Wilcox, Castro, & King, 2006).

Sources of Self-Efficacy Information

Bandura suggested that knowledge of one's self-efficacy is based on four informational sources: (a) enactive attainment, which is the actual performance of a behavior; (b) vicarious experience or visualizing other similar people perform a behavior; (c) verbal persuasion or exhortation; and (d) physiological state or physiological feedback during a behavior, such as pain or fatigue (Bandura, 1982). The cognitive appraisal of these factors results in a perception of confidence in the individual's ability to perform a certain behavior. The performance of this behavior reinforces self-efficacy expectations (Bandura, 1995).

ENACTIVE ATTAINMENT

Enactive attainment has been described as the most influential source of efficacy information (Bandura, 1986; Bandura & Adams, 1977). There has been repeated empirical verification that actually performing an activity strengthens self-efficacy beliefs. Specifically, the impact of enactive attainment has been demonstrated with regard to:

1. Snake phobias (Bandura, 1977; Bandura, Adams, Hardy, & Howells, 1980; Bandura et al., 1982)
2. Smoking cessation (Colletti, Supnick, & Payne, 1985; Condiotte & Lichtenstein, 1981; McIntyre, Lichtenstein, & Mermelstein, 1983)
3. Exercise behaviors and performance of functional activities (Ewart, Taylor, Reese, & DeBusk, 1983; Kaplan, Atkins, & Reinsch, 1984; McAuley, Courneya, & Lettunich, 1991; Resnick, 1998a; 1998b; Robertson & Keller, 1992)
4. Weight loss (Chambliss & Murray, 1979)

Enactive attainment generally results in strengthening self-efficacy expectations better than the other informational sources. However, performance alone does not establish self-efficacy beliefs. Other factors, such as preconceptions of ability, the perceived difficulty of the task, the amount of effort expended, the external aid received, the situational circumstance, and the complex of past successes and failures, all impact the individual's cognitive appraisal of self-efficacy (Bandura, 1995; Gist & Mitchell, 1992). An older adult who strongly believes she is able to independently bathe and dress because she has been doing so for 90 years will not likely alter self-efficacy expectations if she wakes up with severe arthritic changes one morning and is consequently unable to put on a shirt. However, repeated failures to perform the activity will impact self-efficacy expectations. The relative stability of strong self-efficacy expectations is important; otherwise, an occasional failure or setback could severely impact self-efficacy expectations and impact behavior.

VICARIOUS EXPERIENCE

Self-efficacy expectations are also influenced by vicarious experiences or seeing other similar people successfully perform the same activity (Bandura et al., 1980; Kazdin, 1979). There are some conditions, however, that impact the influence of vicarious experience. If the individual has not been exposed to the behavior of interest, or has had little experience with it, vicarious experience is likely to have a greater impact (Takata & Takata, 1976). Additionally, when clear guidelines for performance are not explicated, personal efficacy will be more likely to be impacted by the performance of others.

VERBAL PERSUASION

Verbal persuasion involves verbally telling an individual that he or she has the capabilities to master the given behavior. Empirical support for the influence of verbal persuasion, in addition to the early research of individuals with phobias (Bandura & Adams, 1977), has been demonstrated with regard to adoption of health-promoting behavior (Meyerowitz & Chaiken, 1987), recovery after myocardial infarction (Ewart et al., 1983), performing functional activities (Resnick, 1998b), and exercising (Resnick, 2002). Persuasive health influences lead people with a high sense of efficacy to intensify efforts at self-directed change with regard to engaging in risky health behavior (Meyerowitz & Chaiken, 1987). For example, in patients after a myocardial infarction, verbal persuasion by a physician and a nurse resulted in increasing self-efficacy beliefs in regard to sexual activity, lifting, and general exertion. The counseling, or verbal persuasion, had the greatest impact on the activities that were not actually performed while in the hospital.

PHYSIOLOGICAL FEEDBACK

Individuals rely in part on information from their physiological state in order to judge their abilities. Physiological indicators are especially important in relation to coping with stressors, physical accomplishments, and health functioning. Individuals evaluate their physiological state, or arousal, and if aversive, then they may avoid performing the behavior of interest. For example, if the older adult has a fear of falling or getting hurt when walking, this high arousal state can debilitate performance and make the individual believe that he is not capable of performing the activity. Likewise, if the rehabilitation activities result in fatigue, pain, or shortness of breath, these symptoms may be interpreted as physical inefficacy, and the older adult may not feel that he is capable of performing the activity of interest.

DESCRIPTION OF THEORY: MAJOR COMPONENTS AND THEIR RELATIONSHIPS

The theory of self-efficacy states that perceived self-efficacy, defined as an individual's judgment of his or her capabilities to organize and execute courses of action, is a determinant of performance (Figure 6.1). The theory of self-efficacy must be considered within the context of reciprocal determinism as described above. The four sources of information that can potentially influence self-efficacy and outcome expectations interact with characteristics of the individual and the environment. Ideally, self-efficacy and outcome expectations are

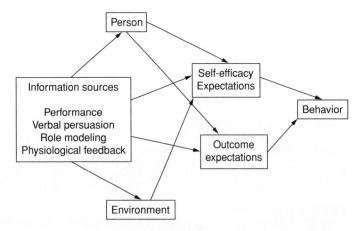

■ **Figure 6.1** Model of theory of self-efficacy.

strengthened by these experiences and thereby influence behavior. It should be recognized that at the core of this theory is the assumption that people can exercise influence over what they do. Based on reflective thought, generative use of knowledge, and skills to perform a specific behavior, as well as other tools of self-influence, a person will decide how to behave. Moreover, in order to determine one's self-efficacy, the individual must have the opportunity for self-evaluation, or the comparison of individual output to some sort of evaluative criterion (White, Kjelgaard, & Harkins, 1995). It is this comparison process that provides the individual with a sense of how likely it is that he or she can achieve a given level of performance.

Utilizing the experiences or informational sources indicated above, it has been suggested that three processes are involved in the ultimate formation of self-efficacy expectations: (a) analysis of task requirements, (b) attributional analysis of experience, and (c) assessment of personal and situational resources/constraints (Gist & Mitchell, 1992). The analysis of task requirements involves consideration of what it takes to perform an activity at various levels. The attributional analysis of experience involves the individual's judgments or attributions about why a particular performance level occurred. For example, an individual might believe that she was able to jog when tired because she had strong muscles. Lastly, the individual considers the specific resources/constraints for performing the task at various levels. This assessment includes consideration of personal factors such as skill level, anxiety, or desire, as well as situational factors, such as competing demands or distractions, that impinge on future performance. All three of these assessment processes are impacted by the individual's familiarity with the behavior and by the nature of the task itself.

RESEARCH APPLICATIONS

General Uses and Specific Examples

The early self-efficacy research by Bandura (1977) was in an ideal controlled setting in that the individuals with snake phobias were unlikely to seek out opportunities to interact with snakes when away from the laboratory setting. Therefore, there was controlled input of efficacy information. While this ideal situation is not possible in the clinical setting, the theory of self-efficacy has been used in nursing research, focusing on clinical aspects of care, education, and nursing competency and professionalism. Over the past 10 years there have been approximately 400 articles in nursing journals that focus on the measurement and use of self-efficacy expectations and/or outcome expectations to predict behavior. While the focus of the studies range from management of chronic illnesses to education of nurses and parental training, the majority have been related to chronic health problems and participation in health-promoting activities such as exercise, smoking cessation, and weight loss (Table 6.1). The majority of these studies are

Table 6.1 USE OF SELF-EFFICACY IN NURSING RESEARCH

AREA OF FOCUS	REFERENCE
Nurse care practices	Ben-Ami, Shaham, Rabin, Melzer, & Ribak, 2001; Dilorio & Price, 2001; O'Brien & Page, 1994; Rabinowitz, Kushnir, & Ribak, 1996
Managing chronic illness	
Asthma and COPD	Scherer & Schmieder, 1996, 1997; Scherer, Schmieder, & Shimmel, 1998; Siela, 1998; Sterling, 1999; Van Der Palen, Klein, Zielhuis, Van Herwaarden, & Seydel, 2001; Zimmerman et al., 1996
Diabetes	Bernal et al., 2000; Bijl et al., 1999; Johnson, 1996; Leonard et al., 1998; Lo, 1998; Remley & Cook-Newell, 1999
Depression	Kurlowicz, 1998; Perraud, 2000
Urinary incontinence	Broome, 1999
Cognitive impairment	McDougall, 1994, 1996, 1999, 2000; Mowat & Laschinger, 1994
Cancer	Boehm et al., 1995; Davis, Busch, Lowe, Taniguchi, & Djkowich, 1994; Hammond et al., 1999; Keefe et al., 1997; Lev, 1997; Lev et al., 1999; Lorig & Holman, 1998
Arthritis	Borsody et al., 1999; Jeng & Braun, 1994; Rejeski, Ettinger, Martin, & Morgan, 1998
Cardiac	Perkins & Jenkins, 1998
Osteoporosis	Ali, 1998; Horan, Kim, Gendler, Froman, & Patel, 1998
Pain	Lin & Ward, 1996
Epilepsy	Dilorio et al., 1992
HIV	Sharts-Hopko, Regan-Kubinski, Lincoln, & Heverly, 1996
Wound healing	Johnson, 1995
Nursing education	
Math	Andrew, 1998; Hodge, 1999
Undergraduate, graduate, and continuing education	Harvey & McMurray, 1994; Murdock & Neafsey, 1995; Nugent et al., 1999; Parsons, 1999
Mentoring	Hayes, 1998
Student	Goldenberg et al., 1997
Transcultural care	Jeffreys & Smodlaka, 1999; Smith, 1998
Health promotion practices	Adderley-Kelly & Green, 1997; Dilorio et al., 2000; Fletcher & Banasik, 2001; Hale & Trumbetta, 1996; Kowalski, 1997; Lindberg, 2000; Moseley, 1999; Plotnikoff et al., 2000; Resnick, 1998a, 1998b; Resnick & Jenkins, 2000; Van Der Plight & Richard, 1994
Pre- and postoperative care	Moon & Backer, 2000; Oetker-Black, 1996; Parent & Fortin, 2000; Pellino et al., 1998
Drug abuse	Washington, 1999, 2001
Maternal–child	Dennis & Faux, 1999; Dilks & Beal, 1997; Drummond & Rickwood, 1997; Gross et al., 1994; Hanson, 1998; Sinclair & O'Boyle, 1999.

descriptive in nature, exploring the relationship between self-efficacy expectations and behavior. A smaller number, however, have tested interventions developed to strengthen efficacy expectations related to the behavior of interest. What is most important with regard to the use of the theory of self-efficacy in nursing research is that the researcher maintains the behavioral specificity of self-efficacy expectations and behavior. That is, measures should be developed to fit specifically with the behavior that is being considered, and efficacy and outcome expectations should be related to a specific behavioral outcome (e.g., exercise, smoking cessation).

SELF-EFFICACY STUDIES RELATED TO MANAGING CHRONIC ILLNESS

Jenkins (1985), based on prior research regarding self-efficacy in cardiac patients (Ewart et al., 1983; Taylor, Bandura, Ewart, Miller, & DeBusk, 1985), did a descriptive study of 40 patients after a myocardial infarction. Self-efficacy measures were completed at four different data collection periods over the course of recovery. Relationships between self-efficacy expectations and behavior were only partially supported for some behaviors. Using a repeated measures analysis of variance (ANOVA), it was noted that magnitude self-efficacy scores increased over time for only two behaviors (walking and resting), and strength self-efficacy scores for each behavior generally increased over time. While this research provided some support for the theory, Jenkins suggested that the results were limited due to the small sample size, and there was limited variance due to a ceiling effect noted in the self-efficacy measures.

Jenkins built on this early research, added new items to the self-efficacy measures for cardiac recovery, and continued to study the impact of self-efficacy expectations on recovery following a cardiac event. Adding to the self-efficacy interventions developed by Gortner, Rankin, and Wolfe (1988), a larger experimental study (Gillis et al., 1993; Gortner & Jenkins, 1990) of the recovery of 156 patients following cardiac surgery was done. During the acute hospital stay, participants were randomized to receive routine information about recovery after cardiac surgery, routine information plus a slide/tape program on family coping and conflict resolution and brief counseling session, and a weekly follow-up telephone call to monitor recovery. Efficacy expectations and behaviors focused on walking, climbing, lifting, and general activity, and follow-up measures were done at 4, 8, 12, and 24 weeks via telephone. Based on repeated measures analyses, main effects of treatment were significant for increasing self-efficacy expectations for walking ($P = 0.013$) and actual walking performance ($P = 0.01$). Post hoc analyses demonstrated significantly higher levels of lifting ($P = 0.001$) and general activity ($P = 0.003$) between 4 and 8 weeks. Significant main effects of time were noted across all aspects of self-efficacy expectations, although there was little increase past week 8. Overall, this study provided some support for the impact of specific interventions to strengthen self-efficacy expectations, as well as the influence of self-efficacy on behavioral outcomes following cardiac surgery.

Allen, Becker, and Swank (1990) considered the impact of self-efficacy expectations on 125 male cardiac patients following cardiac surgery. Patients were tested on the fifth postoperative day and then 4 weeks and 6 months after discharge. Self-efficacy related to performance of activities of daily living at discharge was the best predictor of 6-month functional status. Perkins (1991) in a similar study followed 90 patients after cardiac surgery and measured self-efficacy prior to discharge from the acute care setting and 2 weeks following discharge. Self-efficacy expectations correlated with participation in all cardiac recovery behaviors except work.

Gulanick (1991) studied the impact of self-efficacy on patients after a cardiac event. In this study 40 patients 1 month after cardiac surgery or myocardial infarction were randomly assigned to one of three treatment groups. Treatment group 1 received stress testing, teaching, and exercise training; treatment group 2 received only exercise testing and teaching; and treatment group 3 (control) received only routine care. There were statistically significant differences between the three groups with regard to self-efficacy before the treatments. Following treatment both treatment groups maintained higher, though not significantly greater, self-efficacy expectations than the control group.

Schuster and Waldron (1991) studied the impact of self-efficacy expectations on attendance in a cardiac rehabilitation program. The sample included 101 participants followed over a 4-week period. On admission to rehabilitation, men were significantly better able to tolerate physical activity, had stronger self-efficacy expectations, and were less anxious than the women. Among nonbypass males, those with high self-efficacy and high activity tolerance had fewer days in attendance, and among nonbypass females, those with low self-efficacy had fewer days in attendance. There was no relationship between attendance and anxiety, self-efficacy, or activity tolerance in bypass patients of either sex.

Building on this early work, nurse researchers have also used self-efficacy expectations to increase physical activity in patients with heart failure (Borsody, Courtney, Taylor, & Jairath, 1999) and in those who have had percutaneous transluminal coronary angioplasty (Perkins & Jenkins, 1998). In addition, the impact of self-efficacy expectations on participation in cardiac rehabilitation programs (Jeng & Braun, 1994) has also been considered. Ongoing work continues in the area of recovery after a cardiac event, either acute events or planned cardiac surgery (Hiltunen et al., 2005; Lau-Walker, 2004). Hiltunen et al. (2005) implemented a home-based efficacy intervention to strengthen exercise self-efficacy among other behaviors in older adults recovering from cardiac events. Multiple behaviors related to management of vascular disease, such as medication adherence, exercise, and weight loss, have also been addressed using self-efficacy–based interventions (Sol, Graaf, Bijl, Goessens, & Visseren, 2006). Self-efficacy interventions are also used to teach nurses specific skills related to cardiac care. Specifically, a theory-based intervention was used to increase self-efficacy expectations of nurses to reduce peripherally inserted central catheter occlusion (Ngo & Murphy, 2005).

Several studies have considered self-efficacy expectations in adults with diabetes. In a descriptive study of 142 inpatients with diabetes, Hurley and Shea (1992) reported that self-efficacy expectations with regard to general management of diabetes, insulin, and diet management were predictive of follow-up diabetic self-care behaviors 4 weeks after discharge. An intervention study was done considering self-efficacy expectations with regard to diabetic self-care (diet and exercise activities) in a group of 102 older adults who volunteered to participate in a diabetes self-care program (Glasgow et al., 1992). Although the intervention resulted in an improvement in self-management skills of older diabetic adults, there was no increase in self-efficacy expectations following the intervention. It is possible that there was no increase in self-efficacy beliefs in this study because, similar to the study by Jenkins (1985) of cardiac recovery, there was a ceiling effect in the self-efficacy measure. Specifically, in this study 50% of the subjects had pretest efficacy scores of 90 or higher on the 100-point scale.

Continued research in the area of diabetes management has focused on self-management and self-care issues (Bernal, Woolley, Schensul, & Dickinson, 2000; Bijl, Poelgeest-Eeltink, & Shortridge-Baggett, 1999; Lo, 1998). Specifically, consideration has been given to exploring the relationship between self-efficacy expectations and meal planning for adolescents (Remley & Cook-Newell, 1999), to focusing on maternal self-efficacy related to diabetes management in children (Leonard, Skay, & Rheinberger, 1998), and to encouraging diabetes self-care in rural settings (Bowman & Epp, 2005).

Building off of the early work by Kaplan et al. (1984), nurse researchers have continued to focus on managing chronic obstructive pulmonary disease (COPD). In particular, research has focused on exploring the relationship between self-efficacy expectations and managing the associated shortness of breath in COPD and asthma (Siela, 1998; Scherer & Schmieder, 1996). Interventions such as educational programs and rehabilitation for COPD have been implemented and tested to determine if the interventions result in increased self-efficacy expectations and decreased symptomatology (Nguyen, Carrieri-Kohlman, Rankin, Slaughter, & Stulbarg, 2005; Scherer & Schmieder, 1997; Scherer & Shimmel, 1996; Van der Palen, Klein, & Seydel, 1997; Zimmerman, Brown, & Bowman, 1996) or decrease acute care admissions (Chen & Narsavage, 2006). As with diabetes, consideration has also been given to the impact of parental self-efficacy expectations with regard to the management of childhood asthma (Chiang, Huang, & Chao, 2005; Sterling, 1999).

Self-efficacy theory has been used repeatedly in nursing literature to explore the relationship between self-efficacy expectations and management of chronic musculoskeletal problems including osteoarthritis (Lorig & Holman, 1998), rheumatoid arthritis (Smarr et al., 1997), chronic low back pain (Lin & Ward, 1996), and fibromyalgia (Buckelew et al., 1996; Nelson & Tucker, 2006). Intervention studies have focused on strengthening self-efficacy expectations related to the management of pain (Keefe, Lefebvre, Maixner, Salley, & Caldwell, 1997), joint protection (Hammond, Lincoln, & Sutcliffe, 1999), and medication management and performance of daily activities (Taal, Rasker, & Wiegman, 1996).

Ruiz (1992) studied the impact of self-efficacy expectations of physical functioning following a hip fracture. A sample of 63 older adults (mean age 77.5) who sustained a hip fracture were interviewed once while hospitalized and then followed up by telephone at 4 and 12 weeks after surgery. A series of multiple regression analyses to determine the predictors of physical activity at each follow-up period was done, with different groups of predictors entered on each equation. In-hospital depression accounted for 7% and self-efficacy accounted for 6% of the variance in activities at 4 weeks postsurgery (eight predictors to 37 subjects in this analysis). At week 12, inpatient depression ratings accounted for 10% of the variance and inpatient self-efficacy accounted for 11% of the variance in activity (five predictors to 59 subjects). Lastly, week 4 measures of depression and self-efficacy accounted for 13% and 11%, respectively, of the variance in activity at week 12 (six predictors to 54 subjects). While there are some concerns about sample size and generalizability of these findings, they do lend support to the impact of self-efficacy expectations and mood state on function.

Resnick (1994, 1996, 1998a, 1998b, 1999, 2000a, 2002b), using combined quantitative and qualitative approaches, demonstrated that self-efficacy expectations and outcome expectations influence older adults' participation in functional activities and exercise. Based on these findings, interventions were developed to strengthen self-efficacy and outcome expectations related to these activities (Resnick, 1998a; 1998b, 2002; Resnick, Orwig, Zimmerman, Furstenberg, & Magaziner, 2001; Resnick, Magaziner, Orwig, & Zimmerman, 2002; Resnick, Orwig, Zimmerman, Simpson, & Magaziner, 2005; Resnick et al., 2006).

The relationship between mood and cognition and self-efficacy expectations has also been studied in older adults. Self-efficacy expectations related to coping with depression (Perraud, 2000), as well as the exploration of the self-efficacy for caregivers with regard to coping with individuals with cognitive impairment (Mowat & Laschinger, 1994), has been explored. In addition, interventions to strengthen self-efficacy expectations related to cognition and thereby improve cognitive ability have been tested (McDougall, 2000, 2004).

Nurse researchers in the area of oncology identified relationships between self-efficacy expectations, health promotion and disease prevention behaviors, and adaptation to cancer. Strong self-efficacy expectations, for example, predict intention to quit smoking, increased participation in screening programs, and adjustment to cancer diagnosis (Barta & Stacy, 2005; Boehm et al., 1995; Champion, Skinner, & Menon, 2005; Gaffney, 2006; Ham, 2006; Lev, 1997; Lev, Paul, & Owen, 1999; Park, Chang, & Chung, 2005). Increased self-efficacy is associated with increased adherence to treatment, increased self-care behaviors, and decreased physical and psychological symptoms (Rogers et al., 2004, 2005).

Less frequently studied is the impact of self-efficacy expectations on ulcer healing, particularly leg ulcerations (Johnson, 1995), and urinary incontinence (Broome, 1999; Chen, 2004; Kim, 2004). Self-efficacy beliefs are unlikely to change wound healing or progression of cancer. Rather, the focus of self-efficacy should be on the behavior(s) needed to promote healing of a wound, for example, or management of disease. Beliefs about the ability to perform the required behavior (self-efficacy) are associated with beliefs about a positive health outcome being contingent upon behavior performance (response efficacy).

SELF-EFFICACY STUDIES RELATED TO HEALTH PROMOTION

Self-efficacy theory has directed research in nursing with regard to a variety of health promotion activities. These studies focus on (a) exercise in middle-aged adults (Fletcher & Banasik, 2001), older adults (Resnick, 2000a, 2001, 2004; Resnick et al., 2000; Resnick, Luisi, Vogel, & Junaleepa, 2005; Resnick, Vogel, & Luisi, 2006; Shaughnessy, Resnick, & Macko, 2004), and individuals with diabetes (Plotnikoff, Brez, & Holz, 2000; Sturt, Whitlock, & Hearnshaw, 2006); (b) smoking cessation (Barta & Stacy, 2005; Gaffney, 2006; Kowalski, 1997; Macnee & Talsma, 1995); (c) cancer prevention, specifically related to breast cancer (Adderly, Kelly, & Green, 1997; Champion, Skinner, & Menon, 2005; Ham, 2006) or cervical cancer (Park, Chang, & Chung, 2005); (d) safe sexual activity in adults (Dilorio, Dudley, Soet, Watkins, & Maibach, 2000) and adolescents (van der Pligt & Richard, 1994); (e) education related to pre- and postoperative care for cardiac surgeries (Parent & Fortin, 2000) and orthopedic surgeries (Moon & Backer, 2000; Pellino et al., 1998; Yeh, Chen, & Liu, 2005); and (f) changing behavior related to drug dependence (Washington, 1999, 2001). Self-efficacy theory has likewise driven research in the area of maternal–child nursing specifically related to childbirth activities (Chang, Park, & Chung, 2004; Dilks & Beal, 1997; Drummond & Rickwood, 1997; Sinclair & O'Boyle, 1999), breast feeding (Dennis & Faux, 1999), and maternal self-efficacy expectations for care of infants and toddlers (Barnes & Adamson-Macedo, 2004; Gross, Conrad, Fogg, & Wothke, 1994; Montigny & Lacharite, 2005; Prasopkittikun, Tilokskulchai, Sinsukasai, & Sitthimongkol, 2006) and care of children with chronic illness (Cullen & Barlow, 2004; Hanson, 1998).

In addition to a clinical focus, self-efficacy–based research has guided the exploration of educational techniques for nursing. Studies of undergraduates have focused on self-efficacy expectations related to math and science (Andrew, 1998; Hodge, 1999) and clinical skills (Dilorio & Price, 2001; Ford-Gilboe, 1997; Goldenberg, Iwasiw, & MacMaster, 1997; Madorin & Iwasiw, 1999), and more recently on communication and nursing interactions with patients (Blok et al., 2004; Geanellos, 2005; Goldenberg, Andrusyszyn, & Iwasiw, 2005; Manojlovich, 2005; McConville & Lane, 2006) and cultural sensitivity (Coffman, Shellman, & Bernal, 2004; Hagman, 2004; Joseph, 2004; Lim, Downie, & Nathan, 2004; Shellman, 2006; Jimenez, Contreras, Shellman, Gonzales, & Bernal, 2006). The impact of self-efficacy expectations for the new advanced-practice nurse has also been explored (Berarducci & Lengacher, 1998; Jenkins, Shaivone, Budd, Waltz, & Griffith, 2006), as has teacher and mentor self-efficacy expectations (Nugent, Bradwhaw, & Kito, 1999; Hayes, 1998).

Use of the Theory in Nursing Practice

Translation of research findings into practice is not often done in a timely fashion. This is particularly true of research findings that focus on behavior change. There is, however, evidence to demonstrate that the theory of self-efficacy can help direct care in a variety of areas of relevance to nursing. In particular, the theory of self-efficacy has been particularly helpful with regard to motivating individuals to participate in health-promoting activities such as regular exercise, smoking cessation, weight loss, and going for recommended cancer screenings. Resnick (1999, 2001, 2002) has developed and implemented a variety of clinical programs, based on the theory of self-efficacy, to encourage exercise activity in older adults. The Seven Step Approach to Developing and Implementing an Exercise Program for community dwelling older adults incorporates the theory of self-efficacy. The seven steps are (a) education; (b) exercise pre-screening; (c) setting goals; (d) exposure to exercise; (e) role models; (f) verbal encouragement; and (g) verbal reinforcement/rewards, all of which focus on strengthening self-efficacy and outcome expectations. The theory of self-efficacy also guides the recommended steps for the development and implementation of restorative care nursing programs (Fleishell & Resnick, 2000b; Resnick & Fleishell, 1999; Resnick, 2004; Resnick et al., 2006).

Based on the theory of self-efficacy, a two-tiered approach was developed as a practical way in which to implement a successful restorative care nursing program (Resnick, 2004; Resnick et al., 2006). The two-tiered approach focuses first on teaching nursing assistants how to perform restorative care activities and how to motivate older adults to engage in these activities. The second tier focuses on the residents and the implementation of techniques to motivate these individuals to perform the necessary restorative care tasks. This program, referred to as the ResCare Intervention, includes a 6-week training program. The sessions focus on the philosophy of care that drives a restorative care nursing program, specific benefits of restorative care for the residents and staff, techniques to motivate and strengthen self-efficacy and outcome expectations of residents to perform restorative care activities, and the specific skills and techniques needed to perform restorative care activities. The training sessions are specifically geared toward (a) strengthening self-efficacy expectations and outcome expectations of the nursing assistants to perform restorative care activities; and (b) strengthening self-efficacy and outcome expectations of the residents to engage in restorative care activities with the ultimate goal of maintaining and improving optimal function.

Similarly, self-efficacy theory was used to guide the development of cardiac rehabilitation programs (Hiltunen et al., 2005; Jeng & Braun, 1994). For patients to achieve the greatest benefit from cardiac rehabilitation programs, nurses must help them to modify unhealthy behaviors. The theory of self-efficacy provides a systematic direction that allows the nurse to interpret, modify, and predict the patient's behaviors.

Changes in lifestyle are also commonly needed for individuals who must learn to live with chronic illness. The ease with which such changes occur depends on the individual's self-efficacy and outcome expectations. The self-efficacy theory has also been used to help patients manage chronic disease such as COPD and cancer. A self-management program for COPD, for example, was developed and incorporates a 6-week nurse-directed self-management program geared toward strengthening self-efficacy expectations related to managing dyspnea (Scherer & Shimmel, 1996). Likewise, there are self-efficacy–based interventions for dealing with exacerbations of fibromyalgia (Nelson & Tucker, 2006), for diabetes self-management (Sturt et al., 2006), and for nursing students to learn how to deal with difficult patients (McConville & Lane, 2006).

Instruments Used in Empirical Testing

Self-efficacy is situation specific and dynamic, in that it is focused on beliefs about personal abilities in a specific setting or in regard to a particular behavior such as dieting or exercise. Additionally, self-efficacy varies in magnitude or difficulty, strength or degree of confidence, and generality, which is the ability to generalize self-efficacy from one situation to another. Instruments to measure self-efficacy are developed to include these three parameters (Bandura, 1986; Dilorio, Faherty, & Manteuffel, 1992; O'Leary, 1985). Because self-efficacy is highly context or situation dependent, measurement tools must be developed with respect to a specific task or activity. No single standardized measure of self-efficacy will be appropriate for all studies, and researchers most often need to develop new or significantly revised measures in each investigation.

Generally, operationalization of self-efficacy expectation has been based on Bandura's (1977) early work with snake phobias. This approach included a paper-and-pencil measure with a listing of a series of activities in a specific behavioral domain that were arranged from least to most difficult. The respondents first indicated whether or not they could perform the activity, and then evaluated the degree of confidence they had in performing the given activity. Respondents were given a 100-point scale, divided into 10-unit intervals ranging from 0, which is completely uncertain, to 10, which is completely certain, to identify the extent of confidence they had in performing the activity. Additionally, generality was measured by evaluating the individuals' ability to generalize self-efficacy to other similar behaviors (initially, ability to tolerate snakes was translated to ability to tolerate spiders).

ITEM/SCALE CHARACTERISTICS

The majority of the self-efficacy scales developed have continued to use the format described by Bandura. Most commonly, researchers attempted to measure strength of self-efficacy using the confidence continuum. Vispoel (1990) reported that, when both magnitude and strength measures were included in a study, there was a strong correlation ($r = 0.90$) between the two scores. Therefore, he questioned the need to consider both aspects of self-efficacy. Additionally, the generality aspect of self-efficacy is often neglected. The researchers who have considered generality have done so indirectly by (a) correlating the magnitude or strength scores for two behaviors or (b) assessing the individual's self-efficacy to a different, though similar activity/context.

There have been some alternative-response formats used, which differ from the 0-to-10 (corresponding to 0% through 100%) confidence continuum. These include a rating scale that consists of choices from 1 to 5 or 1 to 4, and in some cases a yes/no format. Bandura, and others working in close association with him, continue to encourage the 0-to-10 format, although this is not based on empirical evidence of its greater accuracy (personal communications, Bertha Ruiz).

Two formats can be used to measure self-efficacy expectations. The dual-judgment format involves having individuals first state whether or not they can execute the given activity (i.e., measuring magnitude of self-efficacy), and if so, then they rate the strength of their perceived efficacy. In the single-judgment format, the individuals simply rate the strength of their perceived efficacy. The single-judgment format is generally used as it provides the same information as the dual-judgment and is easier to use (Bandura, 1995.

Another important issue in the measurement of self-efficacy relates to administration of the measure. The majority of self-efficacy scales have been paper-and-pencil tests (Vispoel, 1990). This type of administration was suggested to afford the participant the most privacy and encourage honesty. Some researchers have developed the scales to be given either as self-administered measures or via an interview (Jenkins, 1985). However, little research has explored whether or not there is a significant difference in using one or the other approach.

Since self-efficacy is dynamic in nature, measurement of self-efficacy is designed to be administered at different points. Additionally, it is important when measuring self-efficacy to be certain to (a) rate self-efficacy expectations before any behavior is measured, or any other scale given that could influence the individual's self-efficacy expectation; (b) include a measure of the behavior of interest that corresponds to the items in the self-efficacy scale; and (c) only measure self-efficacy in respondents who can realistically perform the activity; otherwise, it is a measure of wishful thinking, rather than a belief in one's ability to realistically perform a behavior (Bandura, 1977, 1986).

There are hundreds of different self-efficacy measures that have been identified in the literature, and these measures cover a wide range of content domain. The majority of scales have been associated with school-related and health-related content domains; however, self-efficacy related to careers, military competency, and computer use and general self-efficacy have also been developed. There are, for example, self-efficacy scales for adults with arthritis (Lomi & Nordholm, 1992; Lorig, Chastain, Ung, Shoor, & Holman, 1989) or epilepsy (Dilorio et al., 1992) or those recovering from cardiac events (Gulanick, Holm, & Kim, 1987; Hickey, Owen, & Froman, 1992; Jenkins, 1985) or orthopedic events (Ruiz, unpublished); those that consider overall physical function (Ryckman, Robbins, Thornton, & Cantrell, 1982; Schuster & Waldron, 1991), asthma management (Wigal et al., 1993), and chronic obstructive pulmonary disease (Wigal, Creer, & Kotses, 1991); and outcome expectation scales that focus on functional ability (Resnick, 1998b), exercise (Resnick et al., 2000a, 2001), adherence to osteoporosis medication (Resnick, Wehren, & Orwig 2003), performance of restorative care activities (Resnick & Simpson, 2003), and pelvic floor muscle exercise (Chen, 2004). Self-efficacy measures related to infant and child care have also been developed (Prasopkittikun et al., 2006). There are likewise numerous measures of self-efficacy–related cultural sensitivity and culture care in specific areas such as working with older adults (Shellman, 2006). Since self-efficacy and outcome expectations are behavior specific, it is essential to use an appropriate measure that truly reflects the behavior of interest. Examples of measures developed and used in nursing research are listed in Table 6.2. In-depth examples for how these measures can be developed and tested are provided to serve as a template for how this can be done.

THE SELF-EFFICACY FOR FUNCTIONAL ABILITY SCALE

The Self-Efficacy for Functional Ability (SEFA) scale (Resnick, 1999) is a nine-item measure that asks participants to rate their confidence in their ability to perform functional activities (with or without an assistive device). Specifically, these activities include bathing, dressing, transferring, toileting, ambulating, and climbing stairs. Traditionally, self-efficacy measures are ordered hierarchically from the easiest to the most difficult. There is, however, individual variation with regard to which functional task is the most difficult to perform. Therefore, random ordering of the items in the SEFA scale was done. Empirically, there was no difference in self-efficacy expectations when random ordering was done as opposed to placing items in order of increasing difficulty (Bandura, 1989).

The SEFA scale was administered using an interview format. Participants were instructed to listen to the statement and then use numbers from 0 to 10, with 0 being no confidence and 10 being very confident, to rate present beliefs in their ability to perform functional activities. The scale was scored by summing the numerical ratings for each activity and dividing by the number of activities. Self-efficacy was rated before any other scale was given to participants that might influence their self-efficacy expectations. In addition, only participants who could realistically perform the activity in question were invited to participate in the study. Otherwise, it is a measure of wishful thinking, rather than a belief in one's ability to perform a behavior.

Evidence of reliability and validity of the SEFA scale based on three studies (Resnick, 1998a, 1998b) is described in Table 6.3. These studies provide evidence for the reliability of the SEFA scale based on internal consistency using alpha coefficients and test–retest reliability. Internal consistency of the measure indicated that there was consistency of responses across the items. The high alpha coefficients

Table 6.2 SELF-EFFICACY MEASURES IN NURSING RESEARCH

AUTHOR	MEASURE
Ali, 1998	Hormone Replacement Theory Self-Efficacy Scale
Bijl et al., 1999	Self-Efficacy in New Nurse Educators
Broome, 1999	Self-Efficacy for Pelvic Muscle Exercise
Champion et al., 2005	Self-Efficacy for Mammography
Chen, 2004	Pelvic Floor Muscle Exercise Self-Efficacy Scale
Corbett, 1999	Diabetes Self-Efficacy
De Geest et al., 1994	Long-Term Medication Behavior Scale
Dennis & Faux, 1999	Breast Feeding Self-Efficacy
Dilorio & Price, 2001	Neuroscience Self-Efficacy
Fletcher & Banasik, 2001	Exercise Self-Efficacy
Froman & Owen, 1999	Physical and Mental Self-Efficacy
Hale & Trumbetta, 1996	Women's Self-Efficacy and Sexually Transmitted Disease
Hanson, 1998	Parental Self-Efficacy and Asthma Self-Efficacy
Hayes, 1998	Mentoring NP Student Self-Efficacy
Horan et al., 1998	Osteoporosis Self-Efficacy Scale
Jeffreys & Smodlaka, 1999	Transcultural Self-Efficacy Scale
Lev & Owen, 1996	Self-Care and Self-Agency Self-Efficacy
Lin & Ward, 1996	Self-Efficacy and Outcome Expectation in Coping with Chronic Low Back Pain
Madorin & Iwasiw, 1999	Self-Efficacy of Baccalaureate Nurses
Moseley, 1999	Food Pyramid Self-Efficacy
Oetker-Black, 1996	Preop Self-Efficacy
Perraud, 2000	Depression Coping Self-Efficacy Scale
Prasopkittikun et al., 2006	Self-Efficacy in Infant Care Scale
Remley & Cook-Newell, 1999	Meal Planning Self-Efficacy
Resnick & Jenkins, 2000	Self-Efficacy for Exercise
Resnick, 1999	Self-Efficacy for Functional Activities
Resnick, Wehren, & Orwig, 2003	Self-Efficacy and Outcome Expectations for Osteoporosis Medication Adherence
Resnick & Simpson, 2003	Self-Efficacy for Restorative Care Activities
Resnick, 2005	Outcome Expectations for Exercise-2
Shellman, 2006	Eldercare Cultural Self-Efficacy Scale
Sinclair & O'Boyle, 1999	Childbirth Self-Efficacy

Table 6.3 DESCRIPTIVE STATISTICS OF PILOT SAMPLE

VARIABLE	STUDY I Frequency (%) (*n* = 51 participants in rehabilitation program)	STUDY II Frequency (%) (*n* = 77 participants in rehabilitation program)	STUDY III Frequency (%) (*n* = 44 residents in long-term care facility)
Gender			
Males	11 (22%)	22 (29%)	7 (16%)
Females	40 (78%)	55 (71%)	37 (84%)
Marital status			
Married	20 (39%)	-	8 (12%)
Widowed	30 (59%)	-	50 (73%)
Never married	1 (2%)	-	11 (15%)
Race			
White	44 (86%)	63 (82%)	44 (100%)
Black	7 (14%)	14 (18%)	
Age	77 ± 8	78 ± 7.2	88 ± 6.4
SEFA (admission)	5.9 ± 1	5.6 ± 2	5.6 ± 2.9
SEFA (discharge)	8.3 ± .8	8.8 ± 1.5	
Functional	50 ± 6.8	44 ± 8.5	59 ± 18.5
Performance	65 ± 5.8	63 ± 7.8	

suggested that performance on any one item of the instrument was a good indicator of performance on any other item of the instrument. Test–retest reliability of the SEFA scale suggested that the measure was reliable when given in close temporal proximity.

There was sufficient evidence for the concurrent validity of the SEFA scale, and as anticipated, less consistent support for the predictive validity of the measure. Self-efficacy expectations related to functional activities reflect the individual's motivation to perform these activities, and theoretically will predict behavior, particularly behavior that is measured in *close* temporal proximity to self-efficacy expectations.

There also was support for the construct validity of the measure, suggesting that it can be used to identify those individuals with low self-efficacy expectations related to functional activities. These individuals can then be exposed to interventions to strengthen self-efficacy expectations such as practicing the behavior, verbal persuasion, exposure to role models who successfully perform functional activities, and specific interventions to decrease the unpleasant physical sensations and affective states that are associated with the activity (Bandura, 1997; Resnick, 1996). Ultimately, this will help to improve performance of functional activities.

Additional evidence for the construct validity of the SEFA scale was further supported by hypothesis testing. As hypothesized, there was a statistically significant negative relationship between SEFA and fear of falling with depression, and a statistically significant positive relationship between SEFA and another measure of motivation (the Apathy Evaluation Scale). This work provided evidence that the SEFA measure is appropriate for older adults in a variety of settings.

SELF-EFFICACY FOR EXERCISE SCALE

The Self-Efficacy for Exercise (SEE) scale (Resnick & Jenkins, 2000) is a revision of McAuley's (unpublished) self-efficacy barriers to exercise measure. The self-efficacy barriers to exercise measure is a 13-item measure that focuses on self-efficacy expectations related to the ability to continue to exercise in the face of barriers to exercising. This measure was initially developed for sedentary adults in the community who participated in an outpatient exercise program (including biking, rowing, and walking). Based on previous research, there was sufficient evidence for reliability (alpha coefficient = 0.93) (McAuley, Lox, & Duncan, 1993), and validity with efficacy expectations being significantly correlated with actual participation in an exercise program (McAuley, 1992, 1993).

The revision of McAuley's self-efficacy barriers to exercise measure was based on a combined quantitative and qualitative study exploring factors that influenced adherence to a regular walking program for older adults (Resnick & Spellbring, 2000). A total of 24 older adults living in a continuing care retirement community were included in this study. The average age of the participants in that study was 81 ± 7.2 years, and the majority were female ($n = 21$, 91%) and unmarried ($n = 18$, 88%). All of the participants were Caucasian and had at least completed high school. There was a statistically significant correlation between efficacy expectations related to exercise and adherence to a regular exercise program ($r = 0.42$, $P < 0.05$). Adherence was defined as participating in 20 minutes of walking exercise two to three times per week, and was based on verbal report of the participants confirmed by records kept by the walking program coordinator.

The participants in this exploratory study identified several items on the self-efficacy barriers to exercise measure that were not relevant to them: (a) a question related to the impact of taking a vacation on exercise activity, (b) issues related to getting to the exercise location, (c) feeling self-conscious about one's appearance while exercising, and (d) lack of encouragement from the leader. These questions were therefore removed from the initial measure. There were two questions that participants felt were repetitive (both related to the individuals' interest in the activity), and these questions were combined into a single item (item 5) on the revised measure. Qualitative interviews indicated that past experiences with exercise, identification of goals, personality, sensations associated with exercise such as pain, and mood all influenced exercise activity. Therefore, appropriate items relevant to these issues (items 1, 3, and 9) were added to the SEE measure.

Initial reliability and validity testing was done using a sample of 187 older adults living in a continuing care retirement community. The average age of the participants was 85 ± 6.2 years, and the majority were Caucasian (98%), female (82%), and unmarried (80%). Face-to-face interviews were completed and included the SEE and the Short-Form Health Survey (SF-12) (Ware, Kosinski, & Keller, 1996). Exercise activity was based on verbal report of participation in aerobic exercise (walking, swimming, biking, or jogging). There was sufficient evidence of internal consistency (alpha = 0.92). Using structural equation modeling, R^2 was used to provide further evidence of reliability. This approach is based on a definition of reliability that states that reliability of X (test score) is "the magnitude of the direct relations that all variables have on X" (Bollen, 1989, p. 54). Specifically, R^2 provides a gauge of the systematic variance in the observed score that can be explained by each item in the measurement model (Bollen, 1989; Jagodzinski & Kuhnel, 1987; Reuterberg & Gustafsson, 1992). R^2 ranged from 0.38 to 0.76, with over half of the items being >0.50. There was evidence of validity of the measure based on hypothesis testing: Mental and physical health scores on the SF-12 predicted efficacy expectations, and efficacy expectations predicted exercise activity. Likewise, confirmatory factor analysis provided further evidence of validity. All of the items loaded significantly on the construct self-efficacy and had loadings >0.81.

BOX 6.1   Factors That Influence Adherence to Osteoporosis Medication

Stomach upset
Fear of stomach upset/ulceration
Inconvenience of AM schedule
Cost
Uncertainty about the effects

Lack of knowledge as to need for the
  medication
Constipation
Don't think it is necessary because of low risk
  of disease

THE SELF-EFFICACY FOR OSTEOPOROSIS MEDICATION ADHERENCE SCALE

Previous research exploring the development of long-term medication behavior self-efficacy expectations resulted in the identification of three major categories that influence adherence (De Geest, Abraham, Germoets, & Evers, 1994). These categories are (a) personal attributes, such as emotions, perceived health status, and confidence in the physician; (b) environmental factors such as routine, distraction, cost, and social support; and (c) task-related and behavioral factors such as medication aids, schedules, knowledge about the medication, drug delivery system, and side effects.

Focus groups were held to identify the issues around adherence (particularly the barriers and challenges to adherence) to osteoporosis medication for older adults. Two separate meetings of a total of 50 older men and women were held. These meetings were convened for educational purposes, and included a presentation on osteoporosis. At the end of the presentation, there was open discussion about the issues surrounding medication adherence. Box 6.1 lists the most common challenges identified by the older adults as influencing adherence. Based on these findings, the self-efficacy for osteoporosis medication adherence measures were developed.

The Self-Efficacy for Osteoporosis Medication Adherence (SEOMA) scale (Resnick, Wehren, & Orwig, 2003) is a 14-item measure that addresses the many challenges associated with taking medication for osteoporosis. Examples of these challenges include consideration of adherence in light of side effects such as constipation or stomach upset, or due to the high cost of the treatment. To complete the SEOMA scale, the participant was instructed to listen to a statement and then use numbers from 0 to 10, with 0 being not confident and 10 being very confident, to rate present self-efficacy expectations related to adhering to his or her osteoporosis medication.

Initial reliability and validity testing was based on a study that included 152 older adults with a mean age of 85.7 ± 5.5 years, the majority of whom were Caucasian (99%), female (74%), and unmarried (75%). In addition to the SEOMA scale, demographic information (age, gender, and marital status) and other health behaviors (exercise and osteoporosis medication use) were explored. There was evidence of reliability based on internal consistency (alpha = 0.98). For the SEOMA, there were two items with R^2 values <0.50. These items were item 4, "When you are feeling sick to your stomach," and item 14, "When the medication upsets your stomach, causes constipation, or other side effects."

Confirmatory factor analysis provided evidence of the validity of the SEOMA scale. All factor loadings loaded significantly onto the construct of self-efficacy and a total of 77% of the variance in self-efficacy expectations for medication adherence was accounted for by the measure. There was evidence of criterion-related validity based on a multiple regression analysis. Age, gender, exercise, cognitive status, history of previous fracture, and self-efficacy and outcome expectations related to adherence to osteoporosis medications were entered as predictors of medication adherence. Self-efficacy expectation explained 15% of the variance in medication adherence, gender explained an additional 7% of the variance in adherence to osteoporosis medication, exercise added another 5%, and outcome expectations explained an additional 3% of the variance.

OUTCOME EXPECTATIONS FOR EXERCISE SCALE

The Outcome Expectations for Exercise (OEE) scale is a nine-item scale that was developed based on several previously tested measures that focused on the outcome expectations and benefits associated with exercise in adults (Sechrist, Walker, & Pender, 1987; Steinhardt & Dishman, 1989), as well as qualitative and quantitative studies that identified the specific benefits of exercise to older adults (Conn, 1998; Melillo et al., 1996; Resnick & Spellbring, 2000; Schneider, 1997; Sharon, Hennessy, Brandon, & Boyette, 1997). In these studies, older adults reported that exercise made them feel better and walk better, improved their blood pressure control, and decreased pain. Psychological benefits included feelings of having accomplished something, enjoying the activity, and experiencing an overall sense of well-being. While many of the same concepts were included in earlier versions of measures that focused on the benefits of exercise, the items for the OEE scale were written using the older adults' *own words* to describe the benefits they derived from exercise. Five of the items reflected physical benefits and four focused on mental health benefits. Item 9 was included in the measure as there has been a strong emphasis in the lay literature suggesting that exercise increases bone strength and prevents osteoporosis.

To complete the OEE scale, the participant is asked to listen to a statement about exercise and to strongly agree (1), agree (2), neither agree nor disagree (3), disagree (4), or strongly disagree (5) with the stated outcomes or benefits of exercising. The following nine statements are included:

1. Makes me feel better physically (physical health)
2. Makes my mood better in general (mental health)
3. Helps me feel less tired (physical health)
4. Makes my muscles stronger (physical health)
5. Is an activity I enjoy doing (mental health)
6. Gives me a sense of personal accomplishment (mental health)
7. Makes me more alert mentally (mental health)
8. Improves my endurance in performing my daily activities (physical health)
9. Helps to strengthen my bones (physical health)

The OEE scale was administered using an interview format. The scale was scored by summing the numerical ratings for each response and dividing by the number of responses. OEE scores range from 1 to 5, with 1 indicative of low outcome expectations for exercise and 5 strong outcome expectations for exercise.

Content validity of the OEE scale was established by initially reviewing the items with a group of four researchers who were familiar with the issues related to motivation and exercise adherence in older adults. The four researchers agreed with the items identified and proposed some wording changes so that the measure would be better understood by the older adult. The measure was then sent to two researchers who were familiar with measures that considered the benefits and barriers of exercise for older adults, and two geriatric nurse practitioners. These individuals were asked to rate the relevancy of the items on a scale of 1 (not very relevant) to 4 (very relevant). All four reviewers rated the items as either relevant or very relevant.

Initial reliability and validity testing was based on a sample of 175 community-dwelling older adults (Resnick et al., 2000). Face-to-face surveys were completed that included the OEE scale and demographic information including age, gender, race, education, and marital status; exercise behavior and activity were measured using the Yale Physical Activity Survey (YPAS) (DiPietro, Caspersen, Ostfeld, & Nadel, 1993). There was support for the internal consistency of the OEE scale (alpha coefficient = 0.89). There was some support for reliability based on R^2 estimates, although less than half of these were >0.5. There was evidence of validity of the measure based on a confirmatory factor analysis as all of the items loaded significantly on the construct outcome expectations, and there was a fair fit of the model to the data Normed Fit Index (NFI) = 0.99, Root Mean Square Error of Approximation (RMSEA) = 0.07, χ^2/degrees of freedom [df] = 2.8). Construct validity was also supported based on hypothesis testing. It was hypothesized that those who exercised regularly had higher OEE scores than those who did not (F = 31.3, P <.05, eta squared = 0.15). It was also hypothesized that there would be a statistically significant relationship between outcome expectations and self-efficacy expectations (r = 0.66). Based on a Rasch analysis, this measure has subsequently been revised to include four negative outcomes associated with exercise that were commonly noted to prevent or influence the older adults' willingness to exercise (Resnick, 2005).

THE OUTCOME EXPECTATIONS FOR OSTEOPOROSIS MEDICATION ADHERENCE SCALE

The Outcome Expectations for Osteoporosis Medication Adherence (OEOMA) scale was developed based on findings from the focus groups as described under the SEOMA scale. The measure included five items that focus on the benefits associated with taking medication for osteoporosis. Examples include such things as strengthening bones and preventing fractures, decreasing the fear of falling, and decreasing the risk of developing osteoporosis. Responses to the OEOMA scale ranged from 1 (strongly disagree) to 5 (strongly agree). The scales were scored by summing the numerical ratings for each response and dividing by the number of responses. This score was indicative of the strength of efficacy expectations.

Initial reliability and validity testing was done as described above in the section related to the SEOMA scale. There was evidence of internal consistency with an alpha coefficient of 0.79. There was some evidence for reliability based on estimates of R^2. Specifically, for the OEOMA scale there was only one item that had an R^2 <0.50. This was item 2, "Makes me more confident and less afraid of falling." There was evidence of construct validity based on confirmatory factor analysis. All of the items were statistically significantly loaded onto the construct outcome expectations and together these items explained 73% of the variance in outcome expectations for medication adherence. Model fit, however, of the measurement models was poor: χ^2 was 30, degrees of freedom 5, P <.05, and ratio of χ^2/df 6.0. The NFI was 0.98 and the RMSEA was 0.12 (Bollen, 1989).

As with the SEOMA scale, there was evidence of criterion-related validity of the OEOMA scale based on a multiple regression analysis. Age, gender, exercise, cognitive status, history of prior fracture, and self-efficacy and outcome expectations related to adherence to osteoporosis medications were entered as predictors of medication adherence. Although it was the last variable that was entered into the model, outcome expectations explained an additional 3% of the variance in medication adherence.

SUMMARY

Empirical testing using the theory of self-efficacy has provided significant support for the importance of self-efficacy and outcome expectations with regard to behavior and changing behavior. There is also some support for the effectiveness of specific interventions that have been tested to strengthen both self-efficacy and outcome expectations and thereby improve or change behavior. It is important to note, however, that

ANALYSIS OF THEORY

Using the criteria presented in Chapter 2, critique the theory of self-efficacy. Compare your conclusions about the theory with those found in Appendix A. A researcher who has worked with the theory completed the analysis found in the appendix.

Internal Criticism
1. Clarity
2. Consistency
3. Adequacy

4. Logical development
5. Level of theory development

External Criticism
1. Reality convergence
2. Utility
3. Significance
4. Discrimination
5. Scope of theory
6. Complexity

these studies also serve as a reminder that self-efficacy and outcome expectations may not be the *only* predictors of behavior. Other variables, such as tension/anxiety, barriers to behavior, and other psychosocial constructs, likewise influence behavior. Bandura (1986) recognized that expectations alone will not result in behavior change if there is not incentive to perform, or if there are inadequate resources or external constraints. Certainly, an individual may believe he or she can participate in a rehabilitation program, but may not have the resources (i.e., transportation or money) to do so.

Self-efficacy theory is situation specific. It is difficult, therefore, to generalize an individual's self-efficacy expectations from one type of behavior to another. If an individual has high self-efficacy with regard to diet management, this may or may not generalize to persistence in an exercise program. Consequently, it is essential to utilize appropriate self-efficacy measures or develop an appropriate measure that is relevant to the behavior of interest. This requires the preliminary work of understanding that behavior, particularly the challenges associated with performance and the consequences (both positive and negative) of performance of the behavior.

Self-efficacy and outcome expectation measures should be developed to comprehensively include a series of activities/challenges listed in order of increasing difficulty. It is important to carefully construct these scales and establish evidence of reliability and validity. Since self-efficacy and outcome expectations can be influenced by the many sources of efficacy expectations (e.g., performing a behavior), in most situations it is not appropriate to estimate reliability using test–retest reliability. Although useful in research as either predictors or outcomes of behavior, these scales can be used as the foundation for assessing an individual's self-care abilities in a particular area. Interventions can then be developed that are relevant for that individual.

As with most research findings, use of the theory of self-efficacy, assessments of individual self-efficacy and outcome expectations, and implementation of interventions to strengthen self-efficacy or outcome expectations in real-world settings is slow. Measurement tools can be used clinically to evaluate the individual's efficacy expectations and the health care provider can then implement appropriate interventions to strengthen expectations. For example, if completion of the OEOMA scale indicated that the individual did not believe that taking osteoporosis medication strengthened bones, appropriate interventions would focus on educational sessions that reviewed the impact of osteoporosis medication on bone and bone density.

There are several areas of self-efficacy–based research that have not yet been comprehensively addressed. Consistently, there has been a lack of consideration of outcome expectations and most researchers ignore

CRITICAL THINKING EXERCISES

1. As a nurse on a medical surgical unit you are getting ready to discharge a patient home who has just had a hip fracture and a right hemiorthoplasty to repair the fracture. She is independent with ambulation using her walker and will have some home physical therapy. Of note, however, she had a bone density scan that indicated severe osteoporosis and has been started on a bisphosphonate and calcium. Your goal at discharge is to increase the likelihood that she will adhere to taking these medications. Address the interventions you would do to ensure this.

2. You have just moved to New Mexico and are very concerned about working with a large percentage of Spanish-speaking older adults. You know little about their culture. Address what interventions you might do for yourself to facilitate this transition in your nursing career.

3. You have just started working on a maternity ward and note that the mothers admitted who are younger than 20 years of age have a great deal of difficulty with the idea of breast feeding and how to begin to breast feed. Develop an intervention that you could implement to optimize your nursing interventions with these individuals.

this component of the theory. With regard to exercise in older adults, however, outcome expectations have been noted to be better predictors of exercise behavior than self-efficacy expectations (Resnick et al., 2000; Jette et al., 1998). Increased focus is needed on outcome expectations as this can have a significant influence on the types of interventions developed to strengthen efficacy expectations and alter behavior.

Consideration also needs to be given to the influence of self-efficacy and outcome expectations to not only initiate behavior, but more importantly to adhere to that behavior over time. Most of the current work in this area considers the immediate influence of self-efficacy and outcome expectations, or the impact of these expectations over a relatively short time frame.

WEB RESOURCES

Self-efficacy information and appropriate readings: **http://www.des.emory.edu/mfp/self-efficacy.html**

Manual for Occupational Self-efficacy Scale: **https://www.des.emory.edu/mfp/self-efficacy.**

Diabetes Self-efficacy Scale: **http://patienteducation.stanford.edu/research/sediabetes.html**

Exercise Self-efficacy Scale: **http://www.des.emory.edu/mfp/self-efficacy.html**

Alcohol Self-efficacy Scale: **http://pubs.niaaa.nih.gov/publications/Assesing%20Alcohol/InstrumentPDFs/08_AASE.pdf**

REFERENCES

Adderley-Kelly, B. & Green, P. M. (2000). Health promotion for urban middle school students: a survey of learning needs. *Journal of the National Black Nurses Association, 11*(2), 34–38.

Ali, N. (1998). Hormone replacement therapy self-efficacy scale. *Journal of Advanced Nursing, 28*(5), 1115–1119.

Allen, J. K., Becker, D. M., & Swank, R. T. (1990). Factors related to functional status after coronary artery bypass surgery. *Heart Lung, 19*(4), 337–343.

Andrew, S. (1998). Self-efficacy as a predictor of academic performance in science. *Journal of Advanced Nursing, 27*(3), 596–603.

Bandura, A. (1977). Self-efficacy: Toward a unifying theory of behavioral change. *Psychological Review, 84*, 191–215.

Bandura, A. (1982). The assessment and predictive generality of self-percepts of efficacy. *Journal of Behavior Therapy and Experimental Psychiatry, 13*(3), 195–199.

Bandura, A. (1986). *Social foundations of thought and action*. New Jersey: Prentice Hall.

Bandura, A. (1989). Human agency in social cognitive theory. *American Psychology, 44*(9), 1175–1184.

Bandura, A. (1995). *Self-efficacy in changing societies*. New York: Cambridge University Press.

Bandura, A. (1997). *Self-efficacy: The exercise of control*. New York: W.H. Freeman.

Bandura, A., & Adams, N. (1977). Analysis of self-efficacy theory of behavioral change. *Cognitive Therapy and Research, 1*(4), 287–308.

Bandura, A., Adams, N., & Beyer, J. (1977). Cognitive processes mediating behavioral change. *Journal of Personality and Social Psychology, 35*(3), 125–149.

Bandura, A., Adams, N., Hardy, A., & Howells, G. (1980). Tests of the generality of self-efficacy theory. *Cognitive Therapy and Research, 4*, 39–66.

Bandura, A., Reese, L., & Adams, N. (1982). Microanalysis of action and fear arousal as a function of differential levels of perceived self-efficacy. *Journal of Personality and Social Psychology, 43*, 5–21.

Barnes, C. R., & Adamson-Macedo, E. N. (2004). Perceived Parenting Self-efficacy (PMP S-E) of mothers who are breastfeeding hospitalized preterm neonates. *Neuro Endocrinology Letters, 25*(Suppl 1), 95–102.

Barta, S. K., & Stacy, R. D. (2005). The effects of a theory-based training program on nurses' self-efficacy and behavior for smoking cessation counseling. *Journal of Continuing Education in Nursing, 36*(3), 117–123.

Ben-Ami, S., Shaham, J., Rabin, S., Melzer, A., & Ribak, J. (2001). The influence of nurses knowledge, attitudes and health beliefs on their safe behavior with cytotoxic drugs in Israel. *Cancer Nursing, 24*(3), 192–200.

Berarducci, A., & Lengacher, C. (1998). Self-efficacy: An essential component of advanced practice nursing. *Nursing Connections, 11*(1), 55–67.

Bernal, H., Woolley, S., Schensul, J., & Dickenson, J. (2000). Correlates of self-efficacy in diabetes self-care among Hispanic adults with diabetes. *Diabetes Educator, 26*, 673–680.

Bijl, J., Poelgeest-Eeltink, A., & Shortridge-Baggett, L. (1999). The psychometric properties of the diabetes management self-efficacy scale for patients with type 2 diabetes mellitus. *Journal of Advanced Nursing, 30*(2), 352–359.

Blok, G. A., Morton, J., Morley, M., Kerckhoffs, C. C., Kootstra, G., & Van der Vleuten, C. P. (2004). Requesting organ donation: The case of self-efficacy—effects of the European Donor Hospital Education Programme (EDHEP). *Advances in Health Science Education Theory and Practice, 9*(4), 261–282.

Boehm, S., Coleman-Burns, P., Schlenk, E., Funnell, M. M., Parzuchowski, J., Powel, I. J. (1995). Prostate cancer in African American men: increasing knowledge and self-efficacy. *Journal of Community Health Nursing, 12*(3), 161–169.

Bollen, K. (1989). *Structural equations with latent variables*. New York: Wiley.

Borsody, J., Courtney, M., Taylor, K., & Jairath, N. (1999). Using self-efficacy to increase physical activity in patients with heart failure. *Home Healthcare Nurse, 17*(2), 113–118.

Bowman, A., & Epp, D. (2005). Rural diabetes education: Does it make a difference? *Canadian Journal of Nursing Research, 37*(1), 34–53.

Broome, B. (1999). Development and testing of a scale to measure self-efficacy for pelvic muscle exercises in women with urinary incontinence. *Urology Nursing, 19*(4), 258–268.

Buckelew, S. P., Huyset, B., Hewett, J. E., Parker, J. C., Johnson, J. C., Conway, R., et al. (1996). Self-efficacy predicting outcome among fibromyalgia subjects. *Arthritis Care Research, 9*(2), 82–88.

Chambliss, C., & Murray, E. (1979). Efficacy attribution, locus of control, and weight loss. *Cognitive Therapy and Research, 3*, 349–353.

Champion, V., Skinner, C. S., & Menon, U. (2005). Development of a self-efficacy scale for mammography. *Research in Nursing and Health, 28*(4), 329–336.

Chang, S., Park, S., & Chung, C. (2004). Effect of Taegyo-focused prenatal education on maternal-fetal attachment and self-efficacy related to childbirth. *Taehan Kanho Hakhoe Chi, 34*(8), 1409–1415.

Chen, W. Y. (2004). The development and testing of the pelvic floor muscle exercise self-efficacy scale. *Journal of Nursing Research, 12*(4), 257–266.

Chen, Y. J., & Narsavage, G. L. (2006). Factors related to chronic obstructive pulmonary disease readmission in Taiwan. *Western Journal of Nursing Research, 28*(1), 105–124.

Chiang, L. C., Huang, J. L., & Chao, S. Y. (2005). A comparison, by quantitative and qualitative methods, between the self-management behaviors of parents with asthmatic children in two hospitals. *Journal of Nursing Research 13*(2), 85–96.

Coffman, M. J., Shellman, J., & Bernal, H. (2004). An integrative review of American nurses' perceived cultural self-efficacy. *Journal of Nursing Scholarship, 36*(2), 180–185.

Colletti, G., Supnick, J., & Payne, A. (1985). The smoking self-efficacy questionnaire (SSEQ): Preliminary scale development and validation. *Behavioral Assessment, 6*(3), 234–238.

Condiotte, M., and Lichtenstein, E. (1981). Self-efficacy and relapse in smoking cessation programs. *Journal of Consulting Clinical Psychology, 49*, 648–658.

Conn, V. (1998). Older adults and exercise. *Nursing Research, 47*, 180–189.

Corbett, C. (1999). Research-based practice implications for patients with diabetes. Part II: Diabetes self-efficacy. *Home Healthcare Nurse, 17*(9), 587–596.

Cullen, L. A., & Barlow, J. H. (2004). A training and support programme for caregivers of children with disabilities: An exploratory study. *Patient Education and Counseling, 55*(2), 203–209.

Damush, T. M., Stump, T. E. Saporito, & Clark, D. O. (2001). Predictors of older primary care patients' participation in a submaximal exercise test and a supervise, low-impact exercise class. *Preventive Medicine, 33*(5), 485–494.

Davis, P., Busch, A. J., Lowe, J. C., Taniguchi, J., & Djkowich, B. (1994). Evaluation of a rheumatoid arthritis patient education program: Impact on knowledge and self-efficacy. *Patient Education and Counseling, 24*(1), 55–61.

De Geest, S., Abraham, I., Gemoets, H., & Evers, G. (1994). Development of the long-term medication behavior self-efficacy scale: qualitative study for item development. *Journal of Advanced Nursing, 19*(2), 233–238.

Dennis, C., & Faux, S. (1999). Development and psychometric testing of the breastfeeding self-efficacy scale. *Research in Nursing and Health, 22*(5), 399–409.

Dilks, F., & Beal, J. (1997). Role of self-efficacy in birth choice. *Journal of Perinatal and Neonatal Nursing, 11*(1), 1–9.

Dilorio, C., Dudley, W., Soet, J., Watkins, J., & Maibach, E. (2000). A social cognitive based model for condom use among college students. *Nursing Research, 49*(4), 208–214.

Dilorio, C., Faherty, B., & Manteuffel, B. (1992). Instrument to measure self-efficacy in individuals with epilepsy. *Journal of Neuroscience Nursing, 24*(1), 9–13.

Dilorio, C., & Price, M. (2001). Description and use of the neuroscience nursing self-efficacy scale. *Journal of Neuroscience Nursing, 33*(3), 130–135.

DiPietro, L., Caspersen, C., Ostfeld, A., & Nadel, E. (1993). A survey for assessing physical activity a month older adults. *Medical Science Sports and Exercise, 25,* 628–642.

Drummond, J., & Rickwood, D. (1997). Childbirth confidence: Validating the childbirth self-efficacy inventory (CBSEI) in an Australian sample. *Journal of Advanced Nursing, 26*(3), 613–622.

Ewart, C., Taylor, G., Reese, L., & DeBusk, R. (1983). Effects of early post-myocardial infarction exercise testing on self-perception and subsequent physical activity. *The American Journal of Cardiology, 51,* 1076–1080.

Fletcher, J., & Banasick, J. (2001). Exercise self-efficacy. *Clinical Excellence for Nurse Practitioners, 5*(3), 134–143.

Fleishell, A., & Resnick, B. (1999). *Stayin alive: Minimizing loss and maximizing potential. Manual for restorative care nursing programs.* Laurel, MD: Joanne Wilson's Gerontological Nursing Ventures.

Ford-Gilboe, M. (1997). Family strengths, motivation, and resources as predictors of health promotion behavior in single-parent and two-parent families. *Research in Nursing and Health, 20*(3), 205–217.

Froman, R. D., & Owen, S. V. (1999). American and Korean adolescents' physical and mental health self-efficacy. *Journal of Pediatric Nursing, 14*(1), 51–58.

Gaffney, K. F. (2006). Postpartum smoking relapse and becoming a mother. *Journal of Nursing Scholarship, 38*(1), 26–30.

Geanellos, R. (2005). Undermining self-efficacy: The consequence of nurse unfriendliness on client wellbeing. *Collegian, 12*(4), 9–14.

Gillis, C., Gortner, S., Hauck, W., Shinn, J., Sparacino, P., & Tompkins, C. (1993). A randomized clinical trial of nursing care for recovery from cardiac surgery. *Heart & Lung, 22*(2), 125–133.

Gist, M., and Mitchell, T. (1992). Self-efficacy: A theoretical analysis of its determinants and malleability. *Academy of Management Review, 17*(2), 183–211.

Glasgow, R., Toobert, D., Hampson, S., Brown, J., Lewinston, P., & Donnelly, J. (1992). Improving self-care among older patients with type II diabetes: The Sixty Something study. *Patient Education and Counseling, 19,* 61–70.

Goldenberg, D., Andrusyszyn, M. A., & Iwasiw, C. (2005). The effect of classroom simulation on nursing students' self-efficacy related to health teaching. *Journal of Nursing Education, 44*(7), 310–314.

Goldenberg, D., Iwasiw, C., & MacMaster, E. (1997). Self-efficacy of senior baccalaureate nursing students and preceptors. *Nurse Educator Today, 17*(4), 303–310.

Gortner, S., & Jenkins, L. (1990). Self-efficacy and activity level following cardiac surgery. *Journal of Advanced Nursing, 15,* 1132–1138.

Gortner, S., Rankin, S., & Wolfe, M. (1988). Elders' recovery from cardiac surgery. *Progress in Cardiovascular Nursing, 34*–61.

Grembowski, D., Patrick, D., Diehr, P., Durham, M., Beresford, S., Kay, E., et al. (1993). Self-efficacy and health behavior among older adults. *Journal of Health and Social Behavior, 34,* 89–104.

Gross, D., Conrad, B., Fogg, L., & Wothke, W. (1994). A longitudinal model of maternal self-efficacy, depression, and difficult temperament during toddlerhood. *Research in Nursing and Health, 17*(3), 207–215.

Gulanick, M. (1991). Is phase 2 cardiac rehabilitation necessary for early recovery of patients with cardiac disease? A randomized, controlled study. *Heart & Lung, 20*(1), 9–15.

Gulanick, M., Kim, M.M., & Holm, K. (1991). Resumption of home activities following cardiac events. *Progressions in Cardiovascular Nursing, 6*(1), 21–28.

Hagman, L. W. (2004). New Mexico nurses' cultural self-efficacy: A pilot study. *Journal of Cultural Diversity, 11*(4), 146–149.

Hale, P., & Trumbetta, S. (1996). Women's self-efficacy and sexually transmitted disease preventive behaviors. *Research in Nursing and Health, 19*(2), 101–110.

Ham, O. K. (2006). Factors affecting mammography behavior and intention among Korean women. *Oncology Nursing Forum, 33*(1), 113–119.

Hammond, A., Lincoln, N., & Sutcliffe, L. (1999). A crossover trial evaluating an educational-behavioral joint protection programme for people with rheumatoid arthritis. *Patient Education and Counseling, 37*(1), 19–32.

Hanson, J. (1998). Parental self-efficacy and asthma self-management skills. *Journal of Society of Pediatric Nurses, 3*(4), 146–154.

Harvey, V., & McMurray, N. (1994). Self-efficacy: a means of identifying problems in nursing education and career progress. *International journal of Nursing Studies, 31*(5), 471–485.

Hayes, E. (1998). Mentoring and nurse practitioner student self-efficacy. *Western Journal of Nursing Research, 20*(5), 521–535.

Hickey, M., Owen, S., & Froman, R. (1992). Instrument development: Cardiac diet and exercise self-efficacy. *Nursing Research, 41*(6), 347–351.

Hiltunen, E. F., Winder, P. A., Rait, M. A., Buselli, E. F., Carroll, D. L., & Rankin, S. H. (2005). Implementation of efficacy enhancement nursing interventions with cardiac elders. *Rehabilitation Nursing, 30*(6), 221–229.

Hodge, M. (1999). Do anxiety, math self-efficacy and gender affect nursing students' drug dosage calculations? *Nurse Educator, 24*(4), 36, 41.

Horan, M., Kim, K., Gendler, P., Froman, R., & Patel, M. (1998). Development and evaluation of an osteoporosis self-efficacy scale. *Research in Nursing and Health, 21*(5), 395–403.

Hurley, D., & Shea, C. (1992). Self-efficacy: Strategy for enhancing diabetes self-care. *The Diabetes Educator, 18*(2), 146–150.

Jagodzinski, W., & Kuhnel, S. (1987). Estimation of reliability and stability in single-indicator multiple-wave models. *Sociological Methods & Research, 15,* 219–258.

Jeffreys, M., & Smodlaka, I. (1999). Construct validation of the transcultural self-efficacy tool. *Journal of Nurse Educator, 38*(5), 222–227.

Jeng, C., & Braun, L. T. (1994). Bandura's self-efficacy theory: A guide for cardiac rehabilitation nursing practice. *Journal of Holistic Nursing, 12*(4), 425–436.

Jenkins, L. (1985). Self-efficacy in recovery from myocardial infarction. Unpublished Doctoral Dissertation. University of Maryland, Baltimore, MD.

Jenkins, L. S., Shaivone, K. I., Budd, N., Waltz, C. F., & Griffith, K. A. (2006). Use of genitourinary teaching associates (GUTAs) to teach nurse practitioner students: Is self-efficacy theory a useful framework? *Journal of Nursing Education, 45*(1), 35–37.

Jette, A., Rooks, D., Lachman, M., Lin, T., Levensen, C., Heislein, D., et al. (1998). Effectiveness of home-based, resistance training with disabled older persons. *Gerontologist, 38,* 412–422.

Jimenez, J. A. V., Contreras, J. L. M., Shellman, J., Gonzales, M. L. C., & Bernal, H. (2006). The level of cultural self-efficacy among a sample of Spanish nurses in southeastern Spain. *Journal of Transcultural Nursing, 17*(2), 164–170.

Johnson, J. A. (1996). Self-efficacy theory as a framework for community pharmacy-based diabetes education programs. *Diabetes Educator, 22*(3), 237–241.

Johnson, M. (1995). Healing determinants in older people with leg ulcers. *Research in Nursing and Health, 18*(5), 393–403.

Joseph, H. J. (2004). Attitudes and cultural self-efficacy levels of nurses caring for patients in army hospitals. *Journal of National Black Nurses Association, 15*(1), 5–16.

Kaplan, R., Atkins, C., & Reinsch, S. (1984). Specific efficacy experiences mediate exercise compliance in patients with COPD. *Health Psychology, 3*(3), 223–242.

Kazdin, A. (1979). Behavioral modification and role modeling. *Child Behavior Therapy, 1*(1), 13–36.

Keefe, F. J., Lefebvre, J. C., Maixner, W., Salley, A. N., & Caldwell, D. S. (1997). Self-efficacy for arthritis pain: Relationship to perception of thermal laboratory pain stimuli. *Arthritis Care Research, 10*(3), 177–184.

Kim, J. (2004). The development and evaluation of an incontinence intervention program for the elderly women at elderly welfare center. *Taehan Kanho Hakhoe Chi, 34*(8), 1427–1433.

Kowalski, S. (1997) Self-esteem and self-efficacy as predictors of success in smoking cessation. *Journal of Holistic Nursing, 15*(2), 128–142.

Kurlowica, L. H. (1998). Perceived self-efficacy, functional ability, and depressive symptoms in older elective surgery patients. *Nursing Research, 47*(4), 219–226.

Lau-Walker, M. (2004). Relationship between illness representation and self-efficacy. *Journal of Advanced Nursing, 48*(3), 216–225.

Leonard, B., Skay, C., & Rheinberger, M. (1998). Self-management development in children and adolescents with diabetes: The role of maternal self-efficacy and conflict. *Journal of Pediatric Nursing, 13*(4), 224–233.

Lev, E. L. (1997). Bandura's theory of self-efficacy: Applications to oncology. *Image: Scholarly Inquiry for Nursing Practice, 11*(1), 21–37.

Lev, E. L., & Owen, S. V. (1996). Measure of self-care self-efficacy. *Research in Nursing and Health, 19*(5), 419–421.

Lev, E., Paul, D., & Owen, S. (1999). Age, self-efficacy and change in patients' adjustment to cancer. *Cancer Practitioner, 7*(4), 170–176.

Lim, J., Downie, J., & Nathan, P. (2004). Nursing students' self-efficacy in providing transcultural care. *Nurse Education Today, 24*(6), 428–434.

Lin, C., & Ward, S. (1996). Perceived self-efficacy and outcome expectancies in coping with chronic low back pain. *Research Nursing and Health, 19*(4), 299–310.

Lindberg, C. (2000). Knowledge, self-efficacy, coping and condom use among urban women. *Journal of the Association of Nurses AIDS Care, 11*(5), 80–90.

Lo, R. (1998). A holistic approach in facilitation adherence in people with diabetes. *Australian Journal of Holistic Nursing, 5*(1), 10–18.

Lomi, C., & Nordholm, L. (1992). Validation of a Swedish version of the arthritis self-efficacy scale. *Rheumatology, 21*(5), 231–237.

Lorig, K., Chastain, R., Ung, E., Shoor, S., & Holman, H. (1989). Development and evaluation of a scale to measure perceived self-efficacy in people with arthritis. *Arthritis and Rheumatism, 32*(1), 37–44.

Lorig, K., & Holman, H. (1998). Arthritis self-efficacy scales measure self-efficacy. *Arthritis Care Research, 11*(3), 155–157.

Macnee, C. L., & Talsma, A. (1995). Predictors of progress in smoking cessation. *Public Health Nursing, 12*(4), 242–248.

Madorin, S., & Iwasiw, C. (1999). The effects of computer-assisted instruction on the self-efficacy of baccalaureate nursing students. *Journal of Nurse Educators, 38*(6), 282–285.

Manojlovich, M. (2005). Promoting nurses' self-efficacy: A leadership strategy to improve practice. *Journal of Nursing Administration, 35*(5), 217–219.

McAuley, E. (1992). The role of efficacy cognitions in the prediction of exercise behavior in middle-aged adults. *Journal of Behavioral Medicine, 15*(1), 65–88.

McAuley, E. (1993). Self-efficacy and the maintenance of exercise participation in older adults. *Journal of Behavioral Medicine, 16*(1), 103–113.

McAuley, E., Courneya, K., & Lettunich, J. (1991). Effects of acute and long-term exercise on self-efficacy responses in sedentary, middle-aged males and females. *The Gerontologist, 31*(4), 534–542.

McAuley, E., Lox, C., & Duncan, T. E. (1993). Long-term maintenance of exercise, self-efficacy, and physiological change in older adults. *Journal of Gerontology, 48*(4), 218–224.

McConville, S. A., & Lane, A. M. (2006). Using on line video clips to enhance self-efficacy toward dealing with difficult situations among nursing students. *Nurse Education Today, 26*(3), 200–208.

McDougall, G. J. (1994). Predictors of metamemory in older adults. *Nursing Research, 43*(4), 212–218.

McDougall, G. J. (1996). Predictors of the use of memory improvement strategies by older adults. *Rehabilitation Nursing, 21*(4), 202–209.

McDougall, G. J. (1999). Cognitive interventions among older adults. *Annual Review of Nursing Research, 17*, 219–240.

McDougall, G. (2000). Memory improvement in assisted living elders. *Issues in Mental Health Nursing, 21*(2), 217–233.

McDougall, G. J. (2004). Memory self-efficacy and memory performance among black and white elders. *Nursing Research, 53*(5), 323–331.

McIntyre, K., Lichtenstein, E., & Mermelstein, R. (1983). Self-efficacy and relapse in smoking cessation: A replication and extension. *Journal of Consulting and Clinical Psychology, 51*, 632–633.

Melillo, K., Futrell, M., Williamson, E., Chamberlain, C., Bourque, A., MacDonnell, M., et al. (1996). Perceptions of physical fitness and exercise activity among older adults. *Journal of Advanced Nursing, 23*, 542–547.

Meyerowitz, C., & Chaiken, H. (1987). The impact of self-efficacy on risky health behaviors. *Behavioral Research and Therapy, 25*(5), 267–273.

Montigny, F., & Lacharite, C. (2005). Perceived parental efficacy: concept analysis. *Journal of Advanced Nursing, 49*(4), 387–396.

Moon, L., & Backer, J. (2000). Relationships among self-efficacy, outcome expectancy, and postoperative behaviors in total joint replacement patients. *Orthopedic Nursing, 19*(2), 77–85.

Moseley, J. (1999). Reliability and validity of the Food Pyramid Self Efficacy Scale: Use in coronary artery bypass patients. *Progress of Cardiovascular Nursing, 14*(4), 130–135.

Mowat, J., & Laschinger, H. K. (1994). Self-efficacy in caregivers of cognitively impaired elderly people: A concept analysis. *Journal of Advanced Nursing, 19*(6), 1105–1113.

Murdock, J. E., & Neafsey, P. J. (1995). Self-efficacy measurements: An approach for predicting practice outcomes in continuing education? *Journal of Continuing Education in Nursing, 26*(4), 158–165.

Neff, K., & King, A. C. (1995). Exercise program adherence in older adults: The importance of achieving one's expected benefits. *Medicine and Exercise in Nutrition and Health, 4*, 355–362.

Nelson, P. J., & Tucker, S. (2006). Developing an intervention to alter catastrophizing in persons with fibromyalgia. *Orthopedic Nursing, 25*(3), 205–214.

Ngo, A., & Murphy, S. (2005). A theory-based intervention to improve nurses' knowledge, self-efficacy and skills to reduce PICC occlusion. *Journal of Infusion Nursing, 28*(3), 173–181.

Nguyen, H. Q., Carrieri-Kohlman, V., Rankin, S.H., Slaughter, R. Stulbarg, M. S. (2005). Is internet-based support for dyspnea self-management in patients with chronic obstructive pulmonary disease possible? *Heart & Lung, 34*(1), 51–62.

Nugent, K., Bradwhaw, M., & Kito, N. (1999). Teacher self-efficacy in new nurse educators. *Journal of Professional Nursing, 15*(4), 229–237.

O'Brien, S., & Page, S. (1994). Self-efficacy perfectionism and stress in Canadian Nurses. *Canadian Journal of Nursing Research, 26*(3), 49–61.

Oetker-Black, S. (1996). Generalizability of the preoperative self-efficacy scale. *Applied Nursing Research, 9*(1), 40–44.

O'Leary, A. (1985). Self-efficacy and health. *Behavioral Research and Therapy, 23*(4), 437–450.

Parent, N., & Fortin, F. (2000). A randomized, controlled trial of vicarious experience through peer support for male first time cardiac surgery patients: Impact on anxiety, self-efficacy expectation, and self-reported activity. *Heart Lung, 29*(6), 389–400.

Park, S., Chang, S., & Chung, C. (2005). Effects of a cognition-emotion focused program to increase public participation in Papanicolaou smear screening. *Public Health Nursing, 22*(4), 289–298.

Parsons, L. C. (1999). Building RN confidence for delegation decision-making skills in practice. *Journal of Nurses Staff Development, 15*(6), 263–269.

Pellino, T., Tluczek, A., Collins, M., Trimborn, S., Norwick, H., Engelke, Z., et al. (1998). Increasing self-efficacy through empowerment: preoperative education for orthopaedic patients. *Orthopedic Nursing, 17*(4), 48–51, 54–59.

Perkins, S. (1991). Self-efficacy and mood status in recovery from percutaneous transluminal coronary angioplasty. Unpublished doctoral dissertation. University of Kansas, Kansas City.

Perkins, S., & Jenkins, L. (1998). Self-efficacy expectation, behavior performance and mood status in early recovery from percutaneous transluminal coronary angioplasty. *Heart Lung, 27*(1), 37–46.

Perraud, S. (2000). Development of the Depression Coping Self-efficacy Scale (DCSES). *Archives of Psychiatric Nursing, 14*(6), 276–284.

Plotnikoff, R., Brez, S., & Holz, S. (2000). Exercise behavior in a community sample with diabetes: Understanding the determinants of exercise behavioral change. *Diabetes Educator, 26*(3), 450–459.

Prasopkittikun, T., Tilokskulchai, F., Sinsukasai, N., & Sitthimongkol, Y. (2006). Self efficacy in infant care scale: Development and psychometric testing. *Nursing Health Science, 8*(1), 44–50.

Rabinowitz, S., Kushnir, T., & Ribak, J. (1996). Preventing burnout: Increasing professional self-efficacy in primary care nurses in a Balint Group. *AAOHN Journal, 44*(1), 28–32.

Rejeski, W. J., Ettinger, W. H., Martin, K., & Morgan, T. (1998). Treating disability in knee osteoarthritis with exercise therapy: A central role for self-efficacy and pain. *Arthritis Care Research, 11*(2), 94–101.

Remley, D., & Cook-Newell, M. (1999). Meal planning self-efficacy index for adolescents with diabetes. *Diabetes Educator, 25*(6), 883–886.

Resnick, B. (1994). The wheel that moves. *Rehabilitation Nursing, 19,* 140.

Resnick, B. (1996). Motivation in geriatric rehabilitation. *Image: The Journal of Nursing Scholarship, 28,* 41–47.

Resnick, B. (1998a). Efficacy beliefs in geriatric rehabilitation. *Journal of Gerontological Nursing, 24,* 34–45.

Resnick, B. (1998b). Functional performance of older adults in a long term care setting. *Clinical Nursing Research, 7,* 230–246.

Resnick, B. (1999). Reliability and validity testing of the self-efficacy for functional activities scale. *Journal of Nursing Measurement, 7*(1), 5–20.

Resnick, B. (2000a). Functional performance and exercise of older adults in long-term care settings. *Journal of Gerontological Nursing, 26*(3), 7–16.

Resnick, B. (2000b). A seven step approach to starting an exercise program for older adults. *Patient Education and Counseling, 39,* 243–252.

Resnick, B. (2001). Testing a model of exercise behavior in older adults. *Research in Nursing and Health, 24,* 83–92.

Resnick, B. (2002). Testing the impact of the WALC intervention on exercise adherence in older adults. *Journal of Gerontological Nursing, 28*(6), 32–40.

Resnick, B. (2004). A longitudinal analysis of efficacy expectations and exercise in older adults. *Research and Theory for Nursing Practice, 18*(4), 331–345.

Resnick, B. (2004). *Implementing restorative care nursing in all settings.* New York: Springer Publishing Company.

Resnick, B. (2004, November) Reliability and validity of the outcome expectations for exercise scale-2 (OEE-2). Paper presentation at the Gerontological Society of America, Washington DC. Abstract in *The Gerontologist, 44*(Special Issue II), 8.

Resnick, B. (2005). Across the aging continuum: motivating older adults to exercise. *Advance for Nurse Practitioners, 13*(9), 37–40.

Resnick, B., & Fleishell, A. (1999). Restoring quality of life. *Advance for Nurses, 1,* 10–12.

Resnick, B., & Jenkins, L. (2000). Testing the reliability and validity of the self-efficacy for exercise scale. *Nursing Research, 49*(3), 154–159.

Resnick, B., Magaziner, J., Orwig, D., & Zimmerman, S. (2002). Evaluating the components of the Exercise Plus Program: Rationale, theory and implementation. *Health Education Research, 17*(5), 648–658.

Resnick, B, Luisi, D, Vogel, A., & Junaleepa, P. (2005). Reliability and validity of the Self-Efficacy for Exercise and Outcome Expectations for Exercise Scales with minority older adults. *Journal of Nursing Measurement, 12*(3), 235–247.

Resnick, B., Orwig, D., Zimmerman, S., Simpson, M., & Magaziner, J. (2005). The Exercise Plus Program for older women post hip fracture: Participant perspectives. *The Gerontologist, 45*(4), 539–544.

Resnick, B., Palmer, M. H., Jenkins, L., & Spellbring, A. M. (2000). Path analysis of efficacy expectations and exercise behavior in older adults. *Journal of Advanced Nursing, 31*(6), 1309–1315.

Resnick, B., Simpson, M., Bercovitz, A., Galik, E., Gruber-Baldini, A., Zimmerman, S., & Magaziner, J. (2006). Testing of the Res-Care Pilot Intervention: Impact on residents. *Journal of Gerontological Nursing, 32*(3), 39–47.

Resnick, B., & Simpson, M. (2003). Reliability and validity testing self-efficacy and outcome expectations scales for performing restorative care activities, *Geriatric Nursing, 24*(2), 2–7.

Resnick, B., & Spellbring, A. M. (2000). Understanding what motivates older adults to exercise. *Journal of Gerontologic Nursing, 26*(3), 34–42.

Resnick, B., Vogel, A., & Luisi, D. (2006), Motivating minority older adults to exercise. *Cultural Diversity and Ethnic Minority Psychology, 12*(1), 17–29.

Resnick, B., Wehren, L., & Orwig, D. (2003). Reliability and validity of the self-efficacy and outcome expectations for osteoporosis medication adherence scales. *Orthopedic Nursing, 22*(2), 139–147.

Resnick, B. Zimmerman, S. Orwig, D., Furstenberg, A. L., & Mazaziner, J. (2001). Model testing for reliability and validity of the Outcome Expectations for Exercise Scale. *Nursing Research, 50*(5), 293–299.

Reuterberg, S., & Gustafsson, J. (1992). Confirmatory factor analysis and reliability: Testing measurement model assumptions. *Educational and Psychological Measurement, 52,* 795–811.

Robertson, D., & Keller, C. (1992). Relationship among health beliefs, self-efficacy and exercise adherence in patients with CAD. *Heart and Lung, 21,* 56–63.

Rogers, L. Q., Matevey, C., Hopkins-Price, P., Shah, P., Dunnington, G., & Courneya, K. S. (2004). Exploring social cognitive theory constructs for promoting exercise among breast cancer patients. *Cancer Nursing, 27*(6), 462–473.

Rogers, L. Q., Shah, P., Dunnington, G., Greive, A., Shanmugham, A., Dawson, B., et al. (2005). Social cognitive theory and physical activity during breast cancer treatment. *Oncology Nursing Forum, 32*(4), 807–815.

Rovniak, L. S., Anderson, E. S., Winett, R. A., & Stephens, R. S. (2002). Social cognitive determinants of physical activity in young adults: A prospective structural equation analysis. *Annals of Behavioral Medicine, 24*(2), 149–156.

Ruiz, B. (1992). Hip fracture recovery in older women: The role of self-efficacy and mood. Unpublished doctoral dissertation, University of California, San Francisco.

Ryckman, R., Robbins, M., Thornton, B., & Cantrell, P. (1982). Development and validation of a physical self-efficacy scale. *Journal of Personality and Social Psychology, 42*(5), 891–900.

Scherer, Y., & Schmieder, L. (1996). The role of self-efficacy in assisting patients with chronic obstructive pulmonary disease to manage breathing difficulty. *Clinical Nursing Research, 5*(3), 243–255.

Scherer, Y. K. & Schmieder, L. E. (1997). The effect of a pulmonary rehabilitation program on self-efficacy, perception of dyspnea, and physical endurance. *Heart & Lung, 26*(1), 15–22.

Scherer, Y., Schmieder, L., & Shimmel, S. (1998). The effects of education alone and in combination with pulmonary rehabilitation on self-efficacy in patients with COPD. *Rehabilitation Nursing, 23*(2), 71–77.

Scherer, Y., & Shimmel, L. (1996). The effect of a pulmonary rehabilitation program on self-efficacy, perceptions of dyspnea, and physical endurance. *Heart and Lung, 26*(1), 15–22.

Schneider, J. (1997). Self-regulation and exercise behavior in older women. *Journal of Gerontology, 52,* P235–P241.

Schuster, P., & Waldron, J. (1991). Gender differences in cardiac rehabilitation patients. *Rehabilitation Nursing, 16*(5), 248–253.

Sechrist, K., Walker, S., & Pender, N. (1987). Development and psychometric evaluation of the exercise benefits/barriers scale. *Research in Nursing & Health, 10,* 357–365.

Sharon, B., Hennessy, C., Brandon, L., & Boyette, L. (1997). Older adults' experiences of a strength training program. *The Journal of Nutrition, Health & Aging, 1,* 103–108.

Sharts-Hopko, N., Regan-Kubinski, M., Lincoln, P., & Heverly, M. (1996). Problem-focused coping in HIV-infected mothers in relation to self-efficacy, uncertainty, social support, and psychological disease. *Image: Journal of Nursing Scholarship, 28*(2), 107–111.

Shaughnessy, M. A., Resnick, B., & Macko, R. (2006). Testing a model of exercise behavior post-stroke. *Rehabilitation Nursing, 31*(1), 15–21.

Shellman, J. (2006). Development and psychometric evaluation of the eldercare cultural self-efficacy scale. *International Journal of Nursing Education and Scholarship, 3*(9), Epub February 15.

Siela, D. (1998). Self-efficacy in managing dyspnea in COPD. *Perspectives of Respiratory Nursing, 9*(1), 9, 12.

Sinclair, M., & O'Boyle, C. (1999). The Childbirth Self-efficacy Inventory: A replication study. *Journal of Advanced Nursing, 30*(6), 1416–1423.

Smarr, K. L. Parker, J. C. Wright, G. E. Stucky,-Ropp, R. C., Buckelew, S. P., Hoffman, R. W., et al. (1997). The importance of enhancing self-efficacy in rheumatoid arthritis. *Arthritis Care & Research, 10*(1), 18–26.

Smith, L. (1998). Cultural competence for nurses: Canonical correlation of two culture scales. *Journal of Cultural Diversity, 5*(4), 120–126.

Sol, B. G., Graaf, Y., Bijil, J. J., Goessens, N. B., & Visseren, F. L. (2006). Self-efficacy in patients with clinical manifestations of vascular diseases. *Patient Education and Counseling, 61*(3), 443–448.

Steinhardt, M., & Dishman, R. (1989). Reliability and validity of expected outcomes and barriers for habitual physical activity. *Journal of Occupational Medicine, 31,* 536–546.

Sterling, Y. (1999). Parental self-efficacy and asthma self-management. *Journal of Child and Family Nursing, 2*(4), 280–281.

Sturt, J., Whitlock, S., & Hearnshaw, H. (2006). Complex intervention development for diabetes self-management. *Journal of Advanced Nursing, 54*(3), 293–303.

Taal, E., Rasker, J., & Wiegman, O. (1996). Patient education and self-management in the rheumatic diseases: A self-efficacy approach. *Arthritis Care Research, 9*(3), 229–238.

Takata, C., & Takata, T. (1976). The influence of models on the evaluation of ability: 2 functions of social comparison processes. *Japanese Journal of Psychology, 47*(2), 74–82.

Taylor, C., Bandura, A., Ewart, C., Miller, N., & DeBusk, R. (1985). Exercise testing to enhance wives confidence in their husband's cardiac capability soon after clinically uncomplicated acute MIs. *American Journal of Cardiology, 55,* 635–638.

Van der Palen, J. Klein, J. J., & Seydel. E. R. (1997). Are high generalized and asthma-specific self-efficacy predictive of adequate self-management behavior among adult asthma patients? *Patient Education & Counseling, 32*(1 Suppl), S35–41.

Van der Palen, J., Klein, J., Zielhuis, G., Van Herwaarden, C., & Seydel, E. (2001). Behavioural effect of self-treatment guidelines in a self-management program for adults with asthma. *Patient Education Counseling, 43*(2), 161–169.

Van der Pligt, J., & Richard, R. (1994). Changing adolescents' sexual behavior: Perceived risk, self-efficacy and anticipated regret. *Patient Education and Counseling, 23*(3), 187–196.

Vispoel, W. (1990). Measuring self-efficacy: the state of the art. Paper presented at the Annual Meeting of the American Educational Research Association, Boston, MA, April 16–20, 1990.

Ware Jr., J., Kosinski, M., & Keller, S. D. (1996). SF-12: A 12-item short-form health survey: Construction of scales and preliminary tests of reliability and validity. *Medical Care, 34,* 220–233.

Washington, O. (1999). Effects of cognitive and experiential group therapy on self-efficacy and perceptions of employability of chemically dependent women. *Issues in Mental Health Nursing, 20*(3), 181–198.

Washington, O. (2001). Using brief therapeutic interventions to create change in self-efficacy and personal control of chemically dependent women. *Archives of Psychiatric Nursing, 15*(1), 32–40.

White, P., Kjelgaard, M., & Harkins, S. (1995). Testing the contribution of self-evaluation to goal-setting effects. *Journal of Personality and Social Psychology, 69*(1), 69–79.

Wigal, J. K., Creer, T. L., & Kostes, H. (1991). The COPD Self-Efficacy Scale. *Chest, 99*(5), 1193–1196.

Wigal, J., Stout, C., Brandon, M., Winder, J., McConnaughy, K., Creer, T., et al. (1993). The knowledge, attitude and self-efficacy asthma questionnaire. *Chest, 104*(4), 1144–1148.

Wilcox, S., Castro, C. M., & King, A. C. (2006). Outcome expectations and physical activity participation in two samples of older women. *Journal of Health Psychology, 11*(1), 65–77.

Yeh, M. L., Chen, H. H., & Liu, P. H. (2005). Effects of multimedia with printed nursing guide in education on self-efficacy and functional activity and hospitalization in patients with hip replacements. *Patient Education and Counseling, 57*(2), 217–224.

Zimmerman, B., Brown, S., & Bowman, J. (1996). A self-management program for chronic obstructive pulmonary disease: Relationship to dyspnea and self-efficacy. *Rehabilitation Nursing, 21*(5), 253–257.

Middle Range Theories: Emotional

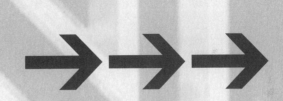

Chronic Sorrow

■ GEORGENE GASKILL EAKES

DEFINITION OF KEY TERMS

Chronic sorrow	Periodic recurrence of permanent, pervasive sadness or other grief-related feelings associated with ongoing disparity resulting from a loss experience
Disparity	A gap between the current reality and the desired as a result of a loss experience
External management methods	Interventions provided by professionals to assist individuals to cope with chronic sorrow
Internal management methods	Positive personal coping strategies used to deal with the periodic episodes of chronic sorrow
Loss experience	A significant loss, either actual or symbolic, that may be ongoing, with no predictable end, or a more circumscribed single-loss event
Trigger event	A situation, circumstance, or condition that brings the negative disparity resulting from the loss into focus, or exacerbates the disparity

INTRODUCTION

The middle range theory of chronic sorrow, first documented in the literature in 1998 by Eakes, Burke, and Hainsworth, offers a framework for explaining how individuals may respond to both ongoing and single-loss events. Moreover, the theoretical model of chronic sorrow provides an alternative way of viewing the experience of grief. The theory of chronic sorrow was inductively derived and subsequently validated from an extensive review of the literature, and from data gathered through 10 qualitative research studies conducted by members of the Nursing Consortium for Research on Chronic Sorrow (NCRCS). Using the Burke/NCRCS Chronic Sorrow Questionnaire (adapted from a guide developed by Burke [1989]) as an interview guide, these nurse researchers interviewed 196 individuals, who shared their loss experiences as people with chronic conditions, as family caregivers of the chronically ill or disabled, or as bereaved family members.

HISTORICAL BACKGROUND

The term *chronic sorrow* was introduced into the literature 40 years ago to characterize the recurring episodes of grief experienced by parents of children with disabilities (Olshansky, 1962). This recurring sadness appeared to persist throughout the lives of these parents, although its intensity varied from time to time, from situation to situation, and from one family member to another. Rather than viewing this phenomenon as pathological, Olshansky described chronic sorrow as a normal response to an ongoing loss situation. Professionals were encouraged to recognize the presence of this phenomenon when working with the parent of a disabled child and to support parents' expressions of feelings. Although the term gained wide use in the professional literature, almost two decades passed before there was any documented research on chronic sorrow.

Initial research conducted in the 1980s validated the occurrence of chronic sorrow among parents of disabled young children. Several investigators suggested that the never-ending nature of the loss of the "perfect" child prevented resolution of grief (Burke, 1989; Damrosch & Perry, 1989; Fraley, 1986; Kratochvil & Devereux, 1988; Wikler, Wasow, & Hatfield, 1981). Moreover, it was this inability to bring closure to the loss experience that was thought to precipitate periodic episodes of re-grief, labeled as chronic sorrow. These early studies refined and operationalized the definition of chronic sorrow as a pervasive sadness that was permanent, periodic, and progressive in nature.

More recent research supports the fact that chronic sorrow is a common experience among family caregivers (Burke, Eakes, & Hainsworth, 1999; Chimarusti, 2002; Clubb, 1991; Copley & Bodensteiner, 1987; Doornbos, 1997; Eakes, 1995; Eakes, Burke, Hainsworth, & Lindgren, 1993; Fraley, 1990; Golden, 1994; Hainsworth, 1995; Hainsworth, Busch, Eakes, & Burke, 1995; Hobdell, 2004; Hobdell & Deatrick, 1996; Hummel & Eastman, 1991; Johsonius, 1996; Kearny & Griffin, 2001; Krafft & Krafft, 1998; Lee, Strauss, Wittman, Jackson, & Carstens, 2001; Lindgren, 1996; Lowes & Lyne, 2000; Mallow & Bechtel, 1999; Matby, Kristjanson, & Coleman, 2003; Northington, 2000; Phillips, 1991; Rosenberg, 1998; Scornaienchi, 2003; Seideman & Kleine, 1995; Shumaker, 1995; Weller Moore, 2002). The caregivers studied represent parents of young children with various disabilities, spouses of individuals diagnosed with chronic illnesses, and parents of adult children with debilitating conditions.

The NCRCS, established in 1989 (Eakes, Hainsworth, Lindgren, & Burke, 1991), expanded research on chronic sorrow and explored the relevance of the concept of chronic sorrow among individuals experiencing a variety of loss situations. This group of nurse researchers not only conducted research on chronic sorrow among family caregivers, but also investigated individuals affected with chronic conditions and bereaved individuals. Among those diagnosed with a chronic condition, 83% evidenced chronic sorrow (Burke, Hainsworth, Eakes, & Lindgren, 1992; Eakes, 1993; Hainsworth, 1994; Hainsworth, Burke, Lindgren, & Eakes, 1993; Hainsworth, Eakes, & Burke, 1994; Lindgren, 1996). The NCRCS also conducted research studies designed to investigate the occurrence of chronic sorrow among individuals who had experienced a single-loss event rather than an ongoing loss. Toward this end, people who had experienced the death of a significant other a minimum of 2 years before the study were interviewed. This time lapse was to allow for acute grief to subside. Findings revealed that a vast majority (97%) of those interviewed evidenced chronic sorrow (Eakes, Burke, & Hainsworth, 1999). These findings led to further modification of the defining characteristics of chronic sorrow, recognizing that it was ongoing disparity associated with the loss, rather than the ongoing nature of the loss experience, as originally thought, that was the antecedent to chronic sorrow. Consequently, chronic sorrow was redefined as permanent, periodic, recurrence of pervasive sadness, or other grief-related feelings associated with ongoing disparity resulting from significant loss (Eakes et al., 1998). The necessary antecedent event is involvement in an experience of significant loss. This loss may be ongoing in nature, with no predictable end, such as the birth of a disabled child or a diagnosis of a debilitating illness, or it may be more circumscribed, such as the death of a loved one. Disparity is created by a loss/situation when an individual's current reality differs markedly from the idealized, or when a gap exists between the desired and the actual. This lack of closure sets the stage for grief to be periodically re-experienced. That is, the chronic sorrow experience is cyclical and continues as long as the disparity created by the loss remains.

DESCRIPTION OF THE THEORY OF CHRONIC SORROW

The middle range theory of chronic sorrow (Eakes et al., 1998) was inductively derived and validated through the qualitative studies described above, as well as through a critical review of existing literature (Figure 7.1). Based on these findings, chronic sorrow was reconceptualized and is now defined as "the periodic recurrence of permanent, pervasive sadness or other grief-related feelings associated with ongoing disparity resulting from a loss experience" (Eakes et al., 1998, p. 180, 1999). Moreover, chronic sorrow is characterized as pervasive, permanent, periodic, and potentially progressive in nature and continues to be viewed as a normal response to loss. Indeed, the theory of chronic sorrow purports that the periodic return of grief among individuals and caregivers whose anticipated life course has been interrupted continues throughout one's lifetime, as long as the disparity created by the loss remains (Lindgren, Burke, Hainesworth, & Eakes, 1992).

The middle range theory of chronic sorrow provides a framework for understanding the reactions of individuals to various loss situations and offers a new way of viewing the experience of bereavement. Although chronic sorrow is viewed as a normal response to the ongoing disparity or void created by significant loss, it is important to note that normalization of the experience in no way diminishes the validity or the intensity of the feelings experienced. At times, feelings can be intense and distressing for the individual experiencing chronic sorrow.

The Development of Chronic Sorrow

Involvement in an experience of significant loss is the necessary antecedent to the development of chronic sorrow. As stated earlier, this may be a loss with no predictable end, such as the birth of a disabled child or diagnosis of a chronic illness, or a more clearly defined loss event, such as the death of a loved one.

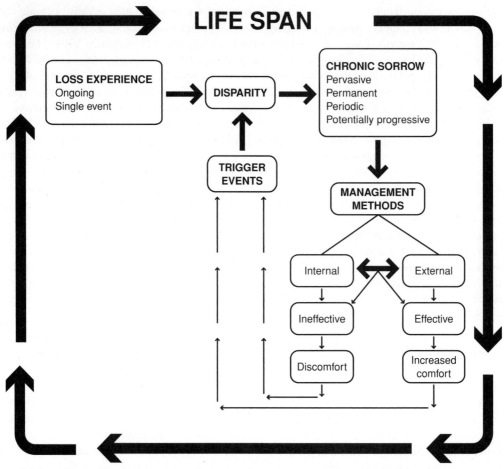

■ **Figure 7.1**   Theoretical model of chronic sorrow. Source: Eakes, G. G., Burke, M. L., & Hainsworth, M. A. (1998). Middle range theory of chronic sorrow. *Image: Journal of Nursing Scholarship, 30*(2), 179–184.

The second antecedent to chronic sorrow is ongoing disparity resulting from the loss. That is, a gap exists between the desired and the actual reality. The lack of closure associated with ongoing disparity sets the stage for chronic sorrow, with the loss experienced in bits and pieces over time. The defining characteristics of chronic sorrow, borne out by the research, are pervasiveness, permanence, periodicity, and the potential for progressivity. As graphically represented in the theoretical model of chronic sorrow (see Figure 7.1), the experience of chronic sorrow may occur at any point across the life span.

Trigger Events

Trigger events, also referred to as milestones, are those situations or circumstances that bring the disparity created by the loss into focus, thereby triggering the grief-related feelings associated with chronic sorrow. Triggers of chronic sorrow vary depending on the nature of the loss experience. For affected individuals, chronic sorrow is most commonly triggered when individuals confront disparity with established norms, whether social, developmental, or personal in nature (Burke et al., 1999; Eakes, 1993; Eakes et al., 1993; Hainsworth, 1994). For example, a trigger may exist when someone diagnosed with a chronic illness is unable to engage in an activity that he once enjoyed due to exacerbation of his condition.

The most frequent trigger of chronic sorrow among parents of young children with disabilities is disparity associated with developmental milestones (Burke, 1989; Clubb, 1991; Damrosch & Perry, 1989; Fraley, 1986, 1990; Golden, 1994; Hummel & Eastman, 1991; Kafft & Krafft, 1998; Mallow & Bechtel, 1999; Olshansky, 1962; Phillips, 1991; Seideman & Kleine, 1995; Shumaker, 1995; Wikler et al., 1981). The chronic sorrow of other family caregivers is often triggered by crises associated with management of the family member's illness and by recognition of the never-ending nature of the caregiving activities (Burke et al., 1999; Eakes, 1995; Eakes et al., 1993; Hainsworth, 1995; Hainsworth et al., 1995; Lindgren, 1996).

The chronic sorrow experience of bereaved individuals is triggered by those situations and circumstances that magnify the "presence of the absence" of the deceased, such as anniversaries and other special occasions (Eakes et al., 1998, p. 182). Also, changes in roles and responsibilities necessitated by the death of a loved one may trigger chronic sorrow.

Management Methods

Another key element of the theoretical model of chronic sorrow is management methods. This term is used to refer to both personal coping strategies used by individuals during the chronic sorrow experience (internal) as well as supportive interventions provided by helping professionals (external). As depicted in the theoretical model, effective internal and external management methods lead to increased comfort and may serve to extend the time between episodes of chronic sorrow.

INTERNAL MANAGEMENT

Effective internal management strategies used by those with chronic sorrow are consistent across the various loss situations. Action-oriented strategies that increase feelings of control are most frequently used to cope with the recurrence of grief-related feelings of chronic sorrow (Burke, 1989; Eakes, 1993, 1995; Hainsworth, 1995; Hainsworth et al., 1994, 1995; Lindgren, 1996). Examples of action-oriented coping include continuing to pursue involvement in interests and activities, gathering information specific to one's loss experience, and seeking out respite opportunities. Cognitive and interpersonal are other types of internal management strategies identified as helpful in dealing with the chronic sorrow. Cognitive strategies include adopting a "can do" attitude and focusing on the positive elements of one's life (Burke, 1989; Eakes, 1993, 1995; Hainsworth, 1995; Hainsworth et al., 1994, 1995). Interpersonal ways of coping include talking with someone close or a trusted professional and interacting with others in a similar situation such as in a support group (Burke, 1989; Eakes, 1993, 1995; Fraley, 1990; Hainsworth, 1995; Hainsworth et al., 1994, 1995; Wikler et al., 1981).

EXTERNAL MANAGEMENT

Interventions provided by health care professionals, referred to as external management methods, and must be based on the premise that chronic sorrow is a normal response to a significant loss situation. As long as disparity created by a loss experience remains, one can anticipate that the individual will likely experience chronic sorrow. Indeed, normalization of the periodic re-grief of chronic sorrow is basic to all other interventions. It is important for professionals to recognize that individuals who have experienced a significant loss may evidence the periodic recurrence of grief-related feelings, defined as chronic sorrow. Armed with this awareness, anticipatory guidance may be provided regarding the situations and circumstances likely to trigger episodes of chronic sorrow. Personal coping mechanisms (internal management methods) can be assessed, strengthened, and supported.

Additionally, specific interventions provided by health care professionals, categorized as roles, have been helpful for those experiencing chronic sorrow (Burke, 1989; Copley & Bodensteiner, 1987; Eakes, 1993, 1995; Eakes et al., 1993; Fraley, 1990; Hainsworth, 1995; Hainsworth et al., 1995; Hummel & Eastman, 1991; Wikler et al., 1981). Family caregivers with chronic sorrow derive the most benefit from professional interventions labeled as the role of "teacher/expert." More specifically, these actions include providing situation-specific information in a manner that can be easily understood and giving practical tips for managing caregiving responsibilities (Burke, 1989; Clubb, 1991; Eakes, 1995; Fraley, 1990; Hainsworth, 1995; Hainsworth et al., 1995; Hummel & Eastman, 1991; Warda, 1992; Wikler et al., 1981). Actions associated with the professional role of "empathetic presence," characterized by taking time to listen, offering support, focusing on feelings, and recognizing uniqueness of each individual, are also helpful to those who were in a caregiver role (Burke, 1989; Clubb, 1991; Eakes, 1995; Fraley, 1990; Hainsworth, 1995; Hummel & Eastman, 1991; Olshansky, 1962; Phillips, 1991; Teel, 1991; Warda, 1992).

For those individuals affected with a chronic or life-threatening condition, as well as bereaved persons, the professional role of "empathetic presence" discussed above is perceived as most helpful in dealing with the periodic episodes of chronic sorrow. In addition, the complementary role of "caring professional," evidenced by sensitivity, respectfulness, nonjudgmental acceptance, and intervention associated with the role of "teacher/expert," is described as beneficial (Burke, 1989; Eakes, 1993; Eakes et al., 1993; Hainsworth et al., 1995).

APPLICATIONS OF THE THEORY

Chronic sorrow has research applications among a variety of populations and across a myriad of loss situations. Identifying the presence of chronic sorrow among family caregivers alerts professionals to potential triggers of the recurrent grief, and leads to the identification and reinforcement of effective coping mechanisms for those experiencing chronic sorrow. See Using Middle Range Theories 7.1 and 7.2 for examples.

INSTRUMENTS USED IN EMPIRICAL TESTING

Historically, research on chronic sorrow has employed qualitative methods with open-ended interview guides, used with study participants both in face-to-face and in telephone interviews. The Burke/NCRCS Chronic Sorrow Questionnaire (Burke, 1989; Eakes, 1993, 1995), with versions adapted for individuals affected with chronic conditions, for family caregivers, and for bereaved individuals, has been used for the majority of studies documented in the literature. This interview guide is composed of 10 open-ended questions that explore feelings experienced at the time of the loss, and whether or not they have been re-experienced. Moreover, questions focus on circumstances or situations that trigger recurrence of the grief-related feeling and identification of effective coping mechanisms. See Research Application 7.1. In her dissertation research, Kendall (2005) tested the Kendall Chronic Sorrow Instrument (KCSI), an 18-item data collection tool designed to screen for and measure the chronic sorrow experience. Results indicate that the KCSI is a valid and reliable instrument, thereby providing the means for quantitative research on chronic sorrow.

7.1 USING MIDDLE RANGE THEORIES

This researcher explored the experience of chronic sorrow among African-American caregivers of school-age children diagnosed with sickle cell disease (SCD). Findings revealed that the process of chronic sorrow was initially triggered by a diagnosis of SCD. Subsequent resurgence of chronic sorrow was triggered by both internal and external events. Internal triggers were found to relate to future-oriented thoughts, including thoughts of the child's death. External factors triggering episodes of chronic sorrow were associated with consequences of the illness itself, as well as concerns about costs of health care and education. Significant others, spirituality, and the strength exhibited by the child with SCD were the primary sources of support for those caregivers studied. The researcher concluded that caregivers of children with SCD engage in a process of readjusting and redefining reality. Thus, the cyclic nature of chronic sorrow they experience assists in the individuals' growth and adjustment. Nurses were encouraged to recognize the existence of chronic sorrow among this population of caregivers so that supportive interventions could be provided.

This study supports the need for reconceptualization of existing grief theories. Indeed, these findings question the expectation purported in traditional grief theories that closure is an expected outcome of the grieving process.

Northington, L. (2000). Chronic sorrow in caregivers of school age children with sickle cell disease: A grounded theory approach. *Issues in Comprehensive Pediatric Nursing, 23*, 141–154.

7.2 USING MIDDLE RANGE THEORIES

Researchers interviewed 34 bereaved individuals who had experienced the death of a loved one. A minimum of 2 years had lapsed since the death occurred, allowing acute grief to subside, with a range from 2 to more than 20 years. The Burke/NCRCS Chronic Sorrow Questionnaire (Bereaved Individual Version), revised from Burke's (1989) original interview guide, was used to gather data about both recurrence of feelings associated with the loss and the triggers of those periodic episodes of re-grief. Findings revealed that 97% of the subjects experienced chronic sorrow. Moreover, common triggers were those situations and circumstances that brought into focus disparity with social norms—parents without children, children without parents, wives without husbands, and husbands without wives. Additionally, memories often associated with anniversaries and special occasions triggered recurrence of the grief-related feelings of chronic sorrow. Normalization of the periodic episodes of chronic sorrow through caring and empathetic professional roles was found to be beneficial to those with chronic sorrow.

Eakes, G., Burke, M., & Hainsworth, M. (1999). Chronic sorrow: The experiences of bereaved individuals. *Illness, Crisis & Loss, 7*(2), 172–182.

7.1 RESEARCH APPLICATION

In 2001, two of the original members of the Nursing Consortium for Research on Chronic Sorrow undertook the development of a quantitative assessment tool (Eakes & Burke, 2002). Questions for the instrument were developed based on the theoretical model and findings from the qualitative studies previously conducted by members of the NCRCS and other researchers. Face and content validity were established by using Lynn's (1986) methodology for establishing validity of an instrument. Once face and content validity of the Burke/Eakes Chronic Sorrow Assessment Tool were established, test–retest reliability studies were conducted. Subjects participating in this aspect of instrument development represented each of the populations previously studied (family caregivers, affected individuals, and bereaved persons). Test–retest correlations for items 4 through 9 (the first three questions assess demographic data) were at acceptable levels, ranging from 0.72 to 0.93. Questions 10 and 11 allow for little variability in responses, and the restricted response range resulted in more marginal test–retest correlations on these items (0.62 and 0.56, respectively).
See Appendix B for a sample of the assessment tool.

SUMMARY

Chronic sorrow has gained increased attention in the past decade, based in large part on the research endeavors of the NCRCS. Increased awareness of the changing nature of grief associated with significant losses, whether ongoing in nature or single-loss events, has spurred interest in this phenomenon. The theory of chronic sorrow provides a framework for understanding and working with individuals who have experienced significant loss. Specifically, situations and circumstances that trigger chronic sorrow are identified, and management methods deemed helpful to those experiencing chronic sorrow are described.

ANALYSIS OF THEORY

Using the criteria presented in Chapter 2, critique the theory of chronic sorrow. Compare your conclusions about the theory with those found in Appendix A. A nurse who has worked with the theory completed the analysis found in the Appendix.

Internal Criticism
1. Clarity
2. Consistency
3. Adequacy

4. Logical development
5. Level of theory development

External Criticism
1. Reality convergence
2. Utility
3. Significance
4. Discrimination
5. Scope of theory
6. Complexity

CRITICAL THINKING EXERCISES

1. You are a case manager for a family with a young child diagnosed with cerebral palsy. Explain how the theory of chronic sorrow can be used as a framework for planning care and identifying resources for this family.
2. Expand the application of the theory of chronic sorrow to a population not yet studied. Describe the strengths and weaknesses of the theory in relation to the population identified and discuss if the theoretical premises apply.
3. Draft a research study designed to measure outcomes for the external management strategies described in the theory.

Adding to its credibility, chronic sorrow has been recognized as a nursing diagnosis (NANDA, 2003) and is included in nursing diagnosis textbooks (Ackly & Ladwig, 2004; Carpenito, 2004).

Moreover, the theoretical model of chronic sorrow, along with the recently constructed Burke/Eakes Chronic Sorrow Assessment Tool and Kendall's Chronic Sorrow Instrument (2005), will facilitate further expansion of research on chronic sorrow and provide opportunities for testing of the theory. The need for exploration of cultural variations in the experience of chronic sorrow has virtually been ignored and must be addressed in future research. Additionally, relevance of the theory of chronic sorrow to types of loss experiences not yet studied (i.e., divorce, abuse) needs to be investigated.

The middle range theory of chronic sorrow has widespread application for nurses and others who strive to better understand individuals' responses to loss and to define effective interventions for those experiencing chronic sorrow. Although chronic sorrow is viewed as a normal response to ongoing disparity resulting from a loss, recognition of the periodic re-grief characteristic of chronic sorrow and provision of supportive interventions can provide an increased level of comfort for those experiencing it.

WEB RESOURCES

1. This site has a nursing theory page, including nursing text and book reviews, plus a variety of nursing-related topics: **www.enursescribe.com**
2. This site contains links to a variety on nursing-related web pages. It has pages on nurse theorists and a special section called Other Nursing Resources: **www.healthsci.clayton.edu**

REFERENCES

Ackly, B. J., & Ladwig, G. B. (2004). *Nursing diagnosis handbook: A guide to planning care* (6th ed.). St. Louis: Mosby.

Burke, M. L. (1989). Chronic sorrow in mothers of school-age children with a myelomeningocele disability (Doctoral dissertation, Boston University, 1989). *Dissertation Abstracts International, 50,* 233–234B.

Burke, M. L., Eakes, G. G., & Hainsworth, M.A. (1999). Milestones of chronic sorrow: Perspectives of affected individuals and family caregivers. *Journal of Family Nursing, 5*(4), 374–387.

Burke, M. L., Hainsworth, M. A., Eakes, G. G., & Lindgren, C. L. (1992). Current knowledge and research on chronic sorrow: A foundation for inquiry. *Death Studies, 16,* 231–245.

Carpenito, L. J. (2004). *Nursing diagnosis: Application to clinical practice.* Philadelphia: Lippincott Williams & Wilkins.

Chimarusti, J. A. (2002). Chronic sorrow: Emotional experiences of parents of children with cerebral palsy (Doctoral dissertation, University of New Mexico). DAI-A 63/02, p. 771.

Clubb, R. L. (1991). Chronic sorrow: Adaptation patterns of parents with chronically ill children. *Pediatric Nursing, 17,* 462–466.

Copley, M. F., & Bodensteiner, J. B. (1987). Chronic sorrow in families of disabled children. *Journal of Child Neurology, 2,* 67–70.

Damrosch, S. P., & Perry, L. A. (1989). Self-reported adjustment, chronic sorrow, and coping of parents of children with Down syndrome. *Nursing Research, 38,* 25–30.

Doornbos, M. M. (1997). The problems and coping methods of caregivers of young adults with mental illness. *Journal of Psychosocial Nursing, 35*(9), 22–26.

Eakes, G. G. (1993). Chronic sorrow: A response to living with cancer. *Oncology Nursing Forum, 20,* 1327–1334.

Eakes, G. G. (1995). Chronic sorrow: The lived experience of parents of chronically mentally ill individuals. *Archives of Psychiatric Nursing, IX,* 77–84.

Eakes, G. G., & Burke, M. L. (2002). Development and validation of the Burke/Eakes chronic sorrow assessment tool. Unpublished raw data. EakesG@mail.ecu.edu.

Eakes, G. G., Burke, M. L., & Hainsworth, M. A. (1998). Middle range theory of chronic sorrow. *Image: Journal of Nursing Scholarship, 30*(2), 179–184.

Eakes, G. G., Burke, M. L., & Hainsworth, M. A. (1999). Chronic sorrow: The lived experience of bereaved individuals. *Illness, Crisis, and Loss, 7*(1), 172–182.

Eakes, G. G., Burke, M. L., Hainsworth, M. A., & Lindgren, C. L. (1993). Chronic sorrow: An examination of nursing roles. In S. G. Funk, E. M. Tornquist, M. T. Champagne, & R. A. Wiese (Eds.), *Key aspects of caring for the chronically ill: Hospital and home* (pp. 231–236). New York: Springer Publishing.

Eakes, G. G., Hainsworth, M. E., Lindgren, C. L., & Burke, M. L. (1991). Establishing a long-distance research consortium. *Nursing Connections, 4,* 51–57.

Fraley, A. M. (1986). Chronic sorrow in parents of premature children. *Children's Health Care, 15,* 114–118.

Fraley, A. M. (1990). Chronic sorrow: A parental response. *Journal of Pediatric Nursing, 5,* 268–273.

Golden, B. (1994). The presence of chronic sorrow in mothers of children with cerebral palsy. Unpublished master's thesis, Arizona State University, Tempe.

Hainsworth, M. A. (1994). Living with multiple sclerosis: The experience of chronic sorrow. *Journal of Neuroscience Nursing, 26,* 237–240.

Hainsworth, M. A. (1995). Chronic sorrow in spouse caregivers of individuals with multiple sclerosis: A case study. *Journal of Gerontological Nursing, 21,* 29–33.

Hainsworth, M. A., Burke, M. L., Lindgren, C. L., & Eakes, G. G. (1993). Chronic sorrow in multiple sclerosis: A case study. *Home Healthcare Nurse, 11,* 9–13.

Hainsworth, M. A., Busch, P. V., Eakes, G. G., & Burke, M. L. (1995). Chronic sorrow in women with chronically mentally disabled husbands. *Journal of the American Psychiatric Association, 1*(4), 120–124.

Hainsworth, M. A., Eakes, G. G., & Burke, M. L. (1994). Coping with chronic sorrow. *Issues in Mental Health Nursing, 15,* 59–66.

Hobdell, E. (2004). Chronic sorrow and depression in parents of children with neural tube defects. *Journal of Neuroscience Nursing, 6*(2), 82–88.

Hobdell, E., & Deatrick, J. (1996). Chronic sorrow: A content analysis of parental differences. *Journal of Genetic Counseling, 5*(2), 57–68.

Hummel, P. A., & Eastman, D. L. (1991). Do parents of premature infants suffer chronic sorrow? *Neonatal Network, 10,* 59–65.

Johnsonius, J. (1996). Lived experiences that reflect embodied themes of chronic sorrow: A phenomenological pilot study. *Journal of Nursing Science, 1*(5/6), 165–173.

Kearney, P., & Griffin, T. (2001). Between joy and sorrow: Being a parent of a child with a developmental disability. *Journal of Advanced Nursing, 34*(5), 582–592.

Kendall, L. C. (2005). The experience of living with ongoing loss: Testing the Kendall chronic sorrow instrument (Doctoral dissertation, Virginia Commonwealth University). DAI-B 66/11, p. 5902.

Krafft, S. K., & Krafft, L. J. (1998). Chronic sorrow: Parents' lived experience. *Holistic Nursing Practice, 13*(1), 59–67.

Kratochvil, M. S., & Devereaux, S. A. (1988). Counseling needs of parents of handicapped children. *Social Casework, 68,* 420–426.

Lee, A. I., Strauss, L., Wittman, P., Jackson, B., & Carstens, A. (2001). The effects of chronic illness on roles and emotions of caregivers. *Occupational Therapy in Health Care 14*(1), 47–60.

Lindgren, C. L. (1996). Chronic sorrow in persons with Parkinson's and their spouses. *Scholarly Inquiry for Nursing Practice, 10,* 351–367.

Lindgren, C. L., Burke, M. L., Hainsworth, M. A., & Eakes, G. G. (1992). Chronic sorrow: A lifespan concept. *Scholarly Inquiry for Nursing Practice, 6,* 27–40.

Lowes, L. L., & Lyne, P. (2000). Chronic sorrow in parents of children with newly diagnosed diabetes: A review of the literature and discussion of the implications for nursing practice. *Journal of Advanced Nursing, 32*(1), 41–48.

Lynn, M. (1986). Determination and quantification of content validity. *Nursing Research, 35*(6), 382–385.

Mallow, G. E., & Bechtel, G. A. (1999). Chronic sorrow: The experience of parents with children who are developmentally disabled. *Journal of Psychosocial Nursing, 37*(7), 31–35.

Matby, H. J., Kristjanson, L., & Coleman, M. (2003). The parenting competency framework: Learning to be a parent of a child with asthma. *International Journal of Nursing Practice, 9*(6), 368–373.

NANDA Diagnoses: Definitions & Classifications. (2003–2004). Philadelphia: North American Nursing Diagnosis Association.

Northington, L. (2000). Chronic sorrow in caregivers of school age children with sickle cell disease: A grounded theory approach. *Issues in Comprehensive Pediatric Nursing, 23,* 141–154.

Olshansky, S. (1962). Chronic sorrow: A response to having a mentally defective child. *Social Casework, 43,* 191–193.

Phillips, M. (1991). Chronic sorrow in mothers of chronically ill and disabled children. *Issues in Comprehensive Pediatric Nursing, 14,* 111–120.

Rosenberg, C. J. (1998). Faculty-student mentoring. A father's chronic sorrow: A daughter's perspective. *Journal of Holistic Nursing, 16*(3), 399–404.

Scornaienchi, J. M. (2003). Chronic sorrow: One mother's experience with two children with lissencephaly. *Journal of Pediatric Health Care, 17*(6), 291–294.

Seideman, R. Y., & Kleine, P. F. (1995). A theory of transformed parenting: Parenting a child with developmental delay/mental retardation. *Nursing Research, 44,* 38–44.

Shumaker, D. (1995). Chronic sorrow in mothers of children with cystic fibrosis. Unpublished master's thesis, University of Tennessee, Memphis.

Teel, C. S. (1991). Chronic sorrow: Analysis of the concept. *Journal of Advanced Nursing, 16,* 1322.

Warda, M. (1992). The family and chronic sorrow: Role theory approach. *Journal of Pediatric Nursing, 7,* 205–210.

Weller Moore, R. M. (2002). The lived experience of a small number of wives caring for a husband with heart failure. (Doctoral dissertation, New York University). DAI-B 62/10, p. 4474.

Wikler, L. M., Wasow, M., & Hatfield, E. (1981). Chronic sorrow revisited: Parents vs. professional depiction of the adjustment of parents of mentally retarded children. *American Journal of Orthopsychiatry, 51,* 63–70.

BIBLIOGRAPHY

Burke, M. L., Eakes, G. G., & Hainsworth, M. A. (1999). Milestones of chronic sorrow: Perspectives of affected individuals and family caregivers. *Journal of Family Nursing, 5*(4), 374–387.

Burke, M. L., Hainsworth, M. A., Eakes, G. G., & Lindgren, C. L. (1992). Current knowledge and research on chronic sorrow: A foundation for inquiry. *Death Studies, 16,* 231–245.

Chang, G. Y. (1999). Room with no flowers. *Clinical Nurse Specialist, 13*(6), 276.

Hainsworth, M. A., Burke, M. L., Lindgren, C. L., & Eakes, G. G. (1993). Chronic sorrow in multiple sclerosis: A case study. *Home Healthcare Nurse, 11,* 9–13.

Hayes, M. (2001). A phenomenological study of chronic sorrow in people with type I diabetes. *Practical Diabetes International, 18*(2), 65–69.

Hobdell, E., & Deatrick, J. (1996). Chronic sorrow: A content analysis of parental differences. *Journal of Genetic Counseling, 5*(2), 57–68.

Johnsonius, J. (1996). Lived experiences that reflect embodied themes of chronic sorrow: A phenomenological pilot study. *Journal of Nursing Science, 1*(5/6), 165–173.

Keamey, P., & Griffin, T. (2001). Between joy and sorrow: Being a parent of a child with a developmental disability. *Journal of Advanced Nursing, 34*(5), 582–592.

Langridge, P. (2002). Reduction of chronic sorrow: A health promotion role for children's community nurses? *Journal of Child Health Care, 6*(3), 157–170.

Lichtenstein, B., Laska, M., & Clair, J. M. (2002). Chronic sorrow in the HIV-positive patient: Issues of race, gender, and social support. *AIDS Patient Care & STDs, 16*(1), 27–38.

Lindgren, C. L., Burke, M. L., Hainsworth, M. A., & Eakes, G. G. (1992). Chronic sorrow: A lifespan concept. *Scholarly Inquiry for Nursing Practice, 6,* 27–40.

Martin, K., & Elder, S. (1993). Pathways through grief: A model of the process. In J. D. Morgan (Ed.), *Personal care in an impersonal world: A multidimensional look at bereavement* (pp. 73–86). Amityville, NY: Baywood Publishing Company, Inc.

Nehring, W. (2001). The child with a chronic condition. Commentary on Todd RD (2000). *Journal of Child & Family Nursing, 4*(4), 289–290.

Stephenson, J. S., & Murphy, D. (1986). Existential grief: The special case of the chronically ill and disabled. *Death Studies, 10,* 135–145.

Middle Range
Theories: Social

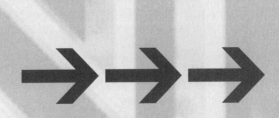

Social Support

■ MARJORIE A. SCHAFFER

DEFINITION OF KEY TERMS

Appraisal support	Affirmation from statements or actions made by another (Kahn & Antonucci, 1980)
Emotional support	Experience of feeling liked, admired, respected, or loved (Norbeck, Lindsey, & Carrieri, 1981)
Formal support	Help from professionals, paraprofessionals, or other service providers from structured community organizations (may be paid or unpaid assistance)
Informal support	Help provided through a person's "lay" social network, such as from family members and friends
Informational support	Knowledge provided to another during a time of stress that assists in problem solving (House, 1981)
Instrumental support	Tangible aid, goods, or services (House, 1981)
Negative support	Interactions that cause stress or are more demanding than helpful (Coyne & DeLongis, 1986)
Perceived support	Generalized appraisal that individuals are cared for and valued, have others available to them, and are satisfied with relationships (Heller, Swindle, & Dusenbury, 1986)
Social network	Structure of the interactive process of persons who give and receive help and protection (Langford, Bowsher, Maloney, & Lillis, 1997)
Social support	(1) An exchange of resources that the provider and recipient perceive to enhance the recipient's well-being (Shumaker & Brownwell, 1984); (2) "A well-intentioned action that is given willingly to a person with whom there is a personal relationship and that produces an immediate or delayed positive response in the recipient" (Hupcey, 1998b, p. 313)

INTRODUCTION

Social support is a middle range theory that addresses structure and interaction in relationships. Related midlevel theories include social exchange, social comparison, coping, attribution, social learning, and social competence theories (Stewart, 1993). Theorists and researchers have experienced challenges in conceptualizing, defining, and measuring social support (Hupcey, 1998a). Disagreement exists about the dimensionality of social support (Bloom, 1990). Some authors give credence to one broad factor (Brown, 1986), while others view social support as multidimensional, with several categories or components (Barrera, 1986; Wandersman, Wandersman, & Kahn, 1980). In addition, there is a need to distinguish between social support and social network, because a social network can contribute to both stress and support (Hutchinson, 1999).

Social support theory is important for middle range theory development in nursing, because social support impacts health status, health behavior, and use of health services (Stewart, 1993). As health professionals, nurses often have access to clients' social networks. Through communication with clients and their family members, nurses can intervene to promote or strengthen social support. The literature identifies many positive consequences of social support, including health-promoting behaviors, personal competence, coping, a sense of well-being, self-worth, and decreased anxiety and depression (Langford et al., 1997). Research on social support interventions can provide nurses with knowledge about the most effective strategies for strengthening social support for clients, which contributes to improved health status.

HISTORICAL BACKGROUND

Cassel (1974), one of the early social support theorists, introduced the term *social support.* Based on animal studies, he theorized that strengthening social supports could improve the health of humans. Studies in the early 1970s suggested that social support mediates the negative effects of stress (Roberts, 1984). The "buffer" theory and attachment theory have been the basis for considerable research on the relationship of social support and health (Callaghan & Morrissey, 1993). The buffer theory suggests that social support protects persons from life stressors (Cassel, 1976; Cobb, 1976). The attachment theory holds that the ability to form socially supportive relationships is related to the secure attachments formed in childhood (Bowlby, 1971). In the mid-1970s to early 1980s, the literature most often described social support in concrete terms, such as an interaction, a person, or a relationship (Veiel & Baumann, 1992). In recent years, the term has been used more abstractly, to include perceptions, quality and quantity of support, behaviors, and social systems. The analysis and testing of social support theory has gained multidisciplinary interest and is prominent in nursing and social–psychological literature. For nurses, social support can connect family assessment, patient needs, and health outcomes (Hupcey, 1998b). Nurses have focused on the client–environment interaction for specific social support situations, such as transition to parenthood, bereavement, and vulnerable children and families (Stewart, 1993).

DEFINITION OF THEORY CONCEPTS

Developers of social support theory have organized definitions of social support by a variety of component labels: aspects, categories, constructs, defining attributes, dimensions, interpersonal transactions, subconcepts, taxonomies, and types (Table 8.1). The variety of definitions of social support provided by

Table 8.1 **THEORETICAL MULTIDIMENSIONAL DEFINITIONS OF SOCIAL SUPPORT**

LABEL	SUPPORT COMPONENTS
Aspects (Cohen, 1992)	Social networks Perceived support Supportive behaviors
Categories (Hupcey, 1998a)	Types of support provided Recipients' perceptions Intentions/behaviors of provider of support Reciprocal support Social networks
Constructs (Vaux, 1988)	Support network resources Support incidents Support behaviors Support appraisals Support or network orientation
Defining attributes (House, 1981)	Emotional support Informational support Instrumental support Appraisal support
Dimensions (Cutrona, 1990)	Emotional Esteem (appraisal) Tangible (instrumental) Information Social integration
Interpersonal transactions (Kahn, 1979)	Affect—feeling liked or loved Affirmation—of behavior, perceptions, and views Affect—feeling respected or admired Aid—material or symbolic
Subconcepts (Barrera, 1981)	Material aid Physical assistance Intimate interaction Guidance Feedback Social participation
Taxonomies (Laireiter & Baumann, 1992)	Social integration Network resources Supportive climate and environment Received and enacted support Perception of being supported
Types (Wortman, 1984)	Expression of positive affect Expression of agreement Encouragement of open expression of feelings Offer of advice and information Provision of material aid Network of reciprocal help and mutual obligation

theorists illustrates the lack of consensus about the nature of social support. This lack of consensus contributes to complexity in evaluating social support interventions and outcomes, comparing research findings, and developing social support theory.

Although multidimensional definitions predominate, positive interaction or helpful behavior is shared by all social support definitions (Rook & Dooley, 1985). In addition, most social support theories have the assumption that support is given and received by members of a social network, leading to social integration or a feeling of belonging (Diamond, 1985; Norbeck & Tilden, 1988). Recipients perceive that social support facilitates coping with stressors in their lives (Pierce, Sarason, & Sarason, 1990). Shumaker and Brownell (1984) defined social support as an exchange of resources that the provider or recipient perceives to enhance the recipient's well-being. Social support can be structural, focusing on who provides the support, or functional, emphasizing the act of providing social support activities (Callaghan & Morrissey, 1993; Norwood, 1996). In addition, there are many characteristics that influence the quality and adequacy of social support, such as the stability, direction, and source of support (Stewart, 1989a). Social networks can be described by the number and categories of persons who provide social support: family members, close friends, neighbors, coworkers, and professionals (Tardy, 1985).

Emotional, Informational, Instrumental, and Appraisal Support

Researchers have often used the conceptualization of social support created by House (1981) and confirmed by others (Barrera, 1986; Tilden & Weinert, 1987). The four theoretical constructs or defining attributes, as labeled by House, are emotional, informational, instrumental, and appraisal support. These four attributes include all possible actions of social support (Langford et al., 1997). Emotional support involves the experience of feeling liked, admired, respected, or loved (Norbeck, 1981). Tangible aid, goods, or services define instrumental support (House, 1981). Providing information during a time of stress is informational support (House, 1981). Appraisal support affirms one's actions or statements (Kahn & Antonucci, 1980).

The following examples from nursing practice illustrate the meaning of emotional, informational, instrumental, and appraisal support. In the first example, a public health nurse can strengthen social support through a comprehensive home visitation program for young mothers (Olds et al., 1999). Through referral to an early childhood parenting program, a young mother can develop friendships with other mothers in the group and receive emotional support from others who are experiencing similar life events. Instrumental support is provided when the pubic health nurse links a young mother to community resources that can provide assistance with child care, education, health care, and financial needs. The public health nurse provides informational support by teaching the young mother about child growth and development. Appraisal support occurs as the young mother engages in positive self-assessment of her parenting abilities based on feedback from the nurse.

In a second example, Ragsdale, Yarbrough, and Lasher (1993) developed a social support protocol for clients who have had a cerebral vascular accident (CVA). By including specific social support interventions in the care plan, nurses can assist a client with a CVA and his wife meet their needs for social support. The nursing care plan can guide nurses to help the wife of the CVA client provide emotional support to her husband by maintaining a positive attitude and listening to her husband when he expresses frustration. The wife can provide tangible assistance or instrumental support when she acts as an interpreter for professional caregivers or helps with suctioning. Nurses can strengthen the ability of the spouse of the CVA client to provide social support to her husband by giving information about how to care for her husband. Nurses can offer appraisal support to the wife, encouraging her and making positive comments about the effectiveness of her caregiving actions.

Negative Social Support

Although often viewed as implying a positive influence, social support may contribute negatively to well-being. The social support activity alone may not be as important as the recipient's perception of the support (perceived support). The perception of or the satisfaction with the support is likely to influence the outcome of the support activity (Heller et al., 1986). The support activity could actually be unrecognized or perceived negatively by the recipient. Negative social support is perceived as unhelpful and may undermine self-esteem. Characteristics of negative social support include stressful or conflicted social networks, misguided or absent support, inappropriate advice, avoidance, and disagreement (Stewart, 1993). Moreover, costs to the provider of social support such as overload, overcommitment, and stressful emotional involvement may occur (Coyne & DeLongis, 1986; La Gaipa, 1990).

In a discussion of the "darker side" of social support, Tilden and Galyen (1987) recommended that the costs of relationships should be addressed in future social support research. They described how social exchange and equity theories explain the costs that may be incurred in social relationships. Social exchanges include both rewards and costs; people behave in ways that maximize their rewards and reduce their costs. The balance of rewards and costs is likely to influence both perceptions and effects of social support. Equity theory addresses this imbalance and suggests that unequal or nonreciprocal social exchanges contribute to stress. Four subdimensions that could be measured to capture the effects of negative aspects of social support are cost, conflict, reciprocity, and equity (Tilden & Galyen, 1987).

DESCRIPTION OF THE THEORY OF SOCIAL SUPPORT

Hupcey (1998b) conducted a concept analysis of social support, based on an examination of 200 studies published from 1978 to 1996, in which social support was one of the variables. Most studies did not include a specific reference to a theoretical definition, and researchers who defined social support often did not use a definition that addressed the interactional nature of social support. According to Hupcey, the four structural factors that help to define social support are precondition, characteristic, outcome, and boundary. The precondition of the provider who perceives a need for social support and is motivated to take action precedes the act of social support. The social support action must be well intentioned and given willingly toward a particular person (characteristic). The outcome is a positive response or change in the recipient. Actions are not considered social support if an organization, the community, or a professional provides them, or if actions have a negative intent or are given grudgingly (boundary). Hupcey (1998b) states that the boundaries of social support help to differentiate it from related concepts. These four structural factors are integrated into Hupcey's definition of social support: "a well-intentioned action that is given willingly to a person with whom there is a personal relationship and that produces an immediate or delayed positive response in the recipient" (p. 313).

Other descriptions of social support in the literature are not consistent with the boundary limitation of personal relationship described by Hupcey. Shumaker and Brownell (1984) stated that acts of social support might also occur during Internet interactions and calling in to radio talk shows or crisis hotlines. Wright and Bell (2003) conceptualized computer-mediated support groups as "weak tie" networks, in which communication occurs between individuals who may not have close relationships.

Participants experience emotional support and informational support as they communicate about health-related experiences they have in common; individuals may be more open in expressing emotions since there is greater anonymity and protection from stigmatization in comparison to face-to-face interactions. However, negative support may occur from hostile messages. Internet-provided social support may limit the full experience of social support through difficulty in forming or investing in long-term relationships and the lack of physical presence. Wright and Bell also raised the concern that the idealized perception of support through electronic communication may diminish reliance on support from family and friends, possibly reducing received support. Scharer (2005) proposed that Internet social support for parents of children with mental illness could meet the additional needs of these parents for social support. Recent evidence suggests that electronic social support may decrease use of health services (Scharer, 2005). Findings about the benefits of social support provided through electronic communication challenge Hupcey's boundary limitation of a personal relationship as a factor that defines social support.

Rook and Dooley (1985) described how social support may be viewed as an environmental or an individual variable. Gottlieb (1978) included environmental action among four classes of helping behaviors. From an ecological perspective, community environments can enhance the likelihood of social support exchanges. Controversy exists about whether professionals can be providers of social support. Although not included as providers of social support in Hupcey's definition, professionals can intervene to strengthen existing social support networks for clients or choose to provide social support when it is lacking. Many researchers have included professionals when measuring sources of social support.

Finfgeld-Connett (2005) investigated the meaning of nurse-provided telephone social support for low-income pregnant women. Although her findings indicated consistency with Oakley's (1994) operational definition of social support (includes behaviors similar to emotional, informational, and instrumental support), Finfgeld-Connett suggested that the telephone-delivered nursing interventions involved something more than the attributes of social support; she reflected that presence may be a sub-concept of social support and that social support may have become the default variable for nursing research studies because of the unavailability of instruments for measuring nursing presence. This is another example of how social support overlaps with related concepts, illustrating a lack of definitional and theoretical clarity.

A number of variables affect the social support that is given and received or experienced. These include perceptions of the need and availability for support; timing; motivation for providing support; duration, direction, and life stage; the source of support; and social network.

Perceptions of the Need for and Availability of Support

The provider of the social support first recognizes another's need for social support before determining the response to the need. If there is a mismatch in the provider's and recipient's perceptions of the need for support or the type of support that is provided, the recipient may not consider the support to be helpful (Dunkel-Schetter & Bennett, 1990; Dunkel-Schetter & Skokan, 1990). The recipient's recognition, desire, and request for the support will influence the perceived helpfulness of the support (Krishnasamy, 1996). Providers of support may assume that the recipient who is experiencing stress needs support. If this assumption is inaccurate, the act of support could result in feelings of dependency, inadequacy, and lower self-esteem (Dunkel-Schetter, Blasband, Feinstein, & Herbert, 1992). Research data suggest that the perception of the availability of support is more important for health and well-being than the actual receiving of the support (Cohen, Gottlieb, & Underwood, 2001).

Timing

Timing is also important, because the support needs of the recipient can change relative to the recipient's appraisal of the situation over time (Jacobson, 1986; Tilden, 1986). The social support provided and the perceived adequacy of the social support vary over time and situations (Norwood, 1996). Social support can be viewed as a contingency rather than a fixed resource, because it is a dynamic process influenced by personal characteristics and situations. Examples of changes affecting both the giving and receiving of social support are (a) the ongoing nature of relationships from a historical perspective, (b) expectations of support based on an assessment of the potential for support from the network, and (c) personal coping skills that range from extreme independence to wanting as much support as could be provided (Lackner, Goldenberg, Arrizza, & Tjosvold, 1994).

Motivation for Providing Support

Motivation for providing social support can affect the quality of the support provided. A sense of obligation on the part of the provider may decrease the recipient's satisfaction with the support (Hupcey, 1998a). Providers of social support are likely to consider the recipient's responsibility and effort relative to the needed support and the costs to the provider that result from the act of support (Jung, 1988). The provider's previous experiences with providing support and previous interactions with the intended recipient will also influence choices of support actions (Hupcey, 1998a).

Duration, Direction, and Life Stage

Duration of the support, referring to length of time or stability of the support, is a consideration for the chronically ill and persons who experience long-term loss (Cohen & Syme, 1985). The long-term effects of stressors on individuals may require ongoing support, as well as support from sources outside the usual social networks. For example, in a longitudinal study of the perceived support and support sources of older women with heart failure, the women identified paid helpers as sources of support at a later time in progression of their illness (Friedman, 1997). If persons requiring care for chronic illness can remain in their community setting, social support from paid caregivers can supplement the available support from informal networks.

The direction of support may be unidirectional or bidirectional. Bidirectional support is characterized by mutuality and reciprocity (Stewart, 1993). Professional support is usually unidirectional. In family and intimate relationships, the roles of "helper" and "helpee" may alternate (Clark, 1983; Rook & Dooley, 1985). Reciprocity in social support is likely to reduce feelings of burden and strain in providers and inadequacy and lack of control in recipients (Albrecht & Adelman, 1987).

The provision and receiving of social support vary over the life span. Some life stages offer more capability for providing social support, while other life stages require more receiving than giving of social support. Social support needs are greater during times of change and additional stress, such as during the birth of a child or with the loss of strength and function associated with aging. Vaux (1988) identified social support resources, social support needs related to growth and development issues, and typical sources of stress for family life cycle stages from infancy to late adulthood.

Sources of Social Support

Individuals are much less likely to identify professionals as sources of support, compared to family members and friends (Hupcey & Morse, 1997; Schaffer & Lia-Hoagberg, 1997). Professionals, who provide formal support, can intervene to enhance the existing social support resources of clients or can act as surrogates to provide support not currently available in the client's social network (Norbeck, 1988). To enhance informal and formal sources of support, professionals can develop and strengthen relationships with personal support networks, mutual aid groups, neighborhood support systems, volunteer programs, and community resources (Froland, Pancoast, Chapman, & Kimboko, 1981).

Nurses may be a source of support for caregivers of family members by facilitating tangible assistance to families (such as provision of transportation, respite care, and caregiving activities), through mobilization of the client's existing social support network, or by linking the client to relevant community resources. Nurses can provide informational support through giving the client knowledge about self-care practices or educating members of the client's network. Finding ways to expand the support network may decrease caregiver burden and increase available emotional and appraisal support for the client. However, assessing the quality of the social support is also important. Research shows there's a negative relationship between the quality of social support and caregiver burden (Vrabec, 1997). In particular, the amount of conflict in the relationship can result in negative social support that contributes to stress rather than well-being.

Newsom, Bookwala, and Schulz (1997) compared differences in formal and informal support sources in a study that described the social support needs and relationships of older adults in nursing homes, residential care facilities, and congregate apartments. The high degree of instrumental support available in institutional settings is provided primarily by professional and nonprofessional paid staff. These formal support sources may also provide a sizeable amount of emotional support for older adults who have physical and cognitive challenges, because paid staff are more often available for older adults in group residences (Pearlman & Crown, 1992). Newsom et al. (1997) discussed four differences in the formal social support provided by paid staff compared to the informal social support provided by family and friends: (a) older adults do not have a choice among staff members for their interactions or when interactions occur; (b) they may experience discomfort in receiving personal care from someone they do not know well; (c) the relationship may still be labeled as a professional relationship, although companionship and emotional support is provided by paid staff; and (d) the relationship is characterized by less reciprocity than would probably occur with informal sources of support.

Social Network

The size of the social network is sometimes considered to be an indicator of social support. Key sources of support, including immediate family members and close friends, are distinguished from sources viewed as less important—other relatives, coworkers, church and community members, and professional caregivers (Griffith, 1985). However, a large social network does not necessarily guarantee that a large amount of support is present (Kahn & Antonucci, 1980). The quality of the relationships and availability of persons in the social network, as well as the number of persons in the network, contribute to the enacted social support.

A variety of network members can better provide the range of needed social support actions. For example, in one study, persons with a cancer diagnosis perceived spouses or partners as helpful for their physical presence, while friends provided practical help (Dakof & Taylor, 1990). In another study with cancer patients, informational support was perceived as helpful from experts but not from friends or families (Dunkel-Schetter, 1984).

The Relationship of Social Support and Health

Heller et al. (1986) posited that two facets of social support, esteem-enhancing appraisal and stress-related, interpersonal transactions, have an effect on health outcomes. They hypothesized that the

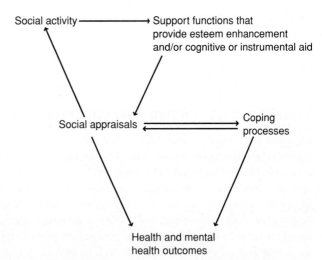

■ **Figure 8.1** Hypothesized relationships between facets of social support, coping, and health outcomes. From Heller, K., Swindle, R. W., & Dusenbery, L. (1986). Component social support processes: Comments and integration. *Journal of Continuing and Clinical Psychology, 54*(4), 466–470. Copyright © 1986 by the American Psychological Association. Reprinted with permission.

appraisal or perception of the social interaction is health protective, rather than the social interaction or support activity itself. Esteem-enhancing appraisal results from an assessment of how one is viewed by others. In stress-related interpersonal transactions, network members provide tangible assistance, which facilitates coping (Figure 8.1).

Cohen et al. (2001) described two models that explain how social support influences health. The stress-buffering model holds that social support contributes to health-promoting behaviors in persons who are experiencing stress. Rather than choosing behaviors that may be harmful to health, the support resources strengthen an individual's perceived ability to cope with a stressful situation (Thoits, 1986). These beliefs lead to a calmer psychological and physiological response to the stressful situation and can decrease negative behavioral responses. In this case, an individual is more likely to have an adaptive response to the stressful situation, thus avoiding a maladaptive response with a greater potential for negative health effects.

The main effect model, the second model described by Cohen et al. (2001), suggests that social support directly impacts psychological and physical health, whether or not an individual is experiencing a stressful situation. Integration into a social network, as contrasted to isolation, can provide social control and peer pressure to engage in health-promoting behaviors and lead to positive psychological states, such as a sense of predictability, stability, purpose, belonging, and security (Cassel, 1976; Hammer, 1981; Thoits, 1983). In addition, social networks can provide multiple sources of information about health care services and may also provide informal health care that prevents progression of illness (Cohen et al., 2001).

Norbeck (1981) proposed a model for using social support as a nursing intervention to improve health outcomes. The social support environment of the client is assessed by determining the need for social support compared to the available social support. An assessment of inadequate social support necessitates developing an intervention plan to increase social support. Possible interventions can focus on strengthening the client's existing social support structure or function or providing direct support during a crisis. According to this nursing process model, adequate social support will result in a positive health outcome; inadequate social support without intervention will result in a negative health outcome.

Manning-Walsh (2005) offers a research-based model (consistent with the stress-buffering model) in which social support is a mediator that contributes to improved health outcomes. In a study of women with breast cancer, personal support provided by family and close friends mediated the negative effects of common symptoms contributing to distress during the breast cancer treatment and resulted in improved scores on quality-of-life measures both general and specific to breast cancer.

Social Support Nursing Assessment and Interventions

Logsdon and Koniak-Griffin (2005) developed a clinical pathway for social support in postpartum adolescents, which outlines assessment of social support; assessment of related variables such as depression, risk for harm, and high-risk behaviors; and health care provider interventions. They give examples of specific assessment questions, suggest relevant instruments for the measurement of social support, and identify professional interventions that strengthen existing social support networks. Identified pathway interventions include counseling and teaching about the reality and demands of the postpartum period, common feelings experienced in the postpartum period, options for social support in their network, and the importance of communication as well as providing social skills training and referral for community services. Such interventions can raise the level of perceived appraisal, emotional, informational, and instrumental support. Beeber and Canuso (2005) offer five critical assessment questions for nurses to help determine effective emotional, information, and instrumental social support interventions: "1) Who helps you get the day-to-day things you need in your life? 2) If you had an emergency, who would you call on for help? 3) Who would lend you money or keep your child(ren) if you needed it? 4) Who gives you advice that is useful? and 5) Who understands your private worries and feelings?" (p. 773).

APPLICATIONS OF THE THEORY

Clinical Applications

Nurses have the knowledge and expertise to assess the interpersonal and social environments of clients, implement health promotion strategies, and facilitate clients in initiating self-care practices (Tilden, 1985). From a prevention perspective, social support can be viewed as "social inoculation" (Pilisuk, 1982). Through "network therapy," nurses can assess social support adequacy, use existing social support measures, determine the roles of professional and nonprofessional providers of social support to move clients to increasing independence, and organize and evaluate community support groups (Roberts, 1984).

One example of preventive support is comprehensive home visitation for vulnerable young mothers provided by public health nurses (Olds et al., 1999). Nurses provided regular home visits to young mothers beginning during their pregnancy and continuing until their children were 2 years of age. The purposes of the visits were to improve pregnancy outcomes, to promote children's healthy development, and to improve the financial self-sufficiency of participating families. Nurses both provided formal support and strengthened informal sources of support. Evaluation of the long-term outcomes through two randomized clinical trials demonstrated an increase in positive self-care practices and child well-being for the mothers who participated in the program.

Additional clinical application examples are described in Table 8.2, which specifies the five social support intervention levels suggested by Stewart (1989b): individual, dyadic, groups, community, and social system. Interventions at these levels include strengthening available social support and providing direct

Table 8.2 CLINICAL APPLICATION: SOCIAL SUPPORT INTERVENTIONS

INTERVENTION LEVEL	SITUATION	SOCIAL SUPPORT INTERVENTIONS	DESIRED HEALTH OUTCOMES
Individual—Modify how individual seeks or perceives support provided by others	A pregnant woman is placed on bed rest for a high-risk pregnancy. She has a 2-year-old son and her husband works long hours. She views her husband as her primary source of social support and does not know how she will manage getting the assistance she needs during her confinement to bed rest. She is receiving care through a hospital-based home care agency that provides nursing care to perinatal clients.	Assess her available components and sources of social support. Educate her about the importance of bed rest for her pregnancy and describe the kind of support she will need (*informational support*). Counsel her about the need to seek social support from other sources during a time of increased stress and need (*appraisal support*). Listen to the client's concerns about her husband's potential reactions to asking the client's mother to assist with household tasks and child care (*emotional support*). The client arranges for help with child care from her mother and several neighborhood families (*instrumental support*).	Reduced family stress Positive coping strategies Healthy infant
Dyadic—Strengthen support from a key network member or introduce outsider to provide support	A 35-year-old woman is having a mastectomy for breast cancer. She states she has a very close relationship with her husband but has not talked with him about how the surgery will affect their sexual relationship.	Assess her available sources of support for talking about her specific concern. Reassure her that this is a common concern that is difficult for couples to discuss (*appraisal support*). Give her information about a program that provides a visitor who has had a breast cancer experience and suggest that referral for couples' counseling is an option (*informational support*). Following a meeting with the visitor from the volunteer program, the client discusses her concerns with her husband and is reassured by his response (*emotional support*).	Maintenance of healthy self-concept Positive couple relationship Reduced complications

(table continued on page 174)

Table 8.2 CLINICAL APPLICATION: SOCIAL SUPPORT INTERVENTIONS (continued)

INTERVENTION LEVEL	SITUATION	SOCIAL SUPPORT INTERVENTIONS	DESIRED HEALTH OUTCOMES
Group—Enlarge existing informal network, improve skills of natural helpers, or refer to or create support groups	A 45-year-old man has MS and recently became wheelchair dependent. His wife has returned to full-time work. The couple has two teenagers. Case management is provided through a home health agency. The wife has become increasingly frustrated with trying to manage her work demands and the needs of her husband.	Assess the family's social support components and sources of family, extended family, friend, community, and professional support. Suggest that a support group for persons with MS and their families could be helpful in providing them with understanding and practical ideas for their situation (*informational support*). Because a local support group does not exist, work with a community service agency to develop a support group (*instrumental support*). The family participates in a local support group (*emotional support*). Re-evaluate the current nursing services. Provide additional services needed to reduce the wife's workload (*instrumental support*).	Reduced caregiver stress level Effective family functioning Increased community resources through provision of a support group for clients with MS and their family members
Community—Promote social support and social network frequency of interaction in neighborhoods, organizations, and communities	Elderly residents in an urban, ethnically diverse, low-income neighborhood are more isolated in the winter. A Block Nurse program has been recently established to address the health care needs of this population. A high percentage of the clients served by the program have diabetes.	Survey a sample of the neighborhood elderly population to determine health concerns and social support needs. Consult and collaborate with a foot-care nurse to offer a foot-care program in a community clinic, as well as through home visits. During the clinic and home visits, assess the social support needs of the elderly persons. Educate them about foot care and community resources that can offer them assistance with house cleaning and maintenance (*instrumental support and informational support*).	Reduction in complications from diabetes in elderly population in neighborhood Elderly residents stay in their own homes for a longer time period Reduction in health care costs for nursing home care

| Systems—Promote policy and structural changes to increase social support in environments and/or remove barriers to social support (in schools, municipalities, hospitals) | The percentage of children who are overweight in an elementary school population has increased. The cafeteria serves highly processed food. The school breakfast program includes sugared cereals. | Collaborate with a local faith-based organization to extend their visitation ministry to isolated elderly persons in the neighborhood for the purpose of increasing their social interaction (*emotional support and appraisal support*).

Educate parents and school staff/administrators about the health concern and collaborate with them to develop a plan to respond to the problem (*informational support*).

Use social marketing in the school setting (posters, announcements, bulletins) to increase awareness of the problem and provide classroom education about health behaviors that influence body mass (*informational support*).

Contribute to development of policy for more nutritional food choices in the breakfast and lunch program (*instrumental support*).

Create a peer support program to encourage positive change in health behavior patterns, such as nutritional food choices and physical activity (*appraisal support*). | Increase in attractive, nutritious food choices and a reduction in the amount of processed food in meals served at the school

Increase in knowledge about the contribution of food choices and exercise to body mass index (BMI) among school children

Increase in percentage of children with a normal BMI |

social support with the goal of improving health status. Table 8-2 provides a summary of the level of intervention based on Stewart's framework, social support intervention examples with the relevant social support theoretical constructs (emotional, informational, instrumental, and appraisal support), and desired health outcomes.

Research Applications

Researchers have explored a great variety of nursing practice issues from a social support perspective including topics such as chronic illness, persons who are grieving, the relationship of social support to acute chest complaints, new mothers in stressful situations, and administrative support for nurses. Researchers have also investigated how social support interacts with other variables, such as pain and loneliness, to predict depression. The majority of studies focus on the individual or family level experience of social support. Few researchers have investigated social support from a community or systems perspective. See the Bibliography at the end of the chapter for citations on social support research on issues relevant to nursing.

MEASURES OF SOCIAL SUPPORT

Although a great number of social support measures have been developed in several disciplines, many measures do not have adequate reliability and validity testing, and many are situation-specific rather than general measures of social support. Available measures address (a) interconnectedness in a social network; (b) received support, based on a person's report of support that was provided; and (c) perceived support, which is support a person believes to be available to him or her (Sarason, Sarason, & Pierce, 1990). Researchers have primarily developed situation-specific measures of social support for groups who encounter a common stressor event, such as pregnancy or chronic illness (Stewart, 1993). Of 21 social support instruments reviewed by Stewart (1989a), only four were applicable on a general level.

Five measures of social support developed by nurse researchers are described in Table 8.3. The selected instruments represent both general and specific measures of social support and have been psychometrically analyzed. The Interpersonal Relationships Inventory (IPRI), the Norbeck Social Support Questionnaire (NSSQ), and the Perceived Resource Questionnaire (PRQ-85) are general measures of social support, which are applicable to any clinical setting where clients have the capacity to respond to a self-report instrument. None of the instruments is applicable to young children. The Support Behaviors Inventory (SBI) is specific for support during pregnancy, and the Social Support in Chronic Illness Survey (SSCII) is specific to social support for persons who are experiencing chronic illness.

The IPRI includes subscales that address reciprocal interaction and conflict in relationships, in addition to social support (Tilden, Nelson, & May, 1990). The inclusion of the reciprocity and conflict subscales can potentially capture the fuller context of relationships, unlike most social support measures. The social support items are consistent with perceived availability of support and the enactment of helping behaviors by members of a person's social network.

On the NSSQ, respondents make a list of up to 24 persons who are important to them. Respondents are given a list of suggested categories to help them identify persons in their social network. Then, each person in the social network is rated on how much social support is provided on several social support components. Although perceived negative aspects of relationships are not addressed, the NSSQ does include an item on loss of persons in the social network and the extent of support that was provided by persons who are no longer available (Norbeck, Lindsey, & Carrieri, 1981, 1983).

Table 8.3 SELECTED SOCIAL SUPPORT INSTRUMENTS DEVELOPED BY NURSE RESEARCHERS

INSTRUMENT	SOCIAL SUPPORT COMPONENTS	DESCRIPTION	SAMPLE ITEM
Interpersonal Relationships Inventory (IPRI) (Tilden et al., 1990)	Social support Reciprocity Conflict	39 items (13 for each subscale) 5-point agree/disagree scale Subscales used separately Internal consistency and test–retest reliability Construct validity for social support and conflict subscales	Someone believes in me (support). I let others know I care (reciprocity). I wish people were more sensitive (conflict).
Norbeck Social Support Questionnaire (NSSQ) (Norbeck, et al., 1981, 1983)	Affect Affirmation Aid Loss Duration of relationship Frequency of contact	Identify persons in network 5-point scale on extent of support provided for 9 questions Internal consistency and test–retest reliability Construct validity	How much does this person make you feel liked or loved?
Perceived Resource Questionnaire (PRQ-85) (Weinert, 1988, 1990)	Intimacy Social integration Nurturance Worth Assistance	Part 1—Identifies resources and satisfaction with help Part 2—25 items on perceived social support; 7-point agree/disagree scale Internal consistency reliability—Part 2 Construct validity—Part 2	If I need advice, there is someone who would assist me to work out a plan for dealing with the situation.
Support Behaviors Inventory (SBI) (Brown, 1986)	Perceived degree of experiential support during pregnancy—satisfaction with partner support and satisfaction with other support	11 items on shortened version 6-point satisfied/dissatisfied scale Internal consistency reliability for total support score on shortened version	Tolerates my ups and downs and unusual behaviors
Social Support in Chronic Illness Survey (SSCII) (Hilbert, 1990)	Intimate interaction Guidance Feedback Maternal aid Behavioral assistance Positive social interaction	38 items 6-point satisfied/dissatisfied scale Internal consistency reliability Content validity	Commented favorably when (s)he noticed me doing something that the health team recommended

Originally designed in 1981, the PRQ has undergone extensive psychometric evaluation (Brandt & Weinert, 1981; Weinert, 1987, 1988). Based on instrument testing with a variety of populations, the authors revised Parts 1 and 2. The nurturance items were extended to include adults as well as younger persons.

Brown (1986) developed the SBI specifically for social support during pregnancy. Although the items were based on the components of emotional, material, informational, and appraisal support, a factor analysis resulted in the identification of one dimension of social support in a sample of pregnant couples. This finding led Brown to question the multidimensional nature of social support. About one-half of the original 45 items in the instrument development stage applied specifically to social support during pregnancy, while the remainder were applicable to general social support situations. Through theoretical analysis, Brown selected 11 items for a shortened version of the SBI. Respondents rate their satisfaction with social support from partners and others for each of the 11 items.

Hilbert (1990) created the SSCII in response to the lack of a social support measure specific to chronic illness. She included items from other measures and added items based on the literature and interviews with myocardial infarction clients. The original 45 items were reduced to 38 items, as a result of a content analysis for relevance to the purpose of the instrument. The finalized instrument includes 29 general social support items and nine items specific to chronic illness.

A six-item general measure of social support (not included in Table 9.3), the Social Support Questionnaire (SSQ6), developed by psychologists (Sarason, Sarason, Shearin, & Pierce, 1987), may be of interest to nurse researchers who are looking for a brief and convenient measure of social support. For each item, the respondent identifies the number of persons available in time of need related to a situation, as well as the satisfaction with the perceived available support, on a six-point scale. Through psychometric evaluation that also involved comparison with other measures of social support, Sarason et al. (1987) determined that the SSQ6 is psychometrically sound and can substitute for the SSQ, the original 27-item instrument. The authors determined the items on the six-item scale were conceptually consistent with the affective component of social support but not with instrumental support. An example of one of the items is, "Whom can you count on to console you when you are very upset?" They hypothesized that people's perceptions about the availability of others to help in times of need may be the most important social support component in relationship to health outcomes.

Most measures of social support are self-reports. Newsom et al. (1997) discussed the challenge of measuring social support for the cognitively impaired. They suggested that proxy and observational measures of social support may be an alternative strategy for determining the adequacy of social support for persons who cannot provide an accurate self-report. Proxies, such as nursing home staff and primary caregivers, can provide information about social network contacts and interactions. Observational methods include recording interaction behaviors and videotaping. A coding system can be used to label the source of the support, the type of support, the recipient response, and other characteristics of the support interaction.

QUALITATIVE METHODS

Some researchers have used qualitative approaches for investigating social support, although quantitative measures appear to be predominant. In Finland, nurse researchers asked one open-ended question to explore perceptions of social support after the death of a spouse: "What helped you cope with your grief?"

(Kaunonen, Tarkka, Paunonen, & Laippala, 1999). The researchers used content analysis to classify the data by the structure of social relationships and the social support functions of aid, affirmation, and affect in relationships (Kahn, 1979).

Lugton (1997) used a strategy called social contact analysis, in addition to interview data, to explore the social support experienced by women treated for breast cancer. Participants drew their social networks, with self at center, using shorter lines for closer relationships and arrows to indicate whether the relationship involved support, strain, or both. The researcher then asked participants to describe how professional and informal persons in the social network had responded to the illness of the participant in supportive and nonsupportive ways. Types of support that facilitated adjustment were emotional support, companionship, practical help, opportunities for confiding, experiential support (from others who had experienced breast cancer), and sexual identity support. See Using Middle Range Theories 8.1 and 8.2 for two examples of how social support has been used in research.

8.1 USING MIDDLE RANGE THEORIES

Adequate social support during pregnancy can mediate the stress of changes related to pregnancy. For pregnant women, social support can contribute to a healthy response to pregnancy if the support encourages women to seek prenatal care and maintain healthy behaviors during the pregnancy, resulting in improved birth outcomes. This study investigated the relationship of social support provided by the partner and others to the adequacy of prenatal care and the prenatal health behaviors of low-income women. Social support was operationalized using the components of affect, affirmation, aid, and loss (Kahn, 1979; Norbeck et al., 1981). The researcher added two pregnancy-specific questions to the Norbeck Social Support Questionnaire: (a) How much does this person talk with you about your pregnancy, and (b) How much does this person give you information that helps you with your pregnancy? The sample included 101 low-income women, ages 18 to 35, from five urban prenatal clinics. Adequacy of prenatal care was determined using Kotelchuck's Adequacy of Prenatal Care Index (1994). Schaffer developed the Prenatal Health Questionnaire (PHQ) to measure behaviors known to contribute to a healthy pregnancy: participation in prenatal education, healthy food choices, and avoidance of tobacco, alcohol, and illegal drugs. Pearson's *r* correlation coefficient was used to determine the relationship of social support variables (source and component of social support) to adequacy of prenatal care and prenatal health behaviors. Social support from the partner was positively related to prenatal care adequacy, while social support from others was positively related to healthy prenatal behaviors. Both sources of support were important, but for different health outcomes. The women in the sample infrequently identified professionals as sources of support in comparison with others from their informal social network. Nurses can provide informational support to the partners and other network members of low-income women to enhance the emotional, instrumental, informational, and appraisal support available in the women's social networks. Social support actions can encourage healthy self-care practices in low-income pregnant women.

Schaffer, M. A., & Lia-Hoagberg, B. (1997). Effects of social support on prenatal care and health behaviors of low-income women. *Journal of Obstetric, Gynecologic, and Neonatal Nursing, 26*(4), 433–440.

8.2 USING MIDDLE RANGE THEORIES

This study addressed the structure, function, and nature of social support. The researchers explored how caregivers of relatives with Alzheimer's disease used formal and informal support. A multidimensional definition of social support was used through the administration of the reciprocity and conflict subscales from the Interpersonal Relationships Inventory (Tilden et al., 1990), in addition to measures of informal and formal support developed by the researchers. The informal support measure included seven items that addressed tangible, emotional, and informational support on a four-point scale of frequency of support. Participants also rated their satisfaction for each informal support item. Formal support was determined by the number and usefulness of formal services provided by structured organizations. The researchers explored characteristics of support sources such as the gender and kinship (adult children or spouses) of the caregivers. The researchers wished to determine whether formal support would substitute for or supplement the informal support based on gender and kinship. The sample, recruited from health and social service agencies in Quebec, consisted of 193 daughters, wives, and husbands who lived with their family member with Alzheimer's disease. Multivariate analyses of variances (MANOVAs) were used to determine differences in support variables among caregiver groups. The researchers used *t*-tests to investigate gender and kinship hypotheses. Gender differences emerged in the use of and response to informal support, while there were kinship differences regarding formal support. In comparison to husbands, wives experienced less satisfaction and a greater level of conflict in situations of less informal support. The researchers commented that women might be socialized to expect more from their informal sources of support. Regarding formal sources of support, the frequency of formal services seemed more important to spouses than to daughters. The researchers found that the support provided by the informal network was not reduced when formal agencies were also providing support. The formal support did not substitute for the informal support. This study demonstrates the importance of exploring social support source characteristics, such as gender and kinship. It is important that the researchers explored negative aspects of social support through use of the conflict subscale of the IPRI. To understand the full context of social support, middle range theory development must also consider the relationship of negative social support actions to health outcomes.

Cossette, S., Levesque, L., & Laurin, L. (1995). Informal and formal support for caregivers of a demented relative: Do gender and kinship make a difference? *Research in Nursing and Health, 18,* 437–451.

CHALLENGES TO SOCIAL SUPPORT THEORY DEVELOPMENT AND RESEARCH

Future efforts in social support theory development and research need to move from a description of the relationship of social support and health outcomes to the investigation of interactional characteristics, negative aspects, gender and cultural contexts, causal relationships in social support, and effective social support interventions. In particular, multilevel interventions that address both interpersonal support and community-level environmental support could contribute to knowledge about cost-effective social support strategies for improving the health status of populations.

Because researchers have used a variety of definitions of social support and have measured different aspects of social support, it is difficult to compare study results (Heitzmann & Kaplan, 1988; Roberts, 1984; Wortman & Dunkel–Schetter, 1987). Hupcey (1998b) commented that many other concepts, such as marital status and frequency of contact, have often been included in definitions of social support. A focus on the interactional nature of social support is missing from many studies. To determine effectiveness of social support, an understanding of the perceptions of the providers of social support as well as those of the recipient merits further exploration (Hupcey, 1998b). The reciprocity of social support is an interactional variable that can contribute to understanding effective social support interventions.

Middle range social support theory development could be enhanced by greater exploration of the negative effects of informal social support. Many social support measures do not include negative aspects of relationships (Krishnasamy, 1996; Stewart, 1993). In a review of 50 studies on social support and caregiver burden, Vrabec (1997) recommended further examination of the amount of conflict in the social support network as a predictor of caregiver burden. The IPRI is one of the few measures that attempts to encompass the full context of relationships through inclusion of reciprocity and conflict subscales (Tilden et al., 1990).

Few authors have discussed the impact of culture in regard to social support theory and measurement. Ducharme, Stevens, and Rowat (1994) acknowledged that few measures consider the personal and contextual factors that can influence social support interactions, such as culture and gender. Higgins and Dicharry (1991) evaluated the Personal Resources Inventory Part 2 (PRQ) for its applicability to Navajo women. They found that 10 of the 25 items were not applicable to Navajo culture. The 10 items were considered too personal because in the Navajo culture family problems and feelings are not discussed with others. Different cultural groups may vary in perceptions of the number of persons they consider to be a part of their social network, as well as the relative importance of the different components of social support. Expectations for independence and help may differ. Some types of assistance could be expected and appreciated by one culture and be interpreted as shameful by another culture. In a study on types of social support in African Americans with cancer, Hamilton and Sandelowski (2004) found that although the broad categories of social support were applicable to the African-American sample, strategies for perceived helpful social support differed from Caucasian populations. African Americans perceived presence and distracting activities as emotional support in contrast to verbal expressions of problems. Instrumental support included offers of prayer and other kinds of assistance that were less often identified in other studies of social support. Martinez-Schallmoser, MacMullen, and Telleen (2005) offer specific assessment questions that are adapted to the social support needs of the Mexican-American pregnant women population. The meaning of social support across cultures needs further exploration. In addition, males are a neglected population in social support research (Langford et al., 1997). Qualitative research approaches could be useful for discovering meanings of social support across cultures.

Causality in social support research needs further exploration. Researchers have conducted many descriptive and correlational studies that link social support to positive health outcomes, but few studies substantiate causal links (Callaghan & Morrissey, 1993). The impact of health status on how people seek and receive support has been explored less often than the effects of social support on health status (Stewart, 1993). Changes in health status are likely to influence the amount of and components of social support that are needed. With increased stress resulting from threats to health, social support actions can facilitate coping. Moreover, the balance of reciprocity in relationships and the amount of conflict present may change in response to health status changes. One question suggested by Cohen et al. (2001) for future study is whether persons with chronic illness decrease their provision of support, resulting in an imbalance in the social network (reciprocity).

To further develop understanding of the linkages of social support to health outcomes, theoretically based social support interventions need to be tested in controlled intervention trials across varied settings and age groups (Ducharme et al., 1994). Cohen et al. (2001) suggested that more intervention research should be conducted on promising interventions, such as support groups and support provided in dyads (partner or peer support). In addition, research on interventions that focus on strengthening the social support environments at a community or systems level can develop knowledge about how to use social support to improve the health status of populations. Multilevel interventions may be the most effective. Rook and Dooley (1985) described two categorical approaches to social support interventions—individual and environmental. Individual interventions are used to change how a person perceives or seeks support, while an environmental approach targets the community to improve the social support climate. Social support is likely to be maximized with the implementation of both approaches. Research methods used to test the effectiveness of social support interventions need to be tailored to the intervention level. Measures for any level should include the potential negative aspects of social support in the person's interactions and environment, which, if not considered, can confound the interpretation of study findings. Evaluation of social support interventions at the individual, dyadic, and group levels is likely to focus on the perceptions of social support actions and available support. Evaluation of social support interventions at the community and systems levels emphasizes analysis of social support available in networks and the environment. The impact of a nurse-initiated program on social support for a group is described in Research Application 8.1.

8.1 RESEARCH APPLICATION

A nurse researcher is evaluating the effectiveness of a parish nursing program to strengthen the social support available to many elderly individuals who live alone in the surrounding low-income, urban community. The goals of the program are to connect elderly residents with needed health care services and make it possible for them to continue living safely in their homes. The program includes bimonthly group meetings of seniors at the church for informational and emotional support, and an outreach program in which congregational members make regular visits and phone calls to elderly residents in the neighborhood who wish to participate in the program. Both program components can strengthen instrumental support by connecting residents to community organizations that provide services needed by the residents, such as health care and home maintenance.

The researcher administers Part 2 of the Personal Resource Questionnaire (PRQ-85) to program participants at the time of initial enrollment and 6 months later to determine any changes in level of perceived social support. In addition, the researcher conducts a focus group with the senior group meeting at the church. Several open-ended questions are used to explore participants' social support experiences related to appraisal, emotional, informational, and instrumental support. For elderly residents who are in the outreach program, the researcher interviews a sample of participants in their homes to collect data on changes in health status and use of health care and community services.

ANALYSIS OF THEORY

The chapter on social support provides several constructs with which to view the phenomenon. Using the criteria presented in Chapter 2, critique the body of knowledge presented in this chapter. You will be using each criterion in a manner different from its use when applied to one specific theory. Specific questions related to the use of each criterion in this new context follow. Compare your conclusions about the constructs across theories with those found in Appendix A. A nurse scholar who has worked with this phenomenon completed the analysis found in the Appendix.

Internal Criticism

1. Clarity (Do we have theories of social support that are clear?)
2. Consistency (Is there consistency in approach, i.e., terms, interpretations, principles, and methods, across theories?)

3. Adequacy (How adequate is the body of theories in accounting for social support?)
4. Level of theory development (At what level of development are the social support theories?)

External Criticism

1. Reality convergence (Do these theories reflect "real world" nursing experiences of social support?)
2. Utility (How useful are present theories when applied in practice and research?)
3. Significance (Do the theories reflect issues essential to nursing?)
4. Discrimination (Do the theories help distinguish social support from other interpersonal processes?)
5. Scope of theory (What seems to be the scope of the theories?)
6. Complexity (As a group, how would you judge the complexity of social support theories?)

CRITICAL THINKING EXERCISES

Compare two options for providing a social support intervention for parents of children diagnosed with a chronic mental illness: (a) a nurse-led monthly face-to-face meeting of parents (with child care provided) and (b) an asynchronous Internet discussion for the parents.

1. Look at the list of definitions of key terms. Use the key terms to analyze the nature of the social support experience that could be expected from each of the two interventions.
2. Analyze how each of the interventions is consistent or inconsistent with Hupcey's definition of social support.
3. Design evaluation studies, using both quantitative and qualitative approaches, to measure the experience of social support and effectiveness of the

intervention for each of the two options. Consider the reliability and validity of suggested measurement strategies.

4. Analyze how the following variables may affect the experience of social support in each of the two options: perceptions of the need for and availability of support; timing; motivation for providing support; duration, direction, and life stage; sources of social support; and social network.
5. Analyze the potential effectiveness (improved health outcomes and coping) resulting from professional or nurse-provided social support versus enhancement of social support provided by personal relationships and social networks for parents of children with a chronic mental illness.

SUMMARY

Social support theory is important to nurses because it can explain and suggest nursing interventions to improve health outcomes. Although a great variety of social support measures have been developed, many are for specific situations. There is a lack of consensus on the definition of social support. Authors disagree on the dimensionality of social support. A major concern is the omission of considering potential negative aspects of social support. The next step for expanding social support theory is knowledge development about effective multilevel social support interventions.

WEB RESOURCES

1. Jane S. Norbeck's web page gives access to downloadable files of the Norbeck Social Support Questionnaire (NSSQ) and scoring instructions at no cost, including a Spanish version. The NSSQ was revised in 1995 to be compatible with Microsoft Windows for data entry and analysis. Her web page can be reached at: **http://nurseweb.ucsf.edu/www/ffnorb.htm**
2. RAND is a nonprofit institute that helps improve policy and decision making through research and analysis. This site includes a brief, self-administered social support survey (18 items) with four subscales that was developed for the Medical Outcomes Study (MOS). The subscales include emotional/informational support, tangible support, affectionate support, and positive social interaction. Scoring instructions are available. This site can be accessed at: **http://www.rand.org/health/surveys_tools/mos /mos_socialsupport.html**
3. Irwin and Barbara Sarason's web site gives access to downloading the Social Support Questionnaire (SSQ): **http://www.measurementexperts.org/instrument/overviews/is_support.asp**

REFERENCES

Albrecht, T., & Adelman, M. (1987). Communication networks as structures of social support. In T. Albrecht & M. Adelman (Eds.), *Communicating social support* (pp. 40–61). Newbury Park, CA: Sage.

Barrera, M. (1981). Social support in the adjustment of pregnant adolescents: Assessment issues. In B. Gottlieb (Ed.), *Social networks and social support* (pp. 69–96). Beverly Hills, CA: Sage.

Barrera Jr., M. (1986). Distinctions between social support concepts, measures, and models. *American Journal of Community Psychology, 14*(4), 413–445.

Beeber, L. S. & Canusao, R. (2005). Strengthening social support for the low-income mother: Five critical questions and a guide for intervention. *Journal of Obstetric, Gynecologic & Neonatal Nursing, 34*(6), 369–376.

Bloom, J. R. (1990). The relationship of social support and health. *Social Science and Medicine, 39*(5), 635–637.

Bowlby, J. (1971). *Attachment.* London: Pelican.

Brandt, P. A., & Weinert, C. (1981). The PRQ—A social support measure. *Nursing Research, 30*(5), 277–280.

Brown, M. A. (1986). Social support during pregnancy: A unidimensional or multidimensional concept? *Nursing Research, 35*(1), 4–9.

Callaghan, P., & Morrissey, J. (1993). Social support and health: A review. *Journal of Advanced Nursing, 18,* 203–210.

Cassel, J. (1974). Psychosocial process and "stress": Theoretical perspectives. *International Journal of Health Services, 4*(3), 471–482.

Cassel, J. (1976). The contribution of the social environment to host resistance. *American Journal of Epidemiology, 104*(2), 107–123.

Clark, J. S. (1983). Reactions to aid in communal and exchange relationships. In J. D. Fisher, D. Nadler, & B. M. DePaulo (Eds.), *New directions in helping: Vol 1. Recipient reactions to aid* (pp. 281–305). New York: Academic Press.

Cobb, S. (1976). Social support as a moderator of life stress. *Psychosomatic Medicine, 38,* 300–314.

Cohen, S. (1992). Stress, social support, and disorder. In H. O. Veiel & U. Baumann (Eds.), *The meaning and measurement of social support* (pp. 109–204). New York: Hemisphere Publishing Corporation.

Cohen, S., Gottlieb, B. H., & Underwood, L. G. (2001). Social relationships and health: Challenges for measurement and intervention. *Advances in Mind–Body Medicine, 17,* 129–141.

Cohen, S., & Syme, S. L. (1985). Issues in the study and application of social support. In S. Cohen & S. L. Syme

(Eds.), *Social support and health* (pp. 3–32). New York: Academic Press.

Cossette, S., Levesque, L., & Laurin, L. (1995). Informal and formal support for caregivers of a demented relative: Do gender and kinship make a difference? *Research in Nursing and Health, 18,* 437–451.

Coyne, J. C., & DeLongis, A. (1986). Going beyond social support: The role of social relationships in adaptation. *Journal of Consulting and Clinical Psychology, 54,* 454–460.

Cutrona, C. E. (1990). Stress and social support: In search of optimal matching. *Journal of Social and Clinical Psychology, 9*(1), 3–14.

Dakof, G., & Taylor, S. (1990). Victim's perception of social support: What is helpful from whom? *Journal of Personality and Social Psychology, 58*(1), 80–89.

Diamond, M. (1985). A review and critique of the concepts of social support. In R. A. O'Brien (Ed.), *Social support and health: New directions for theory and research* (pp. 1–32). Rochester, NY: University of Rochester Press.

Ducharme, F., Stevens, B., & Rowat, K. (1994). Social support: Conceptual and methodological issues for research in mental health nursing. *Issues in Mental Health Nursing, 15,* 373–392.

Dunkel-Schetter, C. (1984). Social support and cancer: Findings based on patient interviews and their implications. *Journal of Social Issues, 40*(4), 77–98.

Dunkel-Schetter, C., & Bennett, T. L. (1990). Differentiating the cognitive and behavioral aspects of social support. In B. R. Sarason, I. G. Sarason, & G. R. Pierce (Eds.), *Social support: An interactional view* (pp. 267–296). New York: Wiley.

Dunkel-Schetter, C., Blasband, D., Feinstein, L., & Herbert, T. (1992). Elements of supportive interactions. When are attempts to help effective? In S. Spacapan & S. Oskamp, (Eds.), *Helping and being helped* (pp. 83–114). New York: Academic Press.

Dunkel-Schetter, C., & Skokan, L. A. (1990). Determinants of social support provision in personal relationships. *Journal of Social and Personal Relationships, 7*(4), 437–450.

Finfgeld-Connett, D. (2005). Telephone social support or nursing presence? Analysis of a nursing intervention. *Qualitative Health Research, 15*(1), 19–29.

Friedman, M. M. (1997). Social support sources among older women with heart failure: Continuity versus loss over time. *Research in Nursing and Health, 20,* 319–327.

Froland, C., Pancoast, D., Chapman, D., & Kimboko, P. (1981). *Helping networks and human services.* Beverly Hills, CA: Sage.

Gottlieb, B. H. (1978). The development and application of a classification scheme of informal helping networks. *Canadian Journal of Behavioral Science, 10,* 105–115.

Griffith, J. (1985). Social support providers: Who are they? Where are they met? And the relationships of network characteristics to psychological distress. *Basic and Applied Social Psychology, 6*(1), 41–60.

Hamilton, J. B., & Sandelowski, M. (2004). Types of social support in African Americans with cancer. *Oncology Nursing Forum, 31*(4), 792–800.

Hammer, M. (1981). "Core" and "extended" social networks in relation to health and illness. *Social Science and Medicine, 17,* 405–411.

Heitzmann, C. A., & Kaplan, R. M. (1988). Assessment of methods for measuring social support. *Health Psychology, 7*(1), 75–109.

Heller, K., Swindle, R. W., & Dusenbury, L. (1986). Component social support processes: Comments and integration. *Journal of Consulting and Clinical Psychology, 54*(4), 466–470.

Hilbert, G. A. (1990). Measuring social support in chronic illness. In O. L. Strickland & C. F. Waltz (Eds.), *Measurement of nursing outcomes,* (Vol. 4, pp. 79–95). New York: Springer Publishing Company.

Higgins, P. G., & Dicharry, E. K. (1991). Measurement issues addressing social support with Navajo women. *Western Journal of Nursing Research, 13*(2), 242–255.

House, J. S. (1981). *Work stress and social support.* Englewood Cliffs, NJ: Prentice Hall.

Hupcey, J. E. (1998a). Clarifying the social support theory–research linkage. *Journal of Advanced Nursing, 27*(6), 1231–1241.

Hupcey, J. E. (1998b). Social support: Assessing conceptual coherence. *Qualitative Health Research, 8*(3), 304–318.

Hupcey, J. E., & Morse, J. M. (1997). Can a professional relationship be considered social support? *Nursing Outlook, 45,* 270–276.

Hutchinson, C. (1999). Social support: Factors to consider when designing studies that measure social support. *Journal of Advanced Nursing, 29*(6), 1520–1526.

Jacobson, D. E. (1986). Types and timing of social support. *Journal of Health and Social Behavior, 27,* 250–264.

Jung, J. (1988). Social support providers: Why do they help? *Basic and Applied Social Psychology, 9,* 231–240.

Kahn, R. L. (1979). Aging and social support. In M. W. Riley (Ed.), *Aging from birth to death: Interdisciplinary perspectives* (pp. 77–91). Boulder, CO: Westview Press.

Kahn, R. L., & Antonucci, T. C. (1980). Convoys over the life course: Attachment, roles, and social support. In P. B. Baltes & G. Brim (Eds.), *Life span development and behavior* (Vol. 3, pp. 253–283). New York: Academic Press.

Kaunonen, M., Tarkka, M., Paunonen, M., & Laippala, P. (1999). Grief and social support after the death of a spouse. *Journal of Advanced Nursing, 30*(6), 1304–1311.

Kotelchuck, M. (1994). An evaluation of the Kessner Adequacy of Prenatal Care Utilization Index. *American Journal of Public Health, 84*(9), 1414–1420.

Krishnasamy, M. (1996). Social support and the patient with cancer: A consideration of the literature. *Journal of Advanced Nursing, 23*(4), 757–762.

La Gaipa, J. J. (1990). The negative effects of informal support systems. In S. Duck (Ed.), *Personal relationships and social support* (pp. 122–139). London: Sage.

Lackner, S., Goldenberg, S., Arrizza, G., & Tjosvold, I. (1994). The contingency of social support. *Qualitative Health Research, 4*(2), 224–243.

Laireiter, A., & Baumann, U. (1992). Network structures and support functions theoretical and empirical analyses. In H. O. Veiel & U. Baumann (Eds.), *The meaning and measurement of social support* (pp. 33–55). London: Hemisphere Publishing Corporation.

Langford, C. P. H., Bowsher, J., Maloney, J. P., & Lillis, P. (1997). Social support: A conceptual analysis. *Journal of Advanced Nursing, 25*(1), 95–100.

Logsdon, M. C., & Koniak-Griffin, D. (2005). Social support in postpartum adolescents: Guidelines for nursing assessments and interventions. *Journal of Obstetric, Gynecologic, and Neonatal Nursing, 34*(6), 761–768.

Lugton, J. (1997). The nature of social support as experienced by women treated for breast cancer. *Journal of Advanced Nursing, 25*(6), 1184–1191.

Manning-Walsh, J. (2005). Social support as a mediator between symptom distress and quality of life in women with breast cancer. *Journal of Obstetric, Gynecologic, and Neonatal Nursing, 34*(4), 482–493.

Martinez-Schallmoser, L., MacMullen, N. J., & Telleen, S. (2005). Social support in Mexican American childbearing women. *Journal of Obstetric, Gynecologic, and Neonatal Nursing, 34*(6), 755–760.

Newsom, J. T., Bookwala, J., & Schulz, R. (1997). Social support measurement in group residences for older adults. *Journal of Mental Health and Aging, 3*(1), 47–66.

Norbeck, J. S. (1981). Social support: A model for clinical research and application. *Advances in Nursing Science, 3*(4), 43–59.

Norbeck, J. S. (1988). Social support. *Annual Review of Nursing Research, 6,* 85–109.

Norbeck, J. S., Lindsey, A. M., & Carrieri, V. L. (1981). The development of an instrument to measure social support. *Nursing Research, 30*(5), 264–269.

Norbeck, J. S., Lindsey, A. M., & Carrieri, V. L. (1983). Further development of the Norbeck social support questionnaire: Normative data and validity testing. *Nursing Research, 32*(1), 4–9.

Norbeck, J. S., & Tilden, V. P. (1988). International research in social support: Theoretical and methodological issues. *Journal of Advanced Nursing, 13,* 173–178.

Norwood, S. L. (1996). The social support Apgar: Instrument development and testing. *Research in Nursing and Health, 19,* 143–152.

Oakley, A. (1994). Giving support in pregnancy: The role of research midwives in a randomized controlled trial. In S. Robinson & A. M. Thompson (Eds.), *Midwives research*

and childbirth (Vol. 3, pp. 30–63). London: Chapman and Hall.

Olds, D. L., Henderson, C. R., Kitzman, H. J., Echenrode, J. J., Cole, R. E., & Tatelbaum, R. C. (1999). Prenatal and infancy home visitation by nurses: Recent findings. *Future of Children, 9*(1), 44–65.

Pearlman, D. N., & Crown, W. H. (1992). Alternative sources of social support and their impacts on institutional risk. *The Gerontologist, 32,* 527–535.

Pierce, G. R., Sarason, B. R., & Sarason, I. G. (1990). Integrating social support perspectives: Working models, personal relationships, and situational factors. In S. Duck (Ed.), *Personal relationships and social support* (pp. 173–189). London: Sage.

Pilisuk, M. (1982). Delivery of social support: The social inoculation. *American Journal of Orthopsychiatry, 52,* 20–31.

Ragsdale, D., Yarbrough, S., & Lasher, A. T. (1993). Using social support theory to care for CVA patients. *Rehabilitation Nursing, 18*(3), 154–172.

Roberts, S. J. (1984). Social support—meaning, measurement, and relevance to community health nursing practice. *Public Health Nursing, 1*(3), 158–167.

Rook, K. S., & Dooley, D. (1985). Applying social support research: Theoretical problems and future directions. *Journal of Social Issues, 41*(1), 5–28.

Sarason, I. G., Sarason, B. R., Shearin, E. N., & Pierce, G. R. (1987). A brief measure of social support: Practical and theoretical implications. *Journal of Social and Personal Relationships, 4,* 497–510.

Sarason, B. R., Sarason, I. G., & Pierce, G. R. (1990). *Social support: An interactional view.* New York: John Wiley.

Schaffer, M. A., & Lia-Hoagberg, B. (1997). Effects of social support on prenatal care and health behaviors of low-income women. *Journal of Obstetric, Gynecologic, and Neonatal Nursing, 26*(4), 433–440.

Scharer, K. (2005). Internet social support for parents: The state of the science. *Journal of Child and Adolescent Psychiatric Nursing, 18*(1), 26–35.

Shumaker, S. A., & Brownell, A. (1984). Toward a theory of social support: Closing conceptual gaps. *Journal of Social Issues, 40*(4), 11–36.

Stewart, M. J. (1993). *Integrating social support in nursing.* Newbury Park, CA: Sage.

Stewart, M. J. (1989a). Social support instruments created by nurse investigators. *Nursing Research, 38*(5), 268–275.

Stewart, M. J. (1989b). Social support intervention studies: A review and prospectus of nursing contributions. *International Journal of Nursing Studies, 26*(2), 93–114.

Tardy, C. H. (1985). Social support measurement. *American Journal of Community Psychology, 13*(2), 187–202.

Thoits, P. A. (1983). Multiple identities and psychosocial well-being: A reformation and test of the social isolation hypothesis. *American Sociological Review, 48,* 174–187.

Thoits, P. A. (1986). Social support as coping assistance. *Journal of Consulting and Clinical Psychology, 54*(4), 416–423.

Tilden, V. P. (1985). Issues of conceptualization and measurement of social support in construction of nursing theory. *Research in Nursing and Health, 81,* 199–206.

Tilden, V. P. (1986). New perspectives on social support. *The Nurse Practitioner, 11,* 60–61.

Tilden, V. P., & Galyen, R. D. (1987). Cost and conflict: The darker side of social support. *Western Journal of Nursing Research, 9*(1), 9–18.

Tilden, V. P., Nelson, C. A., & May, B. A. (1990). The IPR inventory: Development and psychometric characteristics. *Nursing Research, 39*(6), 337–343.

Tilden, V. P., & Weinert, S. C. (1987). Social support and the chronically ill individual. *Nursing Clinics of North America, 22*(3), 613–620.

Vaux, A. (1988). *Social support—theory, research, and intervention.* New York: Praeger.

Veiel, H. O., & Baumann, U. (1992). The many meanings of social support. In H. O. Veiel & U. Baumann (Eds.), *The meaning and measurement of social support* (pp. 1–9). New York: Hemisphere.

Vrabec, N. J. (1997). Literature review of social support and caregiver burden, 1980 to 1985. *Image: Journal of Nursing Scholarship, 29*(4), 383–388.

Wandersman, L., Wandersman, A., & Kahn, S. (1980). Social support in the transition to parenthood. *Journal of Community Psychology, 8,* 332–342.

Weinert, C. (1987). A social support measure: PRQ85. *Nursing Research, 36*(5), 273–277.

Weinert, C. (1988). Measuring social support: Revision and further development of the personal resource questionnaire. In O. L. Strickland & C. F. Waltz (Eds.), *Measurement of nursing outcomes,* (Vol. 1, pp. 309–327). New York: Springer Publishing Company.

Wortman, C. B. (1984). Social support and cancer: Conceptual and methodological issues. *Cancer, 53,* 2339–2360.

Wortman, C. B., & Dunkel-Schetter, C. (1987). Conceptual and methodological issues in the study of social support. In A. Baum & J. E. Singer (Eds.), *Handbook of psychology and health* (pp. 63–108). Hillsdale, NJ: Lawrence Erlbaum Associates.

Wright, K. B., & Bell, S. B. (2003). Health-related support groups on the Internet: Linking empirical findings to social support and computer-mediated communication theory. *Journal of Health Psychology, 8*(1), 39–54.

BIBLIOGRAPHY

Blixen, C., & Kippes, C. (1999). Depression, social support, and quality of life in older adults with osteoarthritis. *Image: Journal of Nursing Scholarship, 31*(3), 221–226.

Bolla, C. D., De Joseph, J., Norbeck, J., & Smith, R. (1996). Social support as road map and vehicle: An analysis of data from focus group interviews with a group of African American women. *Public Health Nursing, 13*(5), 331–336.

Christopher, S. E., Bauman, K. E., & Veness-Meehan, K. (2000). Perceived stress, social support, and affectionate behaviors of adolescent mothers with infants in neonatal intensive care. *Journal of Pediatric Health Care, 14,* 288–296.

Cossette, S., Levesque, L., & Laurin, L. (1995). Informal and formal support for caregivers of a demented relative: Do gender and kinship make a difference? *Research in Nursing and Health, 18,* 437–451.

Friedman, M. M. (1997). Social support sources among older women with heart failure: Continuity versus loss over time. *Research in Nursing and Health, 20,* 319–327.

Hagerty, B. M., & Williams, R. A. (1999). The effects of sense of belonging, social support, conflict, and loneliness on depression. *Nursing Research, 48*(4), 215–219.

Hubbard, P., Muhlenkamp, A. F., & Brown, N. (1984). The relationship between social support and self-care practices. *Nursing Research, 33*(5), 266–270.

Hudson, A. L., & Morris, R. I. (1994). Perceptions of social support of African Americans with acquired immunodefi- ciency syndrome. *Journal of National Black Nurses Association, 7*(1), 36–49.

Ihlenfeld, J. T. (1996). Nurses' perceptions of administrative social support. *Issues in Mental Health Nursing, 17,* 469–477.

Kaunonen, M., Tarkka, M., Paunonen, M., & Laippala, P. (1999). Grief and social support after the death of a spouse. *Journal of Advanced Nursing, 30*(6), 1304–1311.

Kavanaugh, K., Trier, D., & Michelle, K. (2004). Social support following perinatal loss. *Journal of Family Nursing, 19*(1), 70–92.

Logsdon, M. C., Gagne, P., Hughes, T., Patterson, J., & Rakestraw, V. (2005). Social support during adolescent pregnancy: Piecing together a quilt. *Journal of Obstetric, Gynecologic, and Neonatal Nursing, 34*(606–614), 433–440.

Lugton, J. (1997). The nature of social support as experienced by women treated for breast cancer. *Journal of Advanced Nursing, 25*(6), 1184–1191.

Mahon, N. E., Yarcheski, A., & Yarcheski, T. J. (1998). Social support and positive health practices in young adults: Loneliness as a mediating variable. *Clinical Nursing Research, 7*(3), 292–309.

McVeigh, C. A. (2000). Investigating the relationship between satisfaction with social support and functional status after childbirth. *MCN, The American Journal of Maternal/Child Nursing, 25*(1), 25–30.

Norbeck, J. S., De Jospeph, J. F., & Smith, R. T. (1996). A randomized trial of an empirically derived social support intervention to prevent low birthweight. *Social Science and Medicine, 43,* 947–954.

Ostergren, P. O., Hanson, B. S., Isacsson, S. O., & Tejler, L. (1991). Social network, social support and acute chest complaints among young and middle-aged patients in an emergency department—a case control study. *Social Science and Medicine, 33*(3), 257–267.

Reece, S. M. (1993). Social support and the early maternal experience of primiparas over 35. *Maternal-Child Nursing Journal, 21*(3), 91–98.

Roberts, B. L., Matecjyck, M., & Anthony, M. (1996). The effects of social support on the relationship of functional limitations and pain to depression. *Arthritis Care and Research, 9*(1), 67–73.

Schaffer, M. A., & Lia-Hoagberg, B. (1997). Effects of social support on prenatal care and health behaviors of low-income women. *Journal of Obstetric, Gynecologic, and Neonatal Nursing, 26*(4), 433–440.

Tarkka, M., & Paunonen, M. (1996). Social support provided by nurses to recent mothers on a maternity ward. *Journal of Advanced Nursing, 23*(6), 1202–1206.

Weinert, C., & Tilden, V. P. (1990). Measures of social support. *Nursing Research, 39*(4), 212–216.

Caring

■ DANUTA M. WOJNAR

DEFINITION OF KEY TERMS

Caring	A nurturing way of relating to a valued other toward whom one feels a personal sense of commitment and responsibility (Swanson, 1991, p. 165)
Knowing	Striving to understand an event as it has meaning in the life of the other. Knowing involves avoiding assumptions about the meaning of an event to the one cared for, centering on the other's needs, conducting in-depth assessment, seeking verbal and nonverbal cues, and engaging the self of both (Swanson, 1991, p. 163).
Being with	Being emotionally present to the other by conveying ongoing availability, sharing feelings, and monitoring that the one providing care does not burden the one cared for (Swanson, 1991, p. 163)
Doing for	Doing for the other what he or she would do for the self if it were at all possible. Doing for the other means providing care that is comforting, protective, and anticipatory, as well as performing duties skillfully and competently while preserving the person's dignity (Swanson, 1991, p. 164).
Enabling	Facilitating the other's passage through life transitions and unfamiliar events by informing, explaining, supporting, focusing on relevant concerns, thinking through issues, and generating alternatives. Enabling promotes the client's personal healing, growth, and self-care (Swanson, 1991, p. 164).
Maintaining belief	Sustaining faith in the other's capacity to get through an event or transition and face a future with meaning. The goal is to enable the other so that within the constraints of the other's life, he or she is able to find meaning and maintain a hope-filled attitude (Swanson, 1991, p. 165).

INTRODUCTION

Nursing, like other health professions, is based on the ideal of service to humanity. At the core of nursing values lays the ideal of altruistic caring that is guided by theory, research, and a code of ethics. Nursing is focused on creating caring–healing environments that assist individuals, families, and communities to attain or maintain a state of optimal wellness in their life experiences from birth, through adulthood, until the end of life (Swanson & Wojnar, 2004). Most individuals choose nursing as a profession because of their desire to care for others. With advances in nursing science there has been an escalating interest in the concept of caring in nursing. Over the past few decades, philosophical debates, research, and theory development have ensued to define the concept of caring, articulate caring behaviors, and identify outcomes of caring for patients, families, nurses, organizations, and society. Also of deep concern is detecting and eliminating barriers to caring in clinical practice. Among several prominent frameworks, Kristen M. Swanson's middle range Theory of Caring has achieved popularity among practitioners because of its simplicity, elegance, relevance, and ease of application in education, research, and clinical practice.

HISTORICAL BACKGROUND

Nursing has a long legacy as a caring–healing profession. In the 19th century, Florence Nightingale, the matriarch of modern-day nursing, expressed a belief that caring for the sick is based on the understanding of persons and environment. She saw the uniqueness of nursing in creating optimal environments for restoring the health of individuals, a vision that has now been in operation for over 100 years (Chinn & Kramer, 2004).

Nurse theorists, such as Watson (1979, 1988, 1999), Leininger (1981, 1988), Benner (1984), Benner and Wrubel (1989), Boykin (1994), Swanson-Kauffman (1985, 1986, 1988a, 1988b), Swanson-Kauffman and Roberts (1990), and Swanson (1991, 1993, 1998, 1999a, 1999b, 1999c) have reaffirmed the importance of caring for the profession through philosophical debates, theory development, and groundbreaking research. These scholars have led the profession in reminding nurses that caring is essential for delivery of sound nursing care.

Swanson's interest in the caring science has been a rapid process. After graduating from the University of Rhode Island College of Nursing, she began her career as a registered nurse at the University of Massachusetts Medical Center in Worcester. She was drawn to that newly opened clinical facility because the nursing administration had a clearly articulated vision for professional nursing practice and actively supported primary care nursing (Swanson, 2001).

Yet, like most novice nurses, Swanson most desired to become a technically skilled practitioner with an ultimate goal of teaching these skills to others. It wasn't until she enrolled in the Ph.D. in nursing program at the University of Colorado that the concept of caring went to the forefront of Swanson's professional and scholarly activities.

As part of a hands-on health promotion experience during doctoral studies, she participated in a cesarean section support group. During one of the meetings dedicated to miscarriage, she noted that while the physician who facilitated the group discussion focused on the physiological aspects of spontaneous abortion, the women wanted to talk about their personal experiences of miscarriage. From that point on, caring and miscarriage became the foci of Swanson's scholarship (Swanson, 2001).

For her doctoral dissertation, she set out to conduct a descriptive phenomenological investigation of 20 women who had recently miscarried and to identify what types of caring behaviors they considered most helpful (Swanson, 1991). The research question that ultimately guided her analysis was to explore what constituted caring for women who had a miscarriage. As a result of her dissertation research, Swanson developed a model with five caring processes: knowing, being with, doing for, enabling, and maintaining belief (Swanson-Kauffman, 1985, 1986, 1988a; Swanson, 1991, 1993). These caring process provided the foundation for the development of Swanson's middle range Theory of Caring.

In a subsequent investigation, Swanson focused on exploring caring from the perspective of 19 professional caregivers and seven parents of infants hospitalized in the neonatal intensive care unit (NICU) (Swanson, 1990). This study also involved one year of observation of parents and professionals working in the NICU. She discovered that the caring processes she had identified through the miscarriage study were also applicable to parents and professionals who were responsible for taking care of babies in the NICU. As a result of this investigation, Swanson not only was able to retain and refine the definitions describing the acts of caring, but also was able to propose that clinical care in a complex environment requires balance of caring for self and others; attaching to others as well as one's role; managing responsibilities as assigned by self, others, and society; and avoiding bad outcomes for self, others, and society (Swanson, 1990).

The next phase in the development of Swanson's caring theory was the "Caring and the Clinical Nursing Models Project," in which Swanson explored how a group of young mothers who received a long-term public health nursing intervention recalled and described nurse caring (Swanson-Kauffman, 1988b). Based on the findings of this study, Swanson finally defined caring as a concept and further refined the caring processes and subdimensions of caring processes.

The next phase of developing the Theory of Caring involved a meta-analysis of 130 data-based publications about caring (Swanson, 1999c). Through that in-depth analysis of the literature, Swanson proposed that knowledge about caring falls into five domains: the capacity for caring; the concerns and commitments that underline the values or ethics of caring; the nurse-, patient-, or organization-related conditions that support or diminish the likelihood of caring occurring; caring actions; and the consequences of caring and noncaring. This analysis led to a slight refinement of the maintaining belief category, and was particularly fruitful for validation of Swanson's caring processes as having applicability beyond the perinatal contexts from which they were derived.

Subsequently, Swanson's scholarship has focused on making a difference for families experiencing miscarriage. Her work has involved instrument development (Swanson, 1999b), theory testing (Swanson, 2000), and randomized controlled trials of the impact of caring on healing subsequent to miscarriage. She has established psychometric properties of several research measures including the Caring Other Scale (measures support received after miscarriage from one's mate and "others"), the Caring Professional Scale (measures the extent to which health care providers are viewed as competent and compassionate), the Emotional Strength Scale (measures the extent to which individuals view themselves as emotionally strong), and the Impact of Miscarriage Scale (measures key aspects of what it is like to miscarry) (Swanson, 1999b, 1999c, 2000; Swanson, Karmali, Powell, & Pulvermakher, 2003; Swanson, Connor Jolley, Pentinato, & Wang, 2007). Her randomized controlled trials have investigated the impact of delivering caring-based interventions on individuals' and couples' healing after miscarriage. In summary, Swanson's caring processes were and continue to be empirically developed, refined, and tested by Swanson herself.

DEFINITIONS OF THEORY CONCEPTS

In 1993, Swanson refined her theory by making explicit her beliefs about the four phenomena of concern to the discipline of nursing: nursing, person/client, health, and environment. The concepts of caring, central to the

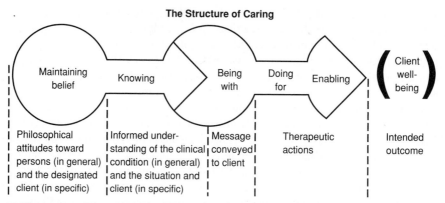

The Structure of Caring

Figure 9.1 The structure of caring as linked to the nurse's philosophical attitude, informed understandings, message conveyed, therapeutic actions, and intended outcome. (From Swanson, K. M. [1993.] Nursing as informed caring for the well-being of others. *Image: The Journal of Nursing Scholarship, 25*[4], 352–357.) Used with permission of Blackwell Publishing, Oxford, United Kingdom.

theory, and caring processes (knowing, being with, doing for, enabling, and maintaining belief) are clearly defined and arranged in a logical sequence (see Figure 9.1, which depicts how caring is delivered). Swanson also made explicit her beliefs about what it means for nurses to practice in a caring manner to promote health and healing of others. Chinn and Kramer (2004) and Meleis (1997) maintain that the simplicity and clarity of a theory refers to a theory with a minimal number of concepts. Simplicity and clarity of language used to define the concepts allow practitioners to understand and apply Swanson's theory in practice.

Nursing

Swanson (1991, 1993) defines nursing as informed caring for the well-being of others. She posits that the discipline is informed by scientific knowledge from nursing and related fields, and by knowledge derived from the humanities, clinical practice, and cultural values and beliefs (Swanson, 1993).

Person

Persons are defined as "unique beings who are in the midst of becoming and whose wholeness is made manifest in thoughts, feelings, and behaviors" (Swanson, 1993, p. 352). Swanson asserts that life experiences of each individual are influenced by a complex interplay of genetics, spiritual endowment, and the person's capacity to exercise free will. Therefore, persons both shape and are shaped by the environment in which they live.

Persons are viewed as dynamic, growing, self-reflecting, yearning to be connected with others, and spiritual beings. Swanson posits that spiritual endowment connects each human being to an eternal and universal source of goodness, mystery, life, creativity, and serenity. The spiritual endowment may be a soul, higher power/holy spirit, positive energy, or, simply, grace; free will equates with choice and the capacity to decide how to act when confronted with a range of possibilities (Swanson, 1993, p. 352). Yet, Swanson also maintains that limitations set by race, class, gender, sociopolitical systems, or access to care might prevent individuals from exercising free will. Hence, acknowledging free will mandates nursing discipline to honor individuality and consideration of a whole range of possibilities that might be acceptable or desirable to the patients, families, and communities for whom nurses care.

According to Swanson, the "other," whose personhood nursing discipline serves, refers to individuals, families, groups, and societies. With this understanding of personhood, nurses are mandated to take on leadership roles in advocating for human rights, equal access to health care, and other humanitarian causes. Lastly, when nurses think about the "other" to whom they direct their caring, they also need to think of self, other, nurses, and the practice of nursing as the designated "other/recipient" of their caring.

Health

According to Swanson (1993), to experience health and well-being is to have a subjective, meaning-filled experience of wholeness that involves a sense of integration and becoming wherein all levels of being are free to be expressed including human spirituality, thoughts, feelings, intelligence, creativity, relatedness, femininity, masculinity, and sexuality, to name just a few. Therefore, re-establishing wholeness involves a complex process of curing and healing at the physical, mental, psychosocial, and spiritual levels.

Environment

Swanson (1993) defines environment as situational rather than physical and views environment as any situation that influences or is influenced by the designated client. Environment is ever changing at the cultural, social, biophysical, political, and economic realms, and by any context that influences or is influenced by the designated client. She believes that the terms *environment* and *person/client* in nursing can be viewed interchangeably since the environment may be specified to the intraindividual level of a specified client, wherein the client may be at the cellular level and the environment may be the tissues or body of which the cell is a component, or the client may be an entire community and its environment includes cultural, social, and political aspects (Swanson, 1993, p. 353). Therefore, when Swanson's theory is used in research or clinical practice, one must remember that what is considered an environment in one situation may be considered a client in another.

Caring

Swanson believes that nurse caring is grounded in a belief in people and their capacities. Therefore, caring is defined as a nurturing way of relating to a valued other toward whom one feels a personal sense of commitment and responsibility. Swanson maintains that caring involves five processes: (a) knowing, (b) being with, (c) doing for, (d) enabling, and (e) maintaining belief. For detailed definitions of the caring processes, refer to the beginning of the chapter, the Definition of Key Concepts section.

DESCRIPTION OF THE THEORY OF CARING

Philosophical Foundation

Swanson has drawn on various philosophical and theoretical sources while developing her Theory of Caring. In the chapter "The Program of Research on Caring," Swanson (2001) recalled that early on in her career knowledge obtained from formal nursing education and clinical practice made her acutely aware of the centrality of caring to preserving human dignity and promoting healing. Swanson also acknowledged several nurse scholars for influencing her beliefs about nursing and caring. She credits Dr. Jacqueline Fawcett for helping her understand the unique role of nursing in caring for others and the importance of altruistic caring for the persons' well-being. Swanson also acknowledges Dr. Jean Watson for encouraging her to inductively study caring. While Drs. Swanson and Watson sustain a deep friendship and respect for each other's scholarship, they both view their scholarship as complementary. They view their programs of research as unique and believe that the congruency of their findings add credibility to each other's work. Yet, both scholars see their Theories of Caring and their programs of research on caring as unique and the congruency of their findings as adding credibility to their individual work (Swanson, 2001). Lastly, Swanson credits Dr. Kathryn M. Barnard for encouraging her to test and apply her Theory of Caring through randomized clinical trials.

Swanson's theory was developed empirically, using inductive methodology. According to Chinn and Kramer (2004), inductive reasoning involves inducing of hypotheses and relationships by observing or living through phenomena and before reaching definite conclusions. Swanson's Theory of Caring was inductively developed through descriptive phenomenological inquiry with women who had miscarried (Swanson-Kauffman, 1985, 1986, 1988a, 1988b), caregivers of vulnerable infants in the NICU (Swanson, 1990), and socially at-risk mothers who had received long-term care from master's-prepared public health nurses (Swanson, 1991).

Theoretical Assumptions

Swanson purports that caring, which she defines as "a nurturing way of relating to a valued other toward whom a nurse feels a sense of commitment and responsibility" (1991, p. 162), is not unique to the domain of perinatal nursing. Instead, she posits, caring is an essential component of the nurse–client relationship in any setting. Swanson also purports that caring occurs in every nurse–client relationship that involves skillful application of caring processes (knowing, being with, doing for, enabling, and maintaining belief). She also posits that regardless of the amount of nursing experience, caring is influenced by the nurse's attitude (maintaining belief), understanding of the client's experience (knowing), verbal and nonverbal interaction with the client (being with), enabling (believing in the client's capacity to live through difficult transitions), and outcomes of caring (intended outcomes of nursing process). Swanson purports that caring processes coexist and overlap, and cannot be delivered in a linear way or in separation from one another. Lastly, Swanson claims that if she had truly identified and defined the universal aspects of caring, then her caring processes should ring true in any situation where caring is a part of an interpersonal relationship.

APPLICATIONS OF THE THEORY IN RESEARCH

Reynolds (1971) suggests that a functional theory is one that can be applied in clinical practice and research. Swanson has persevered in the development of her theory from the point of defining the concept of caring and caring processes in her Caring Model (Swanson-Kauffman, 1985) to the development of the middle range Theory of Caring (Swanson, 1993), based on combining the findings from three phenomenological investigations conducted in various perinatal contexts. Her subsequent works involved instrument development to measure caring, descriptive research to determine human responses to miscarriage over time, and theory testing using intervention designs.

Specifically, in her dissertation research, the theorist analyzed data obtained from in-depth interviews with 20 women who had recently miscarried. Two theoretical models were proposed as a result of this phenomenological investigation: (a) the Human Experience of Miscarriage Model and (b) the Caring Model. In the Caring Model, Swanson proposed that the processes of knowing, being with, doing for, enabling, and maintaining belief give meaning to nursing acts labeled as caring (Swanson-Kauffman, 1985, 1986, 1988a, 1988b). Findings of this investigation provided the foundation for the development of the middle range Theory of Caring at a later time.

As part of her postdoctoral studies, Swanson conducted another phenomenological investigation, in which she explored what it was like to be a provider of care to vulnerable infants in the NICU. As a result of this study, Swanson (1990) found that the caring processes she identified with women who miscarried were also applicable to parents, physicians, and nursing staff responsible for taking care of infants in the NICU. Therefore, Swanson decided to retain the wording describing the acts of caring and propose that wholistic care in a complex environment like the NICU embraces balance of *caring* (for self and the one cared for), *attaching* (to others and roles), *managing responsibilities* (assigned by self, others, and society), and *avoiding bad outcomes* (Swanson, 1990).

In a later investigation, Swanson (1991) explored what it had been like for socially at-risk mothers to receive supportive, long-term nursing interventions. As a result of this study she was finally able to define caring and further refine the definitions of caring processes. Collectively, findings of Swanson's research with women who have miscarried, caregivers in the NICU, and socially at-risk mothers provided the foundation for expanding the Caring Model into the middle range Theory of Caring (Swanson, 1991, 1993).

The subsequent study, conducted to develop the Impact of Miscarriage Scale (IMS), shifted Swanson's work on caring and miscarriage from interpretive to descriptive quantitative design.

Impact of Miscarriage Scale

The development of the IMS was a multiphase instrument development study funded by University of Washington Intramural funds. It consisted of three phases: (a) item derivation using 105 emic quotes taken from earlier research with women who had a miscarriage; (b) a mailed questionnaire completed by 446 women who were within 10 years of miscarrying, which allowed establishing of preliminary psychometric properties; and (c) factor analysis of data obtained from 188 women participating in the Miscarriage Caring project. The scale is a 24-item measure of the overall impact of miscarriage. It has four subscales: Lost Baby, Devastating Event, Personal Significance, and Isolated. Cronbach alphas range from 0.79 to 0.93 (Swanson, Kieckhefer, Powers, & Carr, 1990).

Caring Professional Scale

As a result of later research, Swanson developed the Caring Professional Scale (CPS), which is a self-report survey to rate health care providers' practice relationship styles (Swanson, 2000, 2002). The items of the instrument were derived to reflect Swanson's Theory of Caring, specifically to measure caring acts (knowing, being with, doing for, maintaining belief, and enabling). The scale consists of 15 items constructed on a five-point Likert-type scale and two subscales: compassionate healer and competent practitioner. Psychometric properties of the measure were established with 175 women who had miscarried. Cronbach alphas range from 0.89 to 0.93.

Caring Mate and Caring Other Scale

Based on the items derived from the caring theory, Swanson also developed a 10-item measure called the Caring Mate and Caring Other Scale, which measures supportive behaviors from the partner and others subsequent to unexpected pregnancy loss that range on a scale from 1 (not at all) to 5 (all the time). The instrument has two subscales: mutual caring and caring by doing. Cronbach alphas range from 0.87 to 0.93 (Swanson, 2001). The scale was developed with women who had miscarried and psychometric properties established on 176 women who rated support from their partner or other, usually a female friend, in the Miscarriage Caring Project (Swanson, 1999a).

The self-report measures to assess caring as delivered by practitioners and by couples to each other may serve as a template for delivering caring-based interventions, while the development of research-based measures already used successfully in perinatal contexts opens possibilities for use and further testing with other populations.

Intervention Research

Swanson tested her Theory of Caring with women who had miscarried in several investigations funded by the National Institutes of Health (NIH), National Institutes of Nursing Research, and other funding sources. Swanson's (1999a, 1999b) intervention study with 242 women who had miscarried focused on examining the effects of caring-based counseling sessions on the women's processing of loss and their emotional wellness in the first year after loss. Additional aims of the study were to examine the effects of the passage of time on healing and to design strategies to monitor caring interventions. The main findings of this investigation were that caring was effective in decreasing the participants' overall disturbed mood, depression, and anger. Delayed measurement (with of without treatment) alone affected increased anger and decreased likeliness that participants would say that they had lost a baby. In other words, there was a main effect for delayed measurement that applied to women in both the treated-delayed and the untreated-delayed group. Moreover, all study participants (treated or not) assigned less personal significance to miscarrying and had higher levels of self-esteem and less anxiety, anger, and confusion. In other words, the findings of the study demonstrated that while passing of time had positive effects on women's healing after miscarriage, caring interventions had a positive impact on decreasing the overall disturbed mood, anger, and level of depression.

The second aim of this investigation was to monitor the caring variable and identify whether caring was delivered as intended. In this investigation, caring was monitored in three different ways: (a) approximately 10% of counseling sessions were transcribed and data were analyzed using inductive and deductive content analysis; (b) before each caring session the counselor completed McNair, Lorr, and Droppelman, and Reynold's (1981) Profile of Mood States to monitor whether her own mood was associated with women's ratings of caring after each session, using the investigator-developed Caring Professional Scale; and (c) after each session the counselor completed an investigator-developed Counselor Rating Scale and took narrative notes about the counseling session. The most noteworthy finding of monitoring caring was that the majority of participants were highly satisfied with caring received during counseling sessions, suggesting that caring was delivered as intended.

In the late 1990s, Swanson (1999c) also conducted a literary meta-analysis on caring. An in-depth review of approximately 130 investigations on caring led Swanson to conclude that knowledge about caring may be categorized into five hierarchical levels and that research conducted in any one domain assumes the presence of all previous domains. The first level refers to the persons' capacities to deliver caring; the second level refers to individuals' concerns and commitments that lead to caring actions; the third level refers to the conditions (nurse, client, organizational) that enhance or diminish likelihood of delivering caring; the fourth level includes the actions of caring; and the fifth level refers to the outcomes of caring for both the client and the nurse (Swanson, 1999c). Findings of this literary meta-analysis further clarified the meaning of the concept of caring as it is used in nursing and supported transferability of her middle range Theory of Caring beyond the miscarriage and perinatal contexts, in which she personally studied caring.

Currently, Swanson is in the final stages of data analysis from the NIH-funded intervention research "Couples Miscarriage Healing Project" conducted with ($n = 341$) heterosexual couples over a period of 1 year after loss. The study was conducted to determine the effects of miscarriage on couples in committed heterosexual relationships, and to identify effective ways of helping couples heal both as individuals and as couples subsequent to miscarriage. Study participants (couples) were randomly assigned to one of four groups: (a) nurse caring (three counseling sessions with a nurse), (b) self-caring (three videos and workbooks), (c) combined caring (one nurse caring session and three videos and workbooks), or (d) a control group. The Theory of Caring provided bases for delivering interventions in the study. Data analysis for this intervention study is under way.

Clinicians and other scholars have used Swanson's work extensively. Literature review of computerized databases (MEDLINE, CINAHL, and Digital Dissertations) indicate that Swanson's theory and research has been cited or otherwise used in over 160 data-based publications, while the article "Nursing as Informed Caring for the Well Being of Others" (Swanson, 1993) alone has been cited over 50 times.

Applications of the Theory in Research, Education, and Clinical Practice

Reynolds (1971) asserts that a useful theory provides a sense of understanding and applicability in research, education, and practice. The Theory of Caring has been the theoretical foundation for numerous research studies, master's and doctoral dissertations, and scholarly projects of undergraduate and graduate nursing students. Some recent examples of the applications of Swanson's Theory of Caring in research include Kish and Holder's (1996) exploration of clinical scholarship in practice; Yorkston, Klasner, and Swanson's (2001) guidelines for practitioners working with patients who have multiple sclerosis; Quinn, Smith, Ritenbaugh, and Swanson's (2003) research guidelines for assessing the impact of healing relationships in nursing; Sikma's (2006) study of caring with the elderly population; Kavanaugh, Moro, Savage, and Mehendale's (2006) research with vulnerable populations; Sandblom's (2006) analysis of grief and depression after miscarriage among couples with a history of infertility; and Wojnar's (2007) research with lesbian couples who miscarry, to name only a few. Some recent examples of the applications of Swanson's Theory of Caring in research include Kish and Holder's (1996) exploration of clinical scholarship in practice; Swanson's (1999) investigation of the effects of caring, measurement, and time on women's well being in the first year after miscarriage; and Quinn, Smith, Rittenbaugh, and Swanson's (2003) investigation of the impact of healing relationships in clinical. Swanson's study is summarized in Using Middle Range Theories, 9.1 and Research Application 9.1 suggests an additional research question that could be addressed using Swanson's theory as a framework.

 ### 9.1 USING MIDDLE RANGE THEORIES

Swanson (1999) conducted a repeated measures, randomized Solomon four-group investigation of the effects of caring, measurement, and time on women's well-being in the first year after miscarriage. There were 242 women enrolled into the study and 185 women completed the 1-year-long project. The intervention process was based on the caring theory described earlier. The content for three 1-hour caring-based counseling sessions was derived from Swanson's Human Experience of Miscarriage Model. In this investigation, caring-based interventions were effective ($P < .05$) in reducing overall emotional disturbance, anger, and depression using a valid and reliable measure "Profile of Mood States" (McNair, Lorr, Droppleman, & Reynolds 1981). The passage of time was effective in enhancing study participants' self-esteem and reducing overall emotional disturbance, anger, depression, anxiety, confusion, and the personal significance of miscarriage. Women who did not receive any intervention and for whom measurement was delayed until 16 weeks after loss were more angry and less likely to call their loss a "baby." Swanson concluded that caring-based interventions are an effective strategy for supporting women's healing from spontaneous miscarriage.

Swanson, K. M. (1999). Research-based practice with women who have had miscarriages. *Image: Journal of Nursing Scholarship, 31*(4), 339–345.

9.2 USING MIDDLE RANGE THEORIES

Sikma (2006) conducted a phenomenological study to examine the experience of caring and being cared for as a staff member in a nursing home as well as aspects of the organization that are supportive or unsupportive of caring practice with the residents. Five themes of caring interventions emerged from the perspective of staff caregivers: valuing personhood and the work, belonging, knowing, acting together, and promoting quality. In addition, study participants identified three themes of caring organizational conditions: communicating, providing resources, and trusting. The author concluded that the research-based Model of Caring in the organizational environment can be used to assess and improve the caring environment of nursing homes as well as to develop caring management and staff. These findings provide further evidence that caring theory may be applied beyond the perinatal context in which the concept was first defined and measured. Organizational well-being for nursing homes can be accomplished with the commitment of formal and informal leaders who can create organizational conditions supportive of caring practices, engage in caring interventions with staff, and inspire the synergy of caring.

Sikma, S. (2006). Staff perceptions of caring: The importance of a supportive environment. *Journal of Gerontological Nursing, 32*(6), 22–29.

In recent decades, Swanson's theory has also been successfully adapted as a framework for professional nursing practice by various universities and practice settings across the United States, Canada, and Sweden. One specific example that represents application of Theory of Caring in education is Dalhousie University in Halifax, Nova Scotia, Canada, which embraced Swanson's theory as a framework to guide teaching and professional formation of student nurses. Similarly, nursing care at IWK Health Centre, a

9.1 RESEARCH APPLICATION

Approximately 5 million lesbians in the United States are mothers through donor insemination, adoption, or short-lived heterosexual relationships. Earlier studies concerning lesbian families focused on investigating lesbian mothers' health care experiences and consistently identified a need for improvement in access to health care and the knowledge, skills, and attitudes of practitioners. While later research generally demonstrated advances in the sensitivity of practitioners to the unique needs of lesbian clients, some reports point to the contrary. In a recent literature review, McManus, Hunter, and Renn (2006) provided evidence that health care outcomes for lesbian mothers and their infants are improved by knowledgeable and sensitive care. Yet, large gaps in knowledge exist about the unique caring needs of this minority population in the perinatal context. Swanson's Theory of Caring may be used to guide an investigation aimed at exploring the actual and desired experience of caring and support received by lesbian childbearing families in health care. Using Swanson's caring framework, semi-structured interviews may be carried out with lesbian childbearing families to explore their experiences of actual care and desired caring behaviors from practitioners. In addition, the Caring Professional Scale (CPS) (Swanson, 2000, 2002) may be used to rate health care providers' practice relationship style and the women's perceptions of caring acts (knowing, being with, doing for, maintaining belief, and enabling).

ANALYSIS OF THEORY

Using the criteria presented in Chapter 2, critique the Theory of Caring. Compare your conclusions about the theory with those found in Appendix A. A researcher who has worked with the theory completed the analysis found in the appendix.

Internal Criticism
1. Clarity
2. Consistency
3. Adequacy

4. Logical development
5. Level of theory development

External Criticism
1. Reality convergence
2. Utility
3. Significance
4. Discrimination
5. Scope of theory
6. Complexity

tertiary-level hospital in Halifax, Nova Scotia, Canada, has selected Swanson's theory of caring as representative of the caring–healing legacy of the nursing profession and relevant to the clinical practice. According to Chinn and Kramer (2004), the situations in which the theories may be applied should not be limited. Clearly, it has been demonstrated that Swanson's Theory of Caring may be used effectively to establish therapeutic relationships with diverse populations, far beyond the perinatal context, to promote the individuals' wellness across the lifespan (Swanson, 1999c), making it generalizable to any nurse–client relationship and any clinical setting. Hence, it offers a framework for enhancing contemporary nursing practice while bringing the discipline to its traditional caring–healing roots.

SUMMARY

The usefulness of Swanson's Theory of Caring has been demonstrated in research, education, and clinical practice. The belief that caring has a pivotal role in the practice of professional nursing had its beginning in the theorist's clinical practice, the influence of her mentors, and the findings from her

CRITICAL THINKING EXERCISES

1. Think about a time when you felt that you or someone close to you experienced caring in the health care environment. What was it like to experience caring? What did the practitioner say or do? How consistent were his or her actions with caring processes identified by Swanson? Alternatively, think about a situation when caring was not delivered. What was missing in your interaction with that practitioner?

2. Think about a situation in your clinical practice when your interaction with the client did not go smoothly. Consider key definitions identified in Swanson's theory and reflect on what caring processes were missing from that interaction. In what ways could that interaction be improved?

3. Consider Swanson's Theory of Caring as a theoretical framework for a research study relevant to your clinical practice. In what ways would it be applicable?

phenomenological investigations. Her later works, including a meta-analysis of research on caring (Swanson, 1999), have demonstrated generalizability and applicability of the Theory of Caring in education, clinical nursing practice, and research beyond the perinatal context.

Nurse caring, as demonstrated by Swanson in research with women who miscarried, caregivers in the NICU, and socially at-risk mothers, recognizes the importance of attending to the wholeness of human experiences and needs.

REFERENCES

Benner, P. (1984). *From novice to expert.* Menlo Park, CA: Addison-Wesley.

Benner, P., & Wrubel, J. (1989). *The primacy of caring.* Menlo Park, CA: Addison-Wesley.

Boykin, A. (1994). *Living a caring-based curriculum.* New York: National League for Nursing.

Chinn, P. L., & Kramer, M. K. (2004). *Integrated knowledge development in nursing* (6th ed.). St. Louis: Mosby.

Kavanaugh, K., Moro, T. T., Savage, T., & Mehendale, R. (2006). Enacting a theory of caring to recruit and retain vulnerable participants for sensitive research. *Research in Nursing and Health, 29*(3), 244–252.

Kish, C. P., & Holder, L. M. (1996). Helping to say goodbye: Merging clinical scholarship with community service. *Holistic Nursing Practice, 10*(3), 74–82.

Leininger, M. M. (1981). The phenomenon of caring: Importance of research and theoretical considerations. In M. M. Leininger (Ed.), *Caring: An essential human need.* Thorofare, NJ: Slack.

Leininger, M. M. (1988). Leininger's theory of nursing: Cultural care diversality and universality. *Nursing Science Quarterly, 1*(4), 152–160.

McManus, A. J., Hunter, L. P., & Renn, H. (2006). Lesbian experiences and needs during childbirth: Guidance for health care providers. *Journal of Obstetrical and Neonatal Nursing, 35*(1) 13–23.

McNair, D. M., Lorr, M., Droppleman, L. F., & Reynolds, P. D. (1981). *A primer of theory construction.* Indianapolis: Bobbs-Merrill.

Meleis, A. I. (1997). *Theoretical nursing: Development and progress.* Philadelphia: Lippincott-Raven.

Meleis, A. I. (1981). *Profile of mood states: Manual.* San Diego, CA: Educational and Industrial Testing Service.

Quinn, J., Smith, M., Ritenbaugh, C., & Swanson, K. M. (2003). Research guidelines for assessing the impact of the healing relationship in clinical nursing. *Alternative Therapies, 9*(31), 69–79.

Reynolds, P. D. (1971). *A primer of theory construction.* Indianapolis: Bobbs-Merrill.

Sandblom, S. (2006). Does a history of infertility affect the grief and depression response in couples experiencing a spontaneous miscarriage? Unpublished Master Thesis. University of Washington School of Nursing.

Sikma, S. (2006). Staff perceptions of caring: the importance of a supportive environment. *Journal of Gerontological Nursing, 32*(6), 22–29.

Swanson, K. M. (1990). Providing care in the NICU: Sometimes an act of love. *Advances in Nursing Science, 13*(1), 60–73.

Swanson, K. M. (1991). Empirical development of a middle range theory of caring. *Nursing Research, 40*(3), 161–166.

Swanson, K. M. (1993). Nursing as informed caring for the well-being of others. *Image: Journal of Nursing Scholarship, 25*(4), 352–357.

Swanson, K. M. (1998). Caring made visible. *Creative Nursing Journal, 4*(4), 8–11, 16.

Swanson, K. M. (1999a). Research-based practice with women who have had miscarriages. *Image: Journal of Nursing Scholarship, 31*(4), 339–345.

Swanson, K. M. (1999b). The effects of caring, measurement, and time on miscarriage impact and women's well-being in the first year subsequent to loss. *Nursing Research, 48*(6), 288–298.

Swanson, K. M. (1999c). What's known about caring in nursing: A literary meta-analysis. In A. S. Hinshaw, J. Shaver, & S. Feetham (Eds.), *Handbook of clinical nursing research* (pp. 31–60). Thousand Oaks, CA: Sage.

Swanson, K. M. (2000). Predicting depressive symptoms after miscarriage: A path analysis based on Lazarus' paradigm. *Journal of Women's Health and Gender-based Medicine, 9*(2), 191–206.

Swanson, K. M. (2001). A program of research on caring. In M. E. Parker (Ed.), *Nursing theories and nursing practice* (pp. 411–420). Philadelphia, PA: F. A. Davis.

Swanson, K. M. (2002). Caring Professional Scale. In J. Watson (Ed.), *Assessing and measuring caring in nursing and health science.* New York: Springer Publishing Company.

Swanson, K. M., Connor, S., Jolley, S. N., Pettinato, M., & Wang, T. (2007). Contexts and evolution of women's responses to miscarriage over the first year after loss. *Research in Nursing & Health, 30*(1), 2–16.

Swanson, K. M., Karmali, Z., Powell, S., & Pulvermahker, F. (2003). Miscarriage effects on interpersonal and sexual relationships during the first year after loss: Women's perceptions. *Journal of Psychosomatic Medicine, 65*(5), 902–910.

Swanson, K. M., Kieckhefer, G., Powers, P., & Carr, K. (1990). Meaning of miscarriage scale: Establishment of psychometric properties. (Abstract). *Communicating Nursing Research, 25,* 365.

Swanson, K. M., & Wojnar, D. (2004). Optimal healing environments in nursing. *Alternative Therapies in Health and Medicine, 10*(1), 43–51.

Swanson-Kauffman, K. M. (1985). Miscarriage: A new understanding of the mother's experience. Proceedings of the 50th anniversary celebration of the University of Pennsylvania School of Nursing, pp. 63–78.

Swanson-Kauffman, K. M. (1986). Caring in the instance of unexpected early pregnancy loss. *Topics in Clinical Nursing, 8*(2), 37–46.

Swanson-Kauffman, K. M. (1988a). The caring needs of women who miscarry. In M. M. Leininger (Ed.), *Care, discovery and uses in clinical and community nursing* (pp. 55–71). Detroit, MI: Wayne State University Press.

Swanson-Kauffman, K. M. (1988b). There should have been two: Nursing care of parents experiencing the perinatal death of a twin. *Journal of Perinatal and Neonatal Nursing, 2*(2), 78–86.

Swanson-Kauffman, K. M., & Roberts, J. (1990). Caring in parent and child nursing. In *Knowledge about care and caring: State of the art and future development.* Washington, DC: American Academy of Nursing.

Watson, J. (1979). *Nursing: The philosophy and science of caring.* Boston, MA: Little & Brown.

Watson, J. (1988). New dimensions of human caring theory. *Nursing Science Quarterly, 1,* 175–181.

Watson, J. (1999). *Nursing: Human science and human care: A theory of nursing.* Sudbury, MA: Jones & Barlett.

Wojnar, D. (2007). Miscarriage experiences of lesbian couples. *Journal of Midwifery and Women's Health, 52* (5), 479–485.

Yorkston, K. M., Klasner, E. R., & Swanson, K. M. (2001). Communication in multiple sclerosis: understanding the insider's perspective. *American Journal of Speech Language Pathology, 10,* 126–137.

Interpersonal Relations

■ SANDRA J. PETERSON

DEFINITION OF KEY TERMS

Communication
A skill necessary to understand the nurse–patient relationship; composed of "spoken language, rational and nonrational expressions of wishes, needs, and desires, and the body gesture" (Peplau, 1991, p. 289)

Interpersonal relations
Any process that occurs between two people. The interpersonal processes between nurse and patient are identified as the core of nursing (Forchuk, 1993).

Nursing situation
What occurs between the nurse and the patient, thus the interaction of the individual thoughts, feelings, and actions of both

Observation
A skill necessary to understand the nurse–patient relationship. Its aim, "as an interpersonal process, is the identification, clarification, and verification of impressions about the interactive drama, of the pushes and pulls in the relationship between nurse and patient as they occur" (Peplau, 1991, p. 263).

Personality
". . . Pattern that is relatively stable and that characterizes persisting situations in the life of an individual . . . total assets and liabilities that determine an individual action" (Peplau, 1991, pp. 164–165). Nurses attempt to provide experiences for patients that promote personality development.

Phases of nurse–patient relationship
Four overlapping but generally sequential aspects of the relationship identified as orientation, identification, exploitation, and resolution

Psychobiological experiences
Factors that influence the functioning of personalities, providing energy that is converted into constructive or destructive behavior. The primary source of this energy is anxiety.

(Key Terms continued on next page)

DEFINITION OF KEY TERMS continued

Psychological tasks	"Tasks encountered in the process of learning to live with people as an aspect of formation and development of personality and as an aspect of the tasks demanded of nurses in their relations with patients" (Peplau, 1991, p. 159), for example, counting on others, delaying satisfaction, identifying self, and participating with others
Recording	Methods used to create documents of nurse–patient interactions, primarily for the purpose of student learning
Roles in nursing	Set of functions that nurses use in the context of nurse–patient situations as a means of helping the patient, identified as stranger, resource person, teacher, leader, surrogate, and counselor

INTRODUCTION

"When the history of nursing theory comes to be written few names will be seen to have been more influential than that of Hildegard Peplau" (Welch, 1995, p. 53). Peplau, who developed the Theory of Interpersonal Relations, is identified as the first contemporary nurse theorist (McKenna, 1997). Sills (1978) credits Peplau with clarifying the relationships between nursing theory, practice, and research. "Theory was used to guide nursing practice. Theory was tested in the real world of practice" (Sills, 1978, p. 122).

Though Peplau entitled her work a conceptual frame of reference, she often referred to it as a theory (Peplau, 1992, p. 13). Peplau produced a testable theory, identifying her work as a "source of hypotheses that may be examined with profit in all nursing situations" (Peplau, 1991, p. ix). The Theory of Interpersonal Relations is currently labeled a middle range theory (Armstrong & Kelly, 1995; Fawcett, 2000; O'Toole & Welt, 1989). Peplau, herself, defined the scope of her theory as in the middle range. She referred to it as "a partial theory for the practice of nursing as an interpersonal process" (Peplau, 1991, p. 261).

> Concepts contained within interpersonal relations theory are primarily relevant as [descriptions] of the personal behavior of nurse and patient in nursing situations and of psychological phenomena. Obviously, then for the practice of nursing, a more comprehensive scope of theoretical constructs is needed (Peplau, 1992, p. 13).

Initially developed with a focus on phenomena of most concern to psychiatric nurses, the Theory of Interpersonal Relations is applicable to all nurses (Peplau, 1964, 1992). Peplau (1997) claimed that "the nurse–patient relationship is the primary human contact that is central in a fundamental way to providing nursing care" (p. 163). The stated purpose of her theory is the improvement of nurses' relations with patients. This is achieved through the nurse's understanding of his or her own behavior, helping others identify personally experienced difficulties, and applying principles of human relations to the problems that arise in the context of relationships (Peplau, 1991, p. xi). This process results in a nursing situation in which both the patient and the nurse learn and grow. A growth-producing relationship with others is a goal that transcends any particular nursing specialty and in her description of the theory, Peplau (1952,

1991) used examples of patients with a variety of health issues, for example, a woman diagnosed with lymphosarcoma, a child having surgery on his hand to correct a congenital problem, a woman in labor, and a man with a coronary occlusion.

HISTORICAL BACKGROUND

What makes Peplau's Theory of Interpersonal Relations so remarkable is that it was conceived during a period in nursing's history when nurses had little or no independent role and little or no investment in the development of nursing theory. Peplau was educated and began her nursing practice, as described in her own words, at a time when "we were absolutely not allowed to talk to a patient, because if we did we might say the wrong thing" (Welch, 1995, p. 54). It was not until the late 1930s while working as a staff nurse at Mount Sinai Hospital, New York, that she discovered "there was more to nursing than just this doing activity, because there we were allowed to talk to the patients" (Welch, 1995, p. 54). In the 1940s Peplau found psychiatric nursing still focused on activities, for example, helping patients with tasks of daily living, which included cleaning patients' rooms and doing patients' laundry (Peplau, 1985, p. 31). It was out of her desire to be more useful to patients that the idea of interpersonal relations theory was developed.

Peplau used both deductive and inductive methods in her theory development work (Reed, 1995). Deductively, she integrated ideas from a number of theories into her theory of interpersonal relations. She was influenced by the work of Sigmund Freud, particularly his interest in unconscious motivation. Harry S. Sullivan's theory of interpersonal relations also contributed to her thinking about interpersonal processes in nursing. For example, she refers to his concepts of anxiety, self-system, and modes of experiencing. Also incorporated into her theory are elements from developmental psychology and learning theory (Armstrong & Kelly, 1995; Lego, 1980) and the ideas of the humanistic psychologists, Abraham Maslow, Rollo May, and Carl Rogers (Gastmans, 1998).

Peplau defined her inductive approach both in general and specific terms. The inductive approach for concept naming that she described included several steps:

1. Observing behaviors for which no explanatory concepts are available
2. Seeking to repeat those observations in others, under similar conditions
3. Noting regularities concerning the nature of the data being observed
4. Naming the phenomena (Peplau, 1989, p. 28)

These steps would be followed by further observation, resulting in the phenomenon becoming more clearly defined, which then allowed for testing with additional patients. "Eventually, useful interventions would be derived from the explanation of the phenomenon and the effects of these interventions upon it also tested" (Peplau, 1969, p. 28).

Peplau's specific inductive process of theory development involved using data from student–patient interactions. "I just happened to hit upon the notion of sitting students down with one patient for a long time and then study what they did with patients" (Peplau, 1985, p. 31). It was from these observations that psychotherapy by nurses in the context of the interpersonal relationship emerged.

Her theory of interpersonal relations, first appearing in 1952 in the book *Interpersonal Relations in Nursing*, has been published unchanged several times. During the 1950s and 1960s, her theory was used and tested in the challenging environment of state psychiatric hospitals. Some of this work is reported in *Basic Principles of Patient Counseling* published in 1964 by Smith, Kline, and French (Sills, 1978, p. 124).

In 4 decades since its inception, interpersonal theory has been expanded by Peplau and by other nurse scientists (Peplau, 1991, p. vi). For example, work on therapeutic milieu, crisis, and family therapy has been based on Peplau's theory. Sills (1978) conducted a review of three major nursing journals from 1972 to 1977 (one published for the first time in 1963). She identified 93 citations of Peplau's work and concluded that "it [is] remarkable that twenty-five years after the publication of *Interpersonal Relations in Nursing* that it, with no revisions, is still found useful. And . . . that utilization increases" (Sills, 1978, p. 125).

DEFINITIONS OF THEORY CONCEPTS

Though not specified at the time of the development of the theory in 1952, each domain of the traditional metaparadigm of nursing is addressed by Peplau. Her definitions of these major domain concepts are useful in understanding the rather complex Theory of Interpersonal Relations.

Nursing

The foundation of her theory is her definition of nursing. Perhaps what is unique, but not unexpectedly so, is the primacy of the nurse–patient relationship in her definition. She defines nursing as an interpersonal process, intended to be therapeutic. It "is a human relationship between an individual who is sick or in need of health services" (Peplau, 1991, pp. 5–6) and a nurse who has appropriate preparation to respond to the need. The use of technical procedures in nursing is acknowledged but relegated to a secondary role. Her most frequently quoted definition is:

> Nursing is a significant, therapeutic, interpersonal process. It functions co-operatively with other human processes that make health possible for individuals in communities. . . . Nursing is an educative instrument, a maturing force, that aims to promote forward movement of personality in the direction of creative, constructive, productive, personal, and community living (Peplau, 1952, p. 16).

Persons

In her theory, Peplau includes as components two persons: the nurse and client, or more often, patient (O'Toole & Welt, 1989; Peplau, 1992). Peplau (1952) initially defined Man as:

> An organism that lives in an unstable equilibrium (i.e., physiological, psychological, and social fluidity) and life is the process of striving in the direction of stable equilibrium, i.e. a fixed pattern that is never reached except in death (p. 82).

Forchuk (1991) revised that definition, omitting the terms "organism" and "equilibrium" since they represent a more "mechanical, closed-system perspective" (p. 55) that is inconsistent with Peplau's view of humans as growth seeking. A person is a relational being experiencing "interacting expectations, conceptions, wishes, and desires, as well as feelings when . . . in situations with other persons" (O'Toole & Welt, 1989, p. 5). This perspective on persons as relational beings is fundamental to the theory.

NURSE

The nurse is identified as a professional with definable expertise (Peplau, 1992). This expertise should include the ability to "identify human problems that confront patients, the degrees of skill used to meet situations, and be able to develop with patients the kind of relationships that will be conducive to improvement in skill" (Peplau, 1991, p. xiii). The nurse also possesses "a unique blend of ideals, values, integrity, and commitment to the well-being of others" (Peplau, 1988, p. 10).

PATIENT

The patient is defined first as a person, deserving of "all of the humane considerations: respect, dignity, privacy, confidentiality, and ethical care" (Peplau, 1992, p. 14), but a person who has problems that now require the services of a nurse. Ideally, the patient participates actively in the nurse–patient relationship (O'Toole & Welt, 1989, p. 57).

Health

Peplau (1952) provided a definition of health in her initial description of the theory. "It [health] is a word symbol that implies forward movement of personality and other human processes in the direction of creative, constructive, productive, personal, and community living" (p. 12). In addition, she identified two processes that are necessary for health: (a) biological, for example, absorption and elimination; and (b) social, which promotes physical, emotional, and social well-being (pp. 12–13).

ENVIRONMENT

Peplau focused on the issue of environment as milieu, using the term to describe a therapeutic environment (O'Toole & Welt, 1989, p. 78). The milieu is composed of structured (e.g., ward government) and unstructured components. The unstructured components consist of the complex relationships between patients, staff, visitors, and other patients, which is often neglected and yet has a significant impact on patient outcomes. Milieu ideally involves the creation of an atmosphere conducive to recovery.

DESCRIPTION OF THEORY OF INTERPERSONAL RELATIONS

Peplau implied a philosophical foundation to her Theory of Interpersonal Relations and provided two basic assumptions, which have been expanded by others, using the initial publication of the theory as the primary source. Peplau did not label the propositional statements in her theory as such; instead, they are integrated into her discussion of the components of the theory.

Philosophical Foundations

There are some different perspectives on the nature of the philosophical underpinnings of Peplau's Theory of Interpersonal Relations in Nursing. Sellers (1991) labels the theory:

> . . . a mechanistic, deterministic, persistence ontological view; an epistemology that is consistent with the totality paradigm, with its emphasis on a received view of knowledge and logical positivism; and an axiology that values stability, traditionalism, and nursing's close alignment with medicine (p. 158).

Sellers did not support these conclusions with examples from the theory. Since the complexity of Peplau's theory makes it difficult to categorize, it is not surprising that others have considered it from a different philosophical perspective.

More recently, existential phenomenology has been identified as the philosophical foundation of Peplau's theory (Gastmans, 1998). Consistent with phenomenology, observation of patients as a fundamental task of nursing is seen as contextual and value laden. It requires openness to and involvement with patients' existential situations. "Nursing has a human interpretive character" (Gastmans, 1998, Phenomenology and Nursing Science, para. 5) with the nurse–patient relationship at its core. Interpretations are meaning-seeking activities that arise from a caring relationship between nurse and patient.

These perspectives of nursing are themes found in Peplau's writings. She identifies observation of patients as an essential component of an interpersonal process that is therapeutic and educative for patients (Peplau, 1991, p. 309). Peplau (1992) also believes understanding of the patient best comes from observations of the patient's immediate situation and that participant observation is the preferred form of making observations. This participation with the patient is described as respectful, communicating positive interest and nonjudgmental regard (Peplau, 1991). Peplau uses the term "professional closeness" (Peplau, 1969) to summarize these characteristics that allow the nurse to communicate care when participating with patients. The importance of values is acknowledged by Peplau, as evidenced by her belief that the nurse's self-knowledge of feelings, attitudes, and behaviors is fundamental to understanding the client's situation (Peplau, 1991).

Though most of Peplau's philosophy is imbedded in her writings, she does delineate six "beliefs about patients" (Peplau, 1964). She identifies these as her "philosophy about patients and their care" (p. 30), attributed primarily to psychiatric nurses but applicable to all patients:

1. All behavior is purposeful, has meaning, and can be understood.
2. The nurse must observe what is going on; she must interpret what is observed, and then she must decide action on the basis of her interpretations.
3. The nurse meets the needs of the patient.
4. The nurse–patient interaction—the verbal and nonverbal exchanges in the nursing situation—can influence recovery.
5. The personality of the patient is somehow involved in his illness.
6. There are some ideas about nursing care that relate to the word *anxiety* (pp. 30–35).

Assumptions

In the initial publication of her theory, Peplau (1952) listed two guiding assumptions, emphasizing the importance of the nurse's own growth and development in establishing helpful interpersonal relationships with patients. Others have expanded that list through personal correspondence with Peplau and review of her writings. Table 10.1 provides a list of the assumptions of the Theory of Interpersonal Relations.

These 13 assumptions serve to illustrate the complexity of Peplau's Theory of Interpersonal Relations.

Theory Description with Propositional Statements

The core of the theory, the relationship between nurse and patient, is composed of phases, fulfilled through roles, influenced by psychobiological experiences, and requires attending to certain psychological tasks. Peplau also identified methods that can assist the nurse to develop understanding of the nurse–patient relationship. The description of the theory is presented using the same sequence as Peplau (1952, 1991) did in her seminal work, *Interpersonal Relations in Nursing*.

Table 10.1 ASSUMPTIONS OF THE THEORY OF INTERPERSONAL RELATIONS

SOURCE	ASSUMPTIONS
Identified by Peplau (1952)	1. "The kind of person each nurse becomes makes a substantial difference in what each patient will learn as he is nursed throughout his experience with illness" (p. xii).
	2. "Fostering personality development in the direction of maturity is a function of nursing and nursing education; it requires the use of principles and methods that permit and guide the process of grappling with everyday interpersonal problems or difficulties" (p. xii).
Based on correspondence with Peplau (Forchuk, 1993)	3. Nursing can claim as its uniqueness, the responses of clients to the circumstances of their illnesses or health problems (1989, p. 28).
	4. Because illness provides an opportunity for learning and growth, nurses can assist clients to further develop their intellectual and interpersonal competencies, during the illness experience, by gearing nursing practices to evolving such competencies through nurse–client interactions (1989, p. 28). Peplau references Gregg (1954) and Mereness (1966) in the development of this fourth assumption (Forchuk, 1993, p. 6).
Inferred from Peplau's writings (Forchuk, 1993)	5. Psychodynamic nursing crosses all specialty areas of nursing. It is not synonymous with psychiatric nursing because every nurse–client relationship is an interpersonal situation in which recurring difficulties of everyday life arise (summarized from Peplau, 1952, introduction).
	6. Difficulties in interpersonal relations recur in varying intensities throughout the life of everyone (Peplau, 1952, p. xiv).
	7. The need to harness energy that derives from tension and anxiety connected to felt needs to positive means for defining, understanding, and meeting productively the problem at hand is a universal need (Peplau, 1952, p. 26).
	8. All human behavior is purposeful and goal-seeking in terms of feelings of satisfaction and/or security (Peplau, 1952, p. 26).
	9. The interaction of nurse and client is fruitful when a method of communication that identifies and uses common meanings is at work in the situation (Peplau, 1952, p. 284).
	10. The meaning of behavior to the client is the only relevant basis on which nurses can determine needs to be met (Peplau, 1952, p. 226).
	11. Each client will behave, during crisis, in a way that has worked in relation to crises faced in the past (Peplau, 1952, p. 255).
Inferred from Peplau's writings (Sellers, 1991)	12. The function of personality is to grow and to develop. Nursing is a process that seeks to facilitate development of personality by aiding individuals to use those compelling forces and experiences that influence personality in ways that ensure maximum productivity (p. 73).
	13. Because illness is an event that is experienced along with feelings that derive from older experiences but are re-enacted in the relationship of nurse to patient, the nurse–patient relationship is an opportunity for nurses to help patients to complete the unfinished psychological tasks of childhood to some degree (p. 59).

COMPOSED OF PHASES

Peplau (1991) initially defined four phases of the nurse–patient relationship: orientation, identification, exploitation, and resolution. Forchuk (1991) later reconceptualized these phases into three, with the working phase replacing the identification and exploitation phases. These phases are considered overlapping and interlocking, with each phase possessing characteristic functions. They are experienced in every nursing situation.

Phase of Orientation. There are four functions that nurses use during orientation: (a) *provide the resources* of specific, needed information to help the patient understand the problem and the health care situation; (b) *serve as a counselor* to encourage the patient to express thoughts and feelings related to the problem situation; (c) *act as surrogate* to family members so that the patient can re-enact and examine relevant issues from prior relationships; and (d) *use technical expertise* to attend to concerns or issues that require the use of professional devices. These nursing functions assist the patient to address the needs experienced during the phase of orientation.

The patient needs to recognize and understand the extent of the difficulty and the help that is needed to address it. Orienting the patient to the nature of the problem is a complex task. It requires that the nurse act as both a resource person and a counselor. As a resource person, the nurse provides specific information about the problem confronting the patient and helps the patient see the personal relevance of the information. As a counselor, the nurse encourages the patient to be actively involved in identifying and assessing the problem.

The patient also needs to recognize and use the professional services offered. The nurse serves as a resource person to help the patient identify the range and limitations of services provided. It is important for the patient to know what can be expected from the nurse. It is equally important that the patient understands the limitations in the health care environment, both situational (i.e., related to the routines) and cultural (i.e., related to the standards of conduct).

In order for the patient to move successfully to the next phase in the nurse–patient relationship, he must harness the energy from the tension and anxiety created by felt needs in a constructive fashion to define, understand, and resolve the problem. The counseling role of the nurse is vital in dealing with the patient's anxiety. The nurse must understand the meaning of the situation to the patient and be alert to evidence of anxiety manifested by apathy, dependency, or overaggressiveness. Anxiety can escalate to terror or panic if the patient fails to deal with it. As a resource person, the nurse helps the patient understand the meaning of the anxiety-promoting events he is experiencing in the health care environment. In the counseling role, the nurse encourages the expression of expectations and feelings by responding unconditionally to the patient. This response communicates to the patient that the focus of the relationship is on his needs, not those of the nurse. Through nondirective listening, the nurse encourages the patient to focus on the problem and express related feelings, without offering advice, reassurance, suggestions, or persuasions. This establishes the foundation for the work of the next phase of the relationship.

Phase of Identification. This phase begins after the patient has, to a degree, clarified first impressions and arrived at some understanding of what the situation has to offer. At this time the patient can selectively begin to identify with some of the individuals who are offering help in one of three ways: with interdependence/participation, independence/isolation, or dependence/helplessness. This identification is based on the degree to which the patient believes the nurse will be helpful and on the nature of his past relationships.

The patient who responds interdependently feels less powerless and identifies with and expresses the attitudes of cheerfulness, optimism, and problem solving that he perceives in the nurse. Under these conditions the patient may express feelings that are not normally considered acceptable (e.g., helplessness or self-centeredness). These expressions are seen as potentially growth producing if the nurse accepts the feelings and continues to meet the needs of the patient.

Not all patients can identify with the nurse offering help because of the influence of earlier negative relationships with others. This experience often leads to a response that is independent or isolative. At this time the nurse in the surrogate family member role may provide the patient with the opportunity to have new and more positive relational experiences.

Other patients may identify with the nurse too quickly, which can result in an overly dependent response to the nurse. These patients want all their needs to be met by others with no expectations placed on them. This not uncommon response limits the possibility of growth through the experience.

It is important for the nurse to consider the phenomenon of leadership during the identification phase. The nurse attempts to provide opportunities for the patient to assume responsibility in the situation that promotes more constructive rather than imitative learning. The patient is encouraged to develop the skills to perceive, focus, and interpret cues in the situation, and then respond appropriately, independent of the nurse.

Phase of Exploitation. During this phase the patient feels comfortable enough to take full advantage of the services being offered and experience full value from the relationship with the nurse. Varying degrees of dependence and self-directedness are manifested with vacillation between the states. Ideally, the patient begins to identify and orient self to new goals besides solving the immediate problem, for example, in the case of a hospitalized patient the goal of functioning at home.

Phase of Resolution. As old needs are met, they are replaced by new goals that began to be formulated while the patient engaged in (i.e., exploited) the use of the services provided by the nurse. It is hoped that the patient will experience a sense of security and release that occurs because he received help in the time of need. This security is accompanied by less reliance on and decreasing identification with helping persons and increasing reliance on self to deal with the problem. This is the result of a nurse–patient relationship that is characterized during all phases by (a) an unconditional, patient-focused, and ongoing relationship that provides for the patient's needs; (b) a recognition of and appropriate response to cues that indicate the patient's desire and readiness to grow; and (c) a shift of power from nurse to patient as patient assumes responsibility for achieving new goals (Peplau, 1991, pp. 40–41).

FULFILLED THROUGH ROLES

The roles of nursing are defined by nurses, endorsed by patients, influenced by society, and promoted by the professional literature. Peplau identified the roles that she considered most relevant to nurse–patient situations and delineated principles for the successful fulfilling of those roles. The roles she identified were stranger, resource person, teacher, leader, surrogate, and counselor. Table 10.2 lists principles related to each role.

INFLUENCED BY PSYCHOBIOLOGICAL EXPERIENCES

The psychobiological experiences of needs, frustration, conflict, and anxiety influence the functioning of personalities. These experiences are also sources of energy that can result in both constructive and destructive actions. It is through understanding these experiences that individuals can learn to become more productive human beings (Peplau, 1991).

Needs. Though Peplau identifies needs as both physiological and psychological, her emphasis is on those that are psychological in nature. Security, new experiences, affection, recognition, and mastery are identified as psychological needs.

Table 10.2 ROLES IN NURSING

ROLE	PRINCIPLE	COMMENTS
Stranger	1. "Respect and positive interest accorded a stranger is at first nonpersonal and includes the same ordinary courtesies that are accorded a new guest who has been brought into any situation" (p. 44). 2. "In communicating with a new patient, who is also a stranger, try to say whatever it is that you wish the patient to hear" (p. 46). 3. In a home, "accommodate to the direction of activity in the situation as [the nurse] finds it, await the development of good feeling, and then orient the family of the purpose of the visit and the services offered in a simple manner" (pp. 46–47).	1. The patient is accepted as he or she is and related to as a capable individual, unless there is evidence to the contrary. 2. Inappropriate casual comments by the nurse can interfere with the development of the relationship. 3. Developing rapport promotes the establishment of identification with the nurse and the relationship can proceed to address the problems confronting the patient.
Resource person	1. "A resource person provides specific answers to questions usually formulated with relation to a larger problem" (p. 47).	1. The level of functioning, psychological readiness, psychological atmosphere, and relevance of the question are determinants of the nature of the nurse's response to the questions. The goal of the response is constructive learning.
Teacher	1. "Teaching always proceeds from what the patient knows and it develops around his interest in wanting and being able to use additional medical information" (p. 48).	1. The nurse needs to attempt to develop learning situations that enable the patient to learn through experience.
Leader	1. A goal to pursue is "democratic leadership in nursing situations, [which] implies that the patient will be permitted to be an active participant in designing nursing plans for him" (p. 50). 2. To promote democratic leadership, the nurse needs "to be able to sit at the bedside of any patient, observe, and gather evidence on the way the patient views the situation confronting him, visualize what is happening inside the patient, as well as observe what is going on between them in the interpersonal relations" (p. 50).	1. This also assists the patient to learn problem solving. 2. This allows the nurse to recognize when the patient is overvaluing the nurse.
Surrogate	1. "A nurse helps the patient to learn that there are likenesses and differences between people by being herself" (p. 53). 2. "The nurse and patient relationship moves on a continuum" (p. 55).	1. This requires that the nurse is aware of how he or she behaves in relationships with others. 2. The nurse attempts to move the relationship in the direction of chronological age-appropriate relationships.

(table continued on page 212)

Table 10.2 **ROLES IN NURSING** (continued)

ROLE	PRINCIPLE	COMMENTS
	3. "Surrogate roles are determined by psychological age factors that operate by reason of arrests in development, feelings that have been reactivated on the basis of illness, or demands made by individuals in a situation" (p. 55).	3. The patient psychologically substitutes the nurse for an individual from his or her past. This substitution affects the nursing situation.
	4. ". . . ways of responding, which do not impose goals that the nurse has in mind about how patients should feel, aid the patient in becoming aware of what is actually felt during the experience" (p. 56).	4. By not imposing goals on the patient, the nurse frees him or her to make those judgments. This becomes a growth-producing experience.
	5. "Permitting the patient to re-experience older feelings in new situations of helplessness, but with professional acceptance and attention that provokes personality development, requires a relationship in which the nurse recognizes and responds in a variety of surrogate roles" (p. 57).	5. As the patient deals constructively with these feelings, the nurse may need to assume new surrogate roles that are based on greater patient autonomy.
	6. The nurse needs to consider the "perception of the role in which the patient casts the nurse, identification of the difficulty that is being worked through, and sustaining a working relationship that develops awareness in the patient of how he feels [about] nursing skills" (pp. 57–58).	6. This allows the nurse to develop learning experiences with patients making use of the nurse–patient relationship.
Counselor	1. "All counseling functions in nursing are determined by the purpose of all nurse–patient relationships, namely the promotion of experiences leading to health" (p. 61).	1. The functions include assisting the patient to recognize the conditions necessary for health, providing those when possible, helping the patient identify ongoing threats to health, and using the nurse–patient relationship to promote learning.
	2. "Counseling in nursing has to do with helping the patient to remember and to understand fully what is happening to him in the present situation" (p. 64).	2. This enables the experience to be integrated rather than dissociated from other life experiences.
	3. "Helping a patient to become aware of real feelings related to an event in an immediate way is a counseling function" (p. 67).	3. Feelings not acknowledged will be pushed into the unconscious and can function to distort other feeling experiences and relationships.
	4. "Observation [and listening] precedes interpretation of the collected data" (p. 64).	4. By using nondirective and nonmoralizing listening, the patient can discover aspects of self previously unknown, a process that is quite therapeutic.

Source: Peplau, H. E. (1991). *Interpersonal relations in nursing: A conceptual frame of reference for psychodynamic nursing.* New York: Springer. Reproduced with the permission of Springer Publishing Company, LLC, New York, NY 10036.

Needs create tension, which individuals strive to reduce through the expenditure of energy (behavior). Behavior is directed at meeting the uppermost need, which may leave other needs unrecognized. Underactivity and overactivity are ineffective ways of meeting unrecognized needs. Unmet needs, if persistent, can lead to ever-increasing tension or anxiety. When immediate needs are met others emerge, some of which may be more consistent with promoting health (e.g., recovery and personality development).

Frustration. Frustration occurs when fulfillment of a need or pursuit of a goal is blocked. The primary goal identified by Peplau (1991) is the need for a "feeling of satisfaction and/or security" (p. 86). "Three interacting factors seem to determine the effects of frustration: (1) the degree, (2) the need that is not met, and (3) the personality of the individual [e.g. frustration tolerance]" (Peplau, 1991, p. 94).

Frustration can be manifested as aggression and/or anxiety. Direct expression of aggression occurs when the source is identified and is the recipient of its expression; indirect expression of aggression occurs when the recipient only resembles the original source. The intensity of the expression varies based on the degree to which the recipient resembles the original source. The greater the resemblance, the higher the intensity is. More intense aggression results in a threat to the goals of safety or security and can be directed at self or others.

Anxiety is a result of repeated frustrations that are perceived as failure to accomplish goals. Since the experience of anxiety is difficult to tolerate, the individual defends self from it by (a) modifying the goal to one for which success is more likely, (2) giving up on the goal with the possibility of dissociation of feelings occurring, and/or (3) adopting fixed responses (e.g., stereotyping, delusions).

The nurse may discover that his or her goals and those of the patient are not mutual. In fact, the nurse's goals may be perceived as an obstacle by the patient. It is important for the nurse and patient to communicate to clarify goals and arrive at some mutually acceptable ones.

Conflict. Another issue that the nurse and patient deal with in their interpersonal relationship is conflicting goals. Conflicting goals are often unrecognized and are expressed in the behavioral responses of hesitation, tension, vacillation, or complete blocking.

Blocking occurs when approaching a goal is completely incompatible with avoiding another one (approach–avoidance conflict). The most common example is the desire to go home (approaching goal) that coexists with the desire to not leave the perceived safety of the hospital (avoiding goal). Fear results and intensifies when approaching a goal for which there is a conflicting goal of avoiding. This fear can express itself as withdrawal or avoidance. If that which is feared is external to the patient and can be identified, the nurse can act as a resource person by providing information and experiences that can reduce the strength of avoidance. If the source of the fear cannot be identified, it is referred to as anxiety and is likely an internal conflict that is more difficult to resolve.

Individuals often are required to make choices between two desirable goals (approach–approach conflict). This is manifested with slightly different behavioral responses, for example, ignoring the feelings about the desired goals or keeping them from conscious awareness. The nurse is most helpful by fulfilling the counselor role in this situation. Listening in a way that encourages the expression of feelings allows the individual to recognize the factors that influence the choice to be made.

Unexplained Discomfort/Anxiety. As previously noted, anxiety, or unexplained discomfort, as Peplau sometimes referred to it, can occur when there are unmet needs, obstacles to goals, or conflicting goals. Anxiety is often associated with guilt, doubt, fears, and obsessions. Both patients and nurses experience this feeling state that influences behavior productively or destructively through the energy it produces.

Peplau (1991) identifies two principles that nurses can use to assist patients to use anxiety productively:

1. "When anxiety is held within tolerable limits it can be a 'functionally' effective element in interpersonal relations" (p. 127).
2. As anxiety increases in severity, there is a narrowing of perceptual awareness. Mild anxiety can manifest itself as restlessness, sleeplessness, hostility, misunderstanding, repeated questioning, seeking attention or reassurance, etc. This level of anxiety creates a felt need that can serve as a source of motivation for personality growth. If the nurse provides the help needed, the patient can begin to identify and deal with the anxiety-producing situation. In contrast to mild anxiety, severe anxiety can be crippling and incapacitating. The patient cannot collaborate with the nurse and useful learning cannot take place. The nurse helps reduce the anxiety to a more manageable and useful level by his or her presence as someone who will listen and provide for the patient's physical needs.

The ability of the nurse to be helpful to the patient during the experiences of anxiety is predicated on his or her self-understanding. "If a nurse has developed ability to undergo tension and stress, in order to identify a difficulty that she feels and to take steps that lead to a course of action based on evidence of what is involved, she will be able to help patients to do likewise" (Peplau, 1991, p. 135). Peplau (1991) summarized the responsibility of the nurse in assisting the patient experiencing anxiety in the form of a "hypothesis":

> Nurses face the task of developing experiences with patients that aid them to discriminate aspects of a total experience, to understand what is happening in their relations with nurses, and to develop ways that convert tension and anxiety into purposeful action (p. 130).

REQUIRES ATTENDING TO CERTAIN PSYCHOLOGICAL TASKS

Psychological tasks are those related to learning to live with others. Peplau addresses the tasks of (a) learning to count on others, (b) learning to delay satisfaction, (c) identifying oneself, and (d) developing skills in participation. These tasks occur as an aspect of the development of personality but also as features of nurse–patient relationships. During this relationship the nurse has the opportunity to help patients to develop in areas of task deficit. In order to provide this assistance, the nurse uses the previously discussed roles and understanding of the previously examined psychobiological experiences. In addition, in order to understand his or her own personality and the patient's, the nurse needs to appreciate the "dynamic interaction that occurs in early infancy and childhood as personality is undergoing formation" (Peplau, 1991, p. 162).

Peplau (1991) based her conceptualizations of psychological tasks on the works of Sigmund Freud and Richard Havighurst (p. 166):

> The infant's biological functioning and the need for acculturation set up certain requirements or psychological tasks, which every infant and child must undergo with relative success in order to develop a sound basis for mature functioning of personality as an adult (Peplau, 1991, p. 165).

The acculturation processes of children are general in nature and include both family members' and surrogates' expressions of feelings, attitudes, and ideas.

Counting on Others. This is the first psychological task of the infant. Initially, comfort and discomfort are the only feeling states experienced. If the caregiver (mother) appreciates the feelings of discomfort being communicated and responds unconditionally and in a way consistent with the infant's biological make-up, the infant learns to rely on the mother for help. Dependency is thus learned in an unambiguous fashion. Healthy dependence is not the only possible outcome of a mother's response to the child's needs. If there is maternal rejection and/or overprotection, an ongoing need for dependency may develop. An individual's longing for dependency thus operates as a persistent need that is based on a denial that help is needed or would be useful, or it is based on a belief that others will be able to identify and meet needs without his or her attempts to communicate them.

The nurse encounters varying degrees of both healthy dependency and dependency longings in nursing situations:

> Nurses have two responsibilities in their relations with patients who express longings for dependence: (1) to help the patient to learn that nurses can be counted on for help when needed; . . . (2) to aid the patient to become aware of his wants and to improve his ways of expressing what those wants are (Peplau, 1991, p. 181).

There are a number of positive consequences of having needs met. The patient experiences a feeling of self-worth and as a result begins to collaborate with the nurse in his or her growth. In addition, as needs are met, new, more mature ones can emerge.

Delaying Satisfaction. The socialization of a child includes the lesson of deferring to the wishes of others and delaying gratification of his own wishes, a lesson that is dependent on having already learned that those being deferred to are also those that can also be counted upon. According to Peplau (1991), this lesson takes place primarily during the process of toilet training. A rigorous and rigid form of training may inhibit the child's natural desire to explore this newly developing skill (i.e., producing feces) and can result in a sense of powerlessness. By contrast:

> Every child will learn to accept interference [with his/her own wishes] as inevitable, reasonable, perhaps useful life experience, if personality is not threatened and if anxiety and conflict are not generated through the use of mother love as a barter in the learning process (Peplau, 1991, pp. 193–194).

During the toilet training experience the child has three possible responses: (a) adapt his needs to those of family and gradually learn to behave in a way consistent with family members with whom he identifies, (b) give up feelings of power and comply with other's demands, or (c) refuse to give up power, becoming defiant and resistant. The latter two responses result in distorted relations with others and unresolved personality issues that persist into adulthood. The nurse may note these issues manifested in patients who are exploitive and manipulative; who hoard and withhold, being unable to share (including the inability to share feelings); and who alter their responses to others in a way that indicates a lack of stability and consistency in personality structure.

In order to respond in growth-producing ways to patients exhibiting these behaviors, nurses need insight into their own character traits and the ways they relate to others. With this insight, a nurse can modify her own behavior, a process that once learned can be used to help others modify their behaviors. Peplau (1991) also identifies additional principles that are consistent with healthy toilet training and general socialization activities that help the nurse establish rapport with the patient:

1. Show unconditional interest and acceptance.
2. Encourage expression of needs and feelings.
3. Provide times in which demands are met and times in which they are not met.
4. Promote participation in decision making so patients can become more self-directing.

5. Allow for some "hoarding," which reinforces feelings of security.

6. Encourage sharing, which can only occur when there is freedom from coercion.

When rapport between the nurse and patient has been developed, a rapport that allows them to "understand each other's preconceptions and expectations, it is possible for the nurse anticipatorily to suggest interferences and delays in meeting needs and requests" (Peplau, 1991, p. 206).

Identifying Oneself. Self-identity or concept of self enhances or distorts relationships with others, a fact that is true for both the patient and the nurse. This sense of self develops initially through a child's interactions with adults as he learns to rely on others and delay gratification in relation to needs. The way the child is appraised during these interactions results in three possible views of self: (a) *a sense of competency* to identify wants and needs, communicate them to others, and receive needed assistance; (b) *a sense of helplessness and dependence* on others to provide what is needed and a belief that this helplessness will produce a sense of safety (since making no demands will result in not being deserted); and (c) *a sense of distrust* in others as a source of assistance that results in independently taking what is needed.

This appraisal by others and its significance to the child intensifies during the genital phase of psychosocial development. During this phase the child discovers, explores, and finds pleasure in his genitalia. Ideally, the child is also introduced to other experiences that provide pleasure and is allowed the freedom to make decisions about their pursuit. If this does not occur and instead the child is coerced into certain activities and blocked from others, he will experience frustration.

When a child needs to focus all of his activities in the direction of getting and sustaining approval, or avoiding anxiety connected with disapproval, from parents or surrogates, his concept of self cannot expand beyond what works and is acceptable to the adults upon whom he must count for feelings of safety or security" (Peplau, 1991, p. 219).

These concepts of self are established in childhood but can be reinforced or modified by experiences with others throughout life.

The nurse can provide experiences that help the patient develop a concept of self that facilitates the establishment of interdependent relationships with others. In order to provide the appropriate experiences, the nurse needs to understand the patient's self-perception. Peplau (1992) suggests a number of activities that help the nurse understand a patient's self concept:

1. Consider own response to patient as a source of information about the patient's perceptions of self and situation confronting him.
2. Develop self-awareness of own habits (e.g., regarding cleanliness) and how they are expressed in the nursing situation.
3. Identify patient's patterns of feeling expressions and other behavioral responses as he encounters situational challenges.
4. Consider patient's specific responses to the nursing situation as indicators of needs to be met.

In addition, the nurse can be helpful to the patient by:

1. Being value neutral, ". . . providing merely conditions and acting as a sounding board against which the patient may air his views and give full expression to his feelings in a nonjudgmental relationship" (Peplau, 1991, p. 226)
2. Communicating hope and acceptance
3. Avoiding the problematic responses of praise, blame, and indifference

The nurse who exhibits these characteristics can enhance the patient's whole concept of self, and as a result of this enhanced self-concept, the patient will experience more interdependent and mutually productive relationships with others.

Participating with Others. When individuals participate in making decisions that affect them, they are more likely to understand the decisions, be involved in implementing them, and appreciate the contributions of others to the ultimate decision. The task of learning to participate with others initially occurs during what Sullivan refers to as the "juvenile era" (ages of 6 to 9). This task of participating with others is composed of the abilities to (a) *compromise*, arbitrate and make personal concessions; (b) *compete*, express rivalry and struggle with peers; and (c) *cooperate,* subordinate individual wishes to achieve mutually beneficial goals. The process of developing these skills is influenced by the appraisals of parents and peers. Children will act out in their relationships the lessons about self and others that those appraisals taught.

Following the juvenile era is what Sullivan calls "preadolescence" (8½ to 12 years old). During this time, the abilities to participate with others are consolidated in a process referred to as consensual validation. The view of self becomes more consistent with the views of peers and a more realistic perspective of life and one's role in it develops. It is also at this time that a child begins to be able care for and accept others. This occurs to the degree that he cares for and accepts self.

The nurse attempts to encourage participation with others through collaboration with the patient in addressing his problems. This participatory approach serves to improve the patient's skills in meeting problems. Peplau (1991) describes a three-step process:

1. Assist the patient to identify the problem.
2. Collaborate to "achieve a decision on what is possible, what can be done, and then move into other items that have been mentioned and other *possible courses of action* that can be taken in behalf of and with the co-operation of the patient" (Peplau, 1991, p. 248).
3. Encourage the patient to try out what has been proposed.

As part of the process of identifying the problem, the nurse will need to assess the patient's attitude, since attitude will affect the way the patient will attempt to solve the problem. The two most common attitudes are overconcern or underconcern. If overconcerned, the patient may attempt to arrive at a solution too quickly and the solution will be inadequate. If underconcerned, the patient may not invest sufficient energy in its solution and the solution will be superficial.

In formulating a possible solution to the problem, the nurse needs to allow the patient to determine the pace for working through it. Time pressures are often communicated by the nurse in the form of suggestions about what is wrong and advice as to what needs to be done, leading to premature and ineffective solutions. "The process for recognition and solutions of a problem, like the processes of self-renewal, self-repair, self-awareness, arise within the individual" (Peplau, 1991, p. 251).

Nurses can help patients to experience the process of problem solving and to develop the skills needed to actively participate in its solution. The inability to participate with others in problem solving comes with negative consequences. "Ineffective participation in life impedes the development of a democratic society in which all are free to grow, to change, to mature, and to design a way of life that ensures productive relations among people" (Peplau, 1991, p. 147).

NURSING METHODS USED TO UNDERSTAND INTERPERSONAL PROCESSES

Observation, communication, and recording are three basic skills that are "valuable to the use of nursing as an interpersonal process that is therapeutic and educative for patients" (Peplau, 1991, p. 309). Peplau considered these three operations as integral to the nursing process.

Observation. "The aim of observation in nursing, when it is viewed as an interpersonal process, is the identification, clarification, and verification of impressions about the interactive drama, of the pushes and pulls in the relationship between nurse and patient, as they occur" (Peplau, 1991, p. 263). Observation as described by Peplau is composed of four components: (a) intuitive impressions, (b) hypothesis statements, (c) organized observations, and (d) judgment formations.

Intuitive impressions are hunches or generalizations about what is occurring in an experience. They are an important component of understanding the problems of patients. Impressions are the foundation for the development of hypotheses, and it is hypotheses that provide a means of reducing the risk of concentrating prematurely on details of the situation. Concentrating on details is more likely to lead to rationalization than to understanding of what has been observed. When the impressions or generalizations are formulated as a hypothesis, they serve to provide a useful focus to the observations. The nurse proceeds to gather evidence related to the hypotheses (units of experience) that provides both elaboration of the whole impression and differentiation of the details.

Peplau (1991) provides a classification of types of observer–observed relationships that the nurse can use to gather evidence:

1. Spectator. The patient is unaware of being observed. The nurse is generally engaged in another activity while observing the patient.
2. Interviewer. The patient is aware of being observed as he responds to the situation or to the directive or nondirective questioning of the nurse. The nurse frequently takes notes while observing as an interviewer.
3. Collector. The nurse uses records and reports created by others as a way of determining what has happened in a particular situation. Observations made using this approach can help form partial impressions.
4. Participant. "The nurse engages in ordinary activities connected with nursing a patient and at the same time observes the relationship between the patient and herself" (Peplau, 1991, p. 274). The patient is aware that nursing care is being given but is unaware that his responses are being observed.

Participant observation is further described as composed of three foci: the nurse, the patient, and the relations (Peplau, 1997, p. 162). During participant observation, in addition to noting the behaviors of the patient, the nurse is required to undergo self-scrutiny, observing and analyzing her own behavior. By attending to her own behavior, the nurse can evaluate the usefulness of that behavior in the relationship and modify behaviors if appropriate.

The observations need to be organized. Organization helps provide focus to the multiplicity and complexity of the observations of human behavior in interpersonal relationships. Peplau (1991) suggests hypotheses and the phases of the nurse–patient relationship as two approaches to organizing observations. This organization of observations made through participant observation is the basis of all nursing judgments in practice (p. 283). "Observation and understanding of what is observed are essential operations for making judgments and for designing experiences with patients that aid them in the solution of their problems" (Peplau, 1991, p. 289).

There are two types of judgments—judgments in practice and judgments in fact—that occur during a therapeutic relationship with a patient. The judgments in practice are more situationally specific and based on interpretation of observations; the judgments in fact are less situationally specific and based on objective data. Judgments in practice exist when:

1. Situations demand a decision as to what action a nurse should take.
2. Even though policies exist as a guide to nursing action, nurses need to make appropriate choices between alternative actions.
3. Choices depend upon the interpretation of facts.

Judgments in fact occur when:

1. The facts further limit choices.
2. The facts identify the possibilities and limitations of actions.

Communication. One of the basic tools of nursing is communication, which requires "awareness of means of communication; spoken language, rational and nonrational expressions of wishes, needs, and desires, and the body gesture" (Peplau, 1991, p. 289). Use of words or verbal communication can convey facts, focus on everyday events, and provide interpretations. Spoken language can reveal personal realities or express hidden meanings, but it can also avoid conveying anything meaningful.

There are two main principles for effective verbal communication: clarity and continuity. Clarity occurs when there is a common frame of reference or when specific efforts are made to arrive at mutual understanding. "Clarity is promoted when the meaning to the patient is expressed and talked over and a new view is expanded in awareness" (Peplau, 1991, p. 291). Continuity occurs when the connections between ideas and the related feelings, events, or themes expressed through the ideas are made evident. "Continuity is promoted when the nurse is able to pick up threads of conversation [that occur over time] . . . and when she aids the patient to focus and to expand these threads" (Peplau, 1991, p. 293). Following up on what patients say communicates that what they said is important and that as individuals they are worthwhile.

In the process of promoting clarity and continuity in communication, nurses need to understand more than what the patient communicates directly. The nurse must also be able to interpret symbols to arrive at the hidden meanings of patients' indirect communications. Self-awareness is one of the primary conditions for achieving understanding.

Consciousness of meaning and use of words requires awareness of self. Ability to recognize meaning and the actions implied in words, or concepts, or principles, and to relate them to everyday nursing practices improves practices at the same time leading to sounder personality organization (Peplau, 1991, pp. 297–298).

For a nurse, this awareness enables her to express congruence in the use of words, their relevance, and related actions.

Awareness is also the primary distinction between rational and nonrational expressions. *Rational* attitudes and communication are those of which the participant is aware, recognizing connections between the meaning of an idea and the actions related to it, or between the behavior expressed and the traits of character of the individual whose behavior is being studied. *Nonrational* attitudes and communications are governed by traits of character of which the subject is unaware; they often govern behavior that occurs automatically, without recognition of underlying relationships (Peplau, 1991, p. 298).

Rational expressions more likely occur when individuals see self rather than others as a source of personal security and when they are oriented toward the future in the context of the present rather than oriented to the past.

Nonrational expressions communicate in more ambiguous and indirect ways than do rational expressions. Longings, hopes, and fears are often conveyed in a disguised form. Myths, dreams, rituals, and folk tales are examples of culturally shared nonrational communication. Nonrational expressions can also be specific to an individual. In either case, the nurse attempts to interpret the meaning of the language by considering the symbols being used. Interestingly, Peplau provided interpretations of dreams for her friends and colleagues (Spray, 1999).

In addition to the spoken word, gestures can be considered either rational or nonrational expressions. "The body as a whole, as well as parts of it, act as expressional instruments that communicate to others the feelings, wishes, and aspirations of an individual" (Peplau, 1991, p. 304). Underactivity and overactivity are examples of whole body gestures. Hand gestures (e.g., clenched fist) and facial grimaces (e.g., biting a lip) are examples of more specific gestures. The nurse's responsibility is to observe gestures and attempt to understand both what she and the patient are communicating to each other. Arriving at understanding or meaning is a complicated and ongoing process of observation and communication.

Recording. Peplau focuses primarily on recording for the purpose of student learning. In addition to charting in medical records, students need additional forms for recording what has occurred between student and patient. These additional recordings provide a means of examining the relationship in order to achieve insight into the student nurse's own behavior and the ways the patients responded. They also can help the student develop skills in observation by using hypotheses and units of observation as a structure for the recording. How useful the recording is to the student's development of interpersonal skills is dependent in part on the exactness of the wording of the recording. To produce an exact record, Peplau suggests recall but also "wire recordings," "television and motion pictures," and the use of another student to observe and document the interaction between the student nurse and the patient. The ultimate goal of recordings, as well as observation and communication, is nurse–patient relationships that result in improved health outcomes for the patient.

Applications of the Theory. Peplau is frequently cited in the nursing literature, though the majority of the literature focuses on applications to practice rather than use in nursing research. Sills (1978) found 93 references to Peplau's theory in articles published in three journals: 43 were published in *American Journal of Nursing* (1952 through 1977); 27 were published in *Nursing Outlook* (1952 through 1977); and 23 were published in *Perspectives of Psychiatric Care* (1963 through 1977). A search of the CINAHL database found 260 publications from 1990 through 2007 related to Peplau's Theory of Interpersonal Relations. Articles published in Canada, Spain, Portugal, Italy, Great Britain, Slovenia, and China were among those cited. The articles focused on the life and works of Peplau, her theory, her theory applied to research, and her theory used in practice.

Lego (1980) found similar rates of publication. Of the 166 papers reviewed with a clinical focus on the 1-to-1 nurse–patient relationship, from 1952 through 1979, 78 were written by students or colleagues of Peplau. Most of the work reviewed and analyzed demonstrated little or no linkage to the work of other nursing scientists. If literature was cited, it was most often from other disciplines.

Three types of papers on the 1-to-1 nurse–patient relationship were identified:

1. *Care or case study,* in which the author describes a difficult patient situation, discusses the nursing interventions used, and shares his or her learning from the situation
2. *Concept presentation,* in which the author reviews the relevant literature, provides operational definition, uses vignettes to illustrate the concept, and recommends nursing interventions
3. *Hypothesis testing,* in which the author makes an empirical observation of a clinical phenomenon, generates a hypothesis that is supported through further investigation, and draws conclusions that can be used to guide practice (Lego, 1980, pp. 80–81)

The volume of literature on Peplau's theory reflects its popularity with practicing nurses, particularly those practicing psychiatric–mental health nursing. Surveys of psychiatric nurses in Canada and the United States have found over half of them claiming to use Peplau's theory in their practices (Forchuk, 1993, p. 28). Recent examples of application to practice demonstrate how useful the theory is in a broad range of nursing situations. The theory has been used to (a) promote patient autonomy (Moser, Houtepen, & Widdershoven, 2007), (b) care for patients in end-stage kidney disease (Graham, 2006), (c) educate patients undergoing urinary diversion (Marchese, 2006), (d) promote computer-mediated communication (Hrabe, 2005), (e) educate antepartal patients about prevention of prematurity (Tiedje, 2004), (f) serve as a foundation for assessing needs in a patient with heart failure (Davidson, Cockburn, Daly, & Fisher, 2004), and (g) deal with power struggles (Kozub & Kozub, 2004). Less recent examples of applications to practice include use of the theory (a) in development of relationships in the community (McCann & Baker, 2001), (b) with patients diagnosed with multiple sclerosis (McGuinness & Peters, 1999), (c) in body image care (Price, 1998), (d) with individuals who have problems with alcohol (Buswell, 1997), (e) with families (Forchuk & Dorsay, 1995), (f) with stroke patients (Jones, 1995), (g) with an individual with AIDS (Hall, 1994), and (h) in case management (Forchuk et al., 1989).

Peplau's Theory of Interpersonal Relations has also served as a foundation for the development of other middle range theories applicable to practice. Examples include the Model of Simple Reminiscence (Puentes, 2002) and Cultural Competence (Warren, 2002). But Peplau's contributions to nursing are not limited to the content of her theory. She is credited with promoting the "scholarship of nursing practice" (Reed, 1996), integrating nursing practice with a process for ongoing development of nursing's knowledge base.

> Peplau introduced an approach to knowledge development that was anchored in nursing practice, and in the science and art of the nurse–patient interaction. Development and testing of explanations through the interpersonal process between patient and nurse was done for therapeutic purposes. . . . It can be seen that this interpersonal process is also a strategy for generating nursing knowledge, which can then be examined further and refined through research (Reed, 1996, A Strategy for Linking Knowledge Development and Practice, para. 1).

This approach to converting practice knowledge into nursing knowledge involves a three-step process:

1. *Observation of fundamental units.* The nurse generally assumes the role of participant observer, focusing on relevant units of observation. The units are defined as those that are useful to patients, understandable to all involved in the study, measurable to allow for objective and reliable categorization, and satisfactory to allow for comparison with other data (Peplau, 1991, pp. 270–271).
2. *Peeling out theoretical explanations.* The nurse applies knowledge from practice and relevant theories to interpret what has been observed. The interpretations become hypotheses that are "validated with the patient and tested for their meaningfulness and usefulness in the context of the nurse–patient relationship" (Reed, 1996, Step 2: Peeling Out Theoretical Explanations, para. 2).
3. *Transforming energy and transforming knowledge.* The nurse uses theoretical knowledge in interactions with patients as a means of transforming knowledge that is theoretical into knowledge that is practical. The critical test of this nursing knowledge is not whether it is consistent with theoretical perspectives, but whether it can be used constructively by and with the patient.

These steps initiate what Reed (1996) refers to as a cycle of inquiry in which "nursing knowledge that is generated through practice is further refined through research" (Cycle of Inquiry, para. 1) and then used to enhance nursing practice.

Though Peplau's theory has had a significant impact on nursing practice and has influenced nursing's research methodology, it has not generated a large number of research studies. It is surprising, given the theory's popularity as a topic in clinically based articles and nursing texts, that there is not more empirical testing of Peplau's theory of the nurse–patient relationship. Forchuk has been considered a major exception; she is acknowledged as having the most extensive and sustained research agenda of Peplau's theory (Young, Taylor, & Renpenning, 2001). In recent years researchers have demonstrated increasing interest in Peplau's theory, as Table 10.3 illustrates.

Table 10.3 EXAMPLES OF RESEARCH ON INTERPERSONAL RELATIONS

CITATION	FOCUS
Vogelsang, J. (1990). Continued contact with a familiar nurse affects women's perceptions of the ambulatory surgical experience: A qualitative design. *Journal of Post Anesthesia Nursing, 5*(5), 315–320.	Impact of familiar nurse working with ambulatory surgical patients from preadmission through discharge
Forchuk, C. (1992). The orientation phase of the nurse-client relationship: How long does it take? *Perspectives in Psychiatric Care, 28*(4), 7–10.	The length of the orientation phase of patients in a community health program diagnosed with depression or schizophrenia
Forchuk, C. (1994). The orientation phase of the nurse-client relationship: Testing Peplau's theory. *Journal of Advanced Nursing, 20*(3), 532–537.	Patient and nurse intrapersonal factors (e.g., preconceptions) that influence the development of a therapeutic relationship during the orientation phase
Forchuk, C. (1995). Development of nurse-client relationships: What helps. *Journal of American Psychiatric Nurses Association, 1*(5), 146–151.	Factors (e.g., length of previous hospitalizations, age of nurse and patient, and amount of meeting time) that influence progress of a therapeutic relationship during the orientation phase
Morrison, E. G., Shealy, A. H., Kowalski, C., LaMont, J., & Range, B. A. (1996). Workroles of staff nurses in psychiatric settings. *Nursing Science Quarterly, 9*(1), 17–21.	Role behaviors of psychiatric staff nurses in interactions with adult, child, and adolescent psychiatric patients as compared to those conceptualized by Peplau
Forchuk, C., Westfall, J., Martin, M., Bamber-Azzapardi, W., Kosterewa-Tolman, D., & Hux, M. (1998). Factors influencing movement of chronic psychiatric patients from the orientation to the working phase of the nurse-client relationship of an inpatient unit. *Perspectives in Psychiatric Care, 34*(1), 36–44.	Factors that influence movement from the orientation to working phase of the nurse–client relationship
Peden, A. R. (1998). The evolution of an intervention—the use of Peplau's process of practice-based theory development. *Journal of Psychiatric and Mental Health Nursing, 5*(3), 173–178.	Women's process of recovering from depression and an intervention to reduce negative thinking
Jacobson, G. (1999). Parenting processes: A descriptive explanatory study using Peplau's theory. *Nursing Science Quarterly, 12*, 240–244.	Qualities that were considered examples of positive parenting by recently graduated high school students
Middleton, J., Steward, N., & Richardson, J. (1999). Caregiver distress related to disruptive behaviors on special care units versus traditional long-care units. *Journal of Gerontological Nursing, 2*(3), 11–19.	Perceptions of formal caregivers on units for dementia patients in long-term care facility
Williams, C., & Tappen, R. (1999). Can we create a therapeutic relationship with nursing home residents in the later stages of Alzheimer's disease? *Journal of Psychosocial Nursing, 37*(3), 28–35.	Behaviors exhibited by patients diagnosed with Alzheimer's disease during 1-to-1 interactions over a 16-week period
Edwards, K. (2000). Service users and mental health nursing. *Journal of Psychiatric & Mental Health Nursing, 7*, 555–565.	Views and perceived needs of users of mental health services in the context of the role that users see nurses fulfilling as identified by the users themselves

Table 10.3 **EXAMPLES OF RESEARCH ON INTERPERSONAL RELATIONS** (continued)

CITATION	FOCUS
Forchuk, C., Westfall, J., Martin, M., Bamber-Azzapardi, W., Kosterewa-Tolman, D., & Hux, M. (2000). The developing nurse-client relationship: Nurses' perceptions. *Journal of Psychiatric & Mental Health Nursing, 6*(1), 3–10.	Perspectives of nurses in a tertiary care hospital on the nature and progression of the nurse–client relationship and the factors that facilitate or interfere with the development of the relationship
McNaughton, D. B. (2000). A synthesis of qualitative home visiting research. *Public Health Nursing, 17*(6), 405–414.	The nurse–client relationship during home visits of public health nurses
Forchuk, C., & Reynolds, W. (2001). Clients' reflections on relationships with nurses: Comparisons from Canada and Scotland. *Journal of Psychiatric & Mental Health Nursing, 8*(1), 45–51.	Comparison of what clients from Canada and Scotland want and do not want in relationships with nurses
Kai, J., and Crosland, A. (2002). People with enduring health problems described the importance of communication, continuity of care, and stigma. *Evidence-Based Nursing, 5*(3), 93(1).	Significance of therapeutic relationships in maintaining contacts with primary care and mental health services for individuals with chronic mental illness
Douglass, J. L., Sowell, R. L., & Phillips, K. D. (2003). Using Peplau's theory to examine the psychosocial factors associated with HIV-infected women's difficulty in taking their medications. *The Journal of Theory Construction & Testing, 7*(1), 10–17.	Relationship between the patient and the primary health care provider as it relates to medication adherence of HIV positive women
Carroll, S. M. (2004). Nonvocal ventilated patients' perceptions of being understood. *Western Journal of Nursing Research, 26*(1), 85–112.	Characteristics of nonvocal ventilated patients' communication and the kind of nursing care they desire
Tofthagen, R. (2004). An encounter between two realities: What kind of experiences do psychiatric nurses gain from their efforts to create a helping relationship with psychotic patients? *Nordic Journal of Nursing Research & Clinical Studies, 24*(2) 4–9.	Nature of the relationship between nurses and psychotic patients in acute psychiatric hospital settings
Beebe, L. H. (2004). TIPS: Telephone intervention—problem solving for persons with schizophrenia. *Issues in Mental Health Nursing, 25*(3), 317–329.	Significance of face-to face meetings in the efficacy of telephone intervention with schizophrenic individuals
Mahone, N. E., Yarcheski, A., & Yarcheski, T. J. (2004). Social support and positive health practices in early adolescents: A test of mediating variables. *Clinical Nursing Research, 13*(3), 216–236.	Relationship between social support and positive health practices of young adolescents
Shatell, M. (2005). Nurse bait: Strategies hospitalized patients use to entice nurses within the context of the interpersonal relationship. *Issues in Mental Health Nursing, 26*(2), 205–223.	Patients' experiences of seeking nursing care in the hospital setting
McNaughton, D. B. (2005). A naturalistic test of Peplau's theory in home visiting. *Public Health Nursing, 22*(5), 429–438.	Phases of the nurse–patient relationship identified in home visits to prenatal clients by public health nurses

10.1 USING MIDDLE RANGE THEORIES

This study was a naturalistic test of Peplau's Theory of Interpersonal Relations during home visits. The research was designed to answer the question, "How is the interpersonal relationship between public health nurses and clients during home visits similar or different from the phases of the nurse–client relationship described by Peplau (1952/1991)?" (p. 430).

Purposive sampling was used to recruit five nurse–client dyads from a suburban health department. Inclusion criteria were English speaking, aged 18 to 34 years, sufficient psychosocial or medical risk to warrant multiple nursing contacts, and diverse cultural backgrounds (p. 431). Nurses and clients participating in the study agreed to a minimum of five home visits, beginning with a prenatal visit and ending in early postpartum. The researcher was a passive, nonintrusive observer during the home visits. Data sources included transcripts of audio-recorded interactions and observation notes made during the home visits, in addition to filed notes completed after the visit. The Relationship Form was used to identify behaviors consistent with each of Peplau's stages of the nurse–patient relationship. Within-case and cross-case analyses were performed using NUDIST computer software for consideration of the transcripts.

The findings were supportive of Peplau's theory:

1. Orientation phase. For first home visits, 53% to 72% of dyads were identified as in this phase. Nurses engaged in assessment activities, discussed plans for home visits, and engaged in social conversation. Clients answered nurses' questions, offered additional information, and displayed anxiety.
2. Working phase: Identification. This phase began in the first to third home visit. Nurses provided health information, conducted additional assessments, gave advice, offered affective support, suggested referrals, advocated, and engaged in social conversation. Clients identified problems and asked questions.
3. Working phase: Exploitation. Four of the five dyads entered this phase in the fourth or fifth visit. The primary activity engaged in by the nurse was mutual problem solving. Clients reported using resources or used the nurse as a resource. This was demonstrated through using nurses as sources of information, as confidantes, and as partners in problem solving.
4. Resolution. Only one dyad entered this phase. The client in this dyad was moving out of the service area. In all other dyads, additional but more limited contact between nurses and clients was planned.

McNaughton, D. B. (2005). A naturalist test of Peplau's theory in home visiting. *Public Health Nursing, 22*(5), 429–438.

Though much of the research focuses on issues of interest to psychiatric–mental health nurses, there is a growing body of research that applies the Theory of Interpersonal Relations to a variety of nursing situations. Using Middle Range Theories 10.1 describes one such study.

Consistent with the few research studies of Peplau's theory, only a limited number of instruments have been identified as applicable to the Theory of Interpersonal Relations. Instrument development to study the nurse–patient relationship began in the 1960s and continued into the late 1980s. Table 10.4 provides an overview of those instruments.

ANALYSIS OF THEORY

Using the criteria presented in Chapter 2, critique the Theory of Interpersonal Relations. Compare your conclusions about the theory with those found in the Appendix A. A nurse scholar who has worked with the theory completed the analysis found in the appendix.

Internal Criticism

1. Clarity
2. Consistency
3. Adequacy

4. Logical development
5. Level of theory development

External Criticism

1. Reality convergence
2. Utility
3. Significance
4. Discrimination
5. Scope of theory
6. Complexity

4. What kind of educational and experiential background should the nurse have? What variables affect success? What is success?
5. How does the 1-to-1 relationship fit into the current and the future health care delivery system? (pp. 81–82)

Perhaps the most fundamental and pervasive question that researchers of the nurse–patient relationship can ask and attempt to answer is, What aspects of the nurse–patient relationship contribute to the welfare and well-being of patients (Caris-Verhallen, Kerkstra, & Bensing, 1997)? The promotion of the welfare of patients is core to all nursing theories, but for Peplau the means of achieving that goal focus on the attributes and behaviors of both the nurse and the patient and in the dynamic interaction that occurs between the two of them.

One of the attributes of nurses cited by Peplau (1991) as helpful to patients experiencing anxiety is self-knowledge (p. 135). Research Application 10.1 is designed to examine the relationship between nurses' self-knowledge and relief of patient's anxiety.

CRITICAL THINKING EXERCISES

1. In what ways might Peplau's Theory of Interpersonal Relations need to be revised to be most useful to nurses in a health care environment in which contact time between nurse and client is limited?
2. The surrogate role is not one that is frequently mentioned in recent nursing practice literature. Is that role as defined by Peplau relevant to nursing practice as currently experienced? If so, in what way? If not, why?

3. Peplau's theory focuses on the 1-to-1 therapeutic relationship between a nurse and a patient. Are the phases of relationships, roles of the nurse, psychobiological experiences encountered in the relationship, and psychological tasks described by Peplau relevant in other nursing contexts, for example, in relationships between nurses? If so, what are some examples of these contexts? If not, why?

SUMMARY

Peplau is acknowledged as the first theorist of the modern era of nursing. Her theory of interpersonal relations in nursing focuses on the stages experienced, the nursing roles used, and the issues addressed in the context of the nurse–patient relationship. Though Peplau's work has not attracted the attention of nurse researchers that it would seem to warrant, her Theory of Interpersonal Relations is widely taught in schools of nursing and extensively used in practice. In the nursing profession, the primacy of the nurse–patient relationship is still recognized and Peplau's phenomenological approach to theory development is still valued. Peplau was able to pull together "loose, ambiguous data and put them into systematic terms that could be tested, applied, and integrated into the practice of psychiatric nursing" (Lego, 1980, p. 68). Though because of its complexity research on the theory of interpersonal relations is not a simple undertaking, further testing of Peplau's theory could make significant contributions to nursing's body of knowledge.

WEB RESOURCES

1. This is the primary site for Peplau's work: **http://publish.uwo.ca/~forchuk/peplau/hpcb. html**. The site provides a brief biography of Peplau but is mostly devoted to bibliographies of work about and by Peplau. In addition to the traditional list of journal articles and books authored by Peplau, it includes lists of papers and speeches, audiotapes, and videotapes. It also provides a link to Cheryl Forchuk's web page and an additional link that allows for access to her e-mail address.

2. NurseScribe maintains a nursing theory page that identifies Peplau as one of the early nurse theorists. It provides a brief overview of the theory and links to two other sites devoted to Peplau. The major feature of the site is a direct link to MEDLINE/PubMed, which identifies over 150 citations, including articles about her or by her, as well as those that have used her theory in research or practice. It can be reached at **http://www. enursecribe.com/nurse_theorists.htm.**

3. **http://www.nurses.info/nursing_theory_ midrange_theories_hildegard_peplau.htm.** which includes a brief biography and links to an overview of the interpersonal relations model, a tribute to Peplau published at the time of her death in 1999, the theorist homepage and publications that can be purchased.

REFERENCES

Armstrong, M. E., & Kelly, A. E. (1995). More than the sum of their parts: Martha Rogers and Hildegard Peplau. *Archives of Psychiatric Nursing, 9*(1), 40–44.

Buswell, C. (1997). A model approach to care of a patient with alcohol problems...Peplau's model. *Nursing Times, 93*(3), 34–35.

Caris-Verhallen, W., Kerkstra, A., & Bensing, J. (1997). The role of communication in nursing care for elderly people: A review of the literature. *Journal of Advanced Nursing, 25*, 915–933.

Davidson, P., Cockburn, J., Daly, J., & Fisher, R. S. (2004). Patient-centered needs assessment: Rational for a psychometric measure for assessing needs in heart failure. *Journal of Cardiovascular Nursing, 19*(3), 164–171.

Fawcett, J. (2000). *Analysis and evaluation of contemporary nursing knowledge: Nursing models and theories.* Philadelphia: F. A. Davis.

Forchuk, C. (1991). Peplau's theory: Concepts and their relations. *Nursing Science Quarterly, 4*(2), 54–60.

Forchuk, C. (1993). *Hildegarde E. Peplau: Interpersonal nursing theory.* Park, CA: Sage.

Forchuk, C., Beaton, S., Crawford, L., Ide, L., Voorberg, N., & Bethune, J. (1989). Incorporating Peplau's theory and case management. *Journal of Psychosocial Nursing, 27*(2), 35–38.

Forchuk, C., & Dorsay, J. P. (1995). Hildegard Peplau meets family systems nursing: Innovation in theory-based practice. *Journal of Advanced Nursing, 21*(1), 110–115. Retrieved July, 24, 2002, from http://gateway1.ovid.com/ovidweb.cgi.

Gastmans, C. (1998). Interpersonal relations in nursing: A philosophical-ethical analysis of the work of Hildegard E. Peplau. *Journal of Advanced Nursing, 28*, 1312–1319. Retrieved August 1, 2002, from http://gateway1.ovid.com/ovidweb.cgi.

Graham, J. (2006). Nursing theory and clinical practice: How three nursing models can be incorporated into the care of patients with end stage kidney disease. *Canadian Association of Nephrology Nurses (CANNT) Journal, 16*(4), 28–31.

Haber, J. (2000). Hildegard E. Peplau: The psychiatric nursing legacy of a legend. *Journal of the American Psychiatric Nurses, 6*(2), 56–62.

Hall, K. (1994). Peplau's model of nursing: Caring for a man with AIDS. *British Journal of Nursing, 11,* 418–422.

Hrabe, D. P. (2005). Peplau in cyberspace: An analysis of Peplau's interpersonal relations theory and computer-mediated communication. *Issues in Mental Health Nursing, 26*(4), 397–414.

Jones, A. (1995). Utilizing Peplau's psychodynamic theory for stroke patient care. *Journal of Clinical Nursing, 4*(1), 49–54. Retrieved September 19, 2002, from http://gateway1.ovid.com/ovidweb.cgi.

Kozub, M. L., & Kozub, F. M. (2004). Dealing with power struggles in clinical and educational settings. *Journal of Psychosocial Nursing & Mental Health Services, 42*(2), 22–31.

Lego, S. (1980). The one-to-one nurse-patient relationship. *Perspectives in Psychiatric Care, 18*(2), 67–89.

Marchese, K. (2006). Using Peplau's theory of interpersonal relations to guide the education of patients undergoing urinary diversion. *Urologic Nursing, 26*(5), 363–371.

McCann, T., & Baker, H. (2001). Mutual relating: Developing interpersonal relationships in the community. *Journal of Advanced Nursing, 34,* 530–537. Retrieved September 19, 2002, from http://gateway1.ovid.com/ovidweb.cgi.

McGuinness, S. D., & Peters, S. (1999). The diagnosis of multiple sclerosis: Peplau's interpersonal relations model. *Rehabilitation Nursing, 24*(1), 30–33.

McKenna, H. (1997). *Nursing theories and models.* London: Routledge.

Moser, A., Houtepen, R., & Widdershoven, G. (2007). Patient autonomy in nurse-led shared care: A review of theoretical and empirical literature. *Journal of Advanced Nursing, 57*(4), 357–365.

O'Toole, A. W., & Welt, S. R. (1989). *Interpersonal theory in nursing practice: Selected works of Hildegard E. Peplau.* New York: Springer.

Peplau, H. E. (1952). *Interpersonal relations in nursing.* New York: G.P. Putnam's Sons.

Peplau, H. E. (1964). Psychiatric nursing skills and the general hospital patient. *Nursing Forum, 3*(2), 28–37.

Peplau, H. E. (1969). Professional closeness . . . as a special kind of involvement with a patient, client or family group. *Nursing Forum, 8,* 343–360.

Peplau, H. E. (1985). Help the public maintain mental health. *Nursing Success Today, 2*(5), 30–34.

Peplau, H. E. (1988). The art and science of nursing: Similarities, differences and relations. *Nursing Science Quarterly, 1,* 8–15.

Peplau, H. E. (1989). Theory: The professional dimension. In A. W. O'Toole & S. R. Welt (Eds.), *Interpersonal theory in nursing practice: Selected works of Hildegard E. Peplau* (pp. 21–30). New York: Springer.

Peplau, H. E. (1991). *Interpersonal relations in nursing: A conceptual frame of reference for psychodynamic nursing.* New York: Springer.

Peplau, H. E. (1992). Interpersonal relations: A theoretical framework for application in nursing practice. *Nursing Science Quarterly, 5*(1), 13–18.

Peplau, H. E. (1997). Peplau's theory of interpersonal relations. *Nursing Science Quarterly, 10*(4), 162–167.

Price, B. (1998). Explorations in body image care: Peplau and practice knowledge. *Journal of Psychiatric & Mental Health Nursing, 5*(3), 179–186.

Puentes, W. J. (2002). Simple reminiscence: A stress-adaptation model of the phenomenon. *Issues in Mental Health Nursing, 23*(5), 497–511.

Reed, P. G. (1995). A treatise on nursing knowledge development for the 21st century: Beyond postmodernism [Electronic version]. *Advances in Nursing Science, 17*(3), 70–84.

Reed, P. G. (1996). Transforming practice knowledge into nursing knowledge—A revisionist analysis of Peplau. *Image: The Journal of Nursing Scholarship, 28,* 29–33. Retrieved September 19, 2002, from http://gateway1.ovid.com/ovidweb.cgi.

Sellers, S. C. (1991). A philosophical analysis of conceptual models of nursing. Unpublished doctoral dissertation, Iowa State University, Ames.

Sills, G. M. (1978). Hildegard E. Peplau: Leader, practitioner, academician, scholar, and theorist. *Perspectives in Psychiatric Care, 16*(3), 122–128.

Spray, L. (1999). Living interpersonal theory: The Hildegard Peplau-Suzanne Lego Letters, March 1998-March 1999. *Perspectives in Psychiatric Care, 35*(4), 24ff. Retrieved September 18, 2002, from Health Reference Center-Academic database.

Tiedje, L. B. (2004). Teaching is more than telling: Education about prematurity in a prenatal clinic waiting room. *The American Journal of Maternal Child Nursing, 29*(6), 373–379.

Warren, B. J. (2002). The interlocking paradigm of cultural competence: A best practice approach. *Journal of American Psychiatric Nurses Association, 8*(6), 209–213.

Welch, M. (1995). Hildegard Peplau in a conversation with Mark Welch. Part I. *Nursing Inquiry, 2*(1), 53–56.

Young, A., Taylor, S. G., & Renpenning, K. (2001). *Connections: Nursing research, theory, and practice.* St. Louis: Mosby.

BIBLIOGRAPHY

Selected Works by Peplau

Peplau, H. E. (1984). Help the public maintain mental health (Interview). *Nursing Success, 2*(5), 30–34.

Peplau, H. E. (1986). The nurse as counsellor. *Journal of American College Health, 35*(11), 11–14.

Peplau, H. E. (1987). Interpersonal constructs for nursing practice. *Nurse Education Today, 7*(5), 201–208.

Peplau, H. E. (1989). Future directions in psychiatric nursing from the perspective of history. *Journal of Psychosocial Nursing, 27*(2), 18–21, 25–28, 39–40.

Peplau, H. E. (1994). Quality of life: An interpersonal perspective. *Nursing Science Quarterly, 7*(1), 10–15.

Peplau, H. E. (1995). Some unresolved issues in era of biopsychosocial nursing. *Journal of American Psychiatric Nurses Association, 1*(3), 92–96.

Peplau, H. E. (1996). Fundamental and special – the dilemma of psychiatric mental nursing – commentary. *Archives of Psychiatric Nursing, 10*(4), 162–167.

Selected Works on Peplau's Theory

Armstrong, M. A., & Kelly, A. E. (1993). Enhancing staff nurses' interpersonal skills: Theory to practice. *Clinical Nurse Specialist, 7*(6), 313–317.

Barker, P. J., Reynolds, W., & Stevens, C. (1997). The human science basis of psychiatric nursing theory and practice. *Journal of Advanced Nursing, 25,* 660–667.

Beeber, L. S. (1998). Treating depression through the therapeutic nurse-patient relationship. *Nursing Clinics of North American, 33*(1), 153–157.

Beeber, L., Anderson, C. A., & Sills, G. M. (1990). Peplau's theory in practice. *Nursing Science, 3*(1), 6–8.

Comley, A. L. (1994). A comparative analysis of Orem's self-care model and Peplau's interpersonal theory. *Journal of Advanced Nursing, 20*(4), 755–760.

Feely, M. (1997). Using Peplau's theory in nurse-client relations. *International Nursing Review, 44*(4), 115–120.

Forchuk, C. (1991). A comparison of the works of Peplau and Orlando. *Archives of Psychiatric Nursing, 5*(1), 38–45.

Forchuk, C. (1991). Conceptualizing the environment of the individual with chronic mental illness. *Issues in Mental Health Nursing, 12,* 159–170.

Forchuk, C. (1994). Preconceptions in the nurse-client relationship. *Journal of Psychiatric & Mental Health Nursing, 1*(3), 145–149.

Fowler, J. (1994). A welcome focus on a key relationship: Using Peplau's model in palliative care. *Professional Nurse, 10*(3), 194–197.

Fowler, J. (1995). Taking theory into practice: Using Peplau's model in the care of a patient. *Professional Nurse, 10*(4), 226–230.

Greg, D. E. (1978). Hildegard E. Peplau: Her contributions. *Perspectives in Psychiatric Care, 16*(3), 118–121.

Martin, M. L., Forchuk, C., Santopinto, M., & Butcher, H. K. (1992). Alternatives approaches to nursing practice: Application of Peplau, Rogers, and Parse. *Nursing Science Quarterly, 5*(2) 80–85.

Samhammer, J., & Myers, H. B. (1964). Learning in the nurse-patient relationship. *Perspectives in Psychiatric Care, 2*(3), 20–29.

Schroder, P. J. (1979). Nursing intervention with patients with thought disorders. *Perspectives in Psychiatric Care, 17*(1), 32–39.

Middle Range Theories: Integrative

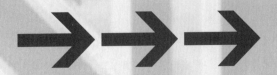

Modeling and Role-Modeling

■ ELLEN D. SCHULTZ

DEFINITION OF KEY TERMS

Adaptation
Adaptation is the "process by which an individual responds to external and internal stressors in a health and growth-directed manner" (Erickson, Tomlin, & Swain, 1983, p. 252).

Affiliated-individuation
Affiliated-individuation is an inherent need to be dependent on support systems while maintaining a sense of autonomy and separateness from those systems.

Environment
The client's environment includes internal and external stressors, as well as internal and external resources. The theorists see the environment in "the social subsystems as the interaction between self and other both cultural and individual" (Erickson, 2002a, p. 452).

Facilitation
Through the interactive process of facilitation, the nurse assists the client to identify, develop, and mobilize personal strengths. The nurse does not effect the outcomes for the client, but, rather, helps the client move toward holistic health.

Health
Health is a "state of physical, mental and social well-being not merely the absence of disease or infirmity. Additionally, it connotes a state of equilibrium within each of the various subsystems of a holistic person" (Erickson, Tomlin, & Swain, 1983, p. 253).

Holism
Holism is the integration of multiple subsystems, unified by spiritual energy that permeates the dimensions of the person. There is a blending of the unconscious and conscious.

Inherent endowment
Inherent endowment includes both the genetic makeup of the person and the inherent characteristics that can result from birth and/or disease, influencing the person's health status.

(Key Terms continued on next page)

DEFINITION OF KEY TERMS (continued)

Lifetime growth and development	Persons change throughout their lifetime, responding to an inherent desire to fulfill their potential in the areas of basic needs and psychological and cognitive stages.
Modeling	Modeling is the process used by the nurse to develop an accurate understanding of the client's perceptions and environment. The nurse seeks to understand the client's world from the perspective and framework of the client.
Nursing	Nursing is a holistic, interactive, and interpersonal process. The nurse nurtures the client's strengths and facilitates the client's self care, with the goal of achieving optimum health.
Nurturance	Nurturance integrates the client's affective, cognitive, and physiological processes to assist the client toward holistic health. To nurture, the nurse must understand the client's model of the world.
Person	"Human beings are holistic persons who have multiple interacting subsystems" including the biophysical, cognitive, psychological, and social subsystems (Erickson, Tomlin, & Swain, 1983, p. 44). Intersecting and permeating these subsystems are the genetic base and spiritual drive.
Role-modeling	In role-modeling, the nurse uses purposeful interventions, based on nursing science, that are unique to the client, to assist the client toward holistic health.
Self-care knowledge	Self-care knowledge is one's personal understanding of what interferes with or what promotes his or her own health and development.
Self-care resources	Self-care resources are internal and external resources that serve as a foundation for growth and can be mobilized to promote holistic health.
Self-care action	Clients demonstrate self-care action when they develop and use self-care knowledge and self-care resources. "Through self-care action the individual mobilizes internal resources and acquires additional resources that will help the individual gain, maintain and promote optimal level of holistic health" (Erickson, Tomlin, & Swain, 1983, p. 48).
Stressor	A stressor is a stimulus experienced by the individual as a challenge that mounts an adaptive response.
Unconditional acceptance	The individual is accepted as a unique and worthwhile human being.

INTRODUCTION

Modeling and Role-Modeling (MRM) is a theory and paradigm for nursing that serves as a foundation for nursing research, education, and practice. It is among the theories "most commonly used by holistic nurses" (Frisch, 2000, p. 176). As a theory that is strongly tied to nursing practice, it is a positive response to the criticism cited by Fawcett (1995, p. 519) that many models and theories are "invented by scholars and academics" and, therefore, may have little relevance for nursing practice.

Chapter 1 of this text describes the hierarchy of nursing knowledge and the classification of nursing theories as grand, middle range, or practice theories. While MRM is included here among the middle range theories, consensus has not been established on this classification. Tomey and Alligood (1998) originally classified MRM as a middle range theory, but later stated that MRM theory is "specific enough to guide nursing practice yet abstract enough for middle-range theories to be derived from it (Alligood & Tomey, 2002, p. 52). McEwen and Wills (2002) consider MRM to be a grand theory, and categorized it as one of the interactive process theories. One system for classifying theory is to consider the scope of the theory. A grand theory includes the nursing metaparadigm concepts of nursing, health, environment, and person, all of which are addressed in MRM. This chapter on MRM is appropriately included in this text because it presents, as components of the grand theory, a number of the middle range concepts that have developed from MRM theory. These concepts are best understood within the context of the grand theory.

Modeling and Role-Modeling is a client-centered nursing theory that places the client's perceptions, or model of the world, at the center of the nurse–client interaction. The theory integrates concepts from several interdisciplinary theories, including psychosocial development (Erikson, 1968), cognitive development (Piaget, 1952), basic human needs (Maslow, 1968), stress adaptation (Selye, 1976; Engel, 1962), and several energy-based concepts (Brekke & Schultz, 2006). These concepts are linked to those unique to MRM theory. Through the processes of modeling and role-modeling, the nurse facilitates and nurtures the client to achieve high-level, holistic wellness.

HISTORICAL BACKGROUND

Modeling and Role-Modeling is a theory "born in practice," as described by Dickoff, James, and Weidenback (1968). "Using nursing practice as a basis for theory development promotes not only a broader view of reality but also an increased relevance of theory to practice" (McClosky & Grace, 1994, p. 78). Through observations made in clinical practice in a variety of nursing settings, Helen Erickson became aware of the nurse's role as a healer. Based on a combination of insights gleaned through personal experience, clinical practice, and discussions with her father-in-law, renowned psychotherapist Milton Erickson, Helen Erickson began, in the mid-1970s, to formulate the ideals that later became MRM theory (Keegan & Dossey, 1998).

During her student experience in both a baccalaureate completion program and graduate education, Erickson began describing the theoretical components of the theory. Challenged by her colleagues Mary Ann Swain and Evelyn Tomlin, Erickson refined the concepts and their linkages. Erickson began testing components of the theory as a graduate student, beginning with research on the Adaptive Potential Assessment Model (Erickson, 2002b; Erickson & Swain, 1982), followed by additional testing of this concept (Barnfather, Swain, & Erickson, 1989) and the concept of self-care resources (Erickson & Swain, 1990).

The process of articulating and researching MRM concepts and the effects of MRM interventions led the way to the publication of *Modeling and Role-Modeling: A Theory and Paradigm for Nursing* (Erickson et al., 1983). This text made the theory more accessible to nurses, thus promoting the use of MRM in practice, education, and research.

In her latest publication, Erickson (2006) articulates beliefs that were implied in the first text on MRM but not specifically described. In addition, the text describes the primary concepts of MRM in greater detail. Erickson discusses beliefs that are central to her model of the world. She states that one's Reason for Being is a means of accomplishing Soul work. People are Soul first, existing in human form for the purpose of accomplishing the continuing work of the Soul. "From this perspective, we have a body so we can have interpersonal relationships, relationships necessary to enhance the growth of the Soul" (p. 7). Erickson describes her Reason for Being in this way:

> "Reflection . . . has led me to conclude that my Life Purpose is to nurture growth in others. . . . Looking back at my life . . . attaching meaning to significant experiences and memories, I've concluded that nurturing growth is tantamount to facilitating self-actualization or finding-of-Self in others. . . . I am satisfied this is my Life Purpose; it is my Soul-work. My Reason for Being is to learn that Unconditional Acceptance of Others precedes nurturing growth. With this in mind, I now understand the Meaning of my life" (p. 28).

Modeling and Role-Modeling serves as a foundation for nursing education. Metropolitan State University, St. Paul, Minnesota, uses MRM as the theoretical foundation for the baccalaureate completion program and teaches the theory in the graduate program. Humboldt State University, Arcata, California, has also selected MRM as the conceptual framework for the nursing program. Students at Bemidji State University (Minnesota) often choose MRM as the theoretical framework for their senior practicum (Scheela, Maple, & Larson, 2006). Perese (2002) describes using MRM as a tool for integrating psychiatric nursing into a nursing curriculum. Other schools that have incorporated MRM into their nursing programs are The College of St. Catherine, Minneapolis; Foo Yin College of Nursing and Medical Technology, Taiwan; the University of Texas at Austin; and the University of Michigan (Erickson, 2002a). Faculty at Lamar University in Beaumont Texas have developed a retention program to promote active learning abilities in nursing students using MRM as the foundation (Curl et al., 2006). In the graduate program at Lamar, graduate students apply MRM using a Case Study Synthesis process (Curl & Blume, 2006). MRM can also be used as a framework for academic advising (Schultz, 1998).

Nurses in many settings who have been exposed to MRM either through the literature or as students in MRM-based programs have introduced the concepts into their practice environments, both informally and in structured ways. Snyder (2006) applied the Adaptive Potential Model to nursing leadership in her thesis. Nurses on a surgical unit at the University of Michigan developed and implemented an assessment tool that is based on MRM (Campbell, Finch, Allport, Erickson, & Swain, 1985; Finch, 1990; Walsh, VandenBosch, & Boehm, 1989); the nurses on the vascular surgery unit use MRM as their practice framework (University of Michigan, 2002); and MRM has been used as the theoretical foundation for the nursing practice model at Brigham and Women's Hospital in Boston, Massachusetts, and the University of Pittsburgh hospitals. In 2003, after implementing MRM in several health care institutions, James (2006) began the process of integrating the theory into nursing practice at the Oregon Health & Science University. This ongoing process has involved orienting 1,600 nurses to the theory. Baker (1999) developed a psychoeducational program based on MRM for parents of children with attention-deficit hyperactivity disorder. MRM has also been the theoretical foundation for the practice of school nursing (Barnfather, 1991).

The Society for the Advancement of Modeling and Role-Modeling was established to advance the development and application of the theory. It promoted the study and integration of the theoretical propositions and philosophical underpinnings, developed a support network, disseminated knowledge and information, and promoted the improvement of holistic health (Bylaws, 2000). The society has sponsored biennial conferences since 1986.

Since the development of the theory, Erickson has conducted research, consulted with schools of nursing and health care institutions, authored several articles, presented papers, and supervised graduate students' research in MRM. Several dissertations completed at the University of Michigan in the late 1980s and at the University of Texas at Austin in the 1990s, under the advisement of Helen Erickson, implement MRM as the theoretical foundation for research. MRM concepts continue to be tested. Examples of MRM-based research are described elsewhere in this chapter.

DEFINITION OF THEORY CONCEPTS

Modeling and Role-Modeling theory is described in terms of its theoretical bases, including how people are alike and how they are different, a philosophy of nursing, and a paradigm for the practice of nursing. To define the major concepts of the theory, they can be categorized into concepts that relate to nursing and those that relate to persons.

Concepts Related to Nursing

Erickson has identified and described several concepts that relate to the discipline of nursing. They include nursing, facilitation, nurturance, unconditional acceptance, modeling, and role-modeling.

NURSING

Modeling and Role-Modeling emphasizes the holistic, interpersonal nature of nursing. Nursing is described as an interactive process that nurtures client strengths to "enable development, release and channeling of resources for coping with one's circumstances and environment. The goal is to achieve a state of perceived optimal health and contentment" (Erickson et al., 1983, p. 49). In the process of assisting clients to achieve holistic health, the nurse must nurture the client; facilitate, not effect, the adaptive process; and accept the client unconditionally.

FACILITATION

Through the activities of facilitation, the nurse assists the client to identify, develop, and mobilize personal strengths as he or she moves toward health. The nurse does not produce the outcomes for the client, but, rather, "aids the client in meeting his or her own needs so that he or she may have the necessary resources" for coping with stressors, growth, development, and self-actualization (Erickson, 1990, p. 13).

NURTURANCE

In the process of nurturance, the nurse promotes the integration of the client's affective, cognitive, and physiological processes as the client moves toward holistic health. For nurturance to occur, the nurse must seek to understand and support the client's model of the world and appreciate the value of the client's self-care knowledge. This understanding can be used to develop nursing interventions that are unique to the client.

UNCONDITIONAL ACCEPTANCE

The nurse accepts the client as a "unique, worthwhile, important individual with no strings attached" (Erickson et al., 1983, p. 255). Empathy is used to communicate nonjudgmental respect with the client.

MODELING

Modeling is a central concept in the theory because understanding the client's viewpoint is the foundation for implementing the nursing process. Modeling is defined as "the process the nurse uses as she develops an image and understanding of the client's world—an image and understanding developed within the client's framework and from the client's perspective" (Erickson et al., 1983, p. 95). The nurse suspends his or her judgment to fully understand the client's perspective.

Both the art and science of nursing are reflected in modeling (Erickson, 1989). The art is demonstrated through the use of therapeutic communication to develop an accurate picture of the client's situation. The science is demonstrated in the data aggregation and analysis based on scientific principles and the concepts from the theory.

ROLE-MODELING

"Role-modeling is the facilitation of the individual in attaining, maintaining, or promoting health through purposeful interventions" (Erickson et al., 1983, p. 95). Role-modeling can occur only after the nurse accurately understands the client's worldview. The art of role-modeling is demonstrated by planning and implementing nursing interventions that are based on the client's model of the world and are, therefore, unique. The science of role-modeling is demonstrated through planning theory-based interventions.

Concepts That Relate to Persons

In describing the concepts that relate to person, Erickson has included concepts formulated for the theory and others that rely on borrowed theories from other disciplines. While nursing seeks to develop "distinctive knowledge" related to the discipline of nursing, the linking of borrowed theory with nursing theory is appropriate if there is congruence between the worldviews of the two (Villarruel, Bishop, Simpson, Jemmott, & Fawcett, 2001). Concepts that have been described in MRM theory that relate to persons include person, health, environment, ways the people are alike, and ways in which they differ.

PERSON

The individual is viewed as holistic, having multiple interacting subsystems. These dynamic subsystems are the biological, cognitive, psychological, and social subsystems. The person's genetic makeup and spiritual drive permeate and intersect the subsystems. The spiritual drive draws energy from the universe, unifies the subsystems, and gives energy back to the universal energy field through a continual energy exchange. When caring for the person, the nurse does not focus on one subsystem but on the integrated, dynamic relationships among the subsystems of the person. His or her internal model of the world determines the person's perceptions and interpretations of the environment.

HEALTH

Health is a "state of physical, mental and social well-being, not merely the absence of disease or infirmity. Additionally, it connotes a state of equilibrium within each of the various subsystems of a holistic person" (Erickson et al., 1983, p. 253). A goal of nursing is to facilitate the client's achievement of perceived optimal health.

ENVIRONMENT

The concept of environment was not defined in Erickson's original work but has been described in later publications. The concept includes the client's internal and external stressors, as well as internal and external resources. "The theorists see environment in the social subsystems as the interaction between self and others both cultural and individual" (Erickson, 2002a, p. 452). The importance of the interpersonal environment is emphasized in the theory.

HOW PEOPLE ARE ALIKE

While recognizing the uniqueness of persons, MRM identifies ways in which people are alike: They are holistic, they experience lifetime growth and development, and they have a need for affiliated-individuation. In understanding how people are alike and how they are different, Erickson synthesizes a number of interdisciplinary theories identified below.

Holism. "The interaction of the multiple subsystems and the inherent bases create holism" (Erickson et al., 1983, p. 45). Dynamic relationships exist among mind, body, emotion, and spirit. Figure 11.1 shows the holistic model. The figure demonstrates the integration of biophysical, psychosocial, cognitive, and social aspects of the person. Both the genetic base and the spiritual drive permeate all of these aspects. While identified as separate parts, the figure shows that the multiple subsystems are integrated. Spiritual energy unifies the dimensions of the holistic person. They interact and function as a total unit.

Lifetime Growth: Basic Needs. People are alike in that they all have basic needs. MRM theory incorporates Maslow's (1968) hierarchy of needs as the framework for understanding basic need satisfaction. Individuals have an inherent desire to fulfill one's potential. Holistic growth is impeded when basic needs are unmet. Consistent with the concept of modeling, the theory supports the view that "all human beings have basic needs that can be satisfied, but only from within the framework of the individual" (Erickson et al., 1983, p. 58).

Lifetime Development. People are also alike because they mature and develop over their lifetimes. The theoretical support for psychosocial development comes from the work of Erik Erikson (1968). As individuals move through the eight developmental stages, they resolve the tasks or crises of that stage. Resolution of the developmental stage results in the acquisition of lasting strengths and virtues.

Piaget's (1952) theory provides the framework for understanding how people are alike in their cognitive development. Individuals progress through a series of stages in which the ability to think and reason becomes more complex.

Affiliated-Individuation. "Individuals have an instinctual need for affiliated-individuation. They need to be able to be dependent on support systems while simultaneously maintaining independence from these support systems" (Erickson et al., 1983, p. 47). The need for affiliation motivates individuals to seek support. As the need for affiliation is met through supportive contacts, an "affiliative resource" is developed. A healthy sense of individuation is developed as individuals make independent choices, feel good about themselves, and feel esteem from others (Acton, 1997).

HOW PEOPLE ARE DIFFERENT

Although people are alike in that they are holistic and share a common process of growth and development, each person is unique. MRM theory identifies these unique aspects of people as the inherent endowment, the ability to adapt, and one's personal model of the world.

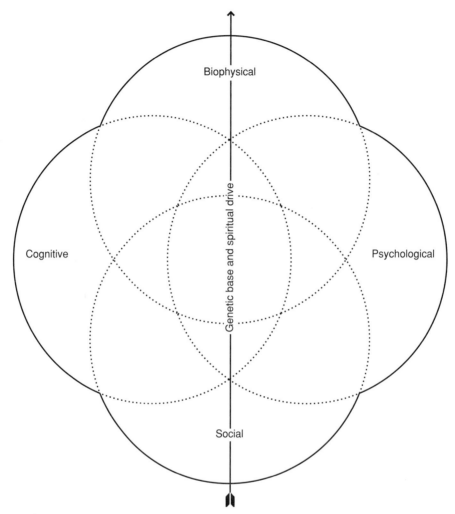

■ **Figure 11.1** Model of the holistic person.
Source: Erickson, HC., Tomlin, E.M. & Swain, M.A. (1983) Modeling and Role - Modeling:
A theory and paradigon for nursing. Englewood Cliffs, NJ: Prentice-Hall, Inc, p45. Used
with permission.

Inherent Endowment. A person's inherent endowment comprises both the genetic base and inherent
characteristics. The genetic base determines, to some extent, how a person progresses through the developmental processes and responds to stressors. Inherent characteristics also influence health and growth
and development. These characteristics include "malformation, brain damage, or other physiological
states secondary to birth, prenatal disease, sicknesses, or other factors" (Erickson et al., 1983, p. 75).

Adaptation. People differ in the ability to adapt. Adaptation is defined as the "process by which an individual responds to external and internal stressors in a health and growth-directed manner" (Erickson
et al., 1983, p. 252). Within MRM theory, adaptation is approached from an integrated perspective. Theoretical

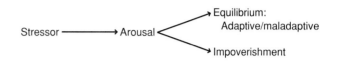

■ **Figure 11.2** Adaptive potential assessment model.
Source: Erickson, HC., Tomlin, E.M. & Swain, M.A. (1983) Modeling and Role - Modeling: A theory and paradigon for nursing. Englewood Cliffs, NJ: Prentice-Hall, Inc, p81. Used with permission.

support for the physiological response to stressors comes from the work of Selye (1976), particularly the general adaptation syndrome. The psychosocial perspective is supported by Engel's (1962) research on the human response to stressors.

Erickson conceptualized a biophysical–psychosocial model, the adaptive potential assessment model (APAM) that identifies states of coping that "reflect an individual's potential to mobilize self-care resources." In Erickson's model, stress states are distinguished from nonstress states. When a stimulus is experienced as a challenge, it is a stressor; when experienced as threatening, it is a distressor and leads to a maladaptive response (Barnfather, Swain, & Erickson, 1989; Erickson & Swain, 1982; Erickson et al., 1983).

Three categories are identified in the adaptive potential assessment model: arousal, equilibrium, and impoverishment. As shown in Figure 11.2, the experience of a stressor leads to a state of arousal. Arousal may be experienced by feelings of tenseness and anxiousness, accompanied by elevations in blood pressure, pulse rate, respirations, and motor–sensory behavior. From arousal, the person may move to a state of equilibrium or impoverishment. In a state of impoverishment, the individual experiences marked feelings of tension and anxiety, with feelings of fatigue, sadness, or depression. In addition to elevated pulse, respiration, blood pressure, and motor–sensory behavior, there is an elevation in verbal anxiety. Equilibrium may be adaptive or maladaptive. In adaptive equilibrium, the individual has normal vital signs and sensory–motor behavior, expresses hope, and has low or absent feelings of tenseness, fatigue, sadness, and depression. In a state of maladaptive equilibrium, one may appear to be coping with stressors, but at the expense of draining energy from another subsystem (Erickson et al., 1983).

Each state is associated with different coping potentials or different abilities to mobilize coping resources. Movement among the states, either to equilibrium or impoverishment, depends on both the ability to mobilize resources and the presence of new stressors. Figure 11.3 shows the relationship among the APAM states. Nursing interventions are directed toward assisting the client to mobilize resources (Erickson et al., 1983).

Person's Model of the World—Self-Care Knowledge, Resources, and Action. Each person has a unique worldview. Nurses use the process of modeling to develop an understanding of how the person perceives the world from her own perspective. One aspect of this "model of the world" that relates to health is self-care knowledge. Each person knows, at some level, what interferes with and what promotes her own health and development. This self-care knowledge makes the client the primary source of information in nurse–client interactions. There are two additional self-care concepts related to self-care knowledge. Self-care resources include both internal and external resources that can be mobilized to promote holistic health. Finally, self-care action is the "development and utilization" of self-care knowledge and self-care resources. Activities include both the acquisition of additional resources and the mobilization of self-care resources toward the goal of achieving optimal holistic health. Nursing intervention can assist the client in acquiring and mobilizing resources (Erickson et al., 1983).

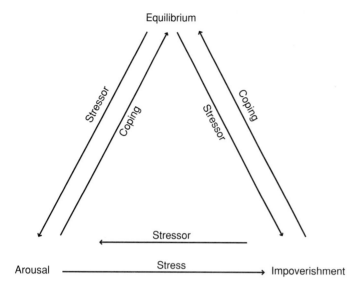

■ **Figure 11.3** Dynamic relationships among states of the adaptive potential assessment model.
Source: Erickson, HC., Tomlin, E.M. & Swain, M.A. (1983) Modeling and Role - Modeling: A theory and paradigon for nursing. Englewood Cliffs, NJ: Prentice-Hall, Inc, p82. Used with permission.

DESCRIPTION OF THE THEORY OF MODELING AND ROLE-MODELING

Theoretical Linkages

Modeling and Role-Modeling theory draws on concepts from several theorists. Each theorist places emphasis on one aspect of the person. However, Erickson's creation of a holistic nursing theory explains the dynamic relationships among basic need satisfaction, growth, developmental processes, loss, grief, and adaptation. The functional relationships among these concepts lead to theoretical linkages. Relationships exist between/among:

- Need satisfaction and developmental task resolution
- Need satisfaction and adaptive potential
- Need satisfaction, object attachment and loss, grief, growth, and development
- Developmental residue and self-care resources (Erickson, 1990, 2002a)

Figure 11.4 shows the relationships among MRM concepts. For example, the figure demonstrates possible outcomes resulting from basic need deficits. Unmet basic needs will interfere with the growth process, which, in turn, limits the person's ability to mobilize resources to adapt to stressors. However, when basic needs are satisfied, the person is able to mobilize resources to contend with new stressors. The figure further demonstrates the relationship between basic needs and attachment. When an object consistently meets one's needs, secure attachments form, leading to a sense of worthiness and the ability to mobilize resources. On the other hand, when objects fail to meet one's needs, insecure attachments form, limiting the ability to mobilize resources to deal with stressors. While the concepts presented in the theory, when viewed individually, may seem simple, the interactions among the factors demonstrate the complexity of the theory.

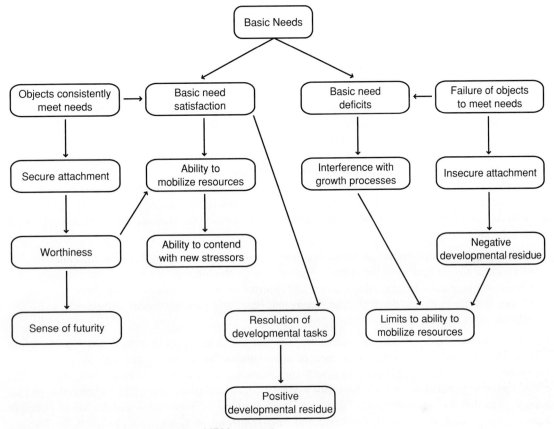

■ **Figure 11.4**   Relationships among MRM concepts.

From these theoretical linkages, Erickson identified 13 propositions that can be used to predict outcomes, direct the planning of nursing care, and evaluate care:

1. Individual's ability to contend with new stressors is directly related to the ability to mobilize resources needed.
2. Individual's ability to mobilize resources is directly related to his or her need deficits and assets.
3. Distressors are related to unmet basic needs; stressors are related to unmet growth needs.
4. Objects that repeatedly facilitate the individual in need of satisfaction take on significance for the individual. Attachment to the object results when this occurs.
5. Secure attachment produces feelings of worthiness.
6. Feelings of worthiness result in a sense of futurity.
7. Real, threatened, or perceived loss of the attachment object results in the grief process.
8. Basic need deficits coexist with the grief process.
9. An adequate alternative object must be perceived available for the individual to resolve the grief process.
10. Prolonged grief due to an unavailable or inadequate object results in morbid grief.
11. Unmet basic and growth needs interfere with growth processes.

12. Repeated satisfaction of basic needs is prerequisite to working through developmental tasks and resolution of related developmental crises.
13. Morbid grief is always related to need deficits (Erickson, 1990, p. 28).

Paradigm for Nursing Practice

The practice paradigm of MRM is presented within the framework of the nursing process, emphasizing the importance of both the interactive, interpersonal nature of nursing and the theoretical and scientific bases of nursing practice. Nursing care begins by determining the client's model of the world and then focusing on the most immediate concerns expressed by the client. The practice paradigm directs data collection, data aggregation, analysis, and synthesis, and provides a framework for planning nursing interventions. Critical thinking is required to implement these activities.

Consistent with the concept of modeling, the client is viewed as the primary data source. Other data sources are included as well, and the nurse looks for congruence between data received from the client and that received from significant others and health care professionals. Data are collected and organized in the following categories:

- Description of the situation—to develop an overview of the client's perspective of the situation
- Expectations—to determine the client's expectations for the future
- Resource potential—to determine internal and external resources available to the client
- Goals and life tasks—to determine developmental status and personal model of the world (Erickson et al., 1983)

The use of standardized nursing interventions is not consistent with modeling and role-modeling beliefs. The theory does provide general aims of interventions that are associated with the principles of the theory and facilitate the planning of systematic interventions. These are to build trust, promote the client's positive orientation, promote the client's control, affirm and promote the client's strengths, and set mutual goals that are health directed. Table 11.1 shows the aims of intervention and the MRM principle associated with each intervention. *Modeling and Role-Modeling: A Theory and Paradigm for Nursing*

Table 11.1 RELATIONSHIP BETWEEN AIMS OF INTERVENTION AND MRM PRINCIPLES

AIM	PRINCIPLE
Build trust	The nursing process requires that a trusting and functional relationship exist between nurse and client.
Promote client's positive orientation	Affiliated-individuation is dependent on the individual's perceiving that he or she is an acceptable, respectable, and worthwhile human being.
Promote client's control	Human development is dependent on the individual's perceiving that he or she has some control over his or her life, while concurrently sensing a state of affiliation.
Affirm and promote client's strengths	There is an innate drive toward holistic health that is facilitated by consistent and systematic nurturance.
Set mutual goals that are health directed	Human growth is dependent on satisfaction of basic needs and facilitated by growth-need satisfaction.

Erickson, H. C., Tomlin, E. M., & Swain, M. A. (1983). *Modeling and role-modeling: A theory and paradigm for nursing* (p. 170). Englewood Cliffs, NJ: Prentice-Hall, Inc.

(Erickson et al., 1983) provides specific examples of how the aims of interventions can be linked to basic need satisfaction. In the implementation of nursing interventions, the goal is to carry out one intervention that reflects each aim during every contact with the client. A single intervention can meet more than one of the general aims of intervention.

APPLICATIONS OF THE THEORY

Modeling and Role-Modeling has been the theoretical foundation for numerous published research studies, master's theses, and doctoral dissertations. Many studies test the middle range concepts found in MRM theory or explore the relationships between or among concepts. The concepts are clearly defined and are used consistently. The relationships among the concepts are complex and have provided the stimulus for several studies.

Affiliated-Individuation

Acton (1997) tested the concept of affiliated-individuation to determine its ability to be a mediator between stress and the burden of caregivers, and caregiver satisfaction with family caregivers of adults with dementia. Acton and Miller (1996) investigated the effects of a theory-based, support-group intervention on affiliated-individuation with a group of caregivers of adults with dementia. This study is summarized in the example found in Using Middle Range Theories 11.1.

Adaptive Potential Assessment Model

The adaptive potential assessment model was first tested by Erickson (1976). Erickson and Swain (1982) studied the model to statistically validate the three categories of the APAM, arousal, equilibrium, and

---

 11.1 USING MIDDLE RANGE THEORIES

The researchers studied the effects of a support-group intervention on affiliated-individuation (AI) in caregivers of persons with dementia. AI was viewed as a self-care resource to help caregivers deal with the stressors associated with their caregiving roles. Twenty-six caregivers were placed in intervention groups of six to seven per group for one year. The support group interventions were based on MRM's five aims of intervention. AI was measured using subscales of the Basic Needs Satisfaction Inventory (BNSI). Data collection consisted of semistructured interviews and participant completion of BNSI and demographic questionnaires. Qualitative data were analyzed for essential meaning. Multivariate analysis of variance was used to analyze the quantitative data. Data analysis indicated that the needs associated with AI were facilitated through the intervention of the support group. In addition, the theoretical definition of AI was supported through this research, and it provided support for the linkage between AI and coping as proposed by MRM theory.

Acton, G. J., & Miller, E. W. (1996). Affiliated-individuation in caregivers of adults with dementia. *Issues in Mental Health Nursing, 17,* 245–260.

11.2 USING MIDDLE RANGE THEORIES

The purpose of this study was to examine predictors of health in undereducated adults, using constructs from Modeling and Role-Modeling theory, psychosocial resources, perceived stress, and health. Subjects studied were 171 individuals without a 12th-grade education, who were enrolled in an adult education program.

Four variables were measured. Psychosocial development was measured using the Modified Eriksonian Psychological Stage Inventory (MEPSI); basic need satisfaction was measured with the Basic Need Satisfaction Inventory (BNSI); subjects were asked to rate their level and frequency of stress and a measure of perceived stress; and health was assessed using the Positive Health Index. Structural equation modeling and latent variables were used to test the relationships among the variables in the model developed by the researchers. This model design reflected the theoretical linkages proposed in MRM theory.

The researchers found that "psychosocial development and basic need satisfaction had significant direct effects on health, with the expected positive signs," with psychosocial development having the strongest direct effect on health (Barnfather & Ronis, 2000, p. 62). No significant relationship between health and perceived stress was found in the study. The researchers recommended that therapeutic nursing interventions "include strengthening psychosocial resources and focusing in the client's perceived needs" (Barnfather & Ronis, 2000, p. 63). This research supported the theoretical linkages delineated in MRM theory.

Barnfather, J. S., & Ronis, D. L. (2000). Test of a model of psychosocial resources, stress and health among undereducated adults. *Research in Nursing and Health*, 23, 55–66.

impoverishment, and to determine whether a relationship existed between the categories and length of hospital stay. Further testing of the validity of the model was conducted by Barnfather, Swain, and Erickson (1989) to determine if subjects could be classified into the three adaptive states, as a measure of ability to mobilize coping resources. Barnfather (1987) applied the adaptive potential assessment model to healthy subjects to test the relationship between basic need satisfaction and the ability to mobilize coping resources. In another study, Barnfather (1993) conducted additional testing of the model and the relationship between basic need status and adaptive potential with male students experiencing stress. Research on perceived stress as one of the predictors of health is reported in the example in Using Middle Range Theories 11.2.

Health/Well-Being

Research conducted by Irvin and Acton (1996) tested a model of caregiver stress mediation to determine if perceived support and self-worth had a mediating effect on well-being. Acton and Malathum (2000) studied the relationship between basic need satisfaction and health-promoting behavior and determined the best predictors of health-promoting self-care behavior.

Self-Care Resources/Actions

Erickson and Swain (1990) conducted a nursing intervention study with hypertensive clients to determine the efficacy of modeling- and role-modeling–based interventions directed toward mobilizing self-care resources. Irvin (1993), identifying social support, self-worth, and hope as self-care resources, studied the relationships among these resources and caregiver stress. Using hope as a self-care resource, Irvin and Acton (1997) studied stress mediation in women caregivers, testing ways that stress and well-being were affected by self-care resources. The purpose of Rosehow's (1992) research was to identify self-care actions perceived as significant for persons 6 months after myocardial infarction. Preferences and rankings of self-care actions were also identified. Baldwin, Hibbein, Herr, Lohner, and Core (2002) investigated the perception of self-care in an Amish community.

Research by Baas (1992) identified the predictor variables related to self-care resources on life satisfaction in persons following myocardial infarction. The concept of self-care resources was also studied in its relationship to quality of life (Bass, Fontana, & Bhat, 1997). The researchers conducted an exploratory pilot study with individuals diagnosed with heart failure to determine potential differences among the groups in measures of self-care needs, resources, and quality of life. Hertz and Rossetti (2006) identified self-care actions of older adults and categorized then into five themes: adapting to life as an older adult, meeting affiliation-individuation needs, promoting holistic health through self-care knowledge, self-managing health concerns, and preventing health problems.

A new concept, perceived enactment of autonomy (PEA), was developed, based on the concept of self-care (Baas, Curl, Hertz, & Robinson, 1994; Hertz, 1991). Perceived enactment of autonomy is conceptually defined as "a state of sensing and recognizing the ability to freely choose behaviors and courses of action on one's own behalf and in accordance with one's own needs and goals" (Hertz, 1995, p. 269). The results of two studies with older adults living in the community "supported a theoretical relationship between PEA and selected self-care health indicators" (Hertz & Anshultz, 2002, p. 179). PEA was shown to be significantly related to self-care knowledge concepts of life satisfaction and perceived control.

The investigation of MRM self-care concepts with children has been the focus of three dissertations. Baldwin (1998) studied the effects of a self-care health curriculum on third-grade students' overall health care characteristics and self-care actions. In this study self-care subconcepts were identified as hope, control, satisfaction with daily living, support, and physical health. The research demonstrated that the group that received the self-care curriculum had higher mean scores on hope and satisfaction with daily living. Nash (2003) studied the impact of the Empowerment program on self-care resources of middle-school-aged children. In another study of middle-school-aged children, Bray (2005) investigated the two theoretical propositions of MRM: the relationship between resolution of developmental tasks and need satisfaction and the relationship of need satisfaction to coping ability. Self-care resources identified in the study included motivation, engagement, and interpersonal relationships. The study supported the relationship between measures of health and self-care resources as well as the significance of self-care resources in explaining variances in health.

Other Studies

Additional studies, not related to the categories of concepts included above, employed MRM as the theoretical foundation. Examples of the concepts researched are comfort (Kennedy, 1991); compassionate visiting (Holl, 1992); psychophysiological processes of stress (Kline, 1988); uncertainty, spiritual well-being, and psychological adjustment to illness (Landis, 1991); unmet needs of persons with chronic mental illness (Perese, 1997); psychological development and coping ability (Miller, 1986); and nurse–patient interactions (Rogers, 2002).

INSTRUMENTS USED IN EMPIRICAL TESTING

Several instruments have been developed to test MRM theory. Two instruments were developed relating to the developmental processes of individuals. Darling-Fisher and Leidy (1988) developed the Modified Erikson Psychosocial Stage Inventory. This tool is designed to measure Erikson's eight stages of the life cycle in adults. The Basic Need Satisfaction Inventory (BNSI) was developed and tested by Leidy (1994). The purpose of the BNSI is to "operationalize Maslow's construct of need satisfaction and for testing many of his theoretical propositions" (p. 293). Each item on the BNSI reflects one of Maslow's five basic needs. Both of these tools are relevant to MRM-based research because of the integration of psychosocial development and basic needs into the theory.

Hertz (1991) designed an instrument, the Hertz Perceived Enactment of Autonomy Scale (HPEAS), to measure the concept, perceived enactment of autonomy, and its attributes: individuality, self-direction, and voluntariness (PEA). The concept of PEA is the potential for self-care action and "links self care knowledge, resources and actions" (Baas et al., 1994, p. 151). Erickson (1996) developed an instrument to measure the bonding–attachment process related to need satisfaction in teenage mothers. The Robinson Self-Appraisal Inventory was developed as a self-reporting instrument to measure the concept of denial (Robinson, 1992). The Health-Promoting Lifestyle Profile II, although not developed from MRM theory, has been used to measure health-promoting self-care behavior in MRM research seeking to study self-care resources (Walker, Sechrist, & Pender, 1995). Research Application 11.1 describes how this concept could be used in a study. However, Baas (1992) developed an instrument based on MRM theory to measure self-care resources, the Self-Care Resource Inventory. This tool provides three scores: resources available, resources needed, and the difference in resources. Table 11.2 lists instruments commonly used in MRM research.

 11.1 RESEARCH APPLICATION

A school nurse, working with a support group for pregnant teenage girls, was concerned about their health-promoting, or self-care, behavior. Based on the MRM proposition that one's ability to mobilize self-care resources is related to need deficits and assets, the nurse was interested in examining the relationship between the girls' basic needs satisfaction and their health-promoting behaviors. A random sample of the 30 teenagers was selected from the 23 high schools located in the nurse's county.

The girls in the study were asked to complete the Basic Need Satisfaction Inventory (Leidy, 1994) that measures need satisfaction; the Health-Promoting Lifestyle Profile II (Walker, Sechrist, & Pender, 1995), used to measure self-promoting self-care behavior; and a demographic questionnaire. Statistical analysis revealed correlations between the subscales of the Basic Need Satisfaction Inventory and the Health-Promoting Lifestyle Profile. In addition, regression analysis could have been used to determine the ability to predict self-care behaviors from basic need subscales (Acton & Malathum, 2000).

Table 11.2 INSTRUMENTS COMMONLY USED IN MRM RESEARCH

INSTRUMENT	VARIABLE(S) MEASURED	SOURCE
Basic Need Satisfaction Inventory	Basic need satisfaction based on Maslow's five basic needs	Leidy, 1994
Health-Promoting Lifestyle Profile II	Health-promoting, self-care behavior	Walker, Sechrist, & Pender, 1995
Modified Erikson Psychosocial Stage Inventory	Erikson's eight stages of the life cycle in adults	Darling-Fisher & Leidy, 1988
Perceived Enactment of Autonomy Scale	Potential for self-care action Perceived enactment of autonomy and its attributes: individuality, self-direction, voluntariness	Hertz, 1991
Robinson Self-Appraisal Inventory	Self-reported denial	Robinson, 1992
Self-Care Resource Inventory	Self-care resources	Baas, 1992

SUMMARY

Modeling and Role-Modeling is a nursing theory and paradigm for nursing practice. MRM synthesizes theories of development, basic needs, stress, and loss, and explains interrelationships among these concepts. These concepts are linked to several concepts specific to MRM theory, such as holism, adaptation, affiliated-individuation, nurturance, facilitation, self-care, and unconditional acceptance. At the heart of the theory is modeling, the process of "stepping into" and understanding the client's thoughts, feelings, and needs. The nurse uses role-modeling to design scientifically based nursing interventions, developed within the understanding of the client's model of the world, to help the client move toward perceived optimal health. MRM serves as a framework for nursing research, education, and practice.

ANALYSIS OF THEORY

Using the criteria presented in Chapter 2, critique the theory Modeling and Role-Modeling. Compare your conclusions about the theory with those found in Appendix A.

Internal Criticism
1. Clarity
2. Consistency
3. Adequacy

4. Logical development
5. Level of theory development

External Criticism
1. Reality convergence
2. Utility
3. Significance
4. Discrimination
5. Scope of theory
6. Complexity

CRITICAL THINKING EXERCISES

1. The adaptive potential assessment model (APAM) identifies states of coping as arousal, equilibrium, and impoverishment. Consider a client for whom you are caring. Given a specific nursing diagnosis, how would your nursing interventions differ depending on the adaptive state of the client?

2. The client's model of the world is a primary concept in MRM. Using the assessment data that you have compiled about a client, write a description of the client's model of the world in the "first person."

3. Modeling and Role-Modeling was developed for application to an individual client. Can MRM be applied to the family? Does a family have a model of the world, an adaptive state, and developmental stages, for example?

WEB RESOURCES

1. The Society for the Advancement of Modeling and Role-Modeling sponsors a site that provides an overview of MRM theory, a description of the society, a reference list, the newsletter, and directions for accessing the society listserve: **http://www.mrmnursingtheory.org.**

2. MRM resources are available on the Sigma Theta Tau Nursing Honor Society Virginia Henderson Library. Select Library Search, and then type Modeling and Role-Modeling in the search box: **http://www.stti.iupui.edu/library/.**

3. MRM is listed on several health care institution and university nursing theory pages. These sites refer to MRM theory and provide a link to the MRM site but offer only limited information about the theory:
   http://www.utmedicalcenter.org/health_ professionals/nursing/modeling_and_role_ modeling
   http://www.ohsu.edu/ohsuedu/central/hr/ nursing/Philosophy.cfm
   http://www.humboldt.edu/~catalog/courses/ nurs_crs.html
   http://www.sandiego.edu/academics/nursing/ theory/
   http://www.healthsci.clayton.edu/eichelberger/ nursing.htm

REFERENCES

Acton, G. J. (1997). Affiliated-individuation as a mediator of stress and burden in caregivers of adults with dementia. *Journal of Holistic Nursing, 15*(4), 336–357.

Acton, G. J., & Malathum, P. (2000). Basic need status and health-promoting self-care behavior in adults. *Western Journal of Nursing Research, 22*(7), 796–811.

Acton, G. J., & Miller, E. W. (1996). Affiliated-individuation in caregivers of adults with dementia. *Issues in Mental Health Nursing, 17,* 245–260.

Alligood, M. R., & Tomey, A. M. (2002). *Nursing theory utilization and application* (2nd ed.). St. Louis: Mosby.

Baas, L. S. (1992). The relationship among self-care knowledge, self-care resources, activity level and life satisfaction in persons three to six months after myocardial infarction. *Dissertation Abstracts International, 53,* 04B.

Baas, L. S., Curl, E. D., Hertz, J. E., & Robinson, K. R. (1994). Innovative approaches to theory-based measurement: Modeling and role-modeling research. In P. L. Chinn, (Ed.), *Advanced methods of inquiry in nursing.* Gaithersburg, MD: Aspen Publication.

Baas, L. S., Fontana, J. A., & Bhat, G. (1997). Relationships between self-care resources and quality of life of persons with heart failure: A comparison of treatment groups. *Progress in Cardiovascular Nursing, 12*(1), 25–38.

Baker, C. (1999). From chaos to order: A nursing-based psycho-educational program for parents of children with attention-deficit hyperactivity disorder. *Canadian Journal of Nursing Research, 31*(2), 7–15.

Baldwin, C. M. (1998). An investigation of health outcomes for urban elementary children utilizing an innovative self-care health curriculum model as compared to the traditional health curriculum. Unpublished doctoral dissertation, Bowling Green State University.

Baldwin, C. M., Hibbein, J., Herr, S., Lohner, L., & Core, D. (2002). Self-care as defined by members of an Amish community utilizing the theory of modeling and role-modeling. *Journal of Multicultural Nursing & Health, 8*(3), 60–64.

Barnfather, J. S. (1987). Mobilizing coping resources related to basic need status in healthy, young adults. *Dissertation Abstracts International, 49,* 02B.

Barnfather, J. S. (1991). Restructuring the role of school nursing in health promotion. *Public Health Nursing, 8*(4), 234–238.

Barnfather, J. S. (1993). Testing a theoretical proposition for modeling and role-modeling: Basic need and adaptive potential status. *Issues in Mental Health Nursing, 14,* 1–18.

Barnfather, J. S., & Ronis, D. L. (2000). Test of a model of psychosocial resources, stress, and health among under-educated adults. *Research in Nursing and Health, 23,* 55–66.

Barnfather, J. S., Swain, M. A., & Erickson, H. C. (1989). Evaluation of two assessment techniques for adaptation to stress. *Nursing Science Quarterly, 2*(4), 172–182.

Barnfather, J. S., Swain, M. A., & Erickson, H. C. (1989). Construct validity of an aspect of the coping process: Potential adaptation to stress. *Issues in Mental Health Nursing, 10,* 23–40.

Bray, C. O. (2005). The relationship between psychosocial attributes, self-care resources, basic need satisfaction and measures of cognitive and psychological health of adolescents: A test of the modeling and role-modeling theory. *Dissertation Abstracts International, 66,* 03B.

Brekke, M., & Schultz, E. D. (2006). Energy theories: Modeling and role-modeling. In H. C. Erickson, (Ed.), *Modeling and role-modeling: A view from the client's world.* Cedar Park, TX: Unicorns Unlimited.

Bylaws. (2000). Society for the Advancement of Modeling and Role Modeling. Retrieved August 6, 2003, from www.mrmnursingtheory.org/Bylaws.htm.

Campbell, J., Finch, D., Allport, C., Erickson, H., & Swain, M. A. (1985). A theoretical approach to nursing assessment. *Journal of Advanced Nursing, 10,* 111–115.

Curl, E. D., & Blume, N. (2006, May). Graduate students' use of modeling and role-modeling theory for advanced practice. Paper presented at the 11th Biennial Conference of the Society for the Advancement of Modeling and Role-Modeling, Portland, OR.

Curl, E. D., Hale, G., Skeels, F., McAfee, N., Hoffmeyer, B., & Patterson, P. (2006, May). Modeling and role-modeling strategies to promote active learning abilities and life-long learning in academically at-risk students. Paper presented at the 11th Biennial Conference of the Society for the Advancement of Modeling and Role-Modeling, Portland, OR.

Darling-Fisher, C. S., & Leidy, N. K. (1988). Measuring Eriksonian development in the adult: The modified Erikson psychosocial stage inventory. *Psychological Reports, 62,* 747–754.

Dickoff, J., James, P., & Weidenback, E. (1968). Theory in a practice discipline: Practice oriented theory. *Nursing Research, 5,* 415–435.

Engel, G. S. (1962). *Psychological development in health and disease.* Philadelphia: W. B. Saunders.

Erickson, H. C. (1976). Identification of state of coping utilizing physiological and psychological data. Unpublished master's thesis, University of Michigan, Ann Arbor, Michigan.

Erickson, H. C. (1989). Looking at patient's needs through new eyes: Modeling and role-modeling. Unpublished manuscript.

Erickson, H. C. (1990). Theory based practice. *Modeling and Role-Modeling: Theory, Practice and Research, 1*(1), 1–27.

Erickson, H. C. (2006). Searching for life purpose: Discovering meaning. In H. C. Erickson (Ed.), *Modeling and role-modeling: A view from the client's world.* Cedar Park, TX: Unicorns Unlimited.

Erickson, H. C., & Swain, M. A. (1982). A model for assessing potential adaptation to stress. *Research in Nursing and Health, 5,* 93–101.

Erickson, H. C., & Swain, M. A. (1990). Mobilizing self-care resources: A nursing intervention for hypertension. *Issues in Mental Health Nursing, 11,* 217–235.

Erickson, H. C., Tomlin, E. M., & Swain, M. A. (1983). *Modeling and role-modeling: A theory and paradigm for nursing.* Englewood Cliffs, NJ: Prentice-Hall, Inc.

Erickson, M. E. (1996). Relationships among support, needs satisfaction and maternal attachment in adolescent mothers. Unpublished doctoral dissertation, University of Texas, Austin.

Erickson, M. E. (2002a). Modeling and role-modeling. In A. M. Tomey & M. R. Alligood (Eds.), *Nursing theorists and their work.* St. Louis: Mosby, Inc.

Erickson, M. E. (2002b). Modeling and role-modeling theory in nursing practice. In M. R. Alligood & A. M. Tomey (Eds.), *Nursing theory utilization & application* (2nd ed.). St. Louis: Mosby, Inc.

Erikson, E. (1968). *Identity, youth and crisis.* New York, NY: Norton.

Fawcett, J. (1995). *Analysis and evaluation of conceptual models of nursing* (3rd ed.). Philadelphia: F. A. Davis Company.

Finch, D. A. (1990). Testing a theoretically based nursing assessment. *Modeling and Role-Modeling: Theory, Practice and Research, 1*(1), 203–213.

Frisch, N. C. (2000). Nursing theory in holistic nursing practice. In B. M. Dossey, L. Keegan, & C. E. Guzzetta (Eds.), *Holistic nursing: A handbook for practice* (3rd ed.). Gaithersburg, MA: Aspen Publishers.

Hertz, J. E. (1991). The perceived enactment of autonomy scale: Measuring the potential for self-care action in the elderly. *Dissertation Abstracts International, 52,* 04B.

Hertz, J. E. (1995). Conceptualization of perceived enactment of autonomy in the elderly. *Issues in Mental Health Nursing, 17,* 261–273.

Hertz, J. E., & Anshultz, C. A. (2002). Relationships among perceived enactment of autonomy, self-care, and holistic health in community-dwelling older adults. *Journal of Holistic Nursing, 20*(2), 166–186.

Hertz, J. E., & Rossetti, J. (2006). Self-care actions reported by older adults. Paper presented at the 11th Biennial Conference of the Society for the Advancement of Modeling and Role-Modeling, Portland, OR.

Holl, R. M. (1992). The effects of role-modeled visiting in comparison to restricted visiting on the well-being of clients who had open heart surgery and their significant family members in the critical care unit. *Dissertation Abstracts International, 53,* 08B.

Irvin, B. L. (1993). Social support, self-worth, and hope as self-care resources for coping with caregiver stress. *Dissertation Abstracts International, 53,* 06B.

Irvin, B. L., & Acton, G. J. (1996). Stress mediation in caregivers of cognitively impaired adults: Theoretical model testing. *Nursing Research, 45*(3), 160–166.

Irvin, B. L., & Acton, G. J. (1997). Stress, hope, and well-being of women caring for family members with Alzheimer's disease. *Holistic Nursing Practice, 11*(2) 69–79.

James, J. (2006, May). Implementing theory in practice: Historical perspectives and future challenges. Paper presented at the 11th Biennial Conference of the Society for the Advancement of Modeling and Role-Modeling, Portland, OR.

Keegan, L., & Dossey, B. M. (1998). *Profile of nurse healers.* Albany, NY: Delmar Publishers.

Kennedy, G. T. (1991). A nursing investigation of comfort and comforting care of the acutely ill patient. *Dissertation Abstracts International, 52,* 12B.

Kline, N. W. (1988). Psychophysiological processes of stress in people with a chronic physical illness. *Dissertation Abstracts International, 49,* 06B.

Landis, B. J. (1991). Uncertainty, spiritual well-being, and psychosocial adjustment to chronic illness. *Dissertation Abstracts International, 52,* 08B.

Leidy, N. K. (1994). Operationalizing Maslow's theory: Development and testing of the basic need satisfaction inventory. *Issues in Mental Health Nursing, 15,* 277–295.

Maslow, A. H. (1968). *Toward a psychology of being.* New York, NY: Van Norstrand Reinhold.

McClosky, J., & Grace, H. (1994). *Current issues in nursing* (4th ed.). St. Louis: C.V. Mosby Company.

McEwin, M., & Wills, E. (2002). *Theoretical basis for nursing.* Philadelphia: Lippincott Williams & Wilkins.

Miller, S. H. (1986). The relationships between psychosocial development and coping ability among disabled teenagers. *Dissertation Abstracts International, 47,* 10B.

Nash, K. (2003). Evaluation of a holistic peer support and education program aimed at facilitating self-care resources in adolescents. Unpublished doctoral dissertation, University of Texas Graduate School of Biomedical Sciences, Galveston.

Perese, E. F. (1997). Unmet need of persons with chronic mental illnesses: Relationship to their adaptation to community living. *Issues in Mental Health Nursing, 18,* 19–34.

Perese, E. F. (2002). Integrating psychiatric nursing into a baccalaureate nursing curriculum. *Journal of the American Psychiatric Nursing Association, 8*(5), 152–158.

Piaget, J. (1952). *The origins of intelligence in children.* New York: International Universities Press, Inc.

Robinson, K. R. (1992). Developing a scale to measure responses of clients with actual or potential myocardial infarctions. *Dissertation Abstracts International, 53,* 12B.

Rogers, S. R. (2002). Nurse-patient interactions: What do patients have to say? Unpublished doctoral dissertation, University of Texas at Austin.

Rosehow, D. J. (1992). Multidimensional scaling analysis of self-care actions for reintegrating holistic health after myocardial infarction. *Dissertation Abstracts International, 53,* 04B.

Scheela, R., Maple, M., & Larson, D. (2006, May). Modeling and role-modeling: Bemidji State University student practicum experience. Paper presented at the 11th Biennial Conference of the Society for the Advancement of Modeling and Role-Modeling, Portland, OR.

Schultz. E. D. (1998). Academic advising from a nursing theory perspective. *Nurse Educator, 23*(2), 22–25.

Selye, H. (1976). *The stress of life.* New York, NY: McGraw-Hill.

Snyder, P. (2006). Respect and its use in the adaptive potential model. *Newsletter, Society for the Advancement of Modeling and Role-Modeling, 16*(1), 3. (Available from the SAMRM website, www.mrmnursingtheory.org.)

Tomey, A. M., & Alligood, M. R. (1998). *Nursing theorists and their work* (4th ed.). Philadelphia: F. A. Davis.

University of Michigan. (2002). 5B Vascular Surgery Unit. Retrieved July 1, 2002, from http://www.med.umich.edu/nursing/5b.htm.

Villarruel, A. M., Bishop, T. L., Simpson, E. M., Jemmott, L. S., & Fawcett, J. (2001). Borrowed theories, shared theories, and the advancement of nursing knowledge. *Nursing Science Quarterly, 14*(2), 158–163.

Walker, S. N., Sechrist, K., & Pender, N. (1995). *The health-promoting lifestyle profile II.* Omaha: University of Nebraska Medical Center, College of Nursing.

Walsh, K. K., VandenBosch, T. M., & Boehm, S. (1989). Modeling and role-modeling: Integrating theory into practice. *Journal of Advanced Nursing, 14,* 755–761.

BIBLIOGRAPHY

Acton, G. J., Irvin, B. L., Jensen, B. A., Hopkins, B. A., & Miller, E. W. (1997). Explicating middle-range theory through methodological diversity. *Advances in Nursing Science, 19*(3), 78–86.

Baldwin, C. M. (1996). Perceptions of hope: Loved experiences of elementary school children in an urban setting. *Journal of Multicultural Nursing and Health, 2*(3), 41–45.

Barnfather, J. S., & Erickson, H. C. (1989). Construct validity of an aspect of the coping process: Potential adaptation to stress. *Issues in Mental Health Nursing, 10,* 23–40.

Erickson, M. E. (1996). Factors that influence the mother-infant dyad relationships and infant well-being. *Issues in Mental Health Nursing, 18,* 185–200.

Kinney, C. K. (1990). Facilitating growth and development: A paradigm case for modeling and role-modeling. *Issues in Mental Health Nursing, 11,* 375–395.

Rogers, S. (1996). Facilitative affiliation: Nurse-client interactions that enhance healing. *Issues in Mental Health Nursing, 17,* 171–184.

Comfort

■ KATHARINE KOLCABA

DEFINITION OF KEY TERMS

Comfort The immediate experience of being strengthened by having needs for relief, ease, and transcendence met in four contexts (physical, psychospiritual, sociocultural, and environmental); much more than the absence of pain or other physical discomforts

ComfortPlace An institution practicing a philosophy of health care that focuses on addressing physical (including homeostatic mechanisms as well as sensations), psychospiritual, sociocultural, and environmental comfort needs of patients and nurses. This type of care has three components: (a) appropriate and timely comfort interventions, (b) delivery of comfort interventions that projects caring and empathy, and (c) the intent to comfort. All components are based on an in-depth understanding of the patient's medical history and current medical problems.

Comfort interventions Skilled actions of the health care team intentionally designed to enhance patients' or families' comfort. Also changes in the health care environment that enhance the comfort of nurses

Comfort needs Patients' or families' desire for or deficit in relief/ease/transcendence in physical, psychospiritual, sociocultural, and environmental contexts of human experience

Health-seeking behaviors (HSBs) Behaviors in which patients, families, or nurses engage consciously or subconsciously moving them toward well-being; HSBs can be internal, external, or dying peacefully (when that is the most realistic option for patients).

(Key Terms continued on next page)

DEFINITION OF KEY TERMS (continued)

Institutional integrity   The values, financial stability, and wholeness of health care organizations at local, regional, state, and national levels. In addition to hospital systems, the definition of "institutions" includes public health agencies, Medicare and Medicaid programs, home care agencies, nursing home consortiums, etc. Examples of variables related to this expanded definition of institutional integrity include cost savings, improved access, decreased morbidity rates, decreased hospitalizations and readmissions, improved health-related outcomes, efficiency of services and billing, and positive cost–benefit ratios. Any health care unit or system that applies Comfort Theory is called a *Comfort Place*.

Intervening variables   Positive or negative factors over which the health care team has little control, but which affect the direction and success of comfort care plans, comfort studies, or comfort interventions. Examples are presence or absence of social support, poverty, positive prognosis, concurrent medical or psychological conditions, health habits, environmental design, administrative philosophy, etc.

INTRODUCTION

The concept of comfort has had a historic and consistent association with nursing. Nurses traditionally provide comfort to patients and their families through actions that, in this theory, are called comfort interventions. The Theory of Comfort, as applied in a *ComfortPlace*, explicates a philosophy of care whereby holistic comfort needs of patients, families, and nurses are identified and addressed. Intervening variables are accounted for in planning and assessment. The desired and immediate outcome is enhanced comfort, an altruistic and patient-centered goal. Recently, Kolcaba expanded this desired outcome as it applies to nurses and other members of health care teams. This application is useful when institutions are applying for national designations, such as Magnet Status from the American Association of Certification for Nurses, the American Association of Critical Care Nurses Beacon Award, or the Gold Seal of Approval from the Joint Commission. In addition, enhanced comfort is related to subsequent desirable outcomes such as higher patient or nurse function, quicker discharge, fewer readmissions, increased satisfaction with care, longevity of employment, and stronger cost–benefit ratios for the institution. These subsequent outcomes provide additional rationales for health care teams to adopt a model of comfort as a unifying framework for care delivery.

HISTORICAL BACKGROUND

Nightingale was perhaps the first health care worker to recognize that comfort was essential for patients. She said, "It must never be lost sight of what observation is for. It is not for the sake of piling up miscellaneous information or curious facts, but for the sake of saving life and increasing health and comfort"

(Nightingale, 1859, p. 70). In this quote, Nightingale seems to imply that the relationship between health and comfort is dependent, and that both are equally important.

At the beginning of the 20th century, the term *comfort* was used in a general sense, much as Nightingale had used it, and comfort was highly valued in nursing. Moreover, the ability to provide comfort determined, to a large degree, the nurse's skill and character (Goodwin, 1935).

At this time, nurses believed that the provision of comfort was their unique mission. Comfort was especially important because curative medical strategies were not yet developed. Enhancing patient comfort was seen as a positive nursing goal that also was nurturing, and, in most cases, should entail an improvement from a previous state or condition. Comfort resulted from physical, emotional, and environmental interventions, but orders for specific comfort measures were under the physician's authority. Some common "comfort orders" in this period were for poultices, heat, and positioning of the patient in the bed (McIlveen & Morse, 1995).

Although emotional care was not one of the specified roles of nurses, physical comfort interventions were intended to bring about mental comfort of patients, indicating that physical and mental comfort were closely related. In early nursing texts, the meaning of comfort was implicit, hidden in context, complex, and general. Many semantic variations, such as comforting, to comfort, in comfort, and comfortable, were used and the term could be in the form of a verb, a noun, an adjective, or an adverb. Comfort also referred to the process of comforting, ("The nurse comforted the patient") or the outcome of comfort ("The patient was comforted by the nurse").

From its general meaning and significant worth in nursing at the beginning of the 20th century, comfort evolved to a less important nursing goal with a connotation more specific to the physical sense. In the 1950s, as analgesics became popular for pain control, few additional treatments for comfort were described (McIlveen & Morse, 1995). At this time, nurses took responsibility for patients' feelings, although nurses were told to refrain from discussing patients' medical conditions with them.

By the 1970s, nurses' autonomy increased and they could implement comfort interventions without a doctor's order. But without doctors' orders for comfort, the motivation, recognition, and documentation for enhancing patient comfort also diminished (McIlveen & Morse, 1995). And, as the use of technology intensified, many traditional comfort interventions were relegated to minor significance or were implemented by assistive personnel. The term remained undefined in the discipline, but now comfort was narrowly interpreted, written about rarely, and of course, not measured or documented. These conditions rendered comfort interventions by nurses, and the results on comfort of patients, invisible.

The 1980s saw many advances in medicine and cures often resulted from surgery, antibiotics, radiation therapy, and chemotherapy. Narcotics were used for treating severe pain. The importance of family comfort began to emerge at this time and families were considered legitimate recipients of care and comfort interventions (McIlveen & Morse, 1995). Interaction between the comfort of patients and the comfort of their families was implied.

During the 1980s, nurses promoted *self*-care for patients whenever possible. Comfort was the *main* goal of nursing only when patients were terminally ill, an observation that supported Glaser and Strauss's earlier suggestion that the goal of nursing reverted to comfort when there were no available cures (1965). Also, where nursing settings were less influenced by technology, such as hospice and long-term care, comfort was more important as a nursing goal. McIlveen and Morse (1995) suggested that this trend had broad implications for nursing in the 21st century, as demographics would shift to large numbers of elders who may wish for less technology and more comfort in their last years of life.

DEFINITIONS OF THEORY CONCEPTS

When a concept is germane to a discipline, as comfort is, but it has not yet been specifically defined, a concept analysis is necessary. Thus, in 1988, this task was undertaken by Kolcaba. It began with a study of several contemporary dictionaries, each of which contained between six and eight definitions of comfort. Those meanings were compared to usages found in an extensive literature search in the journals and textbooks of several disciplines (nursing, medicine, theology, ergonomics, psychology, and psychiatry). From ergonomics came the insight that comfort of persons, for example, in their workplace or their cars, was important for optimum function or productivity (Kolcaba & Kolcaba, 1991).

Also consulted were nursing history books and the Oxford English Dictionary (OED), which traces the origins and evolution of English words. In 1988, the nursing diagnosis (NANDA) for altered comfort was limited to specific physical discomforts such as pain, nausea, and itching. In nursing textbooks, comfort was discussed in terms of pain management. But the origins of comfort supported its later association with strengthening, because the concept itself came from the Latin word *confortare,* meaning "to strengthen greatly." That obsolete meaning of comfort, not included in modern dictionaries, was still very appropriate for nursing! From the OED the following definitions of comfort were explicated: (a) strengthening; encouragement, incitement, aid, succor, support and (b) physical refreshment or sustenance; and (c) refreshing or invigorating influence (Kolcaba & Kolcaba, 1991). These meanings, plus the link to optimum function in the ergonomic literature, provide theoretical significance for comfort in nursing.

From this process, which took 2 years, three technical senses of comfort were derived and labeled relief, ease, and renewal. *Relief* was defined as the experience of a patient who has had a specific comfort need addressed; its theoretical background was consistent with Orlando's need-based philosophy of nursing (1961/1990). *Ease* was defined as a state of calm or contentment; its theoretical background was enriched by the writings of Henderson (1978) about essential human requirements. Renewal was defined as the state in which one rises above problems or pain. Later, the term renewal was changed to *transcendence,* a term already used in the nursing literature by Paterson & Zderad (1976/1988).

[Author's note: Publishing this part of the concept analysis (Kolcaba & Kolcaba, 1991) took one year, as the language was rather complicated. The analysis was comprehensive but not particularly welcomed by American journals. Hence, this first article actually was published at the same time as the second article, described below.]

After presenting these senses or types of comfort at a research conference, audience feedback was so provocative that, in the middle of the night, Kolcaba awoke with the idea that the types of comfort (relief, ease, and renewal) occurred physically and mentally. She sketched out a preliminary grid with *relief, ease, and renewal* across the top and *physical* and *mental* down the side. Thus, there were six cells in this first grid. After presenting this preliminary grid to colleagues and professors at Case Western Reserve University (where she was a doctoral student), Kolcaba was advised that her "physical" and "mental" categories were not holistic, and to go back to the literature to discover how holism was conceptualized for nursing. Doing so took another year. Four contexts of holistic experience were derived from the literature, which were labeled physical, psychospiritual, social, and environmental (Kolcaba, 1991). *Physical comfort* pertained to bodily sensations and homeostatic mechanisms. *Psychospiritual comfort* pertained to the internal awareness of self, including esteem, sexuality, and meaning in one's life; it also encompassed one's relationship to a higher order or being. *Social comfort* pertained to interpersonal, family, and societal relationships (later this term was changed to *sociocultural comfort* and the idea of family and cultural traditions was added to the definition). *Environmental comfort* pertained to the external background of human experience; it encompassed light, noise, ambience, color, temperature, and natural versus synthetic elements.

	Relief	Ease	Transcendence
Physical			
Psychospiritual			
Environmental			
Sociocultural			

■ **Figure 12.1**   Taxonomic structure of comfort.

When the three types of comfort were juxtaposed with the four contexts of experience, a 12-cell grid or taxonomic structure (TS) was created (Figure 12.1) (Kolcaba, 1991). The grid depicted the defining attributes of comfort, and was helpful for deriving the technical definition of *comfort* (provided at the beginning of this chapter): *the immediate experience of being strengthened by having needs for relief, ease, and transcendence met in four contexts (physical, psychospiritual, sociocultural, and environmental)* (Kolcaba, 1992). This grid has been useful for assessing comfort needs of patients, families, and nurses; planning interventions to address those needs; informally evaluating the effectiveness of those interventions to enhance comfort; and measuring the desired outcome of enhanced comfort for research and practice.

DESCRIPTION OF THEORY: MAJOR COMPONENTS AND THEIR RELATIONSHIPS

Assumptions

Assumptions are a theorist's point of view about reality, set forth so future readers know where the theorist is "coming from." Kolcaba's (1994) assumptions are:

- Human beings have holistic responses to complex stimuli.
- Comfort is a desirable holistic state that is germane to the discipline of nursing.

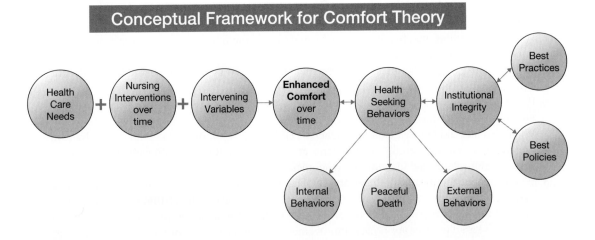

Conceptual Framework for Comfort Theory

© Kolcaba (2007)

■ **Figure 12.2**.   Theoretical framework for Comfort Theory. Source: Kolcaba, K. (2002). Conceptual Framework for Comfort Theory. Retrieved November 11, 2007 from http://thecomfortline.com/conceptualframework.html

- Human beings strive to meet, or to have met, their basic comfort needs. It is an active endeavor.
- Comfort is more than the absence of pain, anxiety, and other physical discomforts.

Concepts

Concepts are ideas that make up the building blocks of specific theories. The concepts for the middle range Theory of Comfort are those listed and defined at the beginning of this chapter: comfort needs, comfort interventions, intervening variables, enhanced comfort, health-seeking behaviors, and institutional integrity. Consistent with middle range theories, these concepts are at a low level of abstraction (easily defined and measured) and are limited in number. All of the above concepts are relative to patients, families, and nurses; the term *family* encompasses significant others as determined by the patient (Kolcaba, 2003; Kolcaba, Tilton, & Drouin, 2006).

Figure 12.2 diagrams the relationship between the concepts that comprise Comfort Theory. Such diagrams are helpful for planning research studies; they are used in many of Kolcaba's articles and on her web site (Kolcaba, 1997).

Propositions

Propositions are relational statements that link concepts together. At the *middle range level* (Figure 14.2, Line 1), the following propositions link those respective variables (Kolcaba, 2001):

1. Nurses and other members of the health care team identify comfort needs of patients and their family members, especially those needs that have not been met by existing support systems. Nurses also identify their own comfort needs in their workplaces, and work constructively for the resolution of these needs.
2. Comfort interventions are designed and coordinated to address those outstanding comfort needs.

3. Intervening variables are taken into account in designing the interventions and determining their probability for success.

4. When interventions are effective, and delivered in a caring manner, the immediate outcome of enhanced comfort is attained.

5. Patients, nurses, and other members of the health care team agree upon desirable and realistic health-seeking behaviors (HSBs).

6. If enhanced comfort is achieved, patients, family members, and/or nurses are strengthened to engage in HSBs, which further enhances comfort.

7. When patients and family members engage in HSBs as a result of being strengthened by comfort interventions, nurses, families, and patients are more satisfied with health care and demonstrate better health-related and institutional outcomes.

8. When patients, families, and nurses are satisfied with health care delivery in a specific institution, system, region, state, or country, public acknowledgement about the institution's contributions to health will lead to those institutions remaining viable and flourishing. Research for best practices (evidence-based practice) or policy improvements at regional, state, or national levels is thus guided by these propositions and this theoretical framework (2001, 2007).

The Comfort Theory can be adapted to any health care setting or age group, whether in the home, hospital, community, region, or state. For research or practice, the concepts can be further defined, at a lower level of abstraction, in terms of specific populations.

RESEARCH APPLICATIONS FOR THE THEORY OF COMFORT

All or parts of the Comfort Theory can be tested for research. The *first part* of the theory, which entails propositions 1 through 4, is the most frequently tested portion to date. Here, the effectiveness of a holistic intervention, targeted to the 12 cells in the taxonomic structure, for enhancing comfort in a specific patient, family, or nurse population over time would be tested. Some holistic interventions that are congruent with the theory are guided imagery, progressive muscle relaxation, hand massage, massage, healing touch, and most environmental interventions.

In an experimental design, patients meeting inclusion criteria are randomly assigned to a treatment group or a comparison group. Researchers use the General Comfort Questionnaire (GCQ) as a starting point, removing items that are not relevant to their research setting or population, and adding items that are relevant. They can plot all items on the taxonomic structure, making sure that the content domain of comfort is evenly represented. Similar numbers of positive and negative items are utilized, unless patients are very frail cognitively. In that case, mostly positive items are used (Cohen & Mount, 1992). Kolcaba usually uses three measurement points, the first being baseline measures of the selected outcomes. Her preferred test statistic is Repeated Measures Multivariate Analysis of Variance (MANOVA) (or if using a covariate, MANCOVA). These are good statistics for comfort research because they capture holistically the interaction between time and the intervention (group assignment) and they have strong power (fewer subjects needed). Accounting for the impact of the interaction between time and the intervention (in other words, does the intervention increase comfort over time?) is congruent with the Comfort Theory because, although comfort is not a stable state, a trend for increased comfort over time can be demonstrated given an effective comfort intervention.

An example where the GCQ was adapted for an intervention study was the test of a new patient-controlled heated gown, as requested by the manufacturer. The gown was designed to be used intraoperatively to enhance patients' comfort and satisfaction with care and reduce anxiety. Kolcaba consulted with the manufacturer to adapt the Thermal Comfort Questionnaire from the GCQ by Kolcaba. Findings of the study, which supported the manufacturer's claims, were recently published in a preeminent nursing journal for operating room nurses (Wagner, Byrne, & Kolcaba, 2006).

The *second part* of the theory is represented by propositions 5 and 6, relating comfort to selected HSBs. The second part provides rationale for *why* nurses and other health care providers should focus on patient, family, and/or nurse comfort, beyond altruistic reasons. Because HSBs include internal and external behaviors, almost any health-related outcome that is deemed important in a given research setting can be classified as an HSB. The task for the investigator is to justify the choice of HSBs and discuss reasons that recipients would want to engage in those HSBs, whether consciously or unconsciously. Kolcaba and colleagues tested propositions 5 and 6 in their studies with persons who have urinary incontinence (UI) (Dowd, Kolcaba, & Steiner, 2000, 2002, 2003). They found that people with higher comfort were more likely to engage in HSBs and be successful in increasing bladder function and management of UI. That is, comfort was a good predictor of engagement in HSBs.

Research with patients near end of life and their family members is in its infancy. Comfort is consistently stated as a desired outcome in hospice standards of care, which makes the Comfort Theory particularly cogent for research with patients near end of life. Making it even more applicable for hospice or palliative research is Schlotfeldt's (1975) inclusion of Peaceful Death as an HSB. Sometimes, a peaceful death is the most realistic outcome in a particular situation and Scholtfeldt's elevating Peaceful Death to an HSB was an example of how her thinking was "ahead of her time." However, recruitment and data collection with patients near end of life is fraught with difficulties. For these reasons, Kolcaba developed a Comfort Behaviors Checklist (CBC), which data collectors can use to rate a patient's *apparent* comfort (Kolcaba, 1997). While not as desirable as actually asking a patient about his or her comfort, the instrument fills a gap regarding data collection in very frail or cognitively limited patients (see instrument section of this chapter for more details). This CBC was recently adapted for clinical documentation of babies' apparent comfort by pediatric nurses from a large western health care system (Kolcaba, 1997).

The *third part* of the Comfort Theory is represented by propositions 7 and 8, relating patients' comfort and their engagement in HSBs to Institutional Integrity (InI). The concept of InI was added to the theory (Kolcaba, 2001, 2007) in order to provide direction for outcomes research that would support the disciplines of nursing and other health professions. Comfort, Patient Satisfaction, and Nurse Satisfaction currently are among the few positive outcomes being utilized for this type of research. Kolcaba believes that future research will show that these positive outcomes are highly correlated. And, because institutions are driven by market competition to produce high patient satisfaction scores, those same institutions will be interested to know that patient and/or nurse comfort are strong predictors of patient satisfaction as well as other positive outcomes such as shorter lengths of stay, fewer hospital readmissions, and lower turnover of health care employees, especially nurses. Achieving sought-after national recognition is another measure of InI.

Perhaps because nursing outcomes research is a newer science, data thus far have largely focused on "absence of" adverse events related to hospitalization, such as new decubiti, medication errors, nosocomial infections, pneumonia, and death. Surely, patients and their family members want and need reassurance about their future hospital admissions beyond statistics about survival and adverse events. They want to get well, avoid future hospitalizations, understand their new health regimen, be treated with respect and care, return to previous levels of function, and, yes, be comforted by their health care team when necessary. Positive outcomes such as patient comfort brought about by sufficiently supported and motivated health professionals, would create "value-added" benefits in contemporary health care situations.

The research examples shown in Using Middle Range Theories 12.1 and 12.2 are published studies that tested the effectiveness of holistic interventions in promoting comfort in specific populations.

12.1 USING MIDDLE RANGE THEORIES

For her dissertation study, Kolcaba developed a Guided Imagery (GI) audiotape for women with breast cancer who were undergoing conservative treatment. Breast-conserving therapy consisted of lumpectomy and radiation therapy (RT). The research question was, Will women who receive GI while going through RT for early-stage breast cancer have greater comfort over time compared to a control group? (see Figure 12.2).

The audiotape medium facilitated the delivery of the same holistic message over and over to all women in the treatment group. In the script for GI, positive statements were directed to every cell in the taxonomic structure of comfort known to be important for this population. Input for construction of the audiotape and design of the study was received from the RT nurses, technicians, and physicians.

The instruments used in this study were the Radiation Therapy Comfort Questionnaire (RTCQ) and four visual analog scales (Total Comfort, Relief, Ease, and Transcendence). The development and psychometric performance of these instruments are discussed in the section "Instruments Used in Empirical Testing." During the pilot test for the methods, the women were asked specifically if there was anything left out of the questionnaire or anything that was forgotten or awkward in the audiotape, and if the instruments were easy to use. When everyone was satisfied with the protocol, the study began.

Nurses told the women about the study during their first appointment in the RT department. When the patients first heard about the study, about half the women burst into tears; the other half wanted to enroll. The nurses faxed the names and phone numbers of those who wanted to enroll to the data collectors, and the intake visit took place before the women's simulation visit. The women in the treatment group were asked to listen to the tape every day, in their own homes, with tape players that the study provided. They indicated in journals and during interviews that they complied with this request diligently for the first 3 weeks of RT, after which some tired of the audiotape. When this occurred, they were encouraged to continue listening to the music side of the tape, which would reinforce recall of the guided imagery script. In this way, the script could be internalized.

Three complete data sets were collected (three visits for each woman) on 53 women, which took a year after IRB approvals were obtained. RM MANOVA was used to test the hypotheses. Alpha was set at 0.10 because the intervention had no risks and the higher alpha reduced Type II error (Lipsey, 1990).

Results. This study was a test of the new Comfort Theory, a test of the effectiveness of the guided imagery intervention, and a test of the ability to show quantitative differences in the complex phenomenon of patient comfort before and after this comfort intervention. Analysis of group differences at baseline on demographic data and comfort revealed that the groups were similar for all baseline variables. This was the desired result for Time 1 data. The result of the MANOVA, which analyzed data from all three time points, was that the groups were significantly different on comfort at Times 2 and 3 ($p = .07$), a second desired result. Then two posttests were conducted. The first was to determine which group had higher comfort (the treatment group did) and the second was to perform a trend analysis, looking at the "slopes" of the

(box continued on page 263)

12.1 USING MIDDLE RANGE THEORIES (continued)

comfort data for both groups. This analysis revealed a linear slope over time, meaning that differences between the groups increased steadily over time. A simplified picture of the trend analysis for this study is in Figure 12.3. All of these results confirmed the efficacy of guided imagery, and supported the Theory of Comfort.

Kolcaba, K., & Fox, C. (1999). The effects of guided imagery on comfort of women with early stage breast cancer undergoing radiation therapy. *Oncology Nursing Forum, 26*(1), 67–72.

12.2 USING MIDDLE RANGE THEORIES

The purpose of this study was to test the effectiveness of audiotaped cognitive strategies for improving comfort related to bladder function. The research question was, Will the group practicing cognitive strategies have higher *comfort* related to bladder function and better actual *bladder function* compared to the control group over time?

A substructed diagram similar to the radiation therapy diagram was used to organize the study. Following this diagram, the known comfort needs of this population were targeted, with the cognitive strategies recorded on a new audiotape. The taxonomic structure was used as a guide to cover the domain of comfort with the recorded statements. Possible covariates (intervening variables) were age, gender, and particulars of bladder health history. To measure comfort in this population, the taxonomic structure was used to develop the Urinary Incontinence and Frequency Comfort Questionnaire (UIFCQ), which was pilottested before using it in this study. The health-seeking behavior that was measured was improved bladder function, operationalized by number of incontinent episodes, number of toileting trips, and the Bladder Function Questionnaire (researcher developed).

Most of the methods from the breast cancer study (described previously) were replicated (because of their success), including having persons in the treatment group listen to the tape daily, having three data collection points, and using the same method of data analysis.

Results indicated that the treatment group had more comfort and improved bladder function over time compared with the comparison group. In addition, a crossover component was added when those in the original comparison group listened to the audiotape for 3 weeks, after which data were collected again from both groups. A significant improvement in bladder function was found in the crossover group, and their comfort had increased to the level of the treatment group after 3 weeks of the intervention.

Another interesting finding was that the UIFCQ predicted which participants ($n = 17$, or 90% of the treatment group) would demonstrate improvement in incontinence. Because comfort was a strong predictor of benefit from treatment for incontinence and frequency, these findings also supported the middle range Theory of Comfort (Dowd, Kolcaba, & Steiner, 2000).

Dowd, T., Kolcaba, K., & Steiner, R. (2000). Using cognitive strategies to enhance bladder control and comfort. *Holistic Nursing Practice, 14*(2), 91–103.

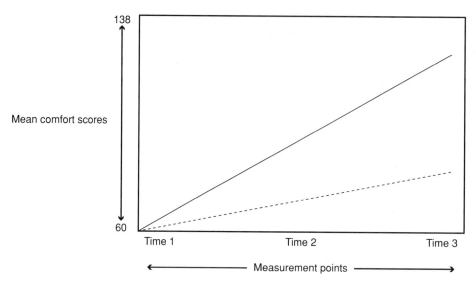

■ **Figure 12.3** Trend analysis for breast cancer study. Source: Kolcaba, K., & Fox, C. (1999). The effects of guided imagery on comfort of women with early stage breast cancer undergoing radiation therapy. *Oncology Nursing Forum, 26*(1), 67–72. Used with permission.

INSTRUMENTS USED IN EMPIRICAL TESTING

General Comfort Questionnaire

If you want to do a comfort study yourself, and a comfort instrument needs to be constructed for your unique population, you can start with the General Comfort Questionnaire and adapt it using your knowledge of the population. Detailed instructions for doing so are on the web (Kolcaba, 1997) and a full discussion of how the GCQ was developed is in Kolcaba (1992, 2003).

As with the other comfort questionnaires available, the GCQ began with the taxonomic structure. For each cell, an equal number of positive and negative items were created. The GCQ contains two positive and two negative items for each of the 12 cells in the taxonomic structure, resulting in 48 items. A four-response Likert-type scale was used for the pilot test, although subsequent questionnaires have six responses, which increases sensitivity of the instrument. An even number of responses also forces the responder to choose one side of the comfort fence or the other.

The GCQ was pilot tested in the community ($n = 30$) and several types of hospital units ($n = 226$). Results of this first instrumentation study were encouraging, as the Cronbach's alpha was 0.88, very high for a new instrument. (Perhaps working from a theoretically driven map of the content domain helped!) Factor analysis, using Principal Components Analysis, extracted 13 factors with eigenvalues above 1.0. The 13th factor had only one item and was collapsed into one of the other factors that was semantically similar, producing 12 factors consistent with the TS. In addition, factors clumped together in three subscales on the scree plot and semantically were similar to the *types of comfort* (Relief, Ease, and Transcendence). This factor structure accounted for 63.4% of the variance in the 48 items (Kolcaba, 1992).

Reliabilities for the subscales (factors) ranged from 0.66 to 0.80, which were lower than for the whole GCQ (0.88). This is because lower numbers of items generally decrease reliability scores. The GCQ revealed significant sensitivity in expected directions between several groups (construct validity). Findings were that (a) the community group had higher comfort than the hospital group, and (b) people with higher comfort demonstrated a higher correlation with their own estimates of progress in rehabilitation.

When researchers adapt the GCQ to fit their population, they can use the psychometric properties and description of the instrumentation study (above) to support their choice of a comfort instrument. If they wish, they can shorten the number of items and remove whole subscales that are not relevant. However, with each of those strategies, reliability scores may decrease. It is important, therefore, to pilot-test adapted instruments with at least 10 subjects who are characteristic of those in the proposed study. A Cronbach's alpha of at least 0.70 is desirable for a new instrument. Kolcaba appreciates your submission of your new instruments to her web site (Kolcaba, 1997) so future researchers do not have to "reinvent the wheel" and the preliminary psychometric statistics that support use of comfort instruments.

Shortened General Comfort Questionnaire (28 Items)

The 28-item GCQ is in the same format as the original GCQ (48 items). That is, both instruments have a Likert-type format, with six responses ranging from strongly agree to strongly disagree. Examples of items relating to the four contexts include, "I have a poor appetite" (physical), "My beliefs give me peace of mind" (psychospiritual), "My friends remember me with their cards and phone calls" (sociocultural), and "These surroundings are pleasant" (environmental). Negatively worded items are reverse scored and a total score is obtained by summing items, with higher scores indicating better comfort levels. The 28-item GCQ had a Chronbach's alpha of 0.86, 0.83, and 0.82 over three measurement points (to measure change over time). Although these were satisfactory alphas for the sample size of 60 frail elders, item number 19 ("The views are soothing") had negative correlations with other items and the total instrument. This item would have had poor congruence with the other comfort items, if views to which the residents were accustomed were *not* pleasing. This instrument is available on Kolcaba's web site as found in Instrument's section (Kolcaba online).

When individuals, especially those who are frail, have difficulty with the length of the instrument, the Likert scale with anchors matching the GCQ is duplicated in large text on 5" × 8" cards. Items then are read by the data collector, as was the procedure used in this study (Kolcaba, Schirm, & Steiner, 2006).

Radiation Therapy Comfort Questionnaire

To adapt the GCQ to women with breast cancer, items that were not relevant for radiation therapy were deleted. The literature identified critical comfort needs specific to this population. From this list of needs, positive and negative items were developed to complete and balance the questionnaire for this population.

A consideration when developing the Radiation Therapy Comfort Questionnaire (RTCQ) was the length of time it would take for the women to answer it. The nurses thought, and it was later confirmed, that many research participants would choose to complete the questionnaires in the RT department rather than in their homes. And, the design of the study was to administer all questionnaires immediately prior to RT. A 48-item questionnaire was deemed too long by the RT staff, and probably too stressful for the women. So, for this study, a 26-item RTCQ was pilot-tested. The instrument performed fairly well in the final study with a Cronbach's alpha of 0.76 ($n = 53$, 26 items).

Visual Analog and Verbal Rating Scales

For the radiation therapy study, visual analog scales (VASs) were developed to measure the three subscales of comfort (Relief, Ease, and Transcendence). Each VAS was a 10-cm vertical line, anchored at the bottom with "strongly disagree" and at the top with "strongly agree." Stems for the VASs were, "I have many discomforts right now" (Relief), "I am feeling at ease right now" (Ease), and "I am feeling motivated, determined, and strengthened right now" (Transcendence). Higher scores, after reverse coding "Relief," meant higher comfort. The VASs were developed, in part, to begin to establish concurrent validity for comfort questionnaires. Concurrent validity is the extent to which a measure correlates with another simultaneously obtained measure of the same trait or state (Goodwin & Goodwin, 1991). There were no other measures available for comfort. Secondly, it was possible that VASs could measure patient comfort more efficiently than the longer questionnaire.

While the statistical performance of the RTCQ was adequate, the performance of the VASs was mixed and required more involved secondary analyses. Hence, these scales were analyzed for a second article (Kolcaba & Steiner, 2000). Findings were that the Total Comfort (TC) line was not sensitive to differences in comfort over time. The scores for Summed Comfort Subscales (Relief, Ease, and Transcendence) provided data that approached significance ($P = .17$) and seemed to be more sensitive to individual perceptions of comfort than the Total Comfort line (Kolcaba & Steiner, 2000). These visual analog scales demonstrated that Total Comfort was greater than the sum of its parts (Relief, Eases, and Transcendence added together). Also, correlations between the VASs and the RTCQ supported preliminary concurrent validity between the two measures of comfort. In view of these limited findings, however, VASs are not recommended for research or clinical purposes.

However, as demonstrated in Research Application 12.1, asking a patient to rate his or her comfort from 0 to 10 can result in meaningful conversations about detractors from comfort in the clinical setting, so that nurses will know how to proceed with comfort care. Findings from the use of verbal rating scales of either total comfort or discomfort can easily be added to documentation forms in health care settings. For example, in a recent study, verbal rating scales of total comfort (and total stress) provided statistically significant data when comparing the effects of two comfort interventions, coaching and healing touch, for the goal of increasing comfort and decreasing stress of college students (Dowd et al., 2007).

Urinary Incontinence and Frequency Comfort Questionnaire

For the comfort study with persons with urinary incontinence, the Urinary Incontinence and Frequency Comfort Questionnaire (UIFCQ) was adapted from the GCQ and contained 23 positive and negative items specific to the experience of living with UI. A six-response Likert-type format, ranging from "strongly agree" to "strongly disagree," was used. After reverse coding negative items, higher scores indicated higher comfort. In this study, 31 women and 9 men participated. The Cronbach's alpha averaged 0.82 across the four measurement points, indicating good reliability. The instrument was sensitive to changes in comfort over time ($P = .01$) (Dowd et al., 2000).

Hospice Comfort Questionnaire (Family and Patient)

For this population, the GCQ was adapted again to create a 49-item Hospice Comfort Questionnaire (HCQ). Family members were asked to rate their *own* comfort, not that of their patient. The adapted instruments were tested in two phases (Novak, Kolcaba, Steiner, & Dowd, 2001). In phase I of the

12.1 RESEARCH APPLICATION

Jim, 75 years old, was apprehensive about his upcoming knee surgery. He was afraid of a general anesthetic, pain, blood loss, loss of mobility, and loss of dignity and independence during the procedure and in the postoperative period. All of these separate fears seemed rather minor when considered objectively and separately; however, when Jim experienced them simultaneously (holistically), sitting in the waiting room, they created panic: "This is MY body, MY surgery, MY unknowns. *I'm* going under the knife!" Jim's whole-person response was greater or stronger than if he thought only about immobility one time, blood loss at another time, etc.

A study was designed where the intake nurse asked Jim to rate his comfort from 0 to 10, 0 being no comfort and 10 being the highest overall comfort possible. From the description of his fears, we were not surprised that Jim was "2" at Time 1. The nurse explored with Jim his detractors from comfort while taking Jim's vital signs (blood pressure, pulse, and respirations were high!). Jim was demonstrating a fight-or-flight response and really just wanted to leave.

The nurse talked with Jim about alternatives to general anesthesia and about patient-controlled analgesia after surgery. The nurse talked about exercises to strengthen his knee and about the minimal blood loss that is usually associated with his surgery. The nurse assured Jim that the surgeon would carefully drape him and that the anesthetist would maintain constant supervision over Jim during the entire procedure. Most reassuring, perhaps, was the fact that Jim's nurse would accompany him into the operating room and stay with him. The nurse fully understood how he felt about his personal dignity and would be his advocate. This type of coaching is called "usual care" in a research study.

The nurse could see that Jim was calming down. Jim now rated his comfort as "5" (Time 2, after usual care) and vital signs were improved. Then the nurse began a guided imagery (GI) exercise with Jim. Jim was asked to close his eyes, picture himself in a favorite place, relax his body incrementally, and then imagine the surgery in the most positive ways as suggested by the nurse: "You will feel no pain upon awaking; you will barely have any bleeding," etc. Kolcaba calls this type of extra intervention "comfort food for the soul." When Jim completed the GI, he was fully relaxed and confident and now rated his comfort at "9" (Time 3), and his vital signs were even better. The nurse documented the GI intervention and Jim's response to it. This is a test of part I of the Comfort Theory (CT).

The nurse quickly looked at Jim's three comfort scores at each time point and noticed that his comfort scores improved considerably at each time point. "Well, coaching improved Jim's comfort but not as much as the guided imagery. And it is interesting that his vital signs improved with each time point, although there was a bigger change between Time 2 and Time 3. Could increased comfort be related to improved vital signs?" The second part of CT proposes that the immediate outcome of comfort is related to the subsequent outcome of improved vital signs. Other subsequent outcomes of interest might have been postoperative bleeding or pain. All of these are HSBs. Institutional outcomes of interest could also be related to Jim's immediate and subsequent outcomes to test the third part of CT. Suggestions for institutional outcomes are patient satisfaction or length of stay in outpatient surgery.

(box continued on page 268)

12.1 RESEARCH APPLICATION (continued)

In this way, concepts such as comfort gain importance when they are related to other concepts. Nurses and other members of the health team have rationale for taking extra time to enhance patient comfort, in addition to the altruistic reason from which nurses usually are motivated. And nurses can demonstrate that guided imagery improves patient outcomes—a quality improvement issue. (Of course, the design of this study would be much stronger with an experimental group [received guided imagery] and comparison group [usual care], each consisting of a large number of patients undergoing a similar surgery.)

study, patient and family member (FM) questionnaires had a six-item Likert scale response set, ranging from "strongly agree" to "strongly disagree," and higher scores indicated higher comfort. Each questionnaire took about 12 minutes for patients to complete and usually less time for FMs. Approximately equal numbers of positive and negative items were created for the FMs' end-of-life questionnaire, and items were worded more simply and with less alternating between positive and negative orientation. This adaptation was necessary because of decreased mental agility in dying patients (Cohen & Mount, 1992).

For phase II of the study, patient and caregiver questionnaires were reduced to a four-item Likert response set, because of concerns of the data collectors that six responses were too confusing. However, results showed that the instrument in phase I (six responses) had the strongest psychometric properties for both FMs and patients. Cronbach's alpha for the FM questionnaire was 0.89 ($n = 38$) and for the patient questionnaire was 0.83 ($n = 48$) (Novak et al., 2001).

In spite of these high reliability scores, nurse researchers working with this population a few years later thought that 49 items was too many, and they asked a panel of experts to prioritize the items that were most important. From that list of priority items, 24 of the highest items were plotted on the taxonomic structure and balanced over the content domain. The result is a 24-item HCQ. This instrument was used in an experiment with hospice patients in which a hand massage protocol was tested with 31 patients over a 3-week period. Despite a lenient alpha of 0.10, the study did not yield significant results overall. However, of clinical significance is that comfort increased somewhat in the treatment group even as patients approached death, while in the comparison group, comfort scores decreased steadily over the three weekly measurement points (Kolcaba, Dowd, Mitzel, & Steiner, 2004).

Healing Touch Comfort Questionnaire

The Healing Touch Comfort Questionnaire (HTCQ) was recently adapted from the GCQ following the same procedure described above. Three experts reviewed it for appropriateness of wording and content, eight HT practitioners distributed the questionnaire to their clients, and 53 persons completed it within several days of the treatment. The questionnaires were returned in self-addressed envelopes provided by the research team. Cronbach's alpha for the HTCQ was 0.94 for Total Comfort. Those who had received five or more HT treatments had comfort scores 13.7 points higher than those who had received one to four treatments. Further analysis showed that there was a trend to a curvilinear relationship between number of treatments and comfort. Comfort seems to increase slightly as the number of treatments increases until about 20 treatments; then comfort levels off and possibly declines. More information is needed about this relationship (Dowd, Kolcaba, & Steiner, 2006).

The HTCQ was used in the study with college students described above (Dowd et al., 2007) to supplement findings from the verbal rating scales. Cronbach's alpha in this study revealed an average of 0.93 over three measurement points. The HTCQ was highly and positively correlated with the verbal rating scales for comfort.

Comfort Behaviors Checklist

Table 12.1 describes several traditional instruments used to measure comfort. However, many nurses who want to do comfort studies have asked about measuring comfort in patients who can't use the traditional comfort questionnaires or rate their comfort from 0 to 10. These patients might be young children or infants, or they might be mentally disabled, brain injured, heavily sedated, or unconscious. Therefore, the Comfort Behaviors Checklist (CBC) was developed on which a nurse or data collector rates the patient's comfort based on observable behaviors. It contains 29 observations with possible responses of Not Applicable, No, Somewhat, Moderate, and Strong (Kolcaba, 1997).

Because scoring of the CBC results in a percent out of 100, a deviation of 20 percentage points between raters for each subject is considered clinically and empirically unreliable. Conversely, a deviation between raters of 10 percentage points for each subject is considered to be acceptable, and of 5 percentage points is a demonstration of very strong inter-rater consistency. Distributions of the differences in

Table 12.1 PSYCHOMETRIC PROPERTIES OF SOME QUANTITATIVE COMFORT INSTRUMENTS

NAME OF INSTRUMENT	RELIABILITY	NO. OF ITEMS	NO. OF SUBJECTS	STRUCTURE ANALYSIS?	REFERENCE
Maternal Comfort Assessment Tool (observer rating)	Inter-rater: 89%	7	40	NA	Andrews & Chrzanowski, 1990
Dementia Comfort Checklist (observer rating)	Correlation coefficient $r = 0.88$	9	82	NA	Hurley, Volicer, Hanrahan, & Volicer, 1992
The Comfort Scale (Distress in Pediatric Intensive Care Units)	Inter-rater: 0.84; internal consistency: 0.90	8 and VAS	50	Correlations between 8 dimensions	Ambuel, Hamlett, Marx, & Blumer, 1992
Physical Bedrest Comfort Measure (patient rating)	Cronbach's alpha: 0.73	19	30	No (not enough subjects)	Hogan-Miller, Rustad, Sendelbach, & Goldenberg, 1995
Radiation Therapy Comfort (position of bed)	Significant differences between groups	1 VAS	17	No	Cox, 1996
Comfort Questionnaire (dehydration/hydration at end of life)	NA	One 4-point Likert scale	31	No	Vullo-Navich et al., 1998
Infant Comfort Behavior (Pain)	Kappa: 0.63–0.93	6 and VAS	158	LISREL	Van Dijk et al., 2000

ratings in 39 data sets were as follows: (a) 36 data sets revealed a 10-point difference or less between rater 1 and rater 2 for each subject ($P = .92$; alpha 0.95), and (b) 31 data sets revealed a 5-point difference or less between rater 1 and rater 2 for each subject ($P = .80$; alpha 0.95). These findings indicate strong inter-rater consistency. However, when correlated with patients' responses on the traditional comfort questionnaire, low correlations were revealed, averaging a Cronbach's alpha of 0.14 over three time points. These disappointing findings seem to indicate that the interior life or feelings of human beings cannot be fully appreciated until they are asked. The stoic demeanors of the long-term care residents, which appeared to indicate comfort, masked many complex and interrelated feelings about their own comfort. However, in the absence of ability to verbalize or indicate specific feelings about comfort, the CBC is, perhaps, better than no comfort assessment at all.

All of these instruments, plus others under development or in different languages, are available on Kolcaba's web site (Kolcaba, 1997). In Table 12.1, Kolcaba (2003) provides a listing of comfort instruments developed by other researchers.

SUMMARY

The Theory of Comfort provides a framework for research in any setting where patients have comfort needs and enhancing their comfort is valued. It can also be used to enhance working environments, especially for nurses, and as a framework for working toward national institutional recognitions. The theory has been used to test the effectiveness of specific holistic interventions for increasing comfort, to demonstrate the correlation between comfort and subsequent HSBs, and to relate HSBs to desirable institutional outcomes. It is important as a framework for interdisciplinary care and research because the focus is on the unifying and positive outcome of patient comfort. It also provides an ethical perspective for decision making in difficult health care situations. For example, when families are faced with difficult choices for their dying loved ones, it is helpful to consider what will make the patient more comfortable (Kolcaba & Kolcaba, 2003).

Comfort Theory has been used in health care institutions nationally and internationally to enhance the working environment for nurses (Kolcaba, Tilton, & Drouin, 2006). In these cases, nurses' comfort is of interest and is theoretically related to the integrity of the institution. Research conducted in such an institution will produce more evidence for best practices and policies in that institution, and hopefully beyond.

ANALYSIS EXERCISES

Using the criteria presented in Chapter 2, critique the Theory of Comfort. Compare your conclusions about the theory with those found in Appendix A. A researcher who has worked with the theory completed the analysis found in the appendix.

Internal Criticism
1. Clarity
2. Consistency
3. Adequacy

4. Logical development
5. Level of theory development

External Criticism
1. Reality convergence
2. Utility
3. Significance
4. Discrimination
5. Scope of theory
6. Complexity

CRITICAL THINKING EXERCISES

1. Nurse leaders attempt to advance practice one unit or agency at a time. In order to bring a philosophy of comfort management to your practice setting, rationale must be developed and presented. Compile logical and compelling rationale for implementing comfort management at your site, and a brief proposal for how you would implement this model.

2. In order to practice comfort management, evidence must be collected about patients'/families' comfort needs, comfort interventions to address those needs, and assessment of baseline comfort compared to comfort after the intervention(s). Design appropriate comfort management documentation for your unit.

3. Research evidence suggests that patients do better when their expectations about specific benefits of nursing care are discussed and met. Design a "comfort contract" whereby patients or their surrogates designate an expected level of postsurgical overall comfort, and also where they can specify chronic discomforts and interventions that they use at home for relief.

WEB RESOURCES

Currently, the only Internet resource about the outcome of patient comfort is Kolcaba's (Kolcaba, 1997) at **www.TheComfortLine.com.** On her web page, references are listed that were instrumental in the development of this theory. A few minor Internet resources (in the area of psychology and religion) refer to comfort, but they don't define it or give instructions for measuring it.

REFERENCES

Ambuel, B., Hamlett, K., Marx, C., & Blumer, J. (1992). Assessing distress in pediatric intensive care environments: The COMFORT scale. *Journal of Pediatric Psychology, 17*(1), 95–109.

Andrews, C., & Chrzanowski, M. (1990). Maternal position, labor, and comfort. *Applied Nursing Research, 3*(1), 7–13.

Cohen, S., & Mount, B. (1992). Quality of life in terminal illness: Defining and measuring subjective well-being in the dying. *Journal of Palliative Care, 8*(3), 40–45.

Cox, J. (1996) Assessing patient comfort in radiation therapy. *Radiation Therapist, 5*(2), 119–125.

Dowd, T., Kolcaba, K., Fashinpaur, D., & Steiner, R. (2007). Comparison of healing touch and coaching on stress and comfort in young college students. *Holistic Nursing Practice, 21*(4), 194–202.

Dowd, T., Kolcaba, K., & Steiner, R. (2000). Using cognitive strategies to enhance bladder control and comfort. *Holistic Nursing Practice, 14*(2), 91–103.

Dowd, T., Kolcaba, K., & Steiner, R. (2002). Correlations among six measures of bladder function. *Journal of Nursing Measurement, 10*(1), 27–38.

Dowd, T., Kolcaba, K., & Steiner, R. (2003). The addition of coaching to cognitive strategies. *Journal of Ostomy and Wound Management, 30*(2), 90–99.

Dowd, T., Kolcaba, K., & Steiner, R. (2006). Development of an instrument to measure holistic client comfort as an outcome of healing touch. *Holistic Nursing Practice. 20*(4), 194–202.

Glaser, C., & Strauss, A. (1965). *Awareness of dying.* Chicago: Aldine.

Goodnow, M. (1935). *The technic of nursing.* Philadelphia: W.B. Saunders.

Goodwin, L., & Goodwin, W. (1991). Focus on psychometrics: Estimating construct validity. *Research in Nursing and Health, 14,* 235–243.

Henderson, V. (1978). *Principals and practice of nursing.* New York: Macmillan.

Hogan-Miller, E., Rustad, D., Sendelbach, S., & Goldenberg, I. (1995). Effects of three methods of femoral site immobilization on bleeding and comfort after coronary angiogram. *American Journal of Critical Care, 4*(2), 143–148.

Hurley, A., Volicer, B., Hanrahan, S., & Volicer, L. (1992). Assessment of discomfort in advanced Alzheimer patient. *Research in Nursing & Health, 15,* 369–377.

Kolcaba, K. (1997). The Comfort Line. Available at: http://www.thecomfortline.com [Copyright, 1997, and updated continuously].

Kolcaba, K. (1991). A taxonomic structure for the concept comfort. *Image: Journal of Nursing Scholarship, 23*(4), 237–239.

Kolcaba, K. (1992). Holistic comfort: Operationalizing the construct as a nurse-sensitive outcome. *Advances in Nursing Science, 15*(1), 1–10.

Kolcaba, K. (1994). A theory of holistic comfort for nursing. *Journal of Advanced Nursing, 19,* 1178–1184.

Kolcaba, K. (2001). Evolution of the mid range theory of comfort for outcomes research. *Nursing Outlook, 49*(2), 86–92.

Kolcaba, K. (2003). *Comfort Theory and practice: A vision for holistic health care and research.* New York: Springer.

Kolcaba, K., Dowd, T., Steiner, R., & Mitzel, A. (2004). Efficacy of hand massage for enhancing comfort of hospice patients. *Journal of Hospice and Palliative Care, 6*(2), 91–101.

Kolcaba, K., & Fox, C. (1999). The effects of guided imagery on comfort of women with early stage breast cancer undergoing radiation therapy. *Oncology Nursing Forum, 26*(1), 67–72.

Kolcaba, K., & Kolcaba, R. (1991). An analysis of the concept of comfort. *Journal of Advanced Nursing, 16,* 1301–1310.

Kolcaba, K., & Kolcaba, R. (2003). Fiduciary decision-making Comfort Care. *Philosophy in the Contemporary World, 10*(1), 81–86.

Kolcaba, K., & Steiner, R. (2000). Empirical evidence for the nature of holistic comfort. *Journal of Holistic Nursing, 18*(1), 46–62.

Kolcaba, K., Schirm, V., & Steiner, V. (2006). Effects of hand massage on comfort of nursing home residents. *Geriatric Nursing, 27*(2), 85–91.

Kolcaba, K., Tilton, C., & Drouin, C. (2006). Use of comfort theory to enhance the practice environment. *Journal of Nursing Administration, 36*(11), 538–544.

Lipsey, M. (1990). *Design sensitivity.* Newbury Park, CA: Sage.

McIlveen, K., & Morse, J. (1995). The role of comfort in nursing care: 1900-1980. *Clinical Nursing Research, 4*(2), 127–148.

Nightingale, F. (1859). *Notes on nursing.* London, Great Britain: Harrison.

Novak, B., Kolcaba, K., Steiner, R., & Dowd, T. (2001). Measuring comfort in caregivers and patients during late end-of-life care. *American Journal of Hospice & Palliative Care, 18*(3), 170–180.

Orlando, I. (1961/1990). *The dynamic nurse-patient relationship.* New York: National League for Nursing.

Paterson, J., & Zderad, L. (1976/1988). *Humanistic nursing.* New York: National League for Nursing.

Schlotfeldt, R. (1975). The need for a conceptual framework. In: P. Verhonic (Ed.), *Nursing research* (pp. 3–25). Boston: Little & Brown.

Van Dijk, M., De Boer, J., Koot, H., Tibboel, D., Passchier, J., & Duivenvoorden, H. (2000). The reliability and validity of the comfort scale as a postoperative pain instrument in 0-3-year-old infants. *Pain, 84*(2–3), 367–377.

Vullo-Navich, K., Smith, S., Andrews, M., Levine, A., Tischler, J., & Veglis, J. (1998). Comfort and incidence of abnormal serum sodium, BUN, creatinine and osmolality in dehydration of terminal illness. *The American Journal of Hospice & Palliative Care, 15*(2), 77–84.

Wagner, D., Byrne, M., & Kolcaba, K. (2006). Effect of comfort warming on preoperative patients. *AORN Journal, 84*(3), 1–13.

Health-Related Quality of Life

- TIMOTHY S. BREDOW
- SANDRA J. PETERSON
- KRISTIN E. SANDAU

DEFINITION OF KEY TERMS

Health-related quality of life (HRQOL)	Subset of quality of life representing satisfaction in areas of life likely to be affected by health status; HRQOL is subjective, multidimensional, and temporal.
Life domains	Basic components of quality of life and HRQOL referring to specific aspects of life, most commonly physical, cognitive, socioeconomic, and psychological/spiritual
Nursing interventions	Although rarely included as a component in formal theoretical models of HRQOL, involve delivering specific care or treatments targeted for an individual or group who have deficits in an identified domain of functioning that disrupts or has the potential to disrupt HRQOL
Quality of life	Satisfaction in areas of life deemed important to the individual

INTRODUCTION

Quality of life (QOL) has been a philosophical and sociopolitical phenomenon for hundreds, if not thousands, of years. In recent years, it has developed into a theory, particularly in response to the growing interest in QOL as expressed by those involved in health care. Because QOL is not clearly identified with one theorist, it is difficult to define and describe. This lack of specificity has not diminished its popularity as an outcome measure among patients tested in hundreds of studies published both nationally and internationally. QOL has been identified as a middle range theory (Meleis, 1997) representing a specific phenomenon, with a limited number of related concepts, that has obvious applications to practice. It may be, however, that the general construct of QOL may be more appropriately labeled a meta-theory because the construct refers to one's perceived status in all areas of life. In contrast, the more limited construct of health-related QOL in the context of health care (often referred to as HRQOL) may be more fitted as a middle range theory because HRQOL is somewhat more limited in focus on areas of life most directly influenced by one's health. Both QOL and HRQOL are developing into explanatory theories.

HISTORICAL BACKGROUND

The concept of QOL, concerned with an individual's personal satisfaction with life, has its roots in classical Greek thought and religious teachings. Aristotle is credited with the initial conceptualization of QOL, defined as happiness, the good life, or the outcome of a life of virtue (Morgan, 1992). In the New Testament (John 10:10), Jesus stated that he came to give life and give it abundantly (The Lockman Foundation, 1995). The 10 stages of enlightenment in Buddhism start out with achieving joy in life (Stryk, 1968).

Pigou has been credited with modern introduction of the term in 1920 in his book on economics and welfare (Wood-Dauphinee, 1999). He discussed the need for governmental support for the lower class as a means of not only directly benefiting them financially, but also promoting the health of the national economy. Pigou's position and the term *quality of life* that he used to express it did not receive much attention. Politically, use of the concept, QOL, was limited until it was reintroduced in remarks made by Presidents Johnson and Nixon in speeches on environmental and social issues (Campbell, 1981; Dalkey, Rourke, Lewis, & Snyder, 1972).

QOL has its academic roots in the disciplines of psychology and sociology (Spranger, 2001). In the 1970s, these disciplines began to consider the issue of QOL. For instance, in 1978, the Ninth World Congress of Sociology introduced the concept as a topic of discussion (Szulai & Andrews, 1980). Also in the 1970s, the business world adopted the term *QOL* to make claims about the ability of a product to enhance a person's life in the milieu of everyday living.

The health care disciplines' recent interest in QOL can be traced to the work of the World Health Organization (WHO). The WHO's more-encompassing definition of health as physical, psychological, and social well-being, and not just the absence of illness or infirmity (World Health Organization, 1948), provided early impetus to the consideration of QOL as a relevant human experience for health care professionals. In 1978, the WHO provided a statement on the application of its definition of health, indicating that individuals have the right "to psychosocial care and adequate QOL in addition to physiologic care" (King & Hinds, 1998, p. xi). The documents "Healthy People 2000" and "Healthy People 2010," consistent with the goals identified by the WHO, have included not only disease- and disability-related issues, but also those concerned with QOL (Baker, 2000).

Nursing's interest in QOL is long standing. Florence Nightingale's involvement with the British military provided multiple examples of how nurses can promote the QOL for individuals. This interest has intensified and become a focus of research in the last 15 to 20 years. In 1991, the Oncology Nursing Society's Research Priority Survey identified QOL as its highest research priority (Mooney, Ferrell, Nail, Benedict, & Haberman, 1991).

Health-related quality of life, a subcategory of global QOL, is a more recent concept. Health care trends have contributed to the emergence of HRQOL as an important phenomenon. In the past 15 to 20 years, the concern for patients has become more inclusive, focusing not just on the treatment of disease, but also on the restoration and promotion of health (Read, 1993). With increased client longevity, health care professionals are attending to the lifestyle issues that accompany chronic disease and often affect QOL.

The Food and Drug Administration (FDA) is reflecting this changing emphasis. It can require documentation of not only the safety and efficacy of new products, but also their effect on a user's QOL (Spilker, 1996). In 1985, the guidelines for approval of antineoplastics included documentation of a favorable response in terms of QOL or survival (Johnson & Temple, 1985).

QOL has emerged as a concept of interest to many disciplines. This multiplicity of discipline-specific perspectives has led to little consensus on a definition. Philosophers consider the nature of existence and what is meant by the "good life." Ethicists are concerned with social utility. Economists pursue cost effectiveness in producing the greatest good. Physicians focus on health- and illness-specific issues, while nurses approach the issue of QOL more holistically (Anderson & Burckhardt, 1999).

DEFINITION OF THEORY CONCEPTS

QOL and the subconstruct HRQOL have suffered from a lack of clarity for both conceptual and operational definitions in research studies. Regrettably, some researchers published results of HRQOL outcome studies without first stating their conceptual definition of HRQOL. Similarly, several researchers have not accurately matched their conceptual definition with their operational definition. For example, researchers have inaccurately stated that they are measuring the broad construct of QOL but have instead operationalized QOL as an objective measure, such as *length of time without return to surgery* (Elkins, Knott-Craig, McCue, & Lane, 1997).

In the 1980s and early 1990s, many researchers reported outcomes as QOL or HRQOL but had only measured one domain, such as physical functional status. However, functional status is not interchangeable with the construct HRQOL and is most appropriately considered only one of several components contributing to overall HRQOL. Functional status has traditionally been defined by degree of disability to perform standard activities in life (Stineman, Lollar, and Ustun, 2005); a more detailed framework of functional status is provided by Leidy (1994). QOL is an even broader construct than HRQOL: inclusive of all life domains important to a person. The construct HRQOL developed as an entity separate from global QOL as a means of specifying health-related domains of particular interest to researchers (Wenger, Naughton, & Furberg, 1996). Its concepts "tend to cross different nursing fields and reflect a wide variety of nursing situations" (Meleis, 1997, p. 18).

Some authors have used the term *subjective health status* interchangeably with HRQOL, considering it a more accurate descriptor of the phenomenon (Staniszewska, 1998). However, Ferrans has recently categorized approaches to HRQOL measurement as *perceived status* or *evaluative* approaches to HRQOL (Ferrans, Zerwic, Wilbur, & Larson, 2005). HRQOL *perceived* status measures ask patients to rate their functional abilities, such as the commonly used SF-36 survey (Ware & Sherbourne, 1992) and the EORTC Quality of Life Questionnaire (Aaronson et al., 1993). Alternatively, HRQOL *evaluation* measures, such as the Ferrans and Power Quality of Life Index (Ferrans, 1990a) and the Quality of Life Scale for Cancer (Padilla et al., 1983) place less emphasis on the specific functional abilities as the patient's perception of how satisfied he or she is with his or her abilities or life domains. Both status and evaluation measures have a purpose in research; perceived status may be helpful in testing specific effects of an intervention, while evaluation may capture more personal judgments of life satisfaction based on internal expectations that are changeable within the individual. Some measures incorporate both status and evaluative approaches. Such is the case with the WHO Quality of Life Assessment, which covers physical, psychological, social, and spiritual domains, and as a result is quite lengthy (World Health Organization, 1995). The McGill Quality of Life Questionnaire uses evaluation approaches for its four domains, with additional status approaches for two of these domains (Cohen, Mount, Strobel, & Bui, 1995).

Despite significant confusion over related terminology, theorists and researchers have increasingly described the constructs of QOL and HRQOL as having three characteristics: HRQOL is multidimensional, temporal, and subjective. The multidimensional aspect of HRQOL (Aaronson et al., 1991; Faden & Leplege, 1992; Staniszewska, 1998) is reflected by the major life domains, commonly identified as physiological, psychological, and sociological (Padilla & Grant, 1985). Other investigators have stated that a spiritual domain is of importance (Ferrans & Powers, 1985; Cella & Tulsky, 1990). Recent publications have featured physical, psychosocial, spiritual, emotional, and cognitive/mental dimensions. Osoba (1994) has suggested that researchers can appropriately refer to their study as measuring HRQOL if at least three life domains received assessment.

HRQOL is temporal in nature—patients can change their self-perceptions as they experience events in everyday life and process what they feel are quality-of-life priorities (Sprangers & Schwartz, 1999; Peplau, 1994). Some scholars state that HRQOL is primarily subjective in nature but may include objective assessments at times (Oleson, 1990; Zhan, 1991). However, most researchers now consider HRQOL as subjective in nature (Cella, 1992; Cooley, 1998; Harrison, Juniper, & Mitchell-DiCenso, 1996; Murdaugh, 1997). Further investigation is needed for practical considerations related to ethical implications of allowing those other than the patients to make treatment decisions based on assumed HRQOL when the patients are unable to speak for themselves, such as those in vegetative states. Work has been done to test the validity of parallel administration of subjective HRQOL with proxy health status measures completed for patients by health care providers or family members (Addington-Hall & Kalra, 2001). Measures obtained by others would be most accurately referred to as proxy subjective health status or evaluation measures rather than HRQOL.

DESCRIPTION OF THE THEORY OF QUALITY OF LIFE AND HEALTH-RELATED QUALITY OF LIFE

There are many models of QOL or HRQOL (Cowan, Graham, & Cochrane, 1992; Ferrell, Grant, Dean, Funk, & Ly, 1996; Ferrans, 1990b; Oleson, 1990; Padilla & Grant, 1985; Zhan, 1992, as found in King & Hinds, 1998), most of which omit the relationship between specific interventions and the factors that affect HRQOL. Three seminal models of QOL were provided in the 1990s. Spilker (1996) provided an introductory framework for QOL in health care by illustrating QOL as a pyramid of three levels (Figure 13.1). A model by Ferrans & Powers (1993) also identified QOL as a main outcomes measure,

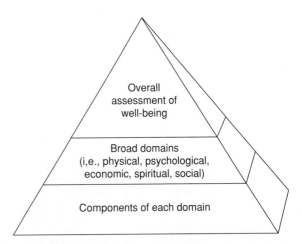

■ **Figure 13.1** Three levels of quality of life. From Spilker, B. (Ed.). (1996). *Quality of life and pharmacoeconomics in clinical trials* (2nd ed., p. 2). Philadelphia: Lippincott-Raven Publishers.

rather than HRQOL (Figure 13.2). However, HRQOL researchers have sometimes chosen to concentrate on specific parts of the model rather than the entire model. Researchers have adapted models for use according to the specific condition or population they wish to study (Sandau, Lindquist, Treat-Jacobson, & Savik, 2008). While technically a model may be designed to illustrate QOL, clinicians wishing to research the more limited construct of HRQOL have made adaptations. Researchers should provide clarity about how any adapted or abbreviated conceptual definition supports their selected operational measures.

Nurses Ferrans and Powers developed a theory in which they provided the seminal definition of QOL as a person's "sense of well-being that stems from satisfaction or dissatisfaction with the areas of life that are important to him/her" (Ferrans & Powers, 1992, p. 29). Because their model encompassed all major life domains, their resulting operational measure, the Ferrans & Powers QOL Index, is a global multidimensional measure designed to represent the comprehensive construct of QOL (Figure 13.2). The listed domains are health and functioning, socioeconomic, psychological/spiritual, and family.

A commonly cited model in health care disciplines is that of Wilson and Cleary (1995). Although both authors are physicians, the model combines the "social" paradigm with the "medical" paradigm. This model represents the relationships between the basic concepts of QOL (Figure 13.3). The model identifies five determinants that exist on a "continuum of increasing biological, social, and psychological complexity" (p. 60). These leveled determinants of QOL are referred to as taxonomy and consist of biological factors, symptoms, functioning, general health perceptions, and overall QOL. They are in turn influenced by characteristics of the individual and environment.

Sousa and colleagues tested the Wilson and Cleary model, using multiple linear regression path analysis to evaluate the variables for empirical linkages to overall QOL (Sousa, Holzemer, Henry, & Slaughter, 1999). They reported that data were consistent with the theory, and reported a 32% variance in overall QOL among their sample of persons with HIV. However, biological and physiological variables provided the weakest correlations with the other variables, suggesting little influence. The authors indicate that further research is necessary into areas such as other potential influences of personality, motivation, and social and economic supports, as well as the influences of time over the model (Sousa et al., 1999). Sousa and Chen (2002) have continued work using structural equation modeling to address conceptual issues of HRQOL. The Wilson and Cleary model encompasses several large constructs as variables, so theory testing the model in its entirety is an intensive feat and is rarely done.

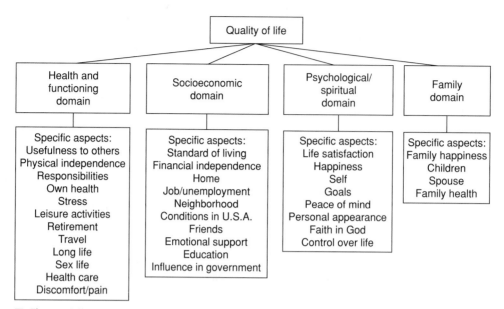

■ **Figure 13.2**   Quality of life framework. From Ferrans, C. E. (1990). Quality of life: Conceptual issues. *Seminars in Oncology Nursing, 6*(4), 248–254.

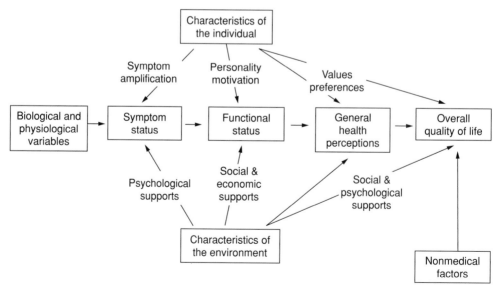

■ **Figure 13.3**   HRQOL conceptual model. From Wilson, I. B., & Cleary, P. D. (1995). Linking clinical variables with health-related quality of life. *JAMA, 273*(1), 60.

Anderson and Burckhardt (1999) suggest that a major limitation of the Wilson and Cleary model is that the medical factors seem central, rather than the nonmedical factors, to the overall QOL. Similarly, Murdaugh (1997) contends that the Wilson and Cleary model may be more accurately referred to as a taxonomy of patient outcomes due to its continuum of intuitively linked pathways with little empirical support. The majority of variance for overall QOL was unexplained, and many questions remain. Further study of relationships between other variables that can be affected by independent nursing interventions affecting QOL and HRQOL (such as resiliency, self-efficacy, and hope) and interventions is encouraged.

Wilson and Cleary have described the arrows in the figure to represent the dominant causal relationships without excluding reciprocal connections between either adjacent or nonadjacent components of the model. Recently, Ferrans and nursing colleagues published a revision to the Wilson and Cleary model (Ferrans, Zerwic, Wilbur, & Larson, 2005), in which they made three major changes: (a) added arrows to show that biological function is influenced by characteristics of the environment and individual, (b) deleted nonmedical factors, and (c) deleted labeling on arrows, which tends to restrict relationships.

Work by Padilla and Grant (1985) occurred as early as the above models, but aside from the oncology realm, appears to have been less recognized among health disciplines. Their work deserves discussion because it offered one of the first QOL models to specifically include independent nursing process interventions as a component in the formal model (Figure 13.4). These include caring attitude, specific nursing interventions, and promotion of self-care. These interventions are perceived by the patient and influence outcome variables that can be categorized by QOL dimensions. For example, the nursing interventions to promote healthy body image in a patient with a new colostomy can influence the patient's

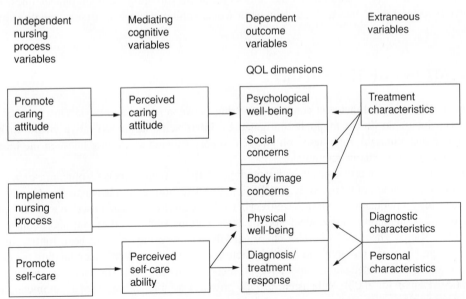

■ **Figure 13.4** A model of the relationship between the nursing process and the dimensions of quality of life. From Padilla, G. V., & Grant, M. M. (1985). Quality of life as a cancer nursing outcome variable. *Advances in Nursing Science, 8*(1), 45–60.

overall QOL by contributing to enhanced or maintained body image. Extraneous variables are recognized in the model, such as the individual's prognosis and personal characteristics, and whether the colostomy is temporary or permanent.

Nurse researchers Haase and colleagues (Haase, Heiney, Ruccione, & Stutzer, 1999) used a mixed-methods approach to first derive a conceptually valid understanding of what QOL is by interviewing adolescents and then develop a measurement tool. Qualitative methods of phenomenology, simultaneous concept analysis, focus groups, and thematic analysis were used to generate their Adolescent Resilience Model. The authors defined QOL as a sense of well-being but measured it based on self-transcendence, mastery, and self-esteem. Testing of the model began by administering existing quantitative instruments and used structural equation modeling. The model consisted of six indirectly measured variables: awareness of condition; ways of coping; relationships with others; spirituality, hope, and spiritual perspective; being courageous; and the outcome variable of QOL. Work continues on this model as the authors study influences of stage of illness and combination of variables into higher-order factors to provide a better fit in the model (Haase et al., 1999).

For their model, nurse researchers Stuifbergen and colleagues (2000) used structural equation modeling to test the selected factors influencing health-promoting behavior or QOL in persons with chronic disabling conditions. QOL was defined as "an individual's overall sense of health, well-being, and satisfaction with life" (2000, p. 124). A complex interaction of contextual factors (severity of illness being most dominant), antecedent variables, and health-promoting behaviors all contributed to QOL in their proposed model. Interventions to enhance mediating factors of social support, acceptance, decreased barriers to self-efficacy, and increased self-efficacy for health behavior can contribute to health-promoting factors and enhanced QOL. The purposeful use of concepts that are currently being tested in nursing makes this model unique to nursing and within the scope of independent nursing interventions. Additionally, Leplege and Hunt (1997) commend the authors for acknowledging the interconnectedness of QOL with other aspects of existence such as changes in work, coping strategies, personal relationships, and self-image.

APPLICATIONS OF THE THEORY

Dudgeon (1992) suggested that past conflicts occurring between nurses and physicians over the care of patients with incurable illness might be mitigated by interdisciplinary cooperative efforts to improve HRQOL. Interdisciplinary efforts based on HRQOL theory provide a bridging between the biomedical and illness models of medicine and nursing.

HRQOL measurement provides an understanding of the patient-perceived outcome experience of chronic illness, evaluation of a procedure, medication, or other intervention between groups, among individuals, or between populations. More recently, HRQOL measures have been used to evaluate efforts of health promotion, including independent nursing interventions such as education and counseling (see Using Middle Range Theories 13.1). Use of formal HRQOL measures has not been routine in clinical practice. The gap between research and clinical practice is fed by the lack of understanding the definition of HRQOL and lack of understanding that HRQOL measures are not "soft" measures but helpful in clinical practice (Rumsfeld, 2002). Rubenstein (1996) provides a table summary of recommendations for incorporating routine and symptom-specific HRQOL screenings into office practice. Mcclane (2006) recommends three specific HRQOL measures for use by clinical nurse specialists in routine clinical assessment of elderly persons.

13.1 USING MIDDLE RANGE THEORIES

Harrison and colleagues conducted a 12-week, prospective, randomized controlled trial to evaluate the effect of transitional care on HRQOL, rates of readmission, and emergency room use of patients with heart failure ($n = 157$). The nurse-led intervention included education and support for self-management for a period of 2 weeks after hospital discharge. HRQOL was operationalized by using both a generic health status (SF-36) and disease-specific measure (Minnesota Living with Heart Failure [MLHFQ]) questionnaire. At 6 weeks after hospital discharge, the overall MLHFQ score was better among the patients randomized to receive the nurse-led intervention than among the usual care patients. However, there was no significant difference in any of the subscales for the SF-36. At 12 weeks after discharge, more of the control group had been readmitted compared to the intervention group (31% vs. 23%); and significantly more of the usual care group visited the emergency department compared with the transitional group (46% vs. 29%). This study provides evidence-based support for nurse-led interventions to successfully improve HRQOL.

The article, like many published in clinical journals, lacked a conceptual definition for HRQOL. However, the authors are to be commended for attempting to address whether or not the statistically significant improvements on the MLHFQ could be considered clinically significant. The authors added a "minimally clinical importance difference" (MCID) analysis, which they defined as a 5-point or greater change in the total MLHFQ score. Relative changes in score between baseline and 12 weeks postdischarge were compared for both groups; the most contrast in scores was with the MLHFQ emotional dimension, where improvement was 36% for the transitional group (vs. <1% for the control group). Finally, the fact that the generic SF-36 scores were not improved, while the MLHFQ scores were improved, highlights the importance of knowing one's sample and selecting a measure that will be sensitive to changes expected by a particular intervention in a select population.

Harrison, M. B., Browne, G. B., Roberts, J., Tugwell, P., Gafni, A., & Graham, A. D. (2002). QOL of individuals with heart failure: A randomized trial of the effectiveness of two models of hospital-to-home transition. *Medical Care, 40*(4), 271–282.

INSTRUMENTS USED IN EMPIRICAL TESTING

Categories of Measurement

Measurement tools for HRQOL can be categorized in a variety of ways. For example, one category of measure is based on the number of life domains that are encompassed within the measure. If a tool is designed to examine a full spectrum of life domains, it may be considered global. Global tools are important because they may show QOL changes in all domains of life. Heart failure, for example, may have a pervasive effect on patients' ability to generate income, socialize, and be sexually intimate. The Minnesota Living with Heart Failure (Rector, Kubo, & Cohen, 1987) questionnaire attempts to capture a global perspective of the impact of a specific disease on various domains of life. In contrast to global measures, another category is that of measures targeting a single domain,

Table 13.1 MEASURES COMMONLY USED TO ASSESS HRQOL

TYPE	EXAMPLES
Generic measures	Ferrans & Powers Quality of Life Index (Ferrans & Powers, 1992) WHOQOL Assessment Tool (World Health Organization, 1995) Nottingham Health Profile (Hunt, McEwan, & McKenna, 1985) SF-36 (Ware & Sherbourne, 1992) EuroQOL (EuroQOL Group, 1990) Sickness Impact Profile (Bergner et al., 1991)
Disease-specific, condition-specific, and treatment-specific measures	Ferrans & Powers Quality of Life Index—Cancer Version (Ferrans, 1990) Minnesota Living With Heart Failure (Rector, Kubo, & Cohen, 1987) Seattle Angina Questionnaire (Spertus et al., 1995) The Arthritis Impact Measurement Scales (Meenan, 1992) Children's Health Survey for Asthma (Sullivan et al., 1995) Quality of Life Index: Hemodialysis (Ferrans & Powers, 1993) QLQ-C30 Version 3.0 is the generic measure that can be supplemented with disease specific modules (Breast, Lung, Head & Neck, Oesophageal, Ovarian, Gastric, and Cervical Cancers, and Multiple Myeloma) (Aaronson et al.,1993)
Symptom-specific measures	McGill Pain Questionnaire (Melzack, 1975) Hospital Anxiety and Depression Scale (Zigmond & Snaith, 1983)
Quality-adjusted life-year (QUALY), health utilities, and time trade-off measures	EQ-5D (Agt, Essink-Bot, Krabbe, & Bonsel, 1990) Time Without Symptoms or Toxicity (Q-TWIST) (Gelber et al., 1996)
Qualitative measures	Interviews Focus groups Preference-based with interview script

such as psychological health, as is offered by the Hospital Anxiety and Depression Scale (Zigmond & Snaith, 1983).

Another method of categorizing HRQOL measures is according to purpose or targeted population of a measure (Table 13.1). Generic tools, while not specific to disease or treatment, are helpful for making comparisons across studies and between populations (Guyatt, Feeny, & Patrick, 1993). The Nottingham Health Profile has been commonly used in the United Kingdom as a generic tool but is also considered global because of its broad coverage of various life domains (Hunt, McEwan, & McKenna, 1985). The

SF-36, which is a generic measure of subjective health status, provides two main summary scores for self-perceived physical and mental functioning, as well as eight more specific health scales (Ware & Sherbourne, 1992).

Recently, researchers have tended toward augmenting general measures with disease- or condition-specific measures in order to capture both overall health status and perceived effects of a certain condition (Bliven, Green, & Spertus, 1998). Disease-, condition-, or symptom-specific tools provide more sensitivity than generic tools for clinicians looking for changes in disease patterns, such as frequency of loose stools or angina. Similarly, use of treatment or therapy-specific tools is helpful to care providers in evaluating specific responses by individual patients to treatments or changes as a result of intervention (see Using Middle Range Theories 13.1).

A quality-adjusted life-year (QUALY) instrument is used by some researchers to measure the extent of health improvement due to an intervention combined with the costs associated with the intervention, resulting in a mathematical formula that is used to assess their relative worth of the intervention from an economic perspective (Phillips & Thompson, 2007). For example, a year of perfect health may be worth a score of 1, but a year of less than perfect health life expectancy may be worth −1 point, and death may be worth 0 points. These measures are somewhat controversial and limited in chronic illness, where QOL is more important than survival, and limited by heterogeneity in the samples being measured (Phillips & Thompson, 2007). They are used most often in pharmacoeconomic studies.

Finally, qualitative measures are valuable for development of theoretical definitions and new HRQOL measures, as well as for validity testing of an existing tool in a new or changing population. Quality measures may be used to augment a quantitative measure. Typically, qualitative methodologies in HRQOL include personal interviews and focus groups, with possible open-ended questions. It must be noted, however, that categorization of measures may vary because some measures can be categorized in more than one way.

Guidelines for Measurement

Investigators selecting measures for HRQOL studies must make sure they have a clear conceptual definition of HRQOL, and their selection of operational measures should match. Unfortunately, this has not always been the case in the early surge of HRQOL studies. An investigator attempting to measure HRQOL among hospice patients should consider which domains are conceptually important, or have been shown in past research or through clinical experience, to be impacted in that population. For example, an HRQOL investigator wishing to assess HRQOL among hospice patients would appropriately select a measure that includes the spiritual domain, or augment a generic measure with assessment of subjective spiritual status. Similarly, if an investigator plans to use a generic HRQOL measure among patients undergoing treatment for prostate cancer, this generic measure would most appropriately be augmented by a subjective measure that includes self-evaluation of the social and sexual dimensions.

Gill and Feinstein (1994) provided guidelines for proper measurement of HRQOL, including allowing patients to rate the importance of domains, as in the Ferrans and Power QOL Index (1992). Gill and Feinstein also recommended allowing patients to supplement standardized measures. While supplementing quantitative measures with qualitative measures may not be feasible in every study, this practice may provide a test of content validity to the quantitative measure. Study participants may alert investigators of important concerns that were not addressed on the quantitative questionnaire. Similarly, qualitative research in HRQOL, such as interviews, focus groups, and journaling, may provide foundational information for researchers striving to measure HRQOL in a previously understudied population. Although Gill and Feinstein encouraged HRQOL investigators to provide an aggregate score so that study results can be compared with others, some debate the conceptual clarity of mathematically combining several measures to produce an artificially aggregated score. However, obtaining a global satisfaction measure in addition to disease-specific measures may be helpful for comparing results for specific interventions in a discrete population.

Researchers studying HRQOL must be prepared to address challenges in psychometric properties among the vast variety of measures available. Challenges to reliability include aberrancies in data collection (such as one research assistant giving more extensive coaching to some participants than others), the absence of a baseline HRQOL measure, and the use of only pieces of HRQOL measures (unless they have been tested for reliability as a subset). Challenges to validity in HRQOL research include potential concurrent life changes. For example, an investigator wishing to study the effect of an intervention for back pain may have confounding results when a generic HRQOL measure is complicated by a life change in a participant (e.g., loss of spouse) that is unrelated to the treatment for back pain. Practical considerations in use of HRQOL measures include timing of study measures. For example, if one is evaluating the effects of a major surgery on HRQOL, it may not be appropriate to obtain measures while the patient is still recovering from postoperative incisional pain, unless the investigator's intention is a purposeful longitudinal assessment. Other practical considerations include subject burden (length of the survey) and clinical relevance (what degree of change in a score will be considered clinically significant). Further discussion of desired psychometric properties of HRQOL measures are provided by DeVon and Ferrans (2003). In summary, selection of a measure includes finding a good match with one's conceptual definition of HRQOL, identifying the life domains and concerns most important to the study population, being clear on the research purpose, investigating past performance of the measure for validity and reliability, and evaluating feasibility of the measure.

HEALTH-RELATED QUALITY OF LIFE AS AN OUTCOME MEASURE IN NURSING

The goal of nursing interventions in HRQOL research is to have a positive impact on a patient's perceived satisfaction with HRQOL (see Research Application 13.1). This is a central component of HRQOL in that the patient provides a subjective and personal expression of both the level of satisfaction (Staniszewska, 1998) and the degree to which the specific nursing interventions contribute to that level (Robinson, Whyte, & Fidler, 1997). Thus, patient-perceived satisfaction with HRQOL becomes a significant indicator of the success of an intervention. Patient satisfaction is conceptualized as a mediating variable, based on the work of Donabedian (1980), who has consistently regarded patient satisfaction as an outcome. He believes that satisfaction with care represents the patient's judgment of quality of care (Yang, Simms, & Yin, 1999, p. 3).

Nursing researchers investigating HRQOL often use approaches and interventions from other models and theories, allowing connections to be made between HRQOL and these models or theories. For instance, Stuifbergen, Seraphine, and Roberts (2000) related health-promoting behaviors from Pender's theory with HRQOL as an outcome. HRQOL as a middle range theory allows for concurrent application of theories that support health within illness, a concept thread that runs through

13.1 RESEARCH APPLICATION

A nurse researcher was interested in determining if the inclusion of a nurse-run education and peer-support group improved the outcomes for elementary-school-aged asthmatics. Using a prospective research design, in an asthma clinic, the researcher matched patients by age, nature and severity of symptoms, and treatment regimens. The patients were randomly assigned to either group involvement or no group involvement. Before treatment began, the nurse researcher administered the Pediatric Asthma Quality of Life Questionnaire (AQOLQ-P, see Appendix B) to a new patient, a 10-year old male. The patient was asked to identify the life domains most affected by the asthma, and he selected "activity limitations" domain, which included riding his bicycle, playing recreational baseball and playing tag with his friends. The patient also chose the "symptoms" domain, and he identified getting a good night's sleep and being disturbed at school with coughing. The nurse then completed the administration of the AQOLQ-P.

The patient, through random selection, was placed in the experimental treatment group. The group met weekly for 3 months. At the end of the 3-month period, the patient returned to the asthma clinic, and the nurse researcher readministered the questionnaire, addressing the same domains that were assessed the first time. Any changes in the ratings fell along a continuum from positive to negative, with positive indicating that a desired outcome relating to HRQOL was achieved. The individual patient data were grouped with other data, and, through statistical analysis, the researcher determined if the group treatment made a statistically significant difference in the quality of life outcomes in elementary-school-aged children diagnosed with asthma.

the work of Peplau, Rogers, Parse, Newman, and others (Moch, 1989; Newman, 1984; Parse, 1994; Peplau, 1994; Rogers, 1970). Ferrans concludes, "A disability that makes life not worth living to one person may only be a nuisance to another" (Ferrans, 1990b, p. 252).

SUMMARY

HRQOL is subjective, multidimensional, and temporal. As an interdisciplinary middle range theory, HRQOL is particularly well matched to nursing because it involves measurement of variables that have traditionally been important to nursing, that is, holistic consideration of the person's responses to real or potential illness. Quality of life is a concept with a long history, which has, in the last 15 to 20 years, become of interest to a number of disciplines. Models of the middle range theory, HRQOL, often comprise three components: 1) *Life domains* refer to the areas of life being affected by a specific condition; 2) *interventions* involve the actions taken to bring about a desired outcome, an improved quality of life; and 3) *perceived satisfaction* is the patient's subjective appraisal of well-being. Nurses wishing to understand the impact of a condition on their patients or to judge the effectiveness of an illness treatment can make use of this middle range theory and the instruments designed to measure it.

ANALYSIS OF THEORY

Using the criteria presented in Chapter 2, critique the theory Health-Related Quality of Life. Compare your conclusions about the theory with those found in Appendix A. A researcher who has worked with the theory completed the analysis found in the appendix.

Internal Criticism
1. Clarity
2. Consistency
3. Adequacy

4. Logical development
5. Level of theory development

External Criticism
1. Reality convergence
2. Utility
3. Significance
4. Discrimination
5. Scope of theory
6. Complexity

CRITICAL THINKING EXERCISES

1. Does HRQOL have subjective and objective components?
2. What are the underlying assumptions and potential ramifications of having proxy subjective health status or evaluation measures for children or those unable to speak for themselves?

3. Should further measurement tools only be accepted if based on commonly accepted conceptual definitions?
4. What are appropriate ways for researchers to test validity of HRQOL measures within their population? (Should an HRQOL measure be tested against an objective health status measure?)

WEB RESOURCES

1. The mission statement included on the official Web site of the International Society for Quality of Life reads: "The scientific study of Quality of Life relevant to health and healthcare is the mission of the International Society for Quality of Life Research (ISOQOL). The Society promotes the rigorous investigation of health-related quality of life measurement from conceptualization to application and practice. ISOQOL fosters the worldwide exchange of information through scientific publications, international conferences, educational outreach, and collaborative support for HRQOL initiatives." The site can be reached at: **http://www.isoqol.org/**.
2. The European Organisation for Research and Treatment of Cancer Group (EORTC) has view-

able portions of its generic HRQOL measure, with validated modular supplements for other diseases, at: **http://www.eortc.be/home/qol/**
3. This site is sponsored by the Sigma Theta Tau Nursing Honor Society Virginia Henderson Library. Type "quality of life" in the search engine box under library search: **http://www.nursinglibrary.org/portal/main. aspx** Included are abstracts of graduate work from nurse researchers, along with their contact information.
4. American Thoracic Society states that "This site was designed for researchers, clinicians, industrial groups, and other interested parties who wish to learn about patient-oriented quality of life (QOL) measures that are useful in the study and management of respiratory disease." This site can be accessed at: **http://www.atsqol.org/**.

5. Maintained by the Public Health Foundation, this site is mainly concerned with providing information about the program "Measuring Healthy Days." It can be found at: **http://www.phf.org/measuringhealthydays.htm.**
6. The official site of the Centers for Disease Control and Prevention offers a search in which one can enter quality of life, yielding many related articles. It can be accessed at: **http://www.cdc.gov/index.htm.**
7. The World Health Organization provides related articles and a broad perspective on cultural influences on QOL. Type "quality of life" in the search engine, which offers articles as well as various editions and language translations of the WHO-QOL tool. They can be accessed at: **http://www.who.int/en/.**

REFERENCES

Aaronson, N. K., Ahmedzai, S., Bergman, B., Bullinger, M., Cull, A., Duez, N., et al. (1993). The European Organization for Research and Treatment of Cancer QLQ-C30: A quality-of-life instrument for use in international clinical trials in oncology. *Journal of the National Cancer Institute, 85,* 365–376.

Addington-Hall, J., & Kalra, J. (2001). Measuring quality of life: Who should measure quality of life? *BMJ, 332,* 1417–1420.

Agt, H. M. V., Essink-Bot, M. L., Krabbe, P. F., & Bonsel, G. J. (1994). Test-retest reliability of health state valuations collected with the EuroQol questionnaire. *Social Science Medicine,* 1537–1544.

Anderson, K. L., & Burckhardt, C. S. (1999). Conceptualization and measurement of quality of life as an outcomes variable for health care intervention and research. *Journal of Advanced Nursing, 29*(2), 298–306.

Baker, F. (2000, Winter). Assessing the quality of life of cancer survivors. *The Behavioral Measurement Letter, 7,* 2–12.

Benner, P. (1985). Quality of life: a phenomological perspective on explanation, prediction, and understanding in nursing science. *Advances in Nursing Science, 8*(1), 1–14.

Bergner, M., Bobbitt, R. A., Carter, W. B., & Gilson, B. S. (1981). The Sickness Impact Profile: Development and final revision of a health status measure. *Medical Care, 19,* 787–805.

Bliven, B. D., Green, P., & Spertus, J. A. (1998). Review of available instruments and methods for assessing QOL in anti-anginal trials. *Drugs & Aging, 13*(4), 311–320.

Campbell, A. (1981). The sense of well being in America. New York: McGraw Hill.

Cella, D. F. (1992). Quality of life: The concept. *Journal of Palliative Care, 8*(3), 40–45.

Cella, D. F., & Tulsky, D. S. (1990). Measuring quality of life today: Methodological aspects. *Oncology, 4*(5), 29–38.

Cohen, S. R., Mount, B. M., Strobel, M., & Bui, F. (1995). The McGill Quality of Life Questionnaire: A measure of quality of life appropriate for people with advanced disease. *Palliative Medicine, 9,* 207–291.

Cooley, M. E. (1998). Quality of life in persons with non-small cell lung cancer: A concept analysis. *Cancer Nursing, 21*(3), 151–161.

Cowan, M. J., Young Graham, K., & Cochrane, B. L. (Jan 1992). Comparison of a theory of quality of life between myocardial infarction and malignant Melanoma: a pilot study. *Progress in Cardiovascular Nursing, 7* (1), 18–21.

Dalkey, N. C., Rourke, D. L., Lewis, R., & Snyder, D. (1972). Studies in the quality of life, delphi and decision making. Toronto: Lexington Books, D.C. Heath and Company.

DeVon, H. A., & Ferrans, C. E. (2003). The psychometric properties of four quality of life instruments used in cardiovascular populations. *J of Cardiopulmonary Rehabilitation, 23*(2), 122–138.

Donabedian, A. (1980). The definition of quality and approaches to its assessment. Ann Arbor, MI: Health Administration Press.

Dudgeon, D. (1992). QOL: A bridge between the biomedical and illness models of medicine and nursing? *Journal of Palliative Care, 8*(3), 14–17.

Elkins, R. C., Knott-Craif, C. J., McCue, C., & Lane, M. M. (1997). Congenital aortic valve disease: Improved survival and quality of life. *Annals of Surgery, 225*(5), 503–511.

European Organisation for Research and Treatment of Cancer Group (EORTC) QOL. QOL questionnaire. *QLQ-C30.* Retrieved January 22, 2007, from http://www.eortc.be/home/qol.

EuroQol Group. (1990). EuroQol-A new facility for the measurement of health-related QOL. *Health Policy, 16,* 199–208.

Faden, R., & Leplege, A. (1992). Assessing quality of life, moral implications for clinical practice. *Medical Care, 30*(5, Supplement), 166–175.

Ferrans, C. E. (1990a). Development of a quality of life index for patients with cancer. *Oncology Nursing Forum, 17,* 15–19.

Ferrans, C. E. (1990b). Quality of life: Conceptual issues. *Seminars in Oncology Nursing, 6*(4), 248–254.

Ferrans, C., & Powers, M. (1985). Quality of Life Index: Development and psychometric properties. *Advances in Nursing Science, 8,* 15–24.

Ferrans, C., & Powers, M. (1992). Psychometric assessment of the Quality of Life Index. *Research in Nursing and Health, 15,* 29–38.

Ferrans, C. E., & Powers, M. J. (1993). QOL of hemodialysis patients. *ANNA Journal, 20*(5), 575–582.

Ferrans, C. E., Zerwic, J. J., Wilbur, J. E., & Larson, J. L. (2005). Conceptual model of health-related QOL. *Journal of Nursing Scholarship, 37*(4), 336–342.

Ferrell, B. R., Grant, M., Dean, G. E., Funk, B., & Ly, J. (1996). "Bone tired": The experience of fatigue and its impact on quality of life. *Oncotology Nursing Forum, 23,* 1539–1547.

Gelber, R. D., Goldhirsch, A., Cole, B. F., Wieand, H. S., Schoeder, G., & Krrok, J. E. (1996). A quality-adjusted time without symptoms or toxicity (Q-TWiST) analysis of adjuvant radiation therapy and chemotherapy for resectable rectal cancer. *Journal of the National Cancer Institute, 88*(15), 1039–1045.

Gill, T., & Feistein, A. (1994). A critical appraisal of the quality-of-life measurements. *JAMA, 272,* 619–620.

Guyatt, G. H., Feeny, D. H., & Patrick, D. L. (1993). Measuring health-related quality of life. *Annals of Internal Medicine, 118,* 622–628.

Haase, J. E., Heiney, S. P., Ruccione, K. S., & Stutzer, C. (1999). Research triangulation to derive meaning-based quality-of-life theory: Adolescent resilience model and instrument development. *International Journal of Cancer, 12,* 125–131.

Harrison, M. B., Juniper, E. F., & Mitchell-DiCenso, A. (1996). Quality of life as an outcomes measure in nursing research: "May you have a long and healthy life." *Canadian Journal of Nursing Research, 28*(3), 49–68.

Hunt, S. M., McEwen, J., & McKenna, S. P. (1985). Measuring health status: A new tool for clinicians and epidemiologists. *Journal of the Royal College of General Practitioners, 35,* 185–188.

Johnson, J. R., & Temple, R. (1985). Food and Drug Administration requirements for approval of new anticancer therapies. *Cancer Reports, 69,* 1115–1157.

King, C., & Hinds, P. (1998). Quality of life. Sudbury, MA: Jones & Bartlett Publishing.

Leidy, N. K. (1994). Functional status and the forward progress of merry-go-rounds: Toward a coherent analytic framework. *Nursing Research, 43,* 196–202.

Leplege, A., & Hunt, S. (1997). The problem of quality of life in medicine. *JAMA, 278,* 47–50.

The Lockman Foundation (Eds.). (1995). New American Standard Bible. Chicago: Moody Press.

McClane, K. S. (2006). Screening instruments for use in a complete geriatric assessment. *Clinical Nurse Specialist, 20*(4), 201–206.

Meenan, R. F., Mason, J. H., Anderson, J. J., Guccione, A. A., & Kazis, L. E. (1992). AIMS2. The content and properties of a revised and expanded Arthritis Impact Measurement Scales Health Status Questionnaire. *Arthritis and Rheumatism, 35*(1), 1–10.

Meleis, A. I. (1997). Theoretical nursing: Development and progress. (3rd ed.). Philadelphia: Lippincott-Raven.

Melzack, R. The McGill Pain Questionnaire: Major properties and scoring methods. *Pain, 1,* 277–299.

Moch, S. D. (1989). Health within illness: Conceptual evolution and practice possibilities. *Advances in Nursing Science, 11*(4), 23–31.

Mooney, K. H., Ferrell, B. R., Nail, L. M., Benedict, S. C., & Haberman, M. R. (1991). 1991 *Oncology Nursing Society Research Priorities Survey. Oncology Nursing Forum,* 18(8), 1381–1388.

Morgan, M. L. (1992). Classics of moral and political theory. Indianapolis, IN: Hacket.

Murdaugh, C. R. (1997). Health-related quality of life as an outcome in organizational research. *Medical Care, 35*(11) Suppl., NS41–N48.

Newman, M. A. (1984). Nursing diagnosis: looking at the whole. *Am J Nsg, 85,* 1496–1499.

Oleson, M. (1990). Subjectively perceived quality of life. *Image: Journal of Nursing Scholarship, 22*(3), 187–190.

Osoba, D. (1994). Lessons learned from measuring health-related quality of life in oncology. *Journal of Clinical Oncology, 12,* 199–220.

Padilla, G. V., & Grant, M. M. (1985). QOL as a cancer nursing outcome variable. *Advances in Nursing Science, 8*(1), 45–60.

Padilla, G. V., Presant, C., Grant, M. M. Metter, G., Lipselt, J., & Heide, F. (1983). Quality of life index for patients with cancer. *Research in Nursing and Health, 6*(3), 117–126.

Parse, R. R. (1994). Quality of life: Sciencing and living the art of human becoming. *Nursing Science Quarterly, 7*(1), 16–20.

Peplau, H. E. (1994). Quality of life: an interpersonal perspective. *Nursing Science Quarterly, 7*(1), 10–15.

Phillips, C., & Thompson, G. (2007). What is a QALY? *Hayward Medical Communications, Vol. 1*(6). Retrieved January 22, 2007, from http://www.evidence-based-medicine.co.uk/what_is_series.html.

Read, J. L. (1993). The new era of quality of life assessment. In S. R. Walker & R. M. Rosser, *Quality of life assessment: Key issues in the 1990s* (pp. 3–10). London: Kluwer Academic Publishers.

Rector, T. S., Kubo, S. H., & Cohen, J. N. (1987). Patients' self-assessment of their congestive heart failure. Part 2: Content, reliability and validity of a new measure, the Minnesota Living with Heart Failure questionnaire. *Heart Failure, Oct./Nov.,* 198–209.

Robinson, D., Whyte, L., & Fidler, I (1997). Quality of life measures in a high security environment. *Nursing Standard, 11*(49), 34–37.

Rogers, M. E. (1970). *An introduction to the theoretical basis of nursing.* Philadelphia: FA Davis Co.

Rubenstein, L. V. (1996). Using QOL tests for patient diagnosis or screening, or to evaluate treatment. In B. Spilker (Ed.), *QOL and pharmocoeconomics in clinical trials* (2nd ed., pp. 362–372). Philadelphia: Lippincott-Raven Publishers.

Rumsfeld, J. S. (2002). Health status and clinical practice: when will they meet? (editorial). *Circulation, 106*(1), 5–7.

Sandau, K. E., Lindquist, R. A., Treat-Jacobson, D., & Savik, K. (2008). Health-related quality of life and subjective neurocognitive function three months after coronary artery bypass graft surgery. *Heart & Lung.*

Sousa, K. H. (1999). Description of a health-related quality of life conceptual model. *Outcomes Management for Nursing Practice, 3*(2), 78–82.

Sousa, K. H. & Chen, F. F. (2002). A theoretical approach to measuring quality of life. *J of Nsg Measurements, 10*(1), Spring/Sumer, 47–58.

Sousa, K. H., Holzemer, W. L., Henry, S. B., & Slaughter, R. (1999). Dimensions of health-related quality of life in persons living with HIV disease. *Journal of Advanced Nursing, 29*(1) 178–187.

Spertus, J. A., Winder, J. A., Dewhurts, T. A., Deyo, R. A., Prodzinski, J., McDonell, M., et al. (1995). Development and evaluation of the Seattle Angina Questionnaire: A new functional status measure for coronary artery disease. *Journal of the American College of Cardiology, 25*(2), 333–341.

Spilker, B. (1996). Quality of life and pharmaco economics in clinical trials. (2nd ed.). New York: Lippincott-Raven.

Spranger, M. J. (2001). International Society of Quality of Life Newsletter 6(1). Retrieved June 15, 2001 from www.ISOQOL.org

Sprangers, M. A. G., & Schwartz, C. E. (1999). Integrating response shift into health-related quality of life research: A theoretical model. *Social Science and Medicine, 48*(11), 1507–1515.

Staniszewska, S. (1998). Measuring quality of life in the evaluation of health care. *Nursing Standard, 12*(17), 36–39.

Stineman, M. G., Lollar, D. J., & Ustun, T. B. (2005). International classification of functioning, disability, and health: ICF empowering rehabilitation through an operational bio-psycho-social model. In J. A. DeLisa (Ed.), *Physical medicine and rehabilitation principles and practice* (pp. 1099–1108). Philadelphia, PA: Lippincott Williams & Wilkins.

Stryk, L. (1968). World of Budha: A reader. Garden City, NY: Doubleday.

Stuifbergen, A. K., Seraphine, A., & Roberts, G. (2000). An explanatory model of health promotion and quality of life

in chronic disabling conditions. *Nursing Research, 49*(3), 122–129.

Sullivan, S. A., & Olson, L. M. (1995). Developing condition-specific measures of functional status and well-being for children. *Clinical Performance and Quality Health Care, 3*, 132–138.

Szulai, A., & Andrews, F. M. (Eds.) (1980). The quality of life. London: Sage Publications.

Ware, J. E., & Sherbourne, C. D. (1992). The MOS 36-item short-form health survey (SF-36). *Medical Care, 20*, 473–483.

Wenger, N. K., Naughton, M. J., & Furberg, C. D. (1996). Cardiovascular disorders. In B. Spilker (Ed.), *Quality of life and pharmacoeconomics in clinical trials* (2nd ed., pp. 883–891). Philadelphia: Lippincott-Raven.

Wilson, I. B., & Cleary, P. D. (1995). Linking clinical variables with health-related quality of life. *JAMA, 273*(1), 59–65.

Wood-Dauphinee, S. (1999). Assessing quality of life in clinical research: From where have we come and where are we going? *Journal of Clinical Epidemiology, 55*, 355–363.

World Health Organization. (1948). Constitution of the World Health Organization. Chronicle of the World Health Organization, 1(1/2), 13.

World Health Organization. (1995). The World Health Organization Quality of Life Assessment (WHOQOL): Position paper from the World Health Organization. *Social Science and Medicine, 41*, 1403–1409.

Yang, K., Simms, L. M., & Yin, J. (1999, August 3). Factors influencing nursing-sensitive outcomes in Taiwanese nursing homes. Journal of Issues in Nursing. Retrieved June 14, 2001 from www. nursingworld.org.

Zhan, L. (1991). Quality of life: Conceptual and measurement issues. *Journal of Advanced Nursing, 17*, 795–800.

Zhan, L. (1992). Quality of life: Conceptual and measurement issues. *Journal of Advanced Nursing, 17*(7) 795–800.

Zigmond, A. S., & Snaith, R. P. (1993). The hospital anxiety and depression scale. *Acta Psychiatrica Scandinavica, 67*, 361–370.

BIBLIOGRAPHY

Ferrans, C. E. (1992). Conceptualizations of QOL in cardiovascular research. *Progress in Cardiovascular Nursing, 2*(7), 2–6.

King, C. R., & Hinds, P. S. (2003). *QOL: From nursing and patient perspective.* Sudbury, MA: Jones and Bartlett Publisher, Inc.

McDowell, I., & Newell, C. (1996). *Measuring health: A guide to rating scales and questionnaires* (2nd ed.). New York: Oxford University Press, Inc.

Health Promotion

■ MARJORIE COOK MCCULLAGH

DEFINITIONS OF KEY TERMS

Activity-related affect	Subjective feelings associated with the health-promoting activity
Commitment to a plan of action	A commitment to carry out a health-promoting behavior. The plan should be specific to time and place, and specify whether it will be with specified persons or alone.
Health-promoting behavior	Behaviors or actions that people carry out with the intention of improving their health
Immediate competing demands	Distracting ideas about other things that must be done (e.g., childcare) immediately prior to the intention to carry out a health-promoting behavior
Immediate competing preferences	Distracting ideas about other attractive activities to engage in (e.g., shopping) immediately prior to engaging in a health-promoting behavior
Interpersonal influences	Beliefs concerning the behaviors, beliefs, or attitudes of others regarding a health-promoting behavior. Ideas include social norms, social support, and modeling.
Perceived benefits of action	Beliefs about the positive or reinforcing consequences of a health-promoting behavior
Perceived barriers to action	Beliefs about the unavailability, inconvenience, expense, difficulty, or time-consuming nature of a health-promoting behavior
Perceived self-efficacy	A person's judgment of his or her own abilities to accomplish a health-promoting behavior
Personal factors: biological, psychological, sociocultural	Factors about the person that influence health-promoting behavior. Examples of biological factors are age, body mass index, and aerobic capacity. Examples of psychological factors are

(Key Terms continued on next page)

DEFINITIONS OF KEY TERMS continued

	self-esteem, self-motivation, and perceived health status. Examples of sociocultural factors are race, ethnicity, acculturation, education, and socioeconomic status. The variables may be specific to each health-promoting activity (i.e., factors influencing healthy dietary behaviors may not be the same as those affecting exercise behavior).
Prior related behavior	Experience with the health-promoting behavior
Situational influences	Beliefs about the situation or context of the health-promoting behavior. These ideas may include perceptions of the available options, demand characteristics, and esthetic features of the environment in which a given behavior is proposed to take place.

INTRODUCTION

Nurses, as well as many other health professionals, are interested in learning more about how they can help their patients, families, and communities improve their lives. In seeking a way to bring greater longevity and a higher quality of life, some nurses are attracted to interventions that enhance health and quality of living. The Health Promotion Model has achieved popularity among nurses as a model that serves this purpose.

Health promotion has many benefits. The benefits of living a healthier lifestyle exceed prevention of disease, and include greater vigor and a subjective feeling of wellness. While these benefits can be enjoyed by the individual, society as a whole also profits from health promotion when people create personal and family lifestyles that are consistent with economic prosperity and interpersonal harmony. Health promotion can decrease social problems, such as violence, suicide, and sexually transmitted diseases. Further, health promotion has the potential to significantly decrease health care costs in the years ahead.

Health promotion is a concept well suited to the needs and interests of nurses and their clients. Nurses commonly work in schools, churches, homes, workplaces, and health care agencies. Many of these settings are ideal locations for the promotion of health. Nurses are skilled in many areas that are necessary for health promotion, such as education, counseling, and advocacy. For example, a parish nurse may offer classes to congregational members in a variety of health-related topics such as parenting and caring for aging family members. A school nurse may facilitate self-help group meetings for bereaved children. An occupational health nurse may advocate for inclusion of mental health services in employee health benefit packages. In addition, clients are likely to be receptive to nursing interventions to promote health, because they trust nurses and are accustomed to seeking the assistance of these professionals in dealing with their health care needs.

HISTORICAL BACKGROUND

During the past century, the major cause of health problems has shifted from infectious diseases to chronic illness. Many chronic illnesses are closely related to lifestyle factors such as diet, exercise, and stress management. In order to improve the health of a population experiencing high rates of chronic illness, it is apparent that changes in lifestyle factors are required.

Nola Pender first published her Health Promotion Model in 1982. It was subsequently revised (Pender, 1996) and published most recently in the fifth edition of *Health Promotion in Nursing Practice* (Pender, Murdaugh, & Parsons, 2006). The revised model incorporates additional concepts and relationships. These revisions to the model (first published in the third edition), based on recent research and theoretical considerations, were made to increase its explanatory power and its potential for use in structuring health-promoting nursing interventions.

PENDER'S DEFINITION OF HEALTH

Nurses are accustomed to assessing their patients for evidence of disease or dysfunction. However, the assessment process commonly reflects a focus on illness, rather than health. This approach is limiting in several ways. First, it risks reducing the patient to a sum of his or her parts (e.g., respiratory, neurological, cardiovascular, etc.). Second, it fails to determine the meaning the client attaches to health and illness. This approach is a negative approach to health in that it views health as an absence of disease. Some consider health and illness to be opposite concepts. This way of thinking suggests that persons with disabilities and chronic illness and those who are near death cannot achieve health. However, many nurses experienced in working with these clients may oppose this view. Negative approaches to health as the absence of illness are inadequate for health professionals at a time that they are increasingly concerned with quality of life and healthy longevity.

Pender's (1990; Pender et al., 2006) definition of health is positive, comprehensive, unifying, and humanistic. She believes that health includes a disease component, but does not make disease its principal element. Her definition of health encompasses the whole person and his or her lifestyle, and includes strengths, resiliencies, resources, potentials, and capabilities. Pender defines health as the actualization of inherent and acquired human potential through goal-directed behavior, competent self-care, and satisfying relationships with others, while adjustments are made as needed to maintain structural integrity and harmony with relevant environments (Pender et al., 2006, p. 23).

A major strength of Pender's definition of health is that it offers an expanded view of health. This expanded view provides for greatly increased opportunities to improve client health, as it is not limited to absence of disease or even limitations in functioning or adaptation. For example, Pender's positive view of health permits the development of nursing interventions that are not limited to decreasing risks for disease, but are aimed at strengthening resources, potentials, and capabilities. This creates broader opportunities for nurses to assist individuals, families, and communities to achieve improved health, enhanced functional ability, and better quality of life.

Health Promotion

Health professionals have long recognized the benefits of early detection and treatment of illness, or secondary prevention. However, recently there has been increased appreciation for the role of primary prevention and health promotion in improving health and quality of life. Primary prevention involves activities aimed at the prevention of health problems before they occur and the avoidance of disease. An example of primary prevention is the administration of tetanus immunization to prevent tetanus infection. Health promotion is intended to increase the level of well-being and self-actualization of an individual or group. Examples of health promotion activities include physical activity and healthy nutrition.

While health promotion and primary prevention are distinct theoretical concepts, in practice they often overlap. Many activities directed toward health promotion will also have preventive effects. Indeed, many adults engage in healthy behaviors with the intent of increasing wellness and avoiding illness. For example, an adult may adopt a low-fat diet with dual purposes in mind. One intention may be to lower blood cholesterol and therefore prevent future cardiovascular problems (primary prevention, also referred to by Pender as health protection). An accompanying intention may be to gain the benefits of weight loss, such as feeling more energetic (health promotion). Other examples of health behaviors that may have both health promotion and preventive benefits include physical activity, adequate rest, and management of stress.

Health promotion is activity directed toward actualization of human potential through goal-directed behavior, competent self-care, and satisfying relationships with others, while adjustments are made as needed to maintain structural integrity and harmony with relevant environments (Pender et al., 2006, p. 7). The concept of health promotion is based on Pender's expanded definition of health that focuses on the whole person and promotes the positive aspects of health. This definition applies to all persons, including persons who are well and those who are experiencing an illness or disability.

Pender advocates the use of health promotion at a variety of levels and settings. Although health promotion is most commonly directed toward the individual, Pender suggests that interventions directed toward the family and community are most likely to be successful in creating a healthy society. Furthermore, Pender discusses health promotion in a variety of settings, including schools, workplaces, homes, and nurse-managed community health centers. In a broad sense, health promotion involves education, food production, housing, employment, and health care. It is multidimensional, encompassing individual, family, community, environmental, and societal health.

DESCRIPTION OF THE HEALTH PROMOTION MODEL

Pender's model is based on theories of human behavior. There is increased recognition of the role of behavior in primary prevention and health promotion, and there is increased attention among health professionals to helping clients adopt healthy behaviors. Motivation for healthy behavior may be based on a desire to prevent illness (primary prevention) or to achieve a higher level of well-being and self-actualization (health promotion). The Pender Health Promotion Model is primarily based on two theories of health behavior: expectancy value theory and social cognitive theory. The first, expectancy value theory, is based on work by Fishbein & Ajzen (1975). The theory explains that people are more likely to work toward goals that are of value to them. This proposition by Feather relates to Pender's proposition that people will engage in "behaviors from which they anticipate deriving personally valued benefits" (Pender et al., 2006, p. 53). Expectancy value theory also explains that people are more likely to invest their effort in goals that they believe are achievable and will result in the desired outcome.

The second parent theory is Bandura's (1986) social cognitive theory. A major tenet of social cognitive theory is self-efficacy. Self-efficacy is the confidence a person has in his or her ability to successfully carry out an action. Bandura's theory proposes that the greater a person's self-efficacy for a behavior, the more likely the person will engage in it, even when faced with obstacles. The concept of self-efficacy is one of the behavior-specific cognitions of Pender's model. Pender's belief is that when a person has high perceived competence or self-efficacy in a certain behavior, it results in a greater likelihood that the person will commit to action and actually perform the behavior.

Some have observed that the Health Promotion Model (HPM) resembles the Health Belief Model (HBM). While it is true that the HPM shares some concepts with the HBM, the HPM differs from the HBM in at least one important way. The HPM is a competence- or approach-oriented model that focuses on attainment of high-level wellness and self-actualization. This is contrasted with the HBM, which was intended for use in explaining patients' use of medical diagnosis and treatment of disease, such as tuberculosis. Further, the HBM incorporates fear or threat of disease as a motivation for action. While this perspective may be valid for diseases that have shorter prodromal periods, the HPM does not consider fear or threat as a powerful motivation for distant threats to health.

The Health Promotion Model has undergone a modification since its initial introduction in 1982. The original model has been examined in a variety of research studies that use model-based hypotheses to test the validity of relationships proposed by the model. These studies of the model have taken place in a variety of settings, health behaviors, and populations. The results of these studies have been mixed. Some studies have demonstrated that the model has been very useful in explaining or predicting health-promoting behavior in a group of research participants. For example, in a study by Kerr, Lusk, and Ronis (2002), Health Promotion Model concepts explained 55% of the variance in use of hearing protection among Mexican American industrial workers. Results of studies in which a large proportion of variance in behavior is explained, such as that by Kerr and colleagues, provide support to the model.

Some study results have been less successful in explaining client behavior. For example, in a study of preadolescents and adolescents, Garcia and colleagues (1995) were able to explain only 19% of the variance in exercise behavior. Garcia suggested the need for addition of concepts to the model in order to increase its predictive power. Pender (1996) analyzed the empirical support provided by each of the studies based on the model. This analysis resulted in the retention of selected model concepts and the deletion of others. In addition, three new concepts and associated relationships have been added to the model. The newly added concepts include prior related behavior, immediate competing demands and preferences, and commitment to a plan of action.

The revised model (Pender, 1996; Pender, Murdaugh, & Parsons, 2002, 2006) consists of individual characteristics and experiences, behavior-specific cognitions and affect, and other factors leading to the behavioral outcome. Pender identifies the behavior-specific cognitions and affect as the major motivational mechanisms for health promotion behavior. These include perceived benefits of action, perceived barriers to action, perceived self-efficacy, activity-related affect, interpersonal influences, and situational influences. Individual characteristics and experiences included in the model include prior related behavior and personal factors. The additional concepts of the model include immediate competing demands and preferences, commitment to a plan of action, and health-promoting behavior. These concepts are briefly described in Definitions of Key Concepts, which appears earlier in this chapter. Relationships of the concepts are described in the model's theoretical propositions (Box 14.1). The schematic representation of the model (Figure 14.1) shows the relationship of model concepts to the behavioral outcome, health-promoting behavior.

The model includes multiple concepts and relationships. However, some concepts and relationships may be more salient than others to a given health behavior. The model does not provide assistance in selecting which concepts and relationships are appropriate for specific behaviors. Therefore, the researcher who seeks to use the model should select concepts and relationships based on previous research, theoretical foundations, clinical experience, or practical limitations in regard to a specific behavior. Indeed, extant research using the Health Promotion Model shows the selectivity of researchers in determining which model concepts to include in their study designs.

BOX 14.1 Theoretical Propositions of the Health Promotion Model

- Prior behavior has "both direct and indirect effects on the likelihood of engaging in health-promoting behaviors. Prior behavior indirectly influences health-promoting behavior through perceptions of self-efficacy, benefits, barriers, and activity-related affect" (p. 52).
- Personal factors (such as age, self-esteem, and socioeconomic status) may influence cognitions, affect, and health behaviors.
- "Perceived benefits directly motivate behavior as well as indirectly motivate behavior through determining the extent of commitment to a plan of action to engage in the behaviors from which the anticipated benefits will result" (p. 53).
- "Perceived barriers to action affect health-promoting behavior directly by serving as blocks to action as well as indirectly through decreasing commitment to a plan of action" (p. 53).
- "The more positive the affect, the greater the perceptions of efficacy is present. Self-efficacy influences perceived barriers to action, with higher efficacy resulting in lowered perception of barriers. Self-efficacy motivates health-promoting behavior directly by efficacy expectations and indirectly by affecting perceived barriers and level of commitment or persistence in pursuing a plan of action" (p. 54).
- "Activity-related affect influences health behavior directly as well as indirectly through self-efficacy and commitment to a plan of action" (p. 54).
- "Interpersonal interaction influences health-promoting behavior directly as well as indirectly through social pressures or encouragement to commit to a plan of action" (p. 55).
- "Situational influences directly influence health behavior, and indirectly influence health behavior through commitment to a plan of action" (p. 56).
- "Commitment to a plan of action propels the individual into and through the behavior unless a competing demand that cannot be avoided or a competing preference that is not resisted occurs" (p. 56).

Source: Pender, N., Murdaugh, C., & Parsons, M. (2006). *Health promotion in nursing practice* (5th ed.). Upper Saddle River, NJ: Prentice Hall. Used with permission.

IMPLICATIONS OF THE MODEL FOR CLINICAL PRACTICE

The Health Promotion Model offers a conceptual framework for the provision of effective nursing care directed at improved health and functional ability. First, the model provides a method for the assessment of client health-promoting behaviors. The model directs nurses to systematically assess clients for their perceived self-efficacy, perceived barriers, perceived benefits, interpersonal influences, and situational influences that are relevant to the selected health behavior.

Second, the model identifies several additional client characteristics as targets for assessment. These client characteristics include prior behavior, demographic characteristics, and perceived health status. While these characteristics are not amenable to alteration, they offer a basis for tailoring of nursing interventions, as discussed below.

Third, the model suggests that nursing interventions can be designed to alter clients' perceptions in these areas. Success in these interventions is expected to result in more frequent health behaviors and resultant improved wellness.

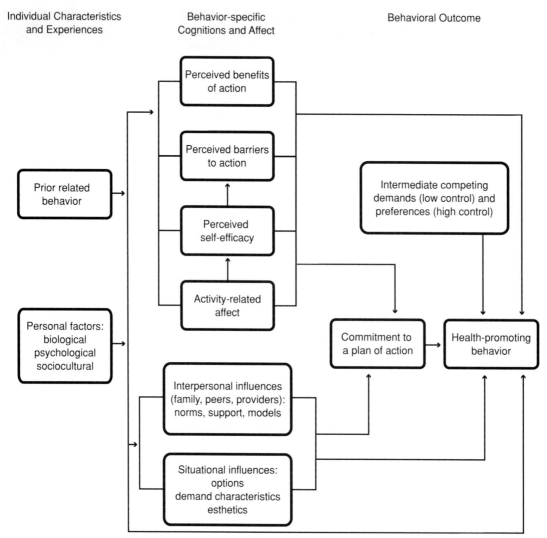

■ **Figure 14.1** Health promotion model. Source: Pender, N., Murdaugh, C., & Parsons, M. (2006). *Health promotion in nursing practice* (5th ed.). © Reprinted by permission of Pearson Education, Inc., Upper Saddle River, NJ.

Although the model identifies foci for nursing interventions, it does not explicitly describe how nurses can effect changes in client perceptions. While these nursing interventions directed at changing client perceptions are proposed by the Health Promotion Model, few studies that test the effectiveness of these proposed interventions have been completed.

Pender prescribes use of the nursing process as the method of producing behavior change. She emphasizes nursing assessment of health, health beliefs, and health behavior using established frameworks, such as North American Nursing Diagnosis Association (NANDA) and Gordon's functional health patterns. In addition, she recommends use of model-based assessments such as the Health Promoting Lifestyles

Profile II (HPLP-II). Pender emphasizes use of the nursing process in empowering self-care across the life span. She outlines a multistep process for health planning that includes reinforcing client strengths, developing a plan based on client preferences and Prochaska and colleagues' (1994) stages of change, addressing facilitators and barriers, and committing to goals.

Areas of intervention for health promotion include exercise, nutrition, stress management, and social support. Pender et al. (2002) review several interventions in each of these areas, many of which are research based, but not model based. These are directed toward increasing the client's capacity for a vigorous and productive life.

Use of the Health Promotion Model in Tailoring Nursing Interventions

Model variables, such as client characteristics, cognitions, and affect, may be used to tailor nursing interventions to clients. Tailoring of interventions involves shaping of health messages based on characteristics unique to that person. Tailoring interventions has been found to increase intervention effectiveness (Strecher et al., 1994, Velicer, Prochaska, & Redding, 2006). The innovative intervention strategy offers exciting opportunities for designing health promotion interventions that are designed to meet the unique needs of each individual client. Once the nurse assesses the client on each of the relevant factors of the model, this information can be used to custom-design a health promotion program for that individual client. Recent applications of the Health Promotion Model have used computers to quickly and accurately assess the health of the client on model-based variables. With the help of computer technology, the nurse has used this information to design a health promotion intervention that is unique to the needs of this individual (Lusk, Kerr, Ronis, & Eakin, 1999). This computer-assisted approach offers nurses the opportunity to provide interventions that are more appropriate to the individual, and may, as a result, greatly enhance intervention effectiveness.

Selecting the Health Promotion Model

Nurses are faced with selecting among a variety of models for use in clinical practice and research. This selection may be based on a variety of factors, including philosophy, research, clarity, and utility.

The Health Promotion Model is appealing to many nurses because it offers a view of health consistent with their motivation for pursing the profession of nursing. Its holistic and humanistic view is congruent with many nurses' own personal philosophy of health and nursing. The model reflects a belief that persons are capable of introspection and are capable of personal change. In turn, the model proposes that health care is more than treatment and prevention of disease, but involves creating conditions where clients can express their unique human potential. The nurse is presented as an agent for creating behavioral and environmental changes.

The Health Promotion Model has been used successfully in several research studies, as discussed earlier in this chapter. While some models have been tested more extensively, the Health Promotion Model does have a body of extant literature that provides support for its use. A more thorough discussion of studies using the Health Promotion Model is presented in Pender's fifth edition (Pender et al., 2006). Examples of research applications of the Health Promotion Model are presented in Research Application 14.1 and Using Middle Range Theories 14.1 and 14.2.

Most nurses will find that the Health Promotion Model is straightforward and easy to understand. It uses terms that are readily comprehended, and its propositional statements are presented clearly. The phenomena addressed by the model are familiar to nurses, and most nurses will require minimal learning of new terms and concepts in order to use and understand the model. The model is clearly presented in graphic form.

The Health Promotion Model has been used in a variety of settings, including schools, workplaces, ambulatory treatment facilities, a rehabilitation center, and a prison. Its use has been with a wide variety of health behaviors, including exercise, nutrition, and use of hearing protection. The studies have involved diverse clients in regard to gender and age. The model has a limited history of application in culturally diverse groups. However, samples of Korean, Taiwanese, Thai, and Japanese individuals have participated in prior studies. It is noteworthy that persons included as study participants have been well or experiencing chronic illness, such as HIV infection.

The Health Promotion Model has been used by nurses working in a variety of community-based settings, such as occupational health and public health. The model is well suited to clients whose health status is stable, and whose basic needs are met. Although Pender's definition of health is broad and encompasses persons who are experiencing illness, application of the Health Promotion Model is untested in acute care settings and with clients whose health concerns are urgent or living conditions are unstable.

14.1 RESEARCH APPLICATION

An occupational health nurse was interested in improving the health status of employees through implementation of a fitness program. A baseline assessment of employee health was offered to a random sample of 397 employees; the Health Promotion Model-based assessment consisted of a survey of health behaviors, personal factors, perceived barriers to exercise, perceived benefits of exercise, self-efficacy, situational influences, and interpersonal influences. The survey was supplemented with selected physical measurements, including height, weight, body mass index, blood pressure, and serum cholesterol. Employee health care claims were also monitored. A review of a summary of employee survey results revealed that the major barrier to fitness for this group included a perception that fitness programs were too time consuming. One situational influence that many employees shared was the lack of year-round access to exercise facilities.

The occupational health nurse planned a multifocal fitness promotion program that featured policy development and health education based on survey responses. The educational interventions included worksite classes, paycheck inserts, and an employee health newsletter. These educational interventions included suggestions for incorporating physical activity into routine activities, such as walking and climbing stairs. The nurse was also successful in obtaining a group discount for employees at a local health club.

After a 6-month period, the survey and physical measures were readministered to employees, and results were compared. Moderate reductions in employee perceptions of barriers to exercise and situational influences on exercise were achieved. Employee participation in exercise was found to increase from an average of 48 to 65 minutes per week. In addition, average serum cholesterol levels were found to drop from 231 to 218 mg/dL, and a 22% difference in health care claims was observed between participants and nonparticipants.

The nurse plans to continue the program, with the goal of improving employee self-efficacy for exercise while continuing to monitor for effects on exercise behavior and health outcomes.

14.1 USING MIDDLE RANGE THEORIES

Although Mexican-American workers are vulnerable to occupationally based noise-induced hearing loss, researchers know little about factors that influence the use of hearing protection among this population. This study was designed to identify the factors that influence Mexican-American workers' use or nonuse of hearing protection devices (HPDs). The Pender Health Promotion Model (HPM) provided the theoretical framework for this study.

A total of 119 noise-exposed workers from three garment manufacturing plants in the southwestern United States completed written questionnaires in English measuring HPM concepts and demographic variables. These concepts included health-related behavior (use of hearing protection), interpersonal influences, situational factors, perceived control of health, perceived self-efficacy, definition of health, perceived health status, perceived benefits, and perceived barriers.

Use of hearing protection among workers ranged from 72% (among workers required to use HPDs) to 27% (among workers not required to use hearing protection). Path analysis using multiple regression was used to estimate the magnitude of relationships between the variables. This resulted in five concepts directly relating to HPD use: health conception, benefits, barriers, self-efficacy, and perceived health status. Indirect influences acting through self-efficacy were education level and interpersonal influences. These results suggest that in order to influence Mexican American workers' use of HPDs, nurses should promote benefits of use, decrease perceived and actual barriers to use, support self-efficacy in use, and relate concept of health to HPD use. Nurses can also influence HPD use by supporting interpersonal influences. These might include role models, social norms in the work setting, and encouraging use. Workers with lower education may particularly be influenced by increased self-efficacy in using hearing protection.

Kerr, M. J., Lusk, L. L., Ronis, D. L. (2002). Explaining Mexican-American workers' hearing protection use with the health promotion model. *Nursing Research, 51*(2), 100–109.

14.2 USING MIDDLE RANGE THEORIES

Improvements in diet and physical activity can significantly modify women's risk for chronic conditions such as obesity, cardiovascular disease, diabetes, osteoporosis, and some cancers. By understanding the determinants of these behaviors, nurses can design interventions to modify these behaviors and subsequently improve women's health. Walker and colleagues sought to describe the cognitive-perceptual determinants of physical activity and healthy eating among midlife and older rural women.

Walker and colleagues studied physical activity and healthy eating among 177 rural women aged 50 to 69. Following recruitment by telephone, participants visited a data collection center to complete computer-based questionnaires and individual health assessments based on the Pender Health Promotion Model.

The researchers found that greater perceived self-efficacy, benefits, and interpersonal support and fewer perceived barriers were associated with better diet and activity. Results of this study are being used to inform the "Wellness for Women" trial intervention. This intervention seeks to compare the effectiveness of tailored and generic newsletters in facilitating the adoption and maintenance of healthy eating and exercise.

Walker, S. N., Pullen, C. H., Hertzog, M., Boeckner, L., & Hageman, P. A. (2006). Determinants of older rural women's activity and eating. *Western Journal of Nursing Research, 28*(4), 449–468.

Table 14.1   **HEALTH PROMOTION MODEL INSTRUMENTS**

INSTRUMENT	FIRST AUTHOR (DATE)	DESCRIPTION
Health-Promoting Lifestyles Profile II (HPLP-II)	Walker, 1997	52-item questionnaire in a 4-point response format measures the frequency of health-promoting behaviors in six domains (health responsibility, physical activity, nutrition, spiritual growth, interpersonal relations, and stress management).
HPLP—Spanish Version	Walker, Kerr, Pender, & Sechrist, 1990	This instrument provides a Spanish language version of the HPLP.
HPLP—Japanese Version	Wei et al., 2000	This instrument provides a Japanese language version of the HPLP.
Exercise Benefits/Barriers Scale (EBBS)	Sechrist, Walker, & Pender, 1987	This Likert scale measures the person's perceived benefits to undertaking preventive behaviors that reduce risk factors in coronary artery disease.
Perceived Self-Efficacy of Hearing Protector Use Scale	Lusk, 1997	This 10-item scale asks respondents to rate the extent to which they have confidence in their ability to use hearing protection. An example of an item from this scale is, "I am sure I can use my hearing protection so it works effectively."
Perception of Accessibility and Availability of Hearing Protectors Scale	Lusk, 1997	This 9-item scale asks respondents to report on this dimension of situational factors influencing health behavior. A sample item from this scale is, "Ear plugs are available to pick up at my job sites."
Interpersonal Influences on Hearing Protector Use Scale	Lusk, 1997	This scale includes three subscales measuring dimensions of these variables: interpersonal norms, interpersonal modeling, and interpersonal support. The Interpersonal Norms Subscale includes 4 items that query respondents about their beliefs as to how much others (family members, friends, supervisors, and coworkers) think they should wear hearing protection. The Interpersonal Support Subscale measures encouragement or praise from family, friends, coworkers, and supervisors about the respondents' use of hearing protection. The Interpersonal Modeling Subscale measures how much they believe others use hearing protection when exposed to noise.

Measurement of Model Concepts

Instruments have been developed to measure a variety of concepts related to the Health Promotion Model. Primary of these is the Health Promoting Lifestyles Profile II (Susan Walker, personal communication, June 24, 2002). Due to the broad nature of the model, many instruments have been developed to measure behavior-specific attitudes and beliefs. A sample of these is described in Table 14.1. Examples of research instruments designed to measure selected model variables can be found on the following web site: http://www.nursing.umich.edu/faculty/penderinstruments/researchinstruments.html.

SUMMARY

Pender has proposed a model of health promotion to guide nurses in helping clients achieve improved health, enhanced functional ability, and better quality of life. The need for behavioral and environmental changes to effect improvements in a society where lifestyle factors account for a large proportion of health problems provides justification for the model. The model is based on established theories of human behavior, including expectancy value theory and social cognitive theory. The Health Promotion Model claims that a variety of client characteristics and cognitive–affective factors combine with competing demands and preferences as well as commitment to a plan of action to explain the likelihood of health-promoting behavior. The model has been tested in several clinical studies using a variety of settings, health behaviors, and client characteristics. It presents exciting possibilities for the creation of interventions that are tailored to the unique characteristics and needs of individual clients.

The model was revised in 1996 following review and analysis of results of model testing and intervention effectiveness research based on the model. While the authors expect the revised model to have greater explanatory and predictive power, this is as yet untested by multiple scientific studies. The model authors acknowledge the need for development of measures of model concepts that fit the target population and the design of robust interventions that can change model beliefs and, subsequently, health outcomes. Interventions that address not only individuals, but also families and communities in creating multilevel interventions employing the Health Promotion Model in combination with community action models are most likely to achieve success.

ANALYSIS OF THEORY

Using the criteria presented in Chapter 2, critique the Health Promotion Model. When you are finished, you can compare your ideas about the model with those of a researcher who has worked with the model (found in Appendix A).

Internal Criticism
1. Clarity
2. Consistency

3. Adequacy
4. Logical development
5. Level of theory development

External Criticism
1. Reality convergence
2. Utility
3. Significance
4. Discrimination

CRITICAL THINKING EXERCISES

The Pender Health Promotion Model identifies benefits and barriers as factors influencing health behavior. Consider clients from your own clinical practice.

1. What are the barriers to and benefits of adopting a selected healthy behavior, such as exercise?

2. Generate several questions designed to elicit specific information about your clients' perceptions of their barriers and benefits.

How can you use this information to improve the effectiveness of your efforts to influence your clients' adaptation of healthy behaviors?

WEB RESOURCES

1. The Canadian Public Health Association, together with Health and Welfare Canada and the World Health Organization, sponsors a page that describes a charter for action to achieve "Health for All" by the year 2000 and beyond. The site can be accessed at: **http://www.hc-sc.gc.ca/hcs-sss/pubs/care-soins/2001-frame-plan-promotion/index_e.html.**

2. This link provides information about the World Health Organization Department of Noncommunicable Diseases and Health Promotion (NCD) and its global conferences on health promotion. The goal of this agency is to reduce the incidence of NCDs and promote positive health and well-being, with particular focus on developing countries. Access this site at: **http://www.who.int/hpr/index.htm#Our department's work.**

3. Healthy People 2010 is the prevention agenda for the nation. It is a statement of national health objectives designed to identify the most significant preventable threats to health and establish national goals to reduce these threats. Find this site at: **http://www.health.gov/healthypeople/.**

4. The Combined Health Promotion Database is a service of the National Center for Chronic Disease Prevention and Health Promotion (part of the Centers for Disease Control and Prevention). The stated goal of this agency is to collect and provide health promotion/health education information emphasizing methodology and the application of effective health promotion and education programs and risk reduction interventions. Find this site at: **http://www.cdc.gov/cdp/he. htm.**

5. The National Council on Aging sponsors the Health Promotion Institute. The Institute accomplishes its mission through advocating for and empowering older adults to achieve health and well-being through a multidisciplinary approach. To find this site, go to: **http://www.ncoa.org/content.cfm?sectionid=37.**

6. Many universities have schools of public health, nursing, medicine, and related fields that offer a variety of resources (e.g., research, teaching, service programs) related to health promotion. An example of one of these is the Center for Health Promotion and Disease Prevention at the University of North Carolina at Chapel Hill (HPDP). Find this site at: **http://www.hpdp.unc.edu/.**

7. The AHRQ's mission includes both "translating research findings into better patient care and providing policymakers and other health care leaders with information needed to make critical health care decisions." This site includes information about improving health care and prevention research. Find this site at: **http://www.ahcpr.gov/news/focus/index.html.**

8. The American Public Health Association (APHA) is a professional association of researchers, health service providers, administrators, teachers, and other health workers. This site includes a rich resource of selected Internet resources for health education and health promotion. Go to: **http://www.apha.org/programs/additional.**

9. Many state health departments sponsor health promotion programs for their residents, and include related information on their home pages. One example is the Minnesota Department of Health, located at: **http://www.health.state.mn.us/index.html.**

10. Dr. Pender maintains a web site of FAQs about the HPM. See it at: **http://www.nursing.umich.edu/faculty/pender_nola.html.**

REFERENCES

Bandura, A. (1997). *Self-efficacy: The exercise of control.* New York: W. H. Freeman.

Fishbein, M., & Ajzen, I. (1975). Belief, attitude, intention and behaviour: An introduction to theory and research. Reading, MA: Addison-Wesley.

Garcia, A., Broda, M., Frenn, M., Coviak, C., Pender, N., & Ronis, D. (1995). Gender and developmental differences in exercise beliefs among youth and prediction of their exercise behavior. *Journal of School Health, 65*(6), 213–219.

Kerr, M., Lusk, S. L., & Ronis, D. L. (2002). Explaining Mexican-American workers' hearing protector use with the health promotion model. *Nursing Research, 51*(2), 100–109.

Lusk, S. L., Ronis, D. L., & Hogan, M. M. (1997). Test of the health promotion model as a causal model of construction workers' use of hearing protection. *Research in Nursing and Health, 20*(3): 183–94

Lusk, S., Kerr, M., Ronis, D., & Eakin, B. (1999). Applying the health promotion model to development of a worksite intervention. *American Journal of Health Promotion, 13*(4), 219–226.

Pender, N. (1990). Expressing health through lifestyle patterns. *Nursing Science Quarterly, 3*(3), 115–122.

Pender, N. (1996). *Health promotion in nursing practice* (3rd ed.). Stamford, CT: Appleton & Lange.

Pender, N., Murdaugh, C., & Parsons, M. (2002). *Health promotion in nursing practice* (4th ed.). Upper Saddle River, NJ: Prentice Hall.

Pender, N., Murdaugh, C., & Parsons, M. (2006). *Health promotion in nursing practice* (5th ed.). Upper Saddle River, NJ: Pearson Prentice Hall.

Prochaska, J., Velicer, W., Rossi, J., Goldstein, M., Marcus, B., Rakowski, W., et al. (1994). Stages of change and decisional balance for 12 problem behaviors. *Health Psychology, 13*(1), 39–46.

Sechrist, K., Walker, W., & Pender, N. (1987). Development and psychometric evaluation of the exercise benefits/barriers scale. *Nursing in Research and Health, 10*(6), 357–365.

Strecher, V. J., Kreuter, M., Den-Boer, D. J., Kobrin, S., Hospers, H. J., & Skinner, C.S. (1994). The effects of computer-tailored smoking cessation messages in family practice settings. *Journal of Family Practice, 39*(3): 262–270.

Velicer, W. F., Prochaska, J. O., & Redding, C. A. (2006). Tailored communications for smoking cessations: Past successes and future directions. *Drug and Alcohol Review, 25*, 49–57.

Walker, S., Sechrist, K., & Pender, N. (1997). The health-promoting lifestyle profile: Development and psychometric characteristics. *Nursing Research, 39*(5), 268–273.

Walker, S. N., Pullen, C. H., Hertzog, M., Boeckner, L., & Hageman, P. A. (2006). Determinants of older rural women's activity and eating. *Western Journal of Nursing Research, 28*(4), 449–468.

Walker, S., Kerr, M., Pender, N., & Sechrist, K. (1990). A Spanish language version of the health-promoting lifestyle profile. *Nursing Research, 39*(5), 268–273.

Wei, C. N., Yonemitsu, H., Harada, K., Miyakita, T., Omori, S., Miyabayashi, T., et al. (2000). Japanese language version of the health-promoting lifestyle profile. *Nippon Eiseigaku Zasshi, 54*(4), 597–606.

Acknowledgment

The author gratefully acknowledges the critical review by Dr. Nola Pender of the first edition of this chapter.

Deliberative Nursing Process

■ MERTIE L. POTTER

DEFINITION OF KEY TERMS

Automatic nursing process	Actions (visible behaviors) the nurse takes based on reasons other than the patient's immediate needs
Deliberative nursing process	Means by which the professional nurse purposefully explores with the patient the nurse's perceptions (stimulation of any one of the five senses), thoughts, and/or feelings related to the patient's immediate need for help
Dynamic nurse–patient relationship	Interactive contact/connection between nurse and patient, when the nurse begins to explore the meaning behind the patient's verbal and nonverbal behaviors
Immediate need for help	Requirement of the patient in a specific situation. Help for the need relieves or diminishes the patient's immediate distress or improves the patient's immediate sense of adequacy or well-being.
Nursing situation	Circumstance that involves a patient's behavior, the nurse's reaction (perceptions, thoughts, and feelings combined together), and the nurse's action (activity the nurse completes with or for the patient)
Patient distress	Feeling experienced by a patient when he or she cannot meet certain needs and is not helped in meeting such needs
Patient outcomes/product	Improved verbal and nonverbal patient behaviors that can result from the nurse's deliberative and effective action(s) with the patient
Validation	Ongoing process of exploring and determining with a patient if the nursing reaction was accurate and if the nursing action was helpful

INTRODUCTION

The birthing of Deliberative Nursing Process by Ida J. Orlando culminated in 1961, after a number of years laboring to define both the function and product of professional nursing (Orlando, 1961). The theory began to take shape through Orlando's experiences within nursing practice and nurse education. Orlando reviewed more than 2,000 anecdotal recordings of faculty, students, and nurses related to their interactions with patients and began to see patterns of effective and ineffective nursing process in various nurse–patient situations (Pelletier, 1976). Emerging from these early experiences, Deliberative Nursing Process since has matured into a significant, enduring, and practical nursing theory.

As a middle range theory, Deliberative Nursing Process has a limited number of variables and is limited in scope (McEwan, 2002; Walker & Avant, 1995). However, it is specific and adequate enough to apply and test in research and practice. Although categorized as a grand theory by some (Walker & Avant, 1995; Wills, 2002), Deliberative Nursing Process demonstrates the following middle range theory characteristics: comprehensive yet focused, generalizable, restricted in its concepts, clear in its propositions, and conducive to testable hypotheses (McEwan, 2002).

An unusual paradox within Deliberative Nursing Process is its proclivity toward both simplicity and complexity as a theory. This paradox partially explains the attractiveness of using this theory. Generally, it is straightforward in its presentation while being multifaceted in its applications. For example, developing a nurse–patient relationship that is dynamic and unique is not complicated. However, the dynamics of the nurse–patient relationship itself may be very complex (Orlando, 1961).

A unique feature related to development of this theory is the inductive manner in which Orlando defined effective nursing (Schmieding, 2002). Orlando determined effective nursing and ineffective nursing from her observations of "good" and "bad" nursing practice (Orlando, 1961, 1972; Pelletier, 1976; Schmieding, 1993a). From her observations of specific phenomena (nurse–patient interactions), Orlando identified relationships with other phenomena to develop propositions that led to the development of larger concepts and, ultimately, the theory (Johnson & Webber, 2001).

Orlando desired that nurses become educated to assist patients to express what help they actually need (Pelletier, 1967). Another distinctive feature of Deliberative Nursing Process is that patient input is critical. It is the nurse's professional responsibility to involve the patient in the process of identifying and meeting the patient's immediate needs for help (Orlando, 1961, 1972, 1990).

HISTORICAL BACKGROUND

The need for nurses to have a distinct body of knowledge to direct and enhance nursing practice and the movement of nursing toward becoming a profession were beginning to take place at the turn of the 20th century (Alligood, 2002). Orlando's Deliberative Nursing Process evolved during an era when nurses were attempting to distinguish nursing from other disciplines, and when psychiatric–mental health nurses were determining their place among nurses of other specialties. Deliberative Nursing Process came into being as Orlando realized that nursing needed to address three areas: "nurse–patient relationships, the nurse's professional role and identity, and the development of knowledge which is distinctly nursing" (Orlando, 1961, p. viii).

Orlando first published work related to this theory after she examined what made nursing interventions effective or ineffective. She asserted early on that effective nursing was "good nursing," and ineffective nursing was "bad nursing" (Orlando, 1976; Schmieding, 1993a). Although this terminology might not be acceptable during today's trend of political correctness and relativity, Orlando was bold in her assertion that nursing was either "good" or "bad." She also stressed that nursing needed to define exactly what "nursing" was, and contended that nursing could not be a profession unless it was able to distinguish what nurses did that was unique (Orlando, 1961).

Orlando was asked to determine what mental health principles were needed in a nursing curriculum. However, she became acutely aware during the project that professional nursing did not have a clear function or product. Nursing was at a crossroads. Orlando understood that nurses were unclear in their attempts to define what nursing was (Orlando, 1961). For someone concerned with meeting patients' immediate needs, here was an immediate need for nurses—to define and to distinguish nursing's function and product. She recognized that the patient and the patient's needs were getting lost in nurses' assumptions of what those needs were. During a project funded by the National Institute of Mental Health, Orlando began to examine nurses' interactions with patients.

Resolute in her mission, Orlando set forth in her later work to assist nurses further in defining what nursing is and what it should entail to distinguish it from other disciplines. Key goals became the following: to define the distinct professional function of nurses; to encourage nurses to assume authority to carry out that function; and to educate nurses to use process discipline (deliberative nursing process) to ensure that the product of nursing function involves the patient and others who impact the patient's care (Orlando, 1972). She developed a user-friendly theory that was readily understandable and broadly applicable.

Orlando held that "to nurse" and "nursing" were very different from "to doctor" and "doctoring" (Orlando, 1961, 1972; Orlando & Dugan, 1989). She asserted that doctors' orders are designed for patients, not nurses, and that nurses keep themselves on a dependent path when they focus on following doctors' orders rather than assisting patients to meet their needs for help, which may include the patient's needing to comply with doctors' orders (Orlando, 1987). Orlando contended that licensure authorizes nurses to fulfill a professional role, but authority is only implicit until the nurse engages in a process with the patient to meet the function of nursing, namely, to help the patient meet immediate needs for help that the patient is unable to meet on his or her own (Orlando, 1972).

Orlando suggested that the concept of "nursing" derives its meaning from the nursing of infants and the need to have someone nurture and assist infants in obtaining what they need from the environment to survive. She postulated that, at times, individuals might need assistance from others to obtain what is needed from the environment to meet their needs when they are unable to nurse themselves (Orlando, 1961, p. 4; Orlando & Dugan, 1989). Orlando (1972, 1987) distinguished the difference between lay and professional nursing by stating that a professional nurse is needed when a lay person cannot ensure that the patient's distress will be identified or relieved.

In some of her works, she questioned whether or not expanded roles of nursing should be considered in the realm of nursing or in the realm of doctoring at a lower cost (Orlando & Dugan, 1989). She used straightforward and uncomplicated language. She contemplated and encouraged nurses to discern what the words "to nurse" meant and referred to a dictionary to emphasize her point of what nursing should entail. She accepted Funk and Wagnall's definition of "to nurse" to mean "to encourage, to look after; to nourish, protect, and nurture; to give curative care to an ailment" (Orlando, 1987, p. 408).

Notably, Orlando was ahead of her time in her concern for and measurement of outcome variables. She promoted progressive ideas, such as defining professional nursing, employing critical thinking within the nursing process, involving the patient in the nursing process, and measuring patient outcomes. Orlando was aware that ineffective nursing activities impacted areas, such as nursing care costs, patient progress, material costs, and medication costs. She was concerned that nursing was acquiring too many nonprofessional tasks that would take the nurse away from helping the patient (Orlando, 1961). Always seeking patient involvement in the provision of nursing care, Orlando looked for a "helpful outcome" as validated with the patient to include "change in the behavior of the object indicating either relief from distress or that a solution to a living or work problem had been found" (Orlando, 1972, p. 61). She addressed work problems involving staff members as well as patient problems in her 1972 reported studies.

Work on Deliberative Nursing Process theory has spanned more than a half-century. Orlando's initial development on this theory began in the early 1950s, and work on the theory's development continues. Her early works referred to the "deliberative nursing process." Orlando began using the term *nursing process discipline* in 1972 because she asserted that nursing process was a discipline that could be learned (Orlando, 1972, p. 2). The term *deliberative nursing process* will be used throughout this chapter for consistency.

It is obvious in both her published and unpublished writings that Orlando is not only an intensely passionate individual about nursing, but also a determined advocate for nursing (Orlando, 1961, 1972, 1976, 1983, 1987). Several basic tenets come through strongly in her work, primarily: (a) the function of nursing is to meet the patient's immediate need for help when the patient is unable to do so without the nurse's help; and (b) that the product of nursing is to relieve the patient's distress caused by the immediate need for help and to be able to observe improvement either verbally or nonverbally (Orlando, 1961, 1972). Furthermore, Orlando's theory promotes the uniqueness of nurses and maintains that patients must be involved in the identification and determination of their immediate needs for help (Orlando, 1961). Orlando was not hesitant to express her grave concern with the definition of nursing promoted in the American Nurses Association Social Policy Statement of 1980—she found "no operational meaning" in it and no differentiation between professional and lay nursing (Orlando, 1983, p. 2). Her passion for nursing continues to be evident, and her assertion that the profession still needs to define nursing persists (I. J. Orlando, personal communication, June 24, 2002).

DEFINITION OF THEORY CONCEPTS

Deliberative Nursing Process

Deliberative Nursing Process remains relevant and significant as a nursing theory due to its patient-focused approach; nurse exploration of nurse perceptions, thoughts, and feelings with patients; and effective outcomes that result from its use. Orlando (1961) proposes a practical approach, with a broad application within nursing education, practice, and research. She focuses on the nurse's unique and deliberative response to the patient who has expressed an immediate need for help. This is accomplished by the nurse's exploration and validation of the nurse's perceptions, thoughts, and feelings about the patient's behavior with the patient. Furthermore, it is the nurse's responsibility in deliberative nursing to see to it that the patient's need for immediate help is met either by the nurse's own activity or by eliciting the help of others (Orlando, 1961).

Orlando acknowledges and affirms the nurse's distinctive interpretation and validation of observations made. Furthermore, she stresses the independent function performed during a deliberative nursing interaction. Orlando recognizes that nurses' continually sharing their unique perceptions, thoughts, and feelings (i.e., their immediate reaction) about patients' unique behaviors within a deliberative process with patients is what makes nurse–patient relationships dynamic (Orlando, 1961, 1972).

Orlando asserts that good nursing initially involves a nurse's determining with the patient a number of elements: (a) What does the patient think is occurring? (b) What does the patient define as the immediate distress? (c) Is the patient's distress related to an immediate need for help? and (d) Is the nurse's help needed for the patient to obtain relief? Orlando also observed that nurse–patient interactions involving Deliberative Nursing Process resulted in positive outcomes, namely both verbal and nonverbal positive changes within the patient (Pelletier, 1976).

Deliberative Nursing Process was renamed Nursing Process Discipline by Orlando (1972). She also refers to Deliberative Nursing Process as Effective Nursing (Orlando, 1961, 1972), or good nursing (Orlando, 1976). She analyzed nurse–patient interactions and determined that effective interactions involved open disclosure of the nurse of perceptions, thoughts, and feelings and validation of the same with the patient. After implementing a nursing action, the nurse validates with the patient if the nursing action met the patient's immediate need for help (Orlando, 1972, p. 26) (Figure 15.1). The figure depicts how the nurse makes an observation (perception) about the patient, thinks about it, and develops a feeling about it. What the nurse shares with the patient in an open reaction is based upon the nurse's perceptions, thoughts, and/or feelings. The nurse will share the nurse's perceptions, thoughts, and/or feelings about the encounter and explore and validate them with the patient to ensure accuracy. As Orlando points out, nurses may encounter the same patient behaviors but perceive, think, and/or feel differently about them (Orlando, 1961). For example, one nurse may think a patient is "slumped" and "sad," while another nurse may think a patient is "sitting quietly" and "reflecting." This is one reason it is important to validate the nurse's perceptions, thoughts, and/or feelings before intervening.

Orlando also noted that ineffective interactions often involved a more secretive style. Both patient and nurse were not aware of each other's perceptions, thoughts, and feelings in such interactions (Orlando, 1972, p. 26) (Figure 15.2). In such situations, it becomes extremely challenging to meet patient needs adequately if either the nurse or the patient is not being open about their perceptions, thoughts, and/or feelings. Such secretive interactions may lead to misinformation and misinterpretation that result in unmet patient needs. For example, a patient may have a painful condition, have recently received pain medication, and not verbalize to the nurse that the pain is not relieved. The nurse may "think" the patient should

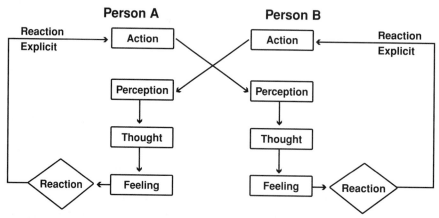

■ **Figure 15.1** The action process in a person-to-person contact functioning by open disclosure. The perceptions, thoughts, and feelings of each individual through the observable action. Used with permission from Orlando, I. J. (1972). *The discipline and teaching of nursing process (an evaluative study)* (p. 26). New York: G. P. Putnam's Sons.

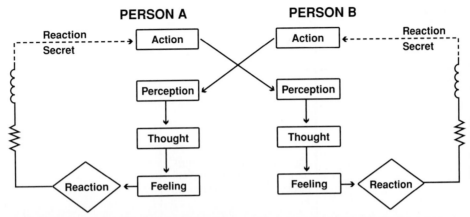

PERSON A   **PERSON B**

■ **Figure 15.2**   The action process in a person-to-person contact functioning in secret. The perceptions, thoughts, and feelings of each individual are not directly available to the perception of the other individual through the observable action. Used with permission from Orlando, I. J. (1972). *The discipline and teaching of nursing process (an evaluative study)* (p. 26). New York: G. P. Putnam's Sons.

be relieved of pain if medications were recently administered and since the patient is not exhibiting any obvious signs indicating pain is present. Subsequently, the nurse may assume the patient has received adequate pain relief and not ask the patient. Thus, the patient's need for effective pain management may not occur.

Orlando (1972, p. 28) developed a Nursing Process Record to assist in learning Deliberative Nursing Process (process discipline) and to be better able to discern nursing process done in secret or using open disclosure (Figure 15.3). Orlando referred to the nurse's perceptions, thoughts, and feelings as part of the nurse's reaction, and whatever the nurse said and/or did to, with, or for the patient as the nurse's action (Orlando, 1972, p. 56).

Automatic Nursing Process

Automatic nursing process refers to any actions or interventions a nurse takes to help a patient that may not be related to the process of helping the patient. Automatic nursing process may be impacted by other influences, such as nursing care costs, patient progress, or additional expenses. Automatic nursing process also is referred to as Nursing Process without Discipline (Orlando, 1972), Ineffective Nursing, (Orlando, 1961, 1972), and bad nursing (Orlando, 1976).

Orlando asserted that automatic nursing process activities were ineffective when they (a) involved nursing action without determining the meaning of the patient's behavior to the patient or the need that caused the behavior; (b) did not assist the patient to inform the nurse how the activity influenced the patient; (c) did not connect the nursing activity to the patient's need; (d) were implemented because of the nurse's inability to explore the nurse's reaction to the patient's behavior; or (e) did not indicate that the nurse was attuned to how the nursing activity influenced the patient (Orlando, 1961, p. 65). Such activities are not necessarily wrong or negative, but they do not determine if the activity is perceived as helpful in relieving the patient's immediate needs. Furthermore, automatic nursing activities indicated to Orlando that nursing care had been given without a disciplined or deliberative professional process (Orlando, 1976).

Nursing Process Record

Perception of or About the Patient	Thought and/or Feeling About the Perception	Said and/or Did to, with, or for the Patient
PROCESS A Mr. G walking back and forth; face red	Looks angry; something must have happened. I'm afraid to ask because he might hit me.	"Good morning, Mr. G."
PROCESS B Mr. G walking back and forth; face red	Looks angry; something must have happened. I'm afraid to ask because he might hit me.	"I'm afraid you will hit me if I ask a question. Should I be afraid?"

■ **Figure 15.3**   Process A illustrates the nursing process functioning in secrecy. Process B illustrates the nursing process functioning by open disclosure. Used with permission from Orlando, I. J. (1972). *The discipline and teaching of nursing process (an evaluative study)* (p. 28). New York: G. P. Putnam's Sons.

An example of the difference between use of an automatic nursing process, which involves nurses' assumptions, and a deliberative nursing process, which involves nurses' exploration of the patients' immediate needs for help, is demonstrated in a study by Bochnak, Rhymes, and Leonard (1962). When two different types of nursing activities to address patients' complaints of pain were examined, statistically significant results occurred at the 0.05 level. In the control group, it was assumed that any complaint of pain indicated a need for pain-relieving medication, and when patients complained of pain, they were given pain-relieving medication. Relief was variable and slow. However, in the experimental group, nurses who used a deliberative approach to determine more accurately what the patients' complaints of pain were about did not automatically administer pain-relieving medication. Their explorations with the patients led to various interventions that provided more extensive relief and quicker relief for the patients (Bochnak, Rhymes, & Leonard, 1962).

Dynamic Nurse–Patient Relationship

According to a recent study, patients are most concerned with personal care issues related to five essential themes: having their needs met, being treated pleasantly, being cared for, having competent nurses, and having care provided promptly (Bolden & Larrabee, 2001). These areas relate to meeting patients' immediate needs for help, which are foundational in Orlando's Theory of Deliberative Nursing Process. Orlando based her ideas about a dynamic nurse–patient relationship on principles from other theories, such as behavioral theory, which postulates that humans are living and behaving organisms who interact continually with one another and within the environment (Orlando, 1961).

Defining the function and product of nursing is explicit in Orlando's definition of the dynamic nurse–patient relationship. Orlando fervently strove to have nurses define the unique function and product of nursing. She defined nursing function as helping the patient and defined nursing product as the improvement or helpful result in the patient's behavior, observable both verbally and nonverbally (Orlando, 1961, 1972, 1983).

Immediate Need for Help

Immediate need for help refers to the patient's inability to fulfill a need for help; the patient may or may not need assistance identifying and/or communicating what the actual need for help is (Orlando, 1961). The observed behavior of the patient is assumed until the meaning behind the behavior is explored (Orlando, 1961, p. 23). Behaviors observed by the nurse may be nonverbal or verbal. Nonverbal behaviors include motor activity, physiological manifestations, and vocalizations. Verbal behaviors take into account complaints, requests, questions, refusals, demands, comments, and statements (Orlando, 1961, pp. 36–37). Immediate needs for help also are referred to simply as "need" in earlier writings (1961).

Therefore, an immediate need for help is any condition in which patients need to have immediate distress relieved or diminished, or their sense of sufficiency or welfare improved (Orlando, 1961, p. 5). Immediate need for help definitely implies that the patient cannot meet the need without professional help.

Patient Distress

Patient distress occurs when a patient's immediate needs are unmet. It is a sense of discomfort that arises when a patient is unable to communicate his or her needs adequately or clearly. Orlando cited physical challenges, unfavorable reactions to the environment, and unfavorable occurrences as examples of circumstances that keep the patient from being able to meet immediate needs (Orlando, 1961, p. 11).

Patient distress is what the patient perceives to be stressful. Orlando holds that behavior has meaning, and that nurses cannot assume what the behavior means without exploring with the patient what the behavior and accompanying distress mean to the patient.

Nursing Situation

According to Orlando (1961, p. 36), a nursing situation encompasses three elements and is dependent upon the nurse's use of them: (a) the patient's behavior, (b) the nurse's reaction, and (c) the nurse's actions intended for the patient's benefit. The interaction of these three elements comprises the nursing process.

Validation

Validation is an ongoing nursing action within the Deliberative Nursing Process. It involves checking with the patient if the nurse's perceptions, thoughts, and/or feelings were accurate in relation to the patient's behavior, and if the nurse's interventions were "correct, helpful, or appropriate" (Orlando, 1961, p. 56). In addition, Orlando sees the nurse as primarily responsible for initiating the process of exploration and discovery in relation to how the patient is responding to any nursing action (Orlando, 1961). Validation safeguards the nurse from operating on assumption resulting in potentially ineffective nursing interventions.

Patient Outcomes/Product

The end result of a nursing action is to "bring about improvement" (Orlando, 1961, p. 6). That improvement should be observable both verbally and nonverbally in the patient's behavior (Orlando, 1972, p. 21). Patient outcomes also should be both "predictable and helpful," and may include such outcomes as "avoidance, relief or diminution of helplessness suffered or anticipated by the individual in an immediate experience" (Orlando, 1972, p. 9). The nurse's activity may result in help or no help, or may be unknown (Orlando, 1961, p. 67). If the outcome does not transpire as predicted, then the nurse must continue to explore what else may be needed to meet the patient's immediate need for help.

DESCRIPTION OF THE THEORY OF DELIBERATIVE NURSING PROCESS

Simple Yet Complex Theory

Deliberative Nursing Process is a theory that is readily understood, has a specific focus (i.e., meeting patients' immediate needs for help), addresses patient problems and probable outcomes (felt distress and lowered distress, respectively), and is explicit to nursing. Its concepts and their relationships are testable and they answer questions about nursing, which are indicators of a middle range nursing theory (Marriner-Tomey, 1998). Orlando's work helped refocus nurses on patients rather than on tasks and on an active, rather than passive, role of patients in their own care.

Complexity refers to the "richness" of a theory to elucidate more variables and their interrelationships (Stevens-Barnum, 1990, p. 97). Part of the theory's complexity involves learning how to use it. Becoming proficient in the use of Deliberative Nursing Process necessitates time, practice, and self-reflection, often in the form of a supervisory experience. Use of Nurse Process Recordings (see Figure 15.3) helps the nurse distinguish between perceptions, thoughts, and feelings—no small task in itself. Learning Deliberative Nursing Process often involves a close supervisory experience in which the learner reconstructs and examines interactions. The process of becoming comfortable in owning one's perceptions, thoughts, and feelings and sharing them with patients is at times difficult and complex.

Function of Nursing

Orlando observed patients in distress and asserted that it was professional nursing's role to determine and meet their immediate needs for help by exploring with the patient the nurse's unique thoughts and feelings resulting from perceptions related to the observed patient behaviors (Orlando, 1961, 1972, 1990).

When the nurse shares perceptions, thoughts, and/or feelings, it is considered to involve open disclosure; by not sharing, the patient is unaware of the nurse's reaction (Orlando, 1972, p. 26). Nurses must not make assumptions, but must explore their perceptions, thoughts, and feelings about the patient's behavior with patients. Orlando's (1961) incorporation of nurses' exploration of their thoughts with patients as part of a deliberative process indicates how critical thinking is an essential part of the deliberative nursing process (Schmieding, 2002).

Major Components and Their Relationships

Nursing is independent, has its own unique professional function, and has its own distinct product (Pelletier, 1976, p. 17). The dynamic nurse–patient relationship involves reciprocity between the nurse and patient; each is influenced by what the other does and says (Marriner-Tomey, 1998). It is dependent upon a nurse-initiated exploration of perceptions, thoughts, and feelings about the patient's behavior, and validation that the nurse's perceptions, thoughts, and feelings are accurate.

The nurse initiates the deliberative process to determine the immediate need for help by helping the patient identify and express the meaning of his or her behavior (Orlando, 1961). Further, the nurse helps the patient explore distress related to the immediate need for help to determine the help needed (p. 29). Within the dynamic nurse–patient relationship, the nurse observes a patient whom the nurse thinks is in distress. This dynamic relationship is dependent upon "what the nurse and patient start with, to the length of their contact and to what they are able to accomplish" (Orlando, 1961, p. 91).

As Schmieding points out, nurses using Deliberative Nursing Process realize "that the patient is the source of the nurse's power" (Schmieding, 2002, p. 327). The nurse uses reflection as part of a critical thinking process to help ascertain the meaning of the patient's behavior according to the patient, and to determine how the behavior relates to the nurse's assumption that an immediate need exists, which is leading to distress for the patient. Nurses obtain information either directly from the patient or indirectly from other sources, such as family, friends, nursing staff, etc. Orlando considers nurses to have access to a tremendous amount of information about the patient (Orlando, 1961).

The nurse using a deliberative process will check what the meaning of the information is with the patient. In an automatic process, the nurse assumes what the information means. Most likely, the outcomes would be significantly different, depending upon which process the nurse uses. Using the deliberative process, the patient partners with the nurse to identify the need, and a successful outcome is more likely. When an automatic process is used, the patient is not included in the assessment or decision-making processes, making a successful outcome less likely (Orlando, 1961, 1972).

Deliberative Nursing Process is a learned and practiced process (Orlando, 1972). The nurse validates with the patient that the patient has an immediate need for help, and that the immediate need for help cannot be met without a professional nurse's help. The nurse intervenes, after exploring with the patient what meaning the patient ascribes to behaviors related to the situation that resulted in an immediate need for help. The nursing situation involves (a) the patient's behavior, (b) the nurse's reaction, and (c) the nurse's activity or actions to assist the patient. Nursing process is the interaction of the three elements contained within a nursing situation (Orlando, 1961, p. 36).

The nurse validates that the immediate need for help has been met by asking the patient and evaluating if the anticipated product or patient outcome of the nursing action, namely improvement and relief of distress, have occurred. If the nursing action has resulted in the patient's relief, the nursing action has been effective in achieving the desired and predicted patient outcome or product. As mentioned, Orlando used

Table 15.1 ASSUMPTIONS AND PROPOSITIONS WITHIN ORLANDO'S (1961) DELIBERATIVE NURSING PROCESS

ASSUMPTIONS	PROPOSITIONS
1. Patients require the expertise of professional nurses to meet certain immediate needs for help.	1. Nurses can determine patients' immediate needs for help by using a deliberative nursing process to ascertain with the patient what the immediate need is.
2. Patients experience distress when they have unmet needs.	2. Nurses can help alleviate patients' distress most effectively when implementing actions based upon a deliberative nursing process because the actions will be designed to meet the need causing distress.
3. Nursing can be evaluated as either good or bad.	3. Good nursing involves open disclosure of and validation with the patient of the nurse's perceptions, thoughts, and/or feelings related to the patient's behavior, and validation with the patient that the nursing action taken met the patient's immediate need for help.
4. It is the responsibility of professional nurses to meet patients' immediate needs for help or to ensure that those needs are met by someone else.	4. Professional nurses using a deliberative nursing process function differently than lay nurses because they are trained in a process whereby they validate with patients (a) what the patients' needs are and (b) if the needs have been met effectively by the nursing actions implemented.
5. Each nursing situation with a patient is unique and dynamic.	5. Patients' individualized needs and nurses' distinctive styles create individually unique nursing situations, and each nursing situation is dynamic because it involves ongoing deliberation by the nurse.
6. The desired outcome of good nursing is that the patient reports or demonstrates (a) relief from distress, (b) experience of less distress, or (c) improvement in "adequacy or well-being" (p. 5).	6. The nurse can determine with the patient if nursing actions based on the deliberative nursing process alleviated or decreased the distress or helped the patient gain a sense of improved "adequacy or well-being" (p. 5).

Nursing Process Recordings to study nursing process and to educate nurses in Deliberative Nursing Process.

Assumptions and propositions will be described, based on Johnson and Webber's (2001) definitions. Assumptions are assumed truths that are associated with the relationships (p. 15). For example, patients becoming distressed when they have an unmet need is an assumption within Deliberative Nursing Process (Orlando, 1961). A more complete listing of assumptions implied within Orlando's Deliberative Nursing Process Theory can be found in Table 15.1.

Propositions direct the relationship between concepts and provide a description of the relationship between concepts (Johnson & Webber, 2001, p. 15). An example that Orlando cited was that "the professional function of nursing is distinct and of central importance to patients in any treatment setting" (Pelletier, 1967, p. 30). Implied propositions within Orlando's Deliberative Nursing Process Theory are listed in Table 15.1.

APPLICATIONS OF THE THEORY

Example of Use of Deliberative Nursing Process in a Group Context

The author supervises nurses in 12-week group leadership training experiences. Nurses receive contact hours for coleading a weekly group session, completing written assignments and readings, and participating actively in supervision throughout the group experience. Each group focuses on meeting patients' immediate needs for help, validating that the nurse coleaders understand that what the group members are stating is their immediate need for help, and sharing with the patients the nurse coleaders' perceptions, thoughts, and/or feelings in response to what behaviors (verbal or nonverbal) that the group members present within the group. Group members often comment when leaving, if not during the group sessions, how helpful they feel the group was. Frequently, members will comment that they feel better. Check-ins and checkouts are extremely helpful in addressing patient immediate needs for help and decreasing patient distress.

Nurses are educated to use a deliberative nursing process within a nursing situation (involving the patient's behavior, the nurse's reaction, and the nurse's action) to identify with the patient what the meaning of the patient's behavior is, so that the patient's immediate need for help can be met and distress can be relieved. Involvement of the patient in discerning the meaning of his or her behavior promotes a dynamic nurse–patient relationship. Validation with the patient that the need has been correctly identified and met results in positive patient outcomes.

Example of Use of Deliberative Nursing Process With Potential Nursing Students

Nursing Camp 2002 was a 2-week camp for eighth-grade students that ran during the summer at Saint Anselm College in Manchester, New Hampshire. Nursing Camp 2002 was a partnership between the Manchester School-to-Careers Partnership, Saint Anselm College, Elliot Hospital, Hanover Hill Healthcare, New Hampshire Hospital, and Visiting Nurses Association Childcare Center. Sylvia Durette, camp director, and this writer introduced the 27 students to Orlando's Deliberative Nursing Process as part of their overview of the nursing profession. Students also participated in an interactive experience related to Deliberative Nursing Process.

Example of Use of Deliberative Nursing Process in a Practice Setting

Nursing staff at an extended care facility requested assistance from their nursing supervisor regarding problematic night behaviors of two older adult patients (Faust, 2002). The supervisor incorporated Deliberative Nursing Process to determine apparent unmet needs of the patients. She met with staff and formulated a plan of action. She assigned an additional nursing assistant to that wing, assumed responsibility for the two patients, observed the patients' behaviors, and validated her perceptions with the two patients. Both patients demonstrated less distress and increased sleep during the nights.

Research Applications

Deliberative Nursing Process has been categorized as a nursing process theory (Orlando, 1990), a prescriptive theory (Wooldridge, Skipper, & Leonard, 1968), and a reflective practice theory (Schmieding, 2002). The inductive, research-based approach Orlando used to develop Deliberative Nursing Process as a theory was unique. Meleis (2007) points out that Orlando used field methodology before it became widely accepted in research use.

Orlando's theory has been widely used as a framework for numerous studies in a variety of settings. Areas studied encompass nursing theory, practice, education, and administration. Both qualitative and quantitative approaches have been employed.

Deliberative Nursing Process has been applied in theory analysis (Alligood & Choi, 1998; Andrews, 1989; Walker & Avant, 1995). A number of patient outcomes have been studied using Deliberative Nursing Process including, but not limited to, pain (Barron, 1966; Bochnak, 1963; Bochnak, Rhymes, & Leonard, 1962); postoperative recovery (Eisler, Wolfer, & Diers, 1972); blood pressure and pulse rates (Mertz, 1963); vomiting (Dumas & Leonard, 1963); and levels of distress (Potter & Bockenhauer, 2000). Additional areas explored using Deliberative Nursing Process include spousal grieving (Dracup & Breu, 1978); breastfeeding (Clausen, 1983); and cancer (Reid-Ponte, 1988). Nursing education (Haggerty, 1987; Orlando, 1972) and nursing administration (Schmieding, 1984, 1992) also have been examined using Deliberative Nursing Process. For additional studies using Deliberative Nursing Process, refer to the Bibliography.

Potter, Dawson, and Vitale-Nolen (2002) have designed a study to determine if implementation of Safety Agreements makes a difference in the rate of patient self-harm incidents and in nurses' feeling more comfortable interacting with patients at risk for self-harm. A Safety Agreement was designed to assist nurses in incorporating Deliberative Nursing Process when interacting with patients at risk for self-harm (see Research Application 15.1).

Bezanson (2002) proposed a theoretical application of Deliberative Nursing Process for an outpatient surgery center of an acute care, community-based hospital. Bezanson asserts that implementation of Deliberative Nursing Process could provide opportunities to improve nursing practice, increase patient satisfaction, and enhance staff satisfaction with their nurse–patient interactions. Bezanson suggests that mechanisms of evaluation might include patient-focused satisfaction surveys, staff self-reports of satisfaction in practice, and improved patient outcomes.

Deliberative Nursing Process can be used as a framework to design research in various settings and to examine specific patient outcomes. The study illustrated in Using Middle Range Theories 15.1 demonstrates patient outcomes related to reduction in levels of distress when Deliberative Nursing Process was implemented in an acute care psychiatric hospital setting.

Olson and Hanchett (1997) carried out a study examining Orlando's assertion that relationships exist between nurse-expressed empathy and several patient outcomes. They used a descriptive, correlational format, described in Using Middle Range Theories 15.2.

Furthermore, Schmieding and Kokuyama (1995) demonstrated the theory's relevance cross-culturally by collaborating in a replication study that compared staff nurse responses. Given that Orlando's theory already was being used in Japan, they postulated that it could be applied in research as well. In addition, they identified the problem as involving staff nurses and head nurses. Orlando's theory involves a problem-solving process or relationship between two individuals. Given the nature of the nursing issue being studied, namely staff nurse perceptions of head nurse actions, the investigators felt Orlando's theory would adapt well. They surveyed 126 staff nurses in an acute care hospital near Tokyo and compared their results with a study done in the United States. The investigators were careful to meet requirements for matching the two samples. Both samples demonstrated significant associations in five of six scenarios surveyed ($P \leq 0.025$) (Schmieding & Kokuyama, 1995, p. 825). In addition, the investigators discussed important points when participating in research across different cultures. These included viewing such research as a partnership, clarifying the purpose of the research, paying close attention to validity and

15.1 USING MIDDLE RANGE THEORIES

A quasi-experimental pilot study was undertaken in a large, university-affiliated state psychiatric facility to determine if implementation of Orlando's nursing theory-based practice (Deliberative Nursing Process) made a difference in patient outcomes when compared with patient outcomes resulting from interventions using nonspecified nursing practice. Two inpatient units were selected that matched most closely in staffing patterns, patient census, and acuity levels. Ten registered nurses (RNs) participated—six in the experimental group and four in the control group. The experimental and control groups of RNs had no significant differences in their demographic composition. Thirty patients were involved in the study—19 in the experimental group and 11 in the control group. Patient experimental and control groups were statistically similar. The RNs were educated in use of the Bockenhauer-Potter Scale of Immediate Distress (BPSID), a 5-point Likert-scaled instrument that quantifies the level of patient-demonstrated distress. The BPSID was developed to control for subjectivity when assessing patients' levels of distress. The two investigators, a consultant in Orlando's theory, and three hospital RN nurse specialists reviewed and enhanced reference points on the scale. Videotaped simulated interactions helped nurses to learn how to use the BPSID, thus increasing inter-rater reliability. RNs in the experimental group received instruction in Deliberative Nursing Process. Data collection took place over a 12-week time frame. Distress levels of patients were measured before and after RN interventions. A greater reduction ($p = .04$) in patients' levels of distress occurred in the group in which RNs used the Deliberative Nursing Process. Interestingly, RNs who used the Deliberative Nursing Process reported that having a "road map" helped them feel more effective in their nursing interventions. Further research is suggested to control for the possible "halo effect" of additional attention provided to the experimental group of RNs via weekly support and education and to obtain verbal feedback from patients who experience nursing interventions that incorporate Deliberative Nursing Process.

Potter, M. L., & Bockenhauer, B. J. (2000). Implementing Orlando's nursing theory: A pilot study. *Journal of Psychosocial Nursing and Mental Health Services*, 38, 14–21.

reliability throughout the process, clarifying responsibilities throughout the research process, and choosing a theory that is culturally compatible to the culture(s) in which the research takes place.

INSTRUMENTS USED IN EMPIRICAL TESTING

There are no set means or tools to measure Deliberative Nursing Process. This is indicative of the nature of the theory because Orlando emphasized that Deliberative Nursing Process involves a nursing situation in which the uniqueness of the nurse is brought to the experience to meet the immediate needs for help, as expressed by the patient, explored by the nurse and patient, and validated by the nurse with the patient. Each circumstance or nursing situation will be unique and different, because each nurse perceives, feels, and thinks differently than any other nurse entering the same nursing situation.

15.2 USING MIDDLE RANGE THEORIES

Relationships between nurse-expressed empathy and two patient outcomes (patient-perceived empathy and patient distress) were explored in a descriptive, correlational study. The hypotheses were (1) a negative relationship will exist between measures of nurse-expressed empathy and measures of patient distress, (2) a positive relationship will exist between measures of nurse-expressed empathy and patient-perceived empathy, and (3) a negative relationship will exist between patient-perceived empathy and measures of patient distress.

One hundred and forty subjects comprised the sample. Seventy staff registered nurses (RNs) were selected from a pool of 50% of all eligible nurses who were invited. Seventy patients for whom the nurses cared during a day shift were randomly selected to participate.

Nurse participants completed the Staff-Patient Interaction Response Scale (SPIRS) and the Behavioral Test of Interpersonal Skills (BTIS). Both measure nurse-expressed empathy. Patient participants completed the Empathy Subscale of the Barrett-Lennard Relationship Inventory (BLRI) to determine patient-perceived empathy measures; their patient distress scores were measured using the Profile of Mood States (POMS) and the Multiple Affect Adjective Check List (MAACL).

Testing of hypothesis was as follows: (a) hypotheses one and three were tested together by means of one canonical correlation and (b) hypothesis three was tested by means of multiple regression analysis. All three hypotheses received statistically significant support with the BTIS measurement. A fuller description of methodology and findings are recorded in a report by Olson (1995). This study supported Orlando's (1961, 1972) assertion that realtionships exist between accurate perceptions of patients' needs (nurse-expressed empathy and patient-expressed empathy) and patient distress.

Olson, J., & Hanchett, E. (1997). Nurse-expressed empathy, patient outcomes, and development of a middle-range theory. *Image: Journal of Nursing Scholarship, 29,* 71–76.

Different tools have been developed and/or used to measure different aspects of Deliberative Nursing Process. These tools facilitate examination of such factors as patient outcomes, nursing process, nurse empathy, and patient-perceived empathy. The instruments have been developed and/or used to test Deliberative Nursing Process qualitatively and quantitatively. Instruments used in different studies explore different aspects of the Deliberative Nursing Process, such as theory description and analysis, use in research, use in clinical practice, and use in administrative practice.

Much of the testing done with Deliberative Nursing Process involves questionnaires and surveys. Examples of tools that have been used for studies involving Orlando's Deliberative Nursing Process are listed in Table 15.2.

One instrument used in the study of Deliberative Nursing Process is the Safety Agreement. The Safety Agreement is an instrument developed by nurses at New Hampshire Hospital (NHH) and is designed to measure patients' risk for self-harm and willingness and ability to agree to remain safe (see Table 15.2). Most of the agreement is designed in Likert-style format. A question related to a patient's perceived ability to remain safe requires a "yes" or "no" response. In addition, a question that seeks to determine how the patient and registered nurse (RN) might work together to manage the current risk for self-harm elicits

Table 15.2 DELIBERATIVE NURSING PROCESS TOOLS

CATEGORY	ABBREVIATION	EXAMPLE
Anxiety		State Anxiety Inventory (Spielberger, Gorsuch, & Lushene, 1970).
Attitude change		Spouse Questionnaire (Silva, 1979) Spouses' Perception Scale (Silva, 1979)
Emotional state	WI	Welfare Inventory (Eisler, Wolfer, & Diers, 1972)
Nurse-expressed empathy	BTIS SPIRS	Behavioral Test of Interpersonal Skills (Gerrard & Bussell, 1980) Staff-Patient Interaction Response Scale (Gallop, 1989)
Patient-perceived empathy	BLRI	Barrett-Lennard Relationship Inventory (Barrett-Lennard, 1962)
Patient distress	POMS MAACL BPSID	Profile of Mood States (McNair, Lorr, & Droppleman, 1981) Nyehuis, Yamamoto, Luchetta, Terrien, & Parmentier (1999) Multiple Affect Adjective Check List (Zuckerman & Lubin, 1965) Bockenhauer/Potter Scale of Immediate Distress (Bockenhauer, 2000)
Patient's self-harm incidents	SA	Safety Agreement (Potter, Vitale-Nolen, & Dawson, 2005)
Nurse-perceived comfort with use of safety agreements		Registered Nurses Evaluation Survey (Potter, Vitale-Nolen, & Dawson, 2005)
Therapeutic effectiveness	EPPS SII	Edwards Personal Preference Schedule (Edwards, 1959) Social Interaction Inventory (Methven & Schlotfeldt, 1962)
Postoperative physical recovery	RI	Recovery Inventory (Eisler, Wolfer, & Diers, 1972)
Social approval	SD Scale	Social Desirability Scale (Crowne & Marlowe, 1964)

a response from a number of given choices with an "other" option included. The intent of the Safety Agreement is to assist the RN in a deliberative process of determining with the patient the patient's risk for self-harm.

A Safety Agreement was implemented nonrandomly, with all patients admitted or considered at risk for self-harm. Patients were asked to self-rate the following areas with the RN: (a) their current harm level, (b) the likelihood of their acting on their thoughts of self-harm, (c) their thoughts about managing the risk with the RN, (d) their willingness to enter an agreement for safety with the RN, and (e) their thoughts about how long they think they can remain safe.

RNs were given the Registered Nurses Evaluation Survey, which also is in Likert-type format except for one question. RNs were asked to evaluate (a) the number of times they used the Safety Agreement in a 3-month period, (b) if the Safety Agreement assisted them in feeling more comfortable while helping patients at risk for self-harm, (c) if they thought self-harming incidents decreased since implementation of Safety Agreements, and (d) if they have any other comments to share related to use of Safety Agreements. Research Application 15-1 describes research on the implementation of Safety Agreements at NHH.

15.1 RESEARCH APPLICATION

Nurses at New Hampshire Hospital (NHH), a university-affiliated, state psychiatric facility, were interested in determining if implementation of Safety Agreements would affect patient outcomes and nursing comfort levels when working with patients at risk for self-harm (Potter, Vitale-Nolen, & Dawson 2005). Registered nurses (RNs) serving on a Continuous Quality Improvement (CQI) committee had examined the use of safety contracts by nurses at the facility and developed a Safety Agreement tool that they thought would facilitate incorporating Orlando's Deliberative Nursing Process when assessing patients at risk for self-harm.

Validity of safety contracts in general has not been tested. Confusion and controversy exist in relation to the definition and use of safety contracts with patients who are suicidal (Potter & Dawson, 2001). It is suspected that this confusion and controversy lead to discomfort and a lack of direction when nurses "contract" with patients for safety.

It has been demonstrated by nurses at NHH that Deliberative Nursing Process can make a difference in patient outcomes (Potter & Bockenhauer, 2000). Hence, these investigators postulated that a more standardized process, using Orlando's Deliberative Nursing Process to enhance communication, might promote patients' agreeing to be safe and, in turn, decrease the rate of self-harm incidents and increase RNs' comfort levels when working with patients at risk for self-harm.

Safety Agreements were implemented as the standard of care on all units in Acute Psychiatric Services (APS). Incidents of self-harm were collected via the organizational-wide data collection system pre- and postimplementation. Instruction for RNs in use of Safety Agreements occurred the month before their implementation. RNs already used Deliberative Nursing Process as a framework for nursing care. The RNs were invited to complete two different surveys on the use of Safety Agreements; one was offered at the end of the first 3-month period, and the second one was offered at the end of 12 months. There were two convenience sample databases: (a) anonymous lists of self-harm incidents (only chart numbers used, not patient names) and (b) all RNs who performed direct patient care (44 RNs responded to Survey I and 49 RNs responded to Survey II) in APS.

The investigators used t-tests to detect differences in pre- and postintervention outcomes and Stat Pac Gold computer software to analyze data for statistical differences. The mean rate of self-harming incidents did not change significantly pre- and postimplementation of Safety Agreements. Registered nurses were equally divided in relation to thinking Safety Agreements enhanced or did not enhance nurse–patient interactions. However, RNs did report improvement in the following areas related to use of Safety Agreements: patient responsibility, nurse contact with patients, guidance for safety concerns, discussions with patients related to safety, and time guidelines around issues of safety.

Potter, M. L., Vitale-Nolen, R., & Dawson, A. M. (2005). Implementation of safety agreements in an acute psychiatric facility. *Journal of the American Psychiatric Association, 11*(3), 144–155.

SUMMARY

Gowan and Morris (1964) speculated that the nursing shortage of that era and the increased expectations upon nurses led to nurses' spending more time designing care than providing care. Results from their study indicated that patients experienced undue delays in receiving care and withheld requests that involved their well-being due to patient perceptions that the nurses were too busy, would disapprove, would not like to be interrupted, or would think the request was not helpful to the patient. Might this same scenario be repeating itself today?

In 1990, the National League for Nursing honored Orlando by reprinting *The Dynamic Nurse–Patient Relationship*. Orlando noted in the Preface to that edition that interest in the United States using her theory had waned (Orlando, 1990, p. viii). Interest and use of the theory may have subsided temporarily, but it never ceased. As noted by Orlando herself, her work has been published in five foreign countries, and there have been numerous publications in recent years related to Deliberative Nursing Process (Potter & Bockenhauer, 2000; Potter & Dawson, 2001; Potter & Tinker, 2000; Rosenthal, 1996; Schmieding, 1993b, 1999, 2002). Many changes have occurred in nursing. However, the essence of nursing, described so simply yet eloquently by Orlando, has not changed— namely that the nurse–patient relationship involves a dynamic and unique process that evolves between nurse and patient when approached deliberatively and validated with the patient on an ongoing basis.

Deliberative Nursing Process is a nursing theory for all times and situations, no matter how complex. Use of Deliberative Nursing Process helps nurses focus on and maintain a patient-centered approach when providing nursing care amidst additional and varied expectations of the nurse. Orlando has kept the message of Deliberative Nursing Process clear throughout the years: "It is the nurse's direct responsibility to see to it that the patient's needs for help are met, either directly by her own activity or indirectly by calling in the help of others" (Orlando, 1961, p. 29). Adopting such a clear function promotes effective and efficient nursing practice as has been demonstrated through empirical studies on Deliberative Nursing Process for more than 40 years.

ANALYSIS OF THEORY

Using the criteria presented in Chapter 2, critique the theory Deliberative Nursing Process. Compare your conclusions about the theory with those found in Appendix A. A nurse scholar who has worked with the theory completed the analysis found in the appendix.

Internal Criticism
1. Clarity
2. Consistency
3. Adequacy

4. Logical development
5. Level of theory development

External Criticism
1. Reality convergence
2. Utility
3. Significance
4. Discrimination
5. Scope of theory
6. Complexity

CRITICAL THINKING EXERCISES

1. Scenario: Upon entering a patient's room on the medical unit, the nurse notices the patient's right hand over her heart. The patient has her head down and is sobbing. Give examples of how you, as the nurse, might share each of the following:
   a. Your perceptions
   b. Your thoughts
   c. Your feelings

2. What is the function of "validation" in Deliberative Nursing Process?
3. State three ways using Deliberative Nursing Process is more beneficial in the nurse–patient relationship than using automatic nursing process.

WEB RESOURCES

The Ida J. Orlando web site gives a brief biography and summary of her theory. There are also many links to additional publications and research studies. This site is sponsored by the University of Rhode Island College of Nursing:
http://www.uri.edu/nursing/schmieding/orlando/index.html

REFERENCES

Alligood, M. R. (2002). The nature of knowledge needed for nursing practice. In M. R. Alligood & A. Marriner-Tomey (Eds.), *Nursing theory—Utilization & application* (2nd ed., pp. 3–14). St. Louis: Mosby, Inc.

Alligood, M. R., & Choi, E. C. (1998). Evolution of nursing theory development. In A. Marriner-Tomey & M. R. Alligood (Eds.), *Nursing theorists and their work* (4th ed., pp. 55–66). St. Louis: Mosby.

Andrews, C. M. (1989). Ida Orlando's model of nursing practice. In J. J. Fitzpatrick & A. L. Whall (Eds.), *Conceptual models of nursing: Analysis & application* (2nd ed., pp. 69–87). Norwalk, CT: Appleton & Lange.

Barrett-Lennard, G. (1962). Dimensions of therapist response as causal factors in therapeutic change. *Psychological Monographs, 76,* (43), Whole No. 562).

Barron, M. A. (1966). The effects varied nursing approaches have on patients' complaints of pain. *Nursing Research, 15,* 90–91.

Bezanson, A. (2002). Theoretical application of Orlando's Theory of Deliberate Nursing Process in an outpatient surgery center. Unpublished manuscript.

Bochnak, M. A. (1963). The effect of an automatic and deliberative process of nursing activity on the relief of patients' pain: A clinical experiment. *Nursing Research, 12,* 191–192.

Bochnak, M. A., Rhymes, J. P., & Leonard, R. C. (1962). The comparison of two types of nursing activity on the relief of pain. In *Innovations in nurse–patient relationships: Automatic or reasoned nurse action* (Clinical Paper No. 6). New York: American Nurses Association.

Bolden, L. V., & Larrabee, J. H. (2001). Defining patient-perceived quality of nursing care. *Journal of Nursing Care Quality, 16,* 34–60.

Clausen [Cameron], J. C. (1983). Clinical nursing research on the science and art of breastfeeding using a deliberative nursing care approach. *Western Journal of Nursing Research, 5,* 29.

Crowne, D. P., & Marlowe, D. (1964). *The approval motive: Studies in evaluative dependence.* New York: John Wiley & Sons.

Dracup, K. A., & Breu, C. S. (1978). Using nursing research findings to meet the needs of grieving spouses. *Nursing Research, 27,* 212–216.

Dumas, R. G., & Leonard, R. C. (1963). The effect of nursing on the incidence of postoperative vomiting. *Nursing Research, 12,* 12–15.

Edwards, A. L. (1959). *Personal preference schedule manual,* rev. ed. New York: Psychological Corporation.

Eisler, J., Wolfer, J. A., & Diers, D. (1972). Relationship between need for social approval and postoperative recovery and welfare. *Nursing Research, 21,* 520–525.

Faust, C. (2002). Orlando's deliberative nursing process theory: A practice application in an extended care facility. *Journal of Gerontological Nursing, 28(7),* 14–18.

Gallop, R. (1989). *The influence of diagnostic labelling on the expressed empathy of nursing staff.* Unpublished doctoral dissertation. University of Toronto, Toronto, Ontario, Canada.

Gerrard, G. B., & Buzzell, M. (1980). *User's manual for the behavioral test of interpersonal skills for health professionals.* Reston, VA: Reston.

Gowan, N. I., & Morris, M. (1964). Nurses' responses to expressed patient needs. *Nursing Research, 13,* 68–71.

Haggerty, L. A. (1987). An analysis of senior nursing students' immediate responses to distressed patients. *Journal of Advanced Nursing, 12,* 451–461.

Johnson, B. M., & Webber, P. B. (2001). *Theory and reasoning in nursing.* New York: Lippincott Williams & Wilkins.

Marriner-Tomey, A. (1998). Introduction to analysis of nursing theories. In A. Marriner-Tomey & M. R. Alligood (Eds.), *Nursing theorists and their work* (4th ed., pp. 3–15). St. Louis: Mosby.

McEwan, M. (2002). Middle-range nursing theories. In M. McEwan & E. M. Wills, (Eds.), *Theoretical basis for nursing* (pp. 202–225). Philadelphia: Lippincott Williams & Wilkins.

McNair, D., Lorr, M., & Dropplemann, L. (1971). *Profile of Mood States.* San Diego, CA: Educational and Industrial Testing Services.

Meleis, A. I. (2007). *Theoretical nursing: Development & progress* (4th ed., pp. 345–356). Philadelphia: Lippincott-Raven.

Mertz, H. (1963). A study of the process of the nurse's activity as it affects the blood pressure readings and pulse rate of patients admitted to the emergency room. *Nursing Research, 12,* 197–198.

Methuen, D. & Schlotfeldt, R. M. (1962). The social inventory. *Nursing Research, 11,* 83–88.

Nyehuis, D. L. Yamamoto, C., Luchetta, T. Terrien, A. & Parmentier, A. (1999). Adult and geriatric normative data and validation of the Profile of Mood States. *Journal of Clinical Psychology, 55,* 79–86.

Olson, J. K. (1995). Relationships between nurse expressed empathy, patient perceived empathy, and patient distress. *Image: Journal of Nursing Scholarship, 27,* 323–328.

Olson, J., & Hanchett, E. (1997). Nurse-expressed empathy, patient outcomes, and development of a middle-range theory. *Image: Journal of Nursing Scholarship, 29,* 71–76.

Orlando, I. J. (1961). *The dynamic nurse–patient relationship.* New York: G. P. Putnam's Sons.

Orlando, I. J. (1972). *The discipline and teaching of nursing process (an evaluative study).* New York: G. P. Putnam's Sons.

Orlando, I. J. (1976, August). The fundamental issue in professional nursing. Paper presented at the University of Tulsa College of Nursing, Tulsa, OK.

Orlando [Pelletier], I. J. (1983, October). Comments on ANA's social policy statement of 1980. Paper presented at Southeastern Massachusetts University, College of Nursing, Honor Society, South Dartmouth, MA.

Orlando, I. J. (1987). Nursing in the 21st century: Alternate paths. *Journal of Advanced Nursing, 12,* 405–412.

Orlando, I. J. (1990, reissue). *The dynamic nurse–patient relationship.* New York: National League for Nursing.

Orlando, I. J., & Dugan, A. B. (1989). Independent and dependent paths: The fundamental issue for the nursing profession. *Nursing and Health Care, 10,* 77–80.

Pelletier, I. O. (1967). The patient's predicament and nursing function. *Psychiatric Opinion, 4,* 25–30.

Pelletier, I. O. (1976). The fundamental issue in professional nursing. Unpublished manuscript, pp. 1–22.

Potter, M. L., & Bockenhauer, B. J. (2000). Implementing Orlando's Nursing Theory: A pilot study. *Journal of Psychosocial Nursing and Mental Health Services, 38,* 14–21.

Potter, M. L., & Dawson, A. M. (2001). From safety contract to safety agreement. *Journal of Psychosocial Nursing and Mental Health Services 39,* 38–45.

Potter, M. L., & Tinker, S. W. (2000). Put power in nurses' hands: Orlando's Nursing Theory supports nurses—simply. *Nursing Management, 31,* 40–41.

Potter, M. L., Vitale-Nolen, R., & Dawson, A. M. (2005). Implementation of safety agreements in an acute psychiatric facility. *Journal of the American Psychiatric Association, 11*(3), 144–155.

Reid-Ponte, P. (1988). The relationship among empathy and the use of Orlando's deliberative process by the primary nurse and the distress of the adult cancer patient. Doctoral dissertation, Boston University, Boston.

Rosenthal, B. C. (1996). An interactionist's approach to perioperative nursing. *Association of Operating Room Nurses Journal, 64,* 254–260.

Schmieding, N. J. (1984). Putting Orlando's theory into practice. *American Journal of Nursing, 84,* 759–761.

Schmieding, N. J. (1992). Relationship between head nurse responses to staff nurses and staff nurse response to patients. *Western Journal of Nursing Research, 13,* 746–760.

Schmieding, N. J. (1993a). *Ida Jean Orlando: A nursing process theory.* London: Sage Publications, Inc.

Schmieding, N. J., (1993b). Successful superior-subordinate relationships require mutual management. *Health Care Supervisor, 11,* 52–63.

Schmieding, N. J. (1999). Reflective inquiry framework for nurse administrators. *Journal of Advanced Nursing, 30,* 631–639.

Schmieding, N. J. (2002). Orlando's nursing process theory. In M. R. Alligood & A. Marriner-Tomey (Eds.), *Nursing theory utilization & application* (2nd ed., pp. 315–337). St. Louis: Mosby.

Schmieding, N. J., & Kokuyama, T. (1995). The need for and process of collaborative internationsl research: A replication study of Japanese staff nurse perceptions of head nurses' actions. *Journal of Advanced Nursing, 21,* 820–826.

Silva, M. C. (1979). Effects of orientation information on spouses' anxieties and attitudes toward hospitalization and surgery. *Research in Nursing and Health, 2,* 127–136.

Spielberger, C. D., Gorsuch, R. L., & Lushene, R. E. (1970). *STAI manual for the state-trait anxiety inventory.* Palo Alto, CA: Consulting Psychologists Press.

Stevens-Barnum, B. J. (1990). *Nursing theory: Analysis, application, evaluation.* Glenview, IL: Scott, Foresman, Little, & Brown.

Walker, L. O., & Avant, K. C. (1995). *Strategies for theory construction in nursing.* (3rd ed.). Norwalk, CT: Appleton & Lange.

Wills, E. M. (2002). Overview of grand nursing theories. In M. McEwan & E. M. Wills (Eds.), *Theoretical basis for nursing* (pp. 111–124). Philadelphia: Lippincott Wilkins & Williams.

Wooldridge, P. J., Skipper, J. K., Jr., & Leonard, R. C. (1968). *Behavioral science, social practice, and the nursing profession.* Cleveland, OH: Case Western Reserve University.

Zuckerman, M., & Lubin, B. (1965). *Manual for the multiple affect adjective check list.* San Diego, CA: Educational and Testing Service.

BIBLIOGRAPHY

Cameron, J. (1963). An exploratory study of the verbal responses of the nurse–patient interactions. *Nursing Research, 12,* 192.

Chapman, J. S. (1969). Effects of different nursing approaches upon psychological and physiological responses of patients. Unpublished doctoral dissertation. Case Western Reserve University, Frances Payne Bolton School of Nursing, Cleveland, Ohio.

Clausen [Cameron], J. C. (1983). Clinical nursing research on the science and art of breastfeeding using a deliberative nursing care approach. *Western Journal of Nursing Research, 5,* 29.

Dumas, R. G., & Johnson [Anderson], B. A. (1972). Research in nursing practice: A review of five clinical experiments. *International Journal of Nursing Studies, 9,* 137–149.

Dumas, R. G., & Leonard, R. C. (1963). The effect of nursing on the incidence of postoperative vomiting. *Nursing Research, 12,* 12–15.

Dye, M. C. (1963a). Clarifying patients' communication. *The American Journal of Nursing, 63,* 56–59.

Dye, M. C. (1963b). A descriptive study of conditions conducive to an effective process of nursing activity. *Nursing Research, 12,* 194.

Elms, R. R., & Leonard, R. C. (1966). Effects of nursing approaches during admission. *Nursing Research, 15,* 39–48.

Farrell, G. A., (1991). How accurately do nurses perceive patients' needs? A comparison of general and psychiatric settings. *Journal of Advanced Nursing, 16,* 1062–1070.

Faulkner, S. A. (1963). A descriptive study of needs communicated to the nurse by some mothers on a postpartum service. *Nursing Research, 4,* 260.

Forchuck, C. (1991). A comparison of the works of Peplau and Orlando. *Archives of Psychiatric Nursing, 5,* 38–45.

Gillis, Sister L. (1976). Sleeplessness: Can you help? *The Canadian Nurse, 72,* 32–34.

Hampe, S. O. (1975). Needs of grieving spouses in a hospital setting. *Nursing Research, 24,* 113.

Kokuyama, T., & Schmieding, N. J. (1995). Responses staff nurses prefer compared with their perception of head nurse responses. *Japanese Journal of Nursing Administration, 5,* 33–38.

Laurent, C. L. (1999). A nursing theory for nursing leadership. *Journal of Nursing Management, 8,* 83–87.

Mahaffy, P. P. (1965). The effects of hospitalization on children admitted for tonsillectomy and adenoidectomy. *Nursing Research, 14,* 12–19.

Nelson, B. (1978). A practical application of nursing theory. *Nursing Clinics of North America, 13,* 157–169.

Peitchinis, J. A. (1972). Therapeutic effectiveness of counseling by nursing personnel. *Nursing Research, 21,* 138–148.

Pride, L. F. (1968). An adrenal stress index as a criterion measure of nursing. *Nursing Research, 17,* 292–303.

Rittman, M. R. (2001). Ida Jean Orlando (Pelletier): The dynamic nurse-patient relationship. In M. E. Parker (Ed.), *Nursing theories and nursing practice* (pp. 125–130). Philadelphia: F. A. Davis Company.

Schmieding, N. J. (1987). Analyzing managerial responses in face-to-face contacts. *Journal of Advanced Nursing, 12,* 357–365.

Schmieding, N. J. (1987). Face-to-face contacts: Exploring their meaning. *Nursing Management, 12,* 82–86.

Schmieding, N. J. (1987). Problematic situations in nursing: Analysis of Orlando's theory based on Dewey's theory of inquiry. *Journal of Advanced Nursing, 12,* 431–440.

Schmieding, N. J. (1988). Action process of nurse administrators to problematic situations based on Orlando's theory. *Journal of Advanced Nursing, 13,* 99–107.

Schmieding, N. J. (1990). A model for assessing nurse administrator's actions. *Western Journal of Nursing Research, 12,* 293–306.

Schmieding, N. J. (1990). Do head nurses include staff nurses in problem solving? *Nursing Management, 21,* 58–60.

Schmieding, N. J. (2006). Ida Jean Orlando (Pelletier): Nursing process theory. In A. M. Tomey & M. R. Alligood (Eds.), *Nursing theorists and their work* (6th ed., pp. 431–451). St. Louis: Mosby, Inc.

Sitzman, K., & Eichelberger, L. W. (2004). *Understanding the work of nurse theorists: A creative beginning.* Sudbury, MA: Jones and Bartlett Publishers.

Tarasuk [Bochnak], M. B., Rhymes, J., & Leonard, R. C. (1965). An experimental test of the importance of communication skills for effective nursing. In J. K. Skipper, Jr., & R. C. Leonard (Eds.), *Social interaction and patient care* (pp. 110–120). Philadelphia: J. B. Lippincott.

Tryon, P. A. (1966). Use of comfort measures as support during labor. *Nursing Research, 15,* 109–118.

Tryon, P. A., & Leonard, R. C. (1964). The effect of patients' participation on the outcome of a nursing procedure. *Nursing Forum, 3,* 79–89.

Williamson, Y. M. (1978). Methodologic dilemmas in tapping the concept of patient needs. *Nursing Research, 27,* 172–177.

Acknowledgments

Much appreciation is expressed to Mimi Dye, MSN, ARNP, who completed the critique on Deliberative Nursing Process in Appendix A and studied Deliberative Nursing Process as a student with the theorist Ida J. Orlando, MS, RN; Joy L. Gabrielli, who served as research assistant in the development of this chapter; and Dorothy Y. Kameoka, MLS, MSW, RN, who provided valuable assistance in seeking out materials for this chapter.

Resilience

■ JOAN E. HAASE

Contributing Authors: Chin-Mi Chen, National Defense Medical Center, Taipei, Taiwan; and Celeste Phillips-Salimi and Cynthia Bell, Indiana University School of Nursing, Indianapolis, IN

DEFINITION OF KEY TERMS

Boundaries of resilience	The contextual influences, dimensions, and assumptions that are considered in determining the attributes of resilience
Meaning-based models	Explanatory models focused on the patterns and experiences of illness from a subjective and holistic perspective
Person-focused research	Research to identify the patterns of variables in which resilience naturally occurs, then examining what might contribute to these outcomes; or using cut-off scores on selected variables to categorize adversity subgroups, then examining outcomes in these groups
Positive health research	Efforts to gain understanding of ways individuals sustain or regain optimal health
Protective factors	The individual, family, social, or other contextual factors that enhance resilience processes and outcomes
Quality of life	A sense of well-being
Resilience	General definition: Positive adjustment in the face of adversity
	Context-derived definition: The process of identifying or developing resources and strengths to flexibly manage stressors to gain a positive outcome, a sense of confidence/mastery, self-transcendence, and self-esteem
Risk factors	The individual, family, social, or other contextual factors that impede development of resilience processes and outcomes
Strengths-based research	Research that focuses on individual, family, or community "promise" rather than on risk

(Key Terms continued on next page)

DEFINITION OF KEY TERMS continued

Triangulation	Use of quantitative or qualitative research approaches either sequentially or simultaneously to refine, evaluate, and/or extend theory
Variable-focused approaches	Use of multivariate statistics to test for linkages to resilience among measures of adversity, outcomes, and environmental or individual qualities that may protect from or compensate for negative consequences.

INTRODUCTION

Researchers and practitioners have long sought answers to questions about psychosocial adjustment to illness, especially chronic conditions. While much research is still guided by pathology and deficit-based models that examine risk, adjustment problems, and developmental delays (Hymovich & Roehnert, 1989), salutogenic, positive health, and strengths-based models are gaining recognition as useful perspectives in nursing and other health care disciplines (Antonovsky, 1979; Hymovich & Roehnert, 1989; Singer & Ryff, 2001; Woodgate, 1999). Theories such as resilience (Rutter, 1979, 1987), hardiness (Kobasa, 1982), self-efficacy, and learned resourcefulness (Bandura, 1977; Rosenbaum, 1983) were developed to explain positive adjustment to illness, based on the belief that such theories may yield information about effective interventions (Forsyth, Delaney, & Gresham, 1984; Garmezy, 1991; Kadner, 1989; Sinnema, 1991). In 2001, the Committee on Future Direction for Behavioral and Social Sciences identified resilience as a research priority for the National Institutes of Health (Singer & Ryff, 2001). The committee highlighted the significance of behavioral and psychosocial processes in disease etiology, well-being, and health promotion. Additionally, the committee recommended increased study of the protective factors that are correlates of resilience, such as optimism, meaning and purpose, social and emotional support, and related neurobiological mechanisms, that promote recovery and increased survival rates (Singer & Ryff, 2001). These recommendations have been accepted to at least some extent, as indicated by the rapidly increasing number of theory and research reports in the literature. Nurses also recognize the importance of positive health concepts and are increasingly seeing an understanding of resilience as potentially useful to (a) guide development of interventions to enhance positive outcomes; (b) improve outcomes for at-risk populations; (c) prevent poor outcomes; and (d) influence public policy related to individuals, families, and communities.

Resilience is broadly defined as a phenomenon of positive adjustment in the face of adversity. Historically, resilience was most frequently studied in children and adolescents and was characterized by attributes usually identified as positive. Examples of such positive attributes found in early research on resilience include competence (Garmezy, Masten, & Tellegen, 1984; Rutter, 1979); self-esteem (Garmezy, 1981); continual growth and "elasticity" in relation to change (Block, 1980); superior coping (Garmezy, 1991; Murphy & Moriarty, 1976); advanced self-help, communication, and problem-solving skills (Garmezy, 1981; Hauser, Vieyra, Jacobson, & Wertlieb, 1985); tendency to perceive experiences constructively (Werner & Smith, 1982); and ability to use spirituality to maintain a positive vision of a meaningful life (Rutter, 1979; Wells & Schwebel, 1987).

HISTORICAL BACKGROUND

Since the 1970s, shifting perspectives on resilience inquiry have occurred. Two authors' descriptions of these shifting perspectives are especially informative. Richardson (2002) describes resilience research as occurring in three waves:

1. Efforts to describe personal qualities that predict success
2. Resilience as a process
3. Resilience as a motivational life force to be fostered in all individuals.

Similarly, Masten (2001) portrays a gradual change in perspectives of resilience, from a view of resilience as an extraordinary occurrence to the current evidence-based perspective that resilience is a commonly occurring phenomenon that is essentially a basic function of adaptational systems.

Positive adaptation research began with studies on the premorbid competence of patients with schizophrenia (Garmezy, 1974; Masten, Best, & Garmezy, 1990). Those studies were precursors to the seminal theoretical and empirical groundwork on resilience done with children of mothers with schizophrenia. The major characteristic of these children was the fact that they thrived despite their high-risk status. After describing children who thrived despite adversity, subsequent studies were directed to understanding individual differences in response to adversity. This effort to understand individual differences was gradually expanded to other contexts, such as childhood exposure to adverse conditions of socioeconomic adversity (Rutter, 1979), abuse (Henry, 2001), urban poverty and community violence (Luthar, Cicchetti, & Becker, 2000), and chronic illness (Wells & Schwebel, 1987). In the early 1990s, researchers began to identify external factors that contributed to development of resilience. Three general classes of protective factors—individual, family, and social—are now generally recognized as influencing resilience development (Rutter, 1987). Currently, in addition to continuing to identify protective factors, researchers are seeking to understand the underlying mechanisms or processes of how the interaction of risk and protective factors influence resilience outcomes (Luthar et al., 2000). There is a strongly emerging priority for research on the biological contributors to or correlates of resilience (Curtis & Cicchetti, 2003). And, there is increasing focus on research examining and fostering resilience with adolescents, while simultaneously on expansion of ages and contexts studied.

DEFINITION OF THEORY CONCEPTS

There is widespread agreement that resilience is a complex, multidimensional construct. Largely because of the complexity of the construct, there is a lack of consensus about terminology, characteristics, or boundaries of resilience. The next sections examine the various perspectives in these three areas from both the general and the nursing literature.

Perspectives on Resilience

TERMINOLOGY AND ATTRIBUTES OF RESILIENCE

To adequately define a construct, terminology needs to be consistent. In the case of resilience, even the labels for the phenomenon have been inconsistently used. Labels variously applied to the phenomenon have included resilience, resiliency, and ego-resilience. Researchers currently recommend the term *resilience,* rather than *resiliency,* to describe positive adjustment in face of adversity (Luthar et al., 2000;

Masten, 1994). "Resiliency" is not recommended, because it implies a personality trait that is difficult to alter, much like hardiness. The term "ego-resilience" characterizes resilience as a distinct personality trait. Hence, ego-resilience decreases the options for intervention and increases the danger of labeling individuals as innately "inadequate."

There are two generally recognized essential attributes of resilience present in most definitions. These are the presence of (a) "good" or positive outcomes that occur in spite of (b) adverse conditions (Masten, 2001).

Good Outcomes. "Good" or positive outcomes are not consistently theoretically or operationally defined in the literature. Debate centers on what constitutes "good" outcomes and who decides. Additional questions include whether external criteria (e.g., academic achievement) or intrapersonal characteristics (e.g., sense of well-being, self-esteem) or a combination of both are defining characteristics of positive outcomes (Masten, 2001).

Paradigmatic approaches also contribute to differences in ways positive outcomes are defined. A pathology-based worldview often defines positive outcomes as the absence of psychopathology or low levels of symptoms or impairments (Masten & Coatsworth, 1998). Developmental and lifespan perspectives usually define positive outcomes as those that meet or exceed expectations. More recently, a subtle shift in worldviews has occurred that emphasizes dynamic ecosystems influenced by complex, ever-changing, and interacting forces (Richardson, 2002; Waller, 2001) and the notion that resilience is possibly a common human characteristic— "ordinary magic" (Masten, 2001).

Adverse Conditions. The theoretical and operational definitions of "adverse conditions" are also inconsistent in the literature. Frequently, definitions infer threats or risk factors that occur in contexts such as war, illness, community deficits, or family adversity. Beyond the requirement that such factors negatively affect resilience outcomes, there is not agreement on how such risks should be operationalized. Options include either (a) current or past occurrence; (b) predictors of poor outcomes or status (moderating) variables such as low socioeconomic status; or (c) single-exposure variables or cumulative combinations of factors. Adding to the inconsistency of defining characteristics, risk factors can be continuous bipolar variables classified as either less or more aversive (e.g., mild to severe symptoms) or as negative to positive assets (e.g., low to high economic status, negative to positive coping) (Masten, 2001). In general, much research indicates that risk factors, however operationalized, often co-occur (Masten, 2001).

BOUNDARIES OF RESILIENCE

Boundaries of resilience are the contextual influences (conditions under which resilience exists/varies/disappears), dimensions (e.g., objective/subjective, physiological/psychological), and underlying assumptions (e.g., growth vs. stability and state vs. trait) that are considered in determining the attributes of resilience. Some boundaries of resilience that need careful explication in theory and research include state/trait/process, psychological/physiological, individual/aggregate, and objective/subjective perspective. Within each of these boundaries, the cross-cultural implications also need thoughtful examination and further research.

Trait/State/Process. Although the definition of resilience as the presence of "good" outcomes that occur in the presence of adverse conditions implies a process, there is no consensus on the issue of resilience as trait, state, or process. Again, the confusion is exacerbated by inconsistent terminology and the inability to draw conclusions of causality (Jacelon, 1997; Pettit, 2000). As indicated above, the term *ego-resiliency,* for example, is frequently used interchangeably with resilience, but the former refers to a set of personal characteristics (traits) that may or may not be specifically linked to adversity (Luthar et al., 2000). In addition, terms such as *resilient children* cause confusion. Although this term implies that resilience is a trait, it is used most often in conjunction with the two coexisting conditions of adversity and positive adaptation, and adaptation is usually conceptualized as a process. Even the terms *outcome* and *process* contribute to the confusion, when researchers do not clearly identify a model of resilience that stipulates how the underlying mechanisms in a resilience process may result in specific resilience outcomes. Luthar and Cicchetti (2000) encourage researchers to clearly specify the context to which resilience outcomes apply and to clearly delineate the outcomes by using terms such as *emotional resilience, behavioral resilience,* or *educational resilience.* It would also be helpful, through staged-model specification, to distinguish proximal resilience outcomes, such as self-transcendence and confidence/mastery, from more distal outcomes, such as quality of life, which result from the resilience process and resilience outcomes.

Psychological/Physiological. Psychological concepts associated with resilience have been more widely studied than physiological concepts. Concepts such as self-esteem, self-perception, personality, temperament, intellect, coping, and problem-solving skills are just a few of the psychological concepts that have been studied in relation to resilience. What is not clear is whether these identified psychological variables influence the process and outcomes associated with resilience or whether they are components of resilience (Jacelon, 1997).

Fewer studies have examined physiological dimensions of resilience. Singer and Ryff (2001) identify several positive physiological mechanisms, including those that involve the hypothalamic-pituitary-adrenal (HPA) axis and the autonomic nervous system, which may be linked to positive health and resilience. They further argue for integrative levels of analysis that include the physiological, behavioral, environmental, and psychosocial systems to better understand how each contributes individually and interactively to resilience. Curtis and Cicchetti (2003) provided a thoughtful perspective of the theoretical and methodological considerations for examining the biological contributors to resilience. Specifically, they discuss a transactional organizational theoretical perspective as a framework for including biological considerations. The recent advances in neurosciences and related technology, such as functional magnetic resonance imaging (fMRI), clearly make this avenue of investigation promising.

Individual/Aggregate. Resilience is most often studied in individuals, but to avoid confusion in yet another boundary, it is important for researchers to clarify the level of analysis. At an individual level, family factors have been identified that influence resilience. For example, Hauser, Vieyra, Jacobson, and Wertlieb (1989) identified both direct and indirect effects of family factors on individual resilience. Family direct effects included household composition and family structure, as well as family atmosphere factors such as patterns of communication, adaptability, and flexibility. Family factors apparently also have an indirect effect on individual and social protective factors, since child personality factors (temperament, attitudes, self-esteem, etc.) and social milieu process are often shaped by family processes.

There are growing bodies of literature focused on additional levels of analysis—resilient families (Hawley & DeHaan, 1996; Patterson, 2002) and resilient communities (Bosworth & Earthman, 2002). At these levels, studies most frequently take a systems approach. The family research on resilience is primarily built on family systems theory, and much of the work was done from a family stress and coping framework. Resilience is equated with family adaptation, that is, the balancing of family demands and capabilities through interaction with family meanings (McCubbin, Balling, Possin, Frierdich, & Bryne,

2002; Patterson, 1995, 2002). Resilience research at the family and community level is increasing and may provide strong significance for public policy decisions.

Objective/Subjective. In a qualitative study of homeless adolescents, Hunter and Chandler (1999) found adolescents who considered themselves resilient. According to the adolescents, being resilient was "surviving." The characteristics self-attributed by the adolescents as being resilient were quite different from the characteristics of resilience found in other literature. Hunter and Chandler's research indicated that resilience in homeless adolescents may be a "process of defense using such tactics as insulation, isolation, disconnecting, denial, and aggression or as a process of survival using such responses as violence" (p. 246). These findings indicate that self-attributed resilience in homeless adolescents seems to lack a positive or good outcome, a key characteristic of resilience in the literature. These findings were further supported in a subsequent study by Hunter (2001) that examined cross-cultural perspectives of resilience in adolescents from New England and Ghana. All the adolescents viewed themselves as resilient, regardless of age, gender, culture, or socioeconomic status. Yet, depending on the presence or absence of consistent, loving, caring, mentoring adults, there were qualitative differences in how the adolescents overcame adversities. Hunter classified these as two different "forms of resilience," self-protective survival resilience or connected resilience.

Hunter and Chandler's findings imply that if the objective and subjective dimensions of resilience are not carefully delineated, much of what determines the process and outcomes of resilience will be difficult to ascertain. For example, the cognitive appraisal of the adversity, the actions that are taken to deal with the adversity, and subsequent evaluation of how one is dealing with the adversity can all influence how resilience as a process proceeds (Fine, 1991). Further, if the objective and subjective appraisal, actions, and evaluation differ, evaluation of outcomes and development of interventions will be more complex.

One potentially helpful way to delineate the objective/subjective dimensions of resilience is to consider whether resilience may be interpersonally assigned to an individual, much like courage is interpersonally assigned (Haase, 1987). Research indicates that individuals usually do not attribute courage to themselves, unless someone else initially indicates that their behavior could be interpreted as courageous (Haase, 1987). Likewise, it is possible that persons who have resilience require time to reflect on the meaning of their actions. That is, resilience may occur through a process that includes deriving meaning from the experience through interaction with others (Haase, Heiney, Ruccione, & Stutzer, 1999). After interviews were conducted, Hunter and Chandler's findings supported this perspective in that the adolescents' resilience scores increased from baseline measures (Hunter, 2001). A second consideration regarding the subjective perspective is the social desirability of being labeled "resilient." It is possible that a label of being resilient parallels a label such as "honest," in that, when asked, one would not readily deny having such a characteristic.

Cross-Cultural Considerations Related to Boundaries. In the midst of adversity, individuals are especially likely to return to cultural tradition to seek solutions (Hwang, 2006, p. 90). Hence, a full understanding of resilience needs to include cultural considerations. Few studies have explicitly examined the cultural boundaries of resilience. As an exemplar of how cultural boundaries may influence resilience, we briefly examine Chinese and Western cultural differences in two concepts that are important to resilience: sense of self and relational self.

The sense of self, a key individual protective factor of resilience, is different in Western society and Chinese society. In Western society, self is individual oriented and reflects the interaction of "I" and "me" (Mead, 1952). "I" is a subjective perception of individual and "me" is an objective evaluation from others about "me" in certain situations. This individualistic perspective that is more prominent in Western society assumes the importance of opportunity to achieve personal goals, irrespective of group goals (Bedford & Hwang, 2003; Triandis, Bontempo, Villareal, Asai, & Lucca, 1988). In contrast, in Chinese culture, self is noted as interdependent self or relational self that is composed of "great self" (social self) and "small self" (physical self) (Ho, Chen, & Chiu, 1991; Hwang, 1997). "Great self" means an individual has obligations to prevent his or her family or group members from any threats; "small self" refers to an individual's physical self that is independent from others (Bedford & Hwang, 2003). "Small self" is similar to the perspective of self in Western society. The Confucian concept of collectivism advocates that one's life is an inheritance from ancestors of the clan and that this ancestral inheritance perspective fosters expectations from families or group members and overrides individual goals (Bedford & Hwang, 2003; Triandis et al., 1988). In the Chinese culture, then, family or community protective factors may have greater influence as pathways to resilience, and individual protective factors, such as sense of self, may require alignment with family goals to actually serve a protective function. In these cases, positive coping strategies, such as confrontive coping from a Western perspective, may be less positive, and strategies that are less effective in Western culture, such as fatalism in deference to ancestors, may actually have a positive influence on resilience.

Interpersonal relationship is another important concept related to resilience. In Western society, interpersonal interactions hold an assumption of respect for the principles of egalitarianism and independence (Triandis et al., 1988). Thus, interpersonal relationships are based on a decisional choice. In Chinese culture, interpersonal relationships are composed of horizontal and vertical relationships. Horizontal relationships are constructed according to intimacy/distance and vertical relationships are built according to superiority/inferiority (Hwang, 1997). Horizontal relationship indicates interaction within equal family or social positions, such as sibling or peer relationships. Vertical relationship means interaction among hierarchal family or social positions, such as child–parent or student–teacher relationships. The vertical relationship is less emphasized in Western society.

Because both sense of self and interpersonal relationships are culturally different in Western and Chinese society, how they work to foster resilience is also likely to be different. In Western society, the presentation of self is based on one's interpretation of interactions in specific social situations (Charon, 1998; Mead, 1952). In contrast, in Chinese society, the self is defined not by any situational interpretation, but by person-in-relation status, which is called the "relational self" (Ho, Chen, & Chiu, 1991). In Chinese society, based on relational self, personal coping strategies, purpose in life, and interpersonal interactions may be more driven by status concerns in social relationships than in Western cultures.

Resilience Perspectives in Nursing

Not surprisingly, information in Table 16.1 indicates that there is no greater consensus on definitions, characteristics, or boundaries of resilience in the nursing literature than there is in the literature from other disciplines. The nursing literature on resilience parallels that of the general literature. Although nurses historically have focused more extensively on individual and family strengths than many disciplines, systematic study of resilience by nurses only began in the mid- to late 1980s. A major contribution to understanding resilience from the nursing literature is the focus on resilience in the context of health, an otherwise neglected area in the resilience literature. The articles included in Table 16.1 provide a representative sample of both theoretical and empirical efforts to understand resilience by nurses, including varied populations and approaches to knowledge development.

TERMINOLOGY AND ATTRIBUTES OF RESILIENCE

Most definitions in Table 16.1 include the characteristic of adversity. Some definitions specifically describe the adversity as stress, loss, or illness, while others use more global terms, such as "challenging life condition" (Drummond, Kysela, McDonald, & Query, 2002) or a "disaster" (Polk, 1997). The "good" varies considerably in the definitions, as well. Although several of the definitions use vague terminology, such as "go on with life" (Dyer & McGuinness, 1996) or "spring back" (Jacelon, 1997), other definitions indicate the "good" reflected in processes of adaptation, positive health, and/or well-being (McCubbin & McCubbin, 1996; Haase et al., 1999; Ahern, 2006; Vinson, 2002). Only a few definitions of resilience provide clear descriptions of outcome variables associated with resilience.

Regarding the essential characteristics of adversity and "good" outcomes, there is the same inconsistency in the nursing literature as was found in the general resilience literature. Risk or adversity factors primarily focus on how protective factors of resilience can deter the impact that risk has on resilience outcomes. In some cases, both protective and vulnerability, or risk, factors were listed together. In these cases one is forced to assume that either the risk factor is the absence of the protective factor identified or that resilience occurs on a continuum of risk to protection. Examples of the risk factors identified in the nursing literature include survival tactics of violence (Hunter & Chandler, 1999); defensive coping and illness-related risks such as uncertainty and symptom distress (Haase et al., 1999); and gender, antisocial behavior, and chronic illness (Stewart, Reid, & Mangham, 1997). Few models specify the mechanisms by which the adversity itself may influence and even contribute to resilience. This is puzzling because individuals often clearly credit the adversity itself as the important factor that influences the outcome. To illustrate, consider Lance Armstrong's quote, "The truth is that cancer was the best thing that ever happened to me. I don't know why I got the illness, but it did wonders for me, and I wouldn't want to walk away from it. Why would I want to change, even for a day, the most important, and shaping event of my life?" (Armstrong, 2000).

The positive factors of resilience reflected in Table 16.1 are numerous. In many cases, where models were specified based on literature synthesis and/or qualitative research to develop a resilience model, the relationship to and among positive factors is clearly described. Taken as a whole, the literature set provides an emerging pattern that may help distinguish positive resilience outcomes from positive outcomes of resilience. Positive resilience outcomes may include:

- Confidence, self-esteem, and self-transcendence (Haase et al., 1999)
- Self-esteem, self-efficacy, trust, connectedness, competence, and ego-resilience (Hunter & Chandler, 1999)
- Maintenance of physiological and psychological health (Stewart et al., 1997)
- Self-esteem, confidence, intelligence, a toughened effect, hope, mastery, and enhanced coping (Dyer & McGuinness, 1996)
- Social competence, global self-worth, and perceived health (Heinzer, 1995)
- Sense of humor (Ahern, 2006)

Positive outcomes of resilience include:

- Enhanced quality of life conceptualized as well-being (Haase et al., 1999; Hockenberry-Eaton, Kemp, & Dilorio, 1994; Vinson, 2002)
- A sense of having overcome that fosters mastery (Dyer & McGuinness, 1996)
- Psychological equilibrium (Kadner, 1989)
- Global psychosocial adjustment (Stewart et al., 1997)
- Health-promoting lifestyles and less risk-taking behavior (Ahern, 2006; Black & Ford-Gilboe, 2004)

(text continues on page 348)

Table 16.1 NURSING LITERATURE ON RESILIENCE

SOURCE	METHODS OF KNOWLEDGE DEVELOPMENT	POPULATIONS STUDIED	DEFINITION OF RESILIENCE	PRIMARY BOUNDARIES
Ahern (2006)	Rodger's Evolutionary Model of Concept Analysis	Adolescents	Process of adaptation to risk that incorporates personal characteristics, family and social support, and community resources	Individual, dynamic psychosocial process
Aronowitz (2005)	Grounded theory	Adolescents who previously engaged in risk behaviors and then stopped	(Borrowed) Values, attitudes, and behavioral dimensions that influence the dynamic, responsive abilities fostering health development and adaptation in the face of normal or unexpected challenges (Luthar et al., 2000; Perkins, Luster, & Villarruel, 1998)	Individual, dynamic psychosocial process
Black & Ford-Gilboe (2004)	Cross-sectional, descriptive correlational design	Adolescent mothers	(Borrowed) Internal strength that develops in the context of adversity (Kadner, 1989) Resilience operationalized by Resilience Scale (Wagnild & Young, 1993)	Individual process influenced by familial experiences

COMPONENTS: ANTECEDENTS/ EXOGENOUS VARIABLES	COMPONENTS: ATTRIBUTES/ PROCESSES	COMPONENTS: OUTCOMES	KEY RELATIONAL STATEMENTS/ FINDINGS

Risks: internal or external factors	Individual protective factors:
	    Competence
	    Positive coping
	    Sense of humor
	    Connectedness with caring adults
	    Knowledge of health behavior and risks
	Sociocultural protective factors:
	    Connectedness with family
	    Community resources
		Resilience is the outcome of triadic influences of risk, protection, and interventions.	A proposed model of resilience includes a continuum of behaviors from risk (internal and external factors) to protection (individual and sociocultural).

Connectedness with caring, competent, and responsible adults
Specific behaviors displayed by adults:
    Modeling
    Monitoring
    Coaching
    Countering
	Feeling competent
	Elevating expectations
		Envisioning a positive future
		Fewer risk behaviors
			Having a connected relationship with a caring, competent, and responsible adult helped the adolescents envision a positive future for themselves and promoted positive health behaviors.

Adversity Income Professional support	Resilience is viewed as an aspect of health potential.	Health-promoting lifestyle practices	Mother's resilience and family health work explained 30.2% of the variance in mother's health-promoting lifestyle practices. Moderate positive correlations were found between mother's resilience and both family health work and mother's health-promoting lifestyle practices.

(table continued on page 336)

Table 16.1 NURSING LITERATURE ON RESILIENCE (continued)

SOURCE	METHODS OF KNOWLEDGE DEVELOPMENT	POPULATIONS STUDIED	DEFINITION OF RESILIENCE	PRIMARY BOUNDARIES
Drummond et al. (2002)	Family Adaptation Model Development, using resilience theory (family protective factors) as underpinnings Survey and posttest-only experimental design	Families of children with special needs and families with children in Head Start	(Borrowed) Maintenance of positive adjustment under challenging life conditions (Luthar et al., 2000a)	Family processes
Dyer & McGuinness (1996)	Concept analysis	Adults	A process whereby people bounce back from adversity and go on with their lives	Individual psychosocial process with outcome on a continuum
Felton & Hall (Felten, 2000; Felten & Hall, 2001)	Concept analysis	Women older than 85 who experienced illness or loss	The ability to achieve, retain, or regain a level of physical or emotional health after devastating illness or loss	Individual psychosocial state influenced by external factors
Haase (Haase et al., 1999; Haase, 2004)	Triangulation using qualitative model and instrument generating and quantitative model evaluating studies	Adolescents with chronic illness, primarily cancer	The process of identifying or developing resources and strengths to manage stressors flexibly and gain a positive outcome (i.e., a sense of confidence or mastery, self-transcendence, and self-esteem)	Individual psychosocial process resulting in specific outcomes

COMPONENTS: ANTECEDENTS/ EXOGENOUS VARIABLES	COMPONENTS: ATTRIBUTES/ PROCESSES	COMPONENTS: OUTCOMES	KEY RELATIONAL STATEMENTS/ FINDINGS
Presence of vulnerability processes in family life that may create demands in maintenance of family protective processes	Ongoing development and successful use of protective family processes (appraisal, support, and coping)	Family adaptation	Normative adaptation is managed mostly through use of supports and through positive appraisals in the families.
Adversity and at least one caring, emotionally available person	Prosocial attitude, Rebounding and carrying on Sense of self-determination	Outcome a continuum of vulnerability to resilience Toughening effect Sense of having overcome that fosters mastery Enhanced coping	Accessed skills and abilities may occur within the individual or interpersonally through a supportive, caring, and responsive environment.
Illness or loss	Environmental factors: frailty, determination, previous experience learning to cope, access to care, cultural-based health beliefs, family support, self-care activities, caring for others and functioning efficiently External factors: structure of the environmental factors and stress		Resilience is conceptualized as a coiled wire enclosed in a box. External factors of resilience are a configuration of environmental factors within the box and stress.
Social protective: Health care resources Social integration Family protective: Family atmosphere Family support/ resources Illness-related risk: Illness perspective Illness-related distress	Individual risk: Defensive coping (sustained over time) Individual protective: Derived meaning Courageous coping	Resilience: Self-esteem, self- transcendence, confidence/mastery Quality of life: Well-being	Illness-related risk and social and family protective factors directly affect individual risk and protective factors. All these factors directly or indirectly affect resilience and quality-of-life outcomes.

(table continued on page 338)

Table 16.1 NURSING LITERATURE ON RESILIENCE (continued)

SOURCE	METHODS OF KNOWLEDGE DEVELOPMENT	POPULATIONS STUDIED	DEFINITION OF RESILIENCE	PRIMARY BOUNDARIES
Heinzer (1995)	Descriptive, model evaluation	Adults who lost a parent when an adolescent	(Borrowed) The dynamic ability or strength (both physiological and psychological in nature) that enables an individual to recover from or adjust easily to loss or misfortune and to mobilize coping resources (Garmezy et al., 1984)	Individual process Psychological variables studied, but physiological recognized in definition
Hockenberry-Eaton et al. (1994)	Quasi-experimental study of physiological and psychosocial variables	Children with cancer	(Inferred) A process of responding to life stressors that involves protective factors	Individual biological and psychological process
Humphreys (2003)	Descriptive correlation design	Sheltered battered women	(Borrowed) An individual's ability in the face of overwhelming adversity to adapt and restore equilibrium to his or her life and to avoid the potentially deleterious effects of stress (Wagnild & Young, 1993)	Individual psychological process

COMPONENTS: ANTECEDENTS/ EXOGENOUS VARIABLES	COMPONENTS: ATTRIBUTES/ PROCESSES	COMPONENTS: OUTCOMES	KEY RELATIONAL STATEMENTS/ FINDINGS
Time since death of parent Age of adolescent at death Gender Circumstances of death (sudden or expected)	Parental attachment as basis for developing social relationships Adaptive coping	Social competence, global self-worth, perceived health	Adaptive coping consistently predicted outcome variables of resilience. Attachment was not significant.
Presence of stressor	Psychological protective: Coping, self-perception, family environment, social support Physiological stress response (endocrine) Psychological stress response (state anxiety)	Well-being	Family environment and global self-worth predict epinephrine levels; social support from friends predicts norepinephrine levels; family environment and social support predict state anxiety.
Battering experience; physical and psychological distress	Resilience is a pattern of successful outcomes in individuals despite challenging or threatening circumstances.	Less physical and psychological distress	Participants who had higher levels of resilience reported significantly fewer symptoms of physical and psychological distress.

(table continued on page 340)

Table 16.1 NURSING LITERATURE ON RESILIENCE (continued)

SOURCE	METHODS OF KNOWLEDGE DEVELOPMENT	POPULATIONS STUDIED	DEFINITION OF RESILIENCE	PRIMARY BOUNDARIES
Hunter & Chandler (Hunter, 2001; Hunter & Chandler, 1999)	Triangulation: Concept clarification through focus groups, phenomenological analysis, and journal writing Cross-cultural comparisons Quantitative analysis using Resilience Scale	Homeless adolescents Adolescents in variety of situational settings across two cultures	State of being that allows a person to overcome adversity without suffering long-term negative consequences	Individual psychological state taking two forms Objective and subjective perspectives on a continuum
Jacelon (1997)	Synthesis of literature on resilience	Children, adolescents, and adults in various circumstances	(Borrowed dictionary definition) Ability of people to "spring back" in the face of adversity	Individual psychological trait and process
Kadner (1989)	Synthesis of literature on resilience in context of mental health services	Vulnerable populations, especially psychiatric	Ability to regain psychosocial equilibrium after a brief fragmentation in response to severe stress	Individual psychological trait, partially physically (genetically) predisposed

COMPONENTS: ANTECEDENTS/ EXOGENOUS VARIABLES	COMPONENTS: ATTRIBUTES/ PROCESSES	COMPONENTS: OUTCOMES	KEY RELATIONAL STATEMENTS/ FINDINGS
Developmental independence Developed competencies Invincibility Mastery Resourcefulness Perseverance Stress	Connected resilience: self-esteem, self-efficacy, connectedness, trust, competence, ego-resilience, sociability OR Survival resilience: psychopathology, maladaption, social and emotional withdrawal, high-risk behaviors, survival tactics of violence		Adolescents without support showed survival and self-protected resilience; those with support showed a connected form of resilience.
Triad of personal, family, and community factors including resources, above-average intelligence, strong sense of self, self-reliance, independence, and positive outlook			Process is labeled "resilition." Trait is labeled resilience.
Stressor as antecedent is implied.	Attributes are psychological resources: ego strength, social intimacy, and resourcefulness.	Outcome implied is psychological equilibrium manifested as coping.	The aggregate of psychological resources promotes coping efficacy.

(table continued on page 342)

Table 16.1 NURSING LITERATURE ON RESILIENCE (continued)

SOURCE	METHODS OF KNOWLEDGE DEVELOPMENT	POPULATIONS STUDIED	DEFINITION OF RESILIENCE	PRIMARY BOUNDARIES
Lee et al. (2004)	Hybrid model of concept development	Parents of a child who had been diagnosed with cancer in Korea	(Inferred) Family resilience is an enduring force that leads a family to change its dynamics of functioning in order to solve problems associated with stresses encountered.	Family dynamic process

COMPONENTS: ANTECEDENTS/ EXOGENOUS VARIABLES	COMPONENTS: ATTRIBUTES/ PROCESSES	COMPONENTS: OUTCOMES	KEY RELATIONAL STATEMENTS/ FINDINGS
Internal or external stressor	*Intrinsic family characteristics*: (e.g., coherence, faith, positive outlook, mature thinking, family self-esteem) *Family member orientation*: (e.g., flexibility in reorganizing, attachment, open communication, mutual understanding, maintaining a balance in the demands of family members) *Responsiveness to stress*: (e.g., adaptability, desire to maintain normal states, patience for attainment of goals, ability to control stress, readiness to accept critical situations, responsibility for causing trouble) *External orientation:* (e.g., economic resources, proactiveness toward information, maintaining cooperative relations with health care providers, ability to maintain good social relations, family member leadership)	Enhanced family functioning and coping	Family resilience identified as a strength that supports family functioning as changes and adaptations are required in response to internal and external stressors

(table continued on page 344)

Table 16.1 NURSING LITERATURE ON RESILIENCE (continued)

SOURCE	METHODS OF KNOWLEDGE DEVELOPMENT	POPULATIONS STUDIED	DEFINITION OF RESILIENCE	PRIMARY BOUNDARIES
Lothe & Heggen (2003)	Ethnography	Young adult famine survivors in Ethiopia	The ability to return to the original form or position after being bent, compressed, or stretched	Individual psychological trait and process
Mandleco & Peery (2000)	Review of relevant literature on resilience from developmental psychology, child psychiatry, and nursing	Children	Tendency to spring back, rebound, or recoil that involves the capacity to respond and endure or develop and master in spite of life stressors or adversity	Individual psychological state influenced by biological trait
McCubbin & McCubbin (1993, 1996)	Triangulation of qualitative and quantitative approaches for model and instrument development	Families experiencing illness of a family member, usually a child	Positive behavioral patterns and functional competencies individuals and the family unit demonstrate under stressful or adverse circumstances, which determine the family's ability to recover by maintaining its integrity as a unit while insuring, and where necessary restoring the well-being of family members and the family unit as a whole	Dynamic family behavioral and functional process
Polk (1997)	Concept synthesis for model development using nursing model as philosophical underpinnings	No specific population	The ability to transform disaster into a growth experience and move forward	Individual pattern that is transformative

COMPONENTS: ANTECEDENTS/ EXOGENOUS VARIABLES	COMPONENTS: ATTRIBUTES/ PROCESSES	COMPONENTS: OUTCOMES	KEY RELATIONAL STATEMENTS/ FINDINGS
Internal and external stressors	Faith Hope Having a living relative Having memories of one's past roots	Adaptation	Participants who managed a successful adaptation had the ability to look at their lives with a balanced perspective.
Internal biological factors: general health, genetic predisposition, temperament, and gender Internal psychological factors: cognitive capacity, coping ability, and personality characteristics External within family factors: home environment, parenting practices, and particular family members External outside family factors: supportive individuals and community resources			Interactional or transactional relationship exists with the internal and external factors affecting resilience and between the internal and external factors.
Family experienced stress and hardship.	Family developed strengths and competencies in adjustment phase including patterns of family functioning, resources, appraisal, coping strategies, and problem solving.	Restoration and adaptation: well-functioning individual members, family sense of balance and harmony in carrying out tasks and responsibilities and in relationship to the community	Resiliency factors that helped families dealing with cancer recovery included internal family rapid mobilization and reorganization; social support from the health care team, extended family, the community, and the workplace; and changes in appraisal to make the situation more comprehensive, manageable, and meaningful.
Human and environmental energy field	Dispositional attributes (e.g., physical and ego-related attributes such as competence and sense of self) Patterns of relationships and roles Situational patterns: characteristic approaches to situations or stressors Philosophical pattern of personal beliefs		Transformation manifested as specific dispositional, relational, situational, and philosophical patterns

(table continued on page 346)

Table 16.1 NURSING LITERATURE ON RESILIENCE (continued)

SOURCE	METHODS OF KNOWLEDGE DEVELOPMENT	POPULATIONS STUDIED	DEFINITION OF RESILIENCE	PRIMARY BOUNDARIES
Rew et al. (2001)	Descriptive/exploratory correlational design	Homeless adolescents	No specific theoretical definition Resilience operationalized by Resilience Scale (Wagnild & Young, 1993)	Individual psychological It is unclear if viewed as state or trait
Rew & Horner (2003)	Author-developed framework	Adolescents	(Borrowed) Resilience represents the interaction between risk factors and protective resources (Rutter, 1987)	Context of health-risk behaviors Dynamic process
Stewart et al. (1997)	Synthesis review of literature on resilience and health	Children	Capability of individuals to cope successfully in the face of significant change, adversity, or risk	Individual physiological and psychological state that changes over time and is influenced by protective factors in the individual and environment
Tusaie & Patterson (2006)	Descriptive, correlational examination of types of optimism to clarify the concept in preparation for developing evidence-based resilience intervention	Rural adolescents	No definition of resilience	Individual Apparently focused on optimism as a mediator

COMPONENTS: ANTECEDENTS/ EXOGENOUS VARIABLES	COMPONENTS: ATTRIBUTES/ PROCESSES	COMPONENTS: OUTCOMES	KEY RELATIONAL STATEMENTS/ FINDINGS
Homelessness as condition Loneliness, hopelessness, life-threatening behaviors, and connectedness	Resilience may be an adaptive or defense strategy, rather than a protective factor.		Loneliness, hopelessness, life-threatening behaviors, and connectedness were negative predictors of resilience as measured by Resilience Scale.
Sociocultural context of interaction among individual risk and protective factors and family and community contexts	Resiliency is process of interaction of the antecedents that can be influenced by interventions.	Reduction of health-risk behaviors/morbidity and mortality	Model developed that proposes interaction between individual risk and family and individual and community protective factors
Transition, increased stressors	*Protective factors:* *Individual level:* Coping, self-help, self-esteem, intelligence, self-efficacy *Family level:* Positive parent–child attachment, future orientation, rules in the household, social support *Community Level:* Positive school experiences	Maintenance of physiological and psychological health, such as: Global psychosocial adjustment Lack of psychopathology Self-esteem Confidence Intelligence Positive immune response	Relationship of resilience and health is clarified in discussions of risk and protective factors and resilient outcomes, in particular psychological and physical health and health behavior.
Age, sex	Trait, situational, and comparative optimism	Expectation of positive outcomes (implied resilience)	Adolescent optimism is expressed differently when examining the trait, situational, and comparative aspects of the concept.

(table continued on page 348)

Table 16.1 **NURSING LITERATURE ON RESILIENCE** (continued)

SOURCE	METHODS OF KNOWLEDGE DEVELOPMENT	POPULATIONS STUDIED	DEFINITION OF RESILIENCE	PRIMARY BOUNDARIES
Vinson (2002)	Inner Core Child Resilience Model Development and Testing based on resilience literature synthesis and data-based findings of descriptive correlational study	School-age children with asthma	A combination of personality characteristics, family influences, and available social and cultural supportive environments that permits the epigenetic unfolding of adaptive processes	Individual psychosocial process
Wagnild & Young (1990, 1993)	Grounded theory and factor analysis of instrument	Older adults	A personality characteristic that moderates the negative effects of stress and promotes adaptation	Individual trait
Woodgate (1999; Woodgate & McClement, 1997)	Synthesis of resilience literature in context of cancer to develop a model	Adolescents with cancer	Dynamic process involving the development of resources within the individual that allows the individual to gain a positive outcome in the face of significant adversity	Individual, dynamic psychological process

BOUNDARIES OF RESILIENCE

With the exception of the psychological dimension that is identified by all authors, all the other boundaries of resilience, either explicit or implied, are inconsistent. There is no consensus on whether resilience is a trait, state, process, or some combination of these dimensions. Most definitions imply that a change occurs, but there is inconsistency as to whether the resilience change is a return to a steady state or is part of a growth-producing process. Jacelon (1997) explicitly distinguishes and labels resilience as the trait and "resilition" as the process. Only one definition explicitly addresses a timeframe (Hunter, 2001; Hunter & Chandler, 1999).

The existence of biological contributions to resilience remains strikingly missing from most of the nursing literature. This gap is reflective of the general state of the science on resilience on biological dimensions. This situation may improve with the advancing technologies that have resulted in a rapidly

COMPONENTS: ANTECEDENTS/ EXOGENOUS VARIABLES	COMPONENTS: ATTRIBUTES/ PROCESSES	COMPONENTS: OUTCOMES	KEY RELATIONAL STATEMENTS/ FINDINGS
Exogenous variables: Child characteristics, Family environment	Coping patterns, threat appraisal	Quality of life, illness indices	Paths are from family to child characteristics, child characteristics to appraisal, appraisal to quality of life, family to child coping, child coping to illness indices, and child perceived quality of life to illness indices.
Personal competence including self-reliance, independence, determination, invincibility, mastery, resourcefulness, and perseverance Acceptance of self and life including adaptability, balance, flexibility, and balanced perspective of life			The Resilience Scale is of potential use as a measure of internal resources and of the positive contribution an individual brings to a difficult life event.
Stressors	*Protective factors:* Self-concept Meaning Coping Social support from family External support from peers	Adaptation (social competence) or maladaptation (depression, low self-esteem)	Resilience is a mediating process initiated by stressors and the results in outcomes on a continuum of adaptation and maladaptation.

developing knowledge base in neuroscience (Curtis & Cicchetti, 2003). In nursing, Hockenberry's and Mandleco's works (Hockenberry-Eaton et al., 1994; Mandleco & Peery, 2000) are among the few that consider biological contributions to resilience. In the context of childhood cancer, Hockenberry argued that activation of the endocrine system as a less adaptive response to stress—as indicated by an elevation of both catecholamine and cortisol—could indicate less resilience to the stressors associated with cancer (Hockenberry-Eaton, Dilorio, & Kemp, 1995). Mandleco and Peery (2000) identified four biological factors as possibly affecting resilience: general health, genetic predisposition, temperament, and gender. Research supports that children with resilience are usually quite healthy and have little hereditary or chronic illness. However, hypotheses about gender and temperament need further exploration. Evidence that temperament is a factor of resilience is derived from studies examining infant temperament; however, it is not clear that temperament is biologically based. Regarding gender, although males are more vulnerable to all risk factors, one cannot assume that more vulnerability equates to less resilience.

Resilience was most frequently studied as an individual dimension rather than as a family or community aggregate. In studies focused on individuals, the family or community variables were often included as protective factors that influence outcomes for the individual. In some ways, the state of knowledge on family resilience is further along than individually focused research, in that the limited number of proposed models is more consistently being used and evaluated, and there is more consistency in the ways that family level measures are used.

Nurses studying resilience seem to assume the importance of obtaining subjective indicators. These subjective indicators were obtained as narratives and as self-reported quantitative measures of resilience-related concepts. As indicated in this chapter's methods section, nurse researchers have also developed creative methods for obtaining the personal meanings associated with resilience. Ways of making sense of combined, simultaneous objective, physiological measures as they relate to subjective ratings is not addressed well in either the nursing or the general literature. Because nurses focus on both physiological and psychosocial aspects of health, it would seem logical that nurse researchers would be well positioned to provide leadership in this area.

DESCRIPTION OF RESILIENCE: THE THEORY

There is agreement that models of resilience should include factors generally characterized as "protective." In addition, "risk" factors are also generally identified as influencing resilience processes and outcomes. A major problem in developing theory about resilience is that these protective and risk factors frequently resemble "laundry lists." That is, they lack an explicit description of underlying assumptions or an explicit theoretical framework that describes the mechanisms by which the protective and risk factors are linked to outcomes. Especially lacking are hypothesized paths or the magnitude of their influence on development of resilience. Additionally, much confusion relates to whether these protective and risk factors are direct ameliorative effects or, rather, they are interactive effects reserved for individuals who have a particular attribute and who were relatively unaffected by high or low levels of adversity (Luthar & Cicchetti, 2000).

Important components that should be considered in all modeling efforts to understand and enhance resilience are context, including culture, psychological and physiological mediating units, and the patterns of mediators in relation to the context (Coyne & Downey, 1991; Freitas & Downey, 1998). Further, there is value in interventions that manipulate mediating variables, such as coping and hope, that have been found to influence resilience outcomes (Singer & Ryff, 2001).

Masten (2001) provides a useful distinction between variable-focused approaches and person-focused approaches to model development. In variable-focused approaches, multivariate statistics are used to test for linkages among measures of adversity, outcomes, and environmental or individual qualities that may protect or compensate for negative consequences. Models may examine direct, indirect, and interaction effects (Luthar et al., 2000; Masten, 2001). Direct-effects models hypothesize direct effects in multivariate correlational analyses. A direct-effects example is when the relationship of high and low scores on outcomes is directly related to high and low scores on measures of adversity, or when a path diagram directly links specific variables with an outcome. Figures 16.1A and B illustrate the direct effects model. Indirect-effect models are those that hypothesize that the effect of variables, such as adversity or personal characteristics, is mediated by another variable, such as parental styles, as seen in Figure 16.1C. Interaction models hypothesize that the effects of adversity can be modified by individual characteristics or the environment. In general, variable-

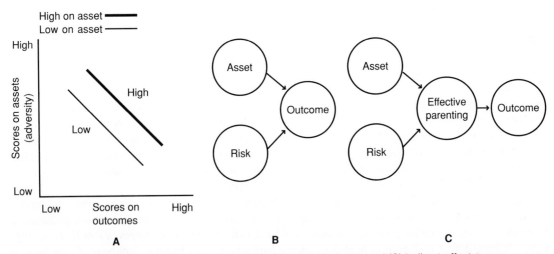

■ **Figure 16.1** Variable-focused research models: **(A)** main, **(B)** direct, and **(C)** indirect effects.

focused research indicates that adversity does not result in lasting or major effects, unless moderating and mediating systems, such as parent or social protective factors, are compromised (Masten, 2001).

Person-focused research attempts to identify and describe the patterns of variables that naturally occur, often identifying persons with either positive or poor functioning and then examining what might contribute to these outcomes, or using cut-off scores on selected variables to categorize adversity subgroups and then examining outcomes in these groups. These types of person-focused designs often lack comparison low-risk groups, which are important to answer questions of whether resilient children differ from children who are doing well but do not have high-risk characteristics. Masten (2001) also argues for more complex person-oriented models that include both health and maladaptive pathways of development in lives studied over time, giving special attention to turning points. These pathway models have a greater potential for providing intervention frameworks.

Approaches to Resilience Knowledge Development in Nursing Literature

Although there is a relatively small amount of research on resilience in the nursing literature, the work accomplished to date has creatively used a variety of approaches to gain a fuller understanding of resilience. In no other discipline is such a rich combination of approaches to studying resilience found. Several of the articles in Table 16.1 include extensive analyses and syntheses of existing literature on resilience (Ahern, 2006; Dyer & McGuinness, 1996; Jacelon, 1997; Kadner, 1989; Polk, 1997; Stewart et al., 1997; Woodgate, 1999; Woodgate & McClement, 1997), and many of these were used to propose models of resilience in specific health contexts. For example, Woodgate (1999) derived the Resilience Model as Applied to Adolescents with Cancer based on her synthesis of the literature on resilience within the context of cancer, and Vinson (2002) proposed a model of resilience in children with asthma. Another synthesis article used a nursing metatheory, the Science of Unitary Human Beings, as the underlying framework for developing a resilience model (Polk, 1997). Ahern

(2006) used evolutionary concept analysis to specify a model of adolescent resilience that includes potential interventions, and Haase et al. (1999) used a combination of methods to develop the Adolescent Resilience Model.

In addition to literature synthesis approaches, several articles were data based. Qualitative research approaches used to gain understanding of resilience included grounded theory and phenomenology. Qualitative methods of data collection included open-ended or phenomenological interviews, focus groups, and free-writing exercises. Some authors used triangulation of qualitative and/or quantitative empirical studies to derive models of resilience in the context of health or a specific illness. As examples, Haase et al. (1999) used a decision-making process to triangulate qualitative and quantitative approaches for instrument identification or development as well as model testing, and Hunter (2001) conducted concept clarification by triangulating qualitative data collection methods, such as free-writing exercises with quantitative measures of resilience, to conduct a cross-cultural comparison of resilience.

The data-based nursing studies in Table 16.1 fall into three categories of design. First are studies describing characteristics of a sample of participants who were designated, a priori, as having resilience. Examples of such studies are resilience in women older than 85 experiencing illness or loss (Felten, 2000; Felten & Hall, 2001); resilience in homeless adolescents (Hunter & Chandler, 1999); resilience in adult daughters of battered women (Humphreys, 2001); modes of comfort used by a resilient survivor suffering multiple losses and severe, excruciating burn pain (Morse & Carter, 1995); and adolescents who had stopped engagement in risky behaviors (Aronowitz, 2005).

Next are studies of resilience conducted with a specific population, but without a priori designation of participants as being resilient. Examples include resilience studies of adolescents with cancer (Haase et al., 1999); resilience in a sample of adults who lost a parent when they were adolescents (Heinzer, 1995); and resilience in children with asthma (Vinson, 2002). The third design type includes studies that did not have resilience as a primary focus, but found resilience as an outcome variable. Examples of these studies include a study of women with a cardiac pacemaker (Beery, Sommers, & Hall, 2002) and a study of risk behavior in adolescents with cancer (Hollen, Hobbie, Finley, & Hiebert, 2001). While these studies fit into Masten's description of variable-focused and person-focused research, they do not reflect the complexity of design Masten recommended, to include both healthy and maladaptive pathways of development in lives studied over time, giving special attention to turning points (Masten, 2001). By their creative approaches to clarify the patterns/processes/components of resilience, it is clear that studies conducted by nurses are headed in the "right" direction. More complex designs would seem to be a logical next phase. Tusaie and Patterson (2006) did not directly study resilience, but examined to clarify factors that may influence resilience prior to developing a resilience intervention.

SPECIFIC NURSING MODELS OF RESILIENCE

The articles in Table 16.1 that describe literature synthesis and concept analysis of resilience indicate the value that nurse scientists place on carefully developing theory. Individual-level resilience models include mastery of chronic illness with resilience as an emergent outcome (White, 1995); a "CARE" framework (containment, awareness, resilience, and engagement) to guide mental health practice (McAllister & Walsh, 2003); the Adolescent Resilience Model for adolescents with cancer and other chronic conditions (Haase et al., 1999); the Inner Core Child Resilience Model for children with asthma (Vinson, 2002); the Resiliency Model applied to adolescents with cancer (Woodgate, 1999); a model of resilience in the context of loss of a parent (Heinzer, 1995); a model of resilience in community-dwelling women older than 85, overcoming adversity from illness or loss

(Felten, 2000; Felten & Hall, 2001); and a model of adolescent resilience focused on the outcome of reduction of risk behaviors (Aronowitz, 2005). Also, a model of resilience in adolescents was proposed by Rew & Horner (2003) and adapted by Ahern (2006). Both of these models propose a continuum of risk and protective factors. Many of these models were thoughtfully developed, with underlying assumptions or philosophical perspectives explicated, and the perspectives of those experiencing the adversity taken into consideration. Potential interventions are proposed in three models (Ahern, 2006; Haase, 2004; Rew & Horner, 2003). These models differ in specificity of targeted factors and in potential timing of interventions. All recognize the importance of longitudinal studies to detect patterns of change with and without intervention. Although there is less nursing literature on family or community resilience models, the work that has been done has made significant contributions to knowledge. The Family Resilience Model developed by McCubbin and McCubbin (1996) is increasingly supported in the literature on family resilience (Board & Ryan-Wenger, 2000; Smith, 1997; Svavarsdottir, McCubbin, & Kane, 2000; White, Bichter, Koeckeritz, Lee, & Munch, 2002). Other family models are also being proposed. Drummond, Kysela, McDonald, and Query (2002) proposed and tested a model of family adaptation that identified family protective factors of appraisal, support, and coping as mediators of adaptation. Appraisal was a key variable predicting adaptation. These authors identify the need for further concept clarification of the mediating variables and suggest narrative analysis as a possible method.

Across the models of resilience, the many adversity and positive concepts were inconsistently identified as antecedents, critical components, and outcomes of resilience. Antecedents usually included adversity (e.g., death, loss, illness, stressor[s], and homelessness). Protective factors were modeled as antecedents in only a few studies (Haase et al., 1999; Hunter & Chandler, 1999; Polk, 1997). Across several studies, especially those that viewed resilience as a trait, it was difficult to discern the role or order of resilience-related concepts, such as coping, hope, or mastery. These concepts were alternatively viewed as antecedent and critical component protective factors or as outcomes of resilience. For example, in some articles, coping is viewed as a mediating protective factor, while in other studies, it is an outcome of resilience. Reflective of the general literature, many protective factors do fall into broad classes of factors classified as individual, social, or family.

It is clear that more work needs to be done to clarify the relationship among concepts that are correlated with resilience and those that influence resilience. To increase explanatory power, this work will most productively be done in longitudinal studies, with models that attempt to capture the full, integrative perspective of resilience.

APPLICATIONS OF THE THEORY

Research to Develop a Model and Guide the Development of Intervention

The Adolescent Resilience Model (ARM) provides one example of how a theoretical model that is grounded in contextual experiences can guide interventions. The context for the ARM was chronic illness in adolescents. Most of the work was done from the perspective of adolescents with cancer; some studies included parent and health care provider perspectives.

To develop the ARM, two series of studies were conducted: (a) model generation studies, using inductive approaches, and (b) model evaluation studies, involving instrumentation and exploratory model testing (Haase et al., 1999). The qualitative, model-generating studies provided a basis for development of the ARM through identification and clarification of salient concepts to be included in the model, and as a qualitative means of evaluating subsequent model testing results. These studies were also guided by the Haase Decision-Making Process for Model and Instrument Development (Haase et al., 1999).

Research to Evaluate Instruments

The quantitative model and instrument evaluation studies for the ARM were primarily done using latent variable structural-equation modeling approaches. The studies were done to evaluate the psychometric properties of the instruments used to measure each latent variable, and to develop an appropriate measurement model. Based on the exploratory studies of the theoretical model, factors were identified that affect the development of resilience. The resulting ARM, as it is being studied longitudinally and guiding interventions, is found in Figure 16.2.

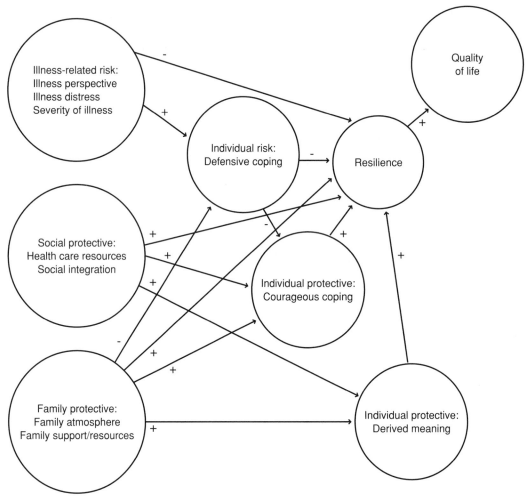

■ **Figure 16.2** The adolescent resilience model.

Both protective and risk factors are included in the ARM. These factors with their related variables are highlighted in Table 16.2. Three classes of ARM protective factors are hypothesized to positively affect resilience outcomes. Class I Individual Protective Factors include courageous or positive coping and derived meaning. Class II Family Protective Factors include family atmosphere and support/resources available to the family. Class III Social Protective Factors include health care resources and social integration. Two classes of ARM risk factors are hypothesized to negatively affect resilience. The Class IV Individual Risk Factor is sustained defensive coping. The Class V Illness-Related Factors include illness perspective and illness distress. The outcome factors of resilience include self-esteem, mastery/confidence, and self-transcendence, as well as quality of life, defined as a sense of well-being.

Table 16.2 ADOLESCENT RESILIENCE MODEL LATENT AND MANIFEST VARIABLES

LATENT FACTOR	MANIFEST VARIABLES
I Individual Protective	
Courageous coping	Confrontive coping
	Optimistic coping
	Supportant coping
Derived meaning	Hope
	Spiritual perspective
II Family Protective	
Family atmosphere	Adaptability and cohesion
	Parent–adolescent communication
	Perceived social support—family
Family support/resources	Family strengths
	Socioeconomic status variables
III Social Protective	
Health care resources	Perceived social support—health care provider
	Adolescent support program participation and satisfaction
	Adolescent support program site evaluation
Social integration	Perceived social support—friends
IV Individual Risk	
Defensive coping	Evasive coping
	Emotive coping
V Illness-related Risk	
Illness perspective	Uncertainty in illness
Illness distress	Symptom distress
	Severity of illness
VI Resilience	
	Confidence/mastery
	Self-transcendence
	Self-esteem
Quality of life	Sense of well-being

INSTRUMENTS USED IN EMPIRICAL TESTING

Measurement is an approach to knowledge development for resilience that is gaining more attention (Ahern, Kiehl, Sole, & Byers, 2006). The lack of instruments to directly measure resilience may be connected with the lack of a consistent view as to whether resilience is a state, trait, or process. The first measure of resilience developed by Wagnild and Young addressed concerns regarding the lack of empirical support for the relationships between resilience and psychosocial adaptation (Wagnild & Young, 1993). Resilience was conceptualized as a personality characteristic rather than a process. The instrument was developed from a grounded theory study of 24 older women who had adapted successfully to a major life event (Wagnild & Young, 1990). Five components of resilience were identified from that study. These components were validated via a review of literature and developed into a theoretical definition of resilience. In psychometric analysis of the factors in the Resilience Scale (RS), a two-factor structure—personal competence and acceptance of self and life—was found (Wagnild & Young, 1993). This scale has been used in other studies that represent different cultural and age samples (Aroian, Schappler-Morris, Neary, Spitzer, & Tran, 1997; Humphreys, 2003; Hunter & Chandler, 1999; Rew, Taylor-Seehafer, Thomas, & Yockey, 2001). Nygren, Randstrom, Lejonklou, and Lundman (2004) have tested the reliability and validity of the Swedish language version of the RS on 142 adults. Heilemann, Lee, and Kury (2003) tested the reliability and validity of a Spanish version of the RS. Modifications were made from 25 items to 23 items with internal consistency reliability. Construct validity was determined for both the Swedish and Spanish translations (Heilemann et al., 2003; Nygren et al., 2004). Two other scales were tested on persons in other cultures, the Adolescent Resilience Scale (Oshio, Kaneko, Nagamine, & Nakaya, 2003) and the Multidimensional Trauma Recovery and Resilience (MTTR) scale (Haz, Castillo, & Aracena, 2003). Construct validity of the Adolescent Resilience Scale was assessed and supported on Japanese undergraduate students ($n = 207$). The MTTR was tested on Chilean mothers ($n = 80$) who were all physically abused as children. Half of the sample went on to abuse their offspring, while half did not. The MTTR instrument was reliable in discriminating between the two groups.

The Resilience Scale for Adults (RSA) (Friborg, Hjemdal, Rosenvinge, & Martinussen, 2003) was given to a small sample ($n = 59$) once and to a larger sample of normal controls ($n = 259$) twice. The RSA differentiated between patients and healthy controls. Further cross-validation of the RSA (Friborg, Barlaug, Martinussen, Rosenvinge, & Hjemdal, 2005) revealed that items of personal strength were associated with emotional stability. RSA items of social competence were associated with extroversion, agreeableness, and social skills. RSA items of structured style were associated with conscientiousness. Family cohesion and social resource items were related to personality. Convergent and discriminative validity of the scale were supported (Friborg et al., 2005).

Lastly, the development of the Connor-Davidson Resilience Scale (CD-RISC) has had promising results among six demographic groups (Connor & Davidson, 2003).

Most studies using quantitative methods in the Table 16.1 literature used existing instruments or developed instruments to measure numerous variables in proposed models. However, in many cases, it is not clear whether the instruments were derived from theories that are congruent with the conceptual frameworks or philosophical approaches being used in the studies. Haase et al. (1999) describe one approach to identifying and/or developing instruments that is clearly linked to the emerging ARM theory. Methods triangulation was done in a series of studies to develop and test the ARM and to identify or develop the instruments used to evaluate the model (Haase, 1987; Haase, Britt, Coward, Leidy, & Penn, 1992; Haase et al., 1999; Haase & Rostad, 1994). Decision trees were used to

16.1 RESEARCH APPLICATION

Using the Adolescent Resilience Model, interventions can be designed to target specific protective or risk factors to enhance resilience outcomes. Several studies were developed and tested using the Adolescent Resilience Model. In one study, the Adolescent Resilience Model was used to guide a music video production (Haase, 2004).

The study aims were to (a) test the efficacy of a therapeutic music video (TMV) intervention for adolescents and young adults (AYAs) during the acute phase of stem cell transplant (SCT), and (b) qualitatively examine the self-reported benefits of the TMV intervention for AYAs.

For AYAs undergoing SCT, participation in the TMV intervention was hypothesized to directly:

- Decrease illness-related distress
- Improve family environment
- Increase perceived social support
- Decrease defensive coping
- Increase positive coping
- Increase derived meaning

Through improved family environment and perceived social support, the TMV was also hypothesized to indirectly affect:

- Positive coping
- Derived meaning

As a consequence of enhancing these variables, the intervention was expected to:

- Increase resilience
- Increase quality of life

In addition to the efficacy of the intervention for AYAs, it was hypothesized that the TMV intervention was helpful and meaningful to family caregivers. This aim was qualitatively evaluated.

The multisite study design was a two-group, randomized clinical trial. Study participants in the treatment group received the TMV intervention over six sessions, conducted by a board-certified music therapist. In the sessions, participants in the music group selected music and engaged in song writing, music recording, and developing the visual content for a music video. Study participants randomized to the low-dose control group also received six sessions conducted by a board-certified music therapist, focused on discussing content of self-selected audio-recorded books. Sites in five states participated in the study to increase sample ethnic, cultural, and economic diversity.

decide on labels and definitions for each model factor, and to decide whether to use existing instruments or ones developed to measure the model factors. This iterative process of decision making sought to retain the inductively derived meanings from the qualitative studies while taking advantage of existing theory and instruments. The result was a set of 15 instruments to measure manifest variables—eight existing instruments meeting established criteria for reliability and validity and seven new instruments. To test the ARM and instruments, latent variable instrument and model-testing studies were done (Haase et al., 1999).

It is clear that additional measurement work is essential to further the science of resilience from a nursing perspective. Cultural considerations in measurement are not well addressed. Measurement in nursing research on resilience needs to consider the issues of boundaries, including trait/process and physiological/psychological. Measurement also needs to focus on differences in resilience based on developmental factors, including age (Research Application 16.1).

SUMMARY

The work of nurse scientists to add to the body of knowledge on resilience is considerable, but much work still needs to be accomplished. Areas of strength within the nursing literature include the careful attention to theory, both by clarifying concepts through literature analysis and synthesis and by using qualitative methods that explore experiences of resilience from the perspectives of those who have experienced adversity. The recognition of resilience as a positive health concept and the recognition of resilience as a dynamic process are strengths. To advance the science, much work remains for nurses in collaboration with scientists from other disciplines. Some specific recommendations can be made: (a) continue efforts on measurement issues, so that instruments are context and culturally sensitive, meaning based, and time sensitive; (b) conduct longitudinal, prospective studies of resilience to test integrative models; (c) develop and test interventions planned to manipulate targeted variables that are promising to influence resilience outcomes; and (d) take advantage of the rapid advancements in neurocognitive sciences to include biological markers that may contribute to existing knowledge of resilience.

ANALYSIS EXERCISES

Using the criteria presented in Chapter 2, critique the theory of resilience. Compare your conclusions about the theory with those found in Appendix A. A nurse scholar who has worked with the theory completed the analysis found in the appendix.

Internal Criticism
1. Clarity
2. Consistency
3. Adequacy

4. Logical development
5. Level of theory development

External Criticism
1. Reality convergence
2. Utility
3. Significance
4. Discrimination
5. Scope of theory
6. Complexity

CRITICAL THINKING EXERCISES

1. The Adolescent Resilience Model (ARM) has primarily been developed for use in adolescents/young adults with cancer. Identify other populations where this model could be used to guide further research. What issues would you need to consider before applying the model to another population?
2. Develop a potential intervention targeted at one or more of the protective factors in the ARM that

may influence resilience and quality of life in adolescents and young adults.
3. Describe how the middle range theory proposed in this chapter helps to refine your previous conceptualization of resilience.
4. Describe the benefits of meaning-based models or strengths-based research in your area of interest.

WEB RESOURCES

1. This site provides information, education, and training materials on strengths-based approaches to resilience. It features the work of Wolin and Wolin, two prominent researchers who focus on resilience: **http://www.projectresilience.com.**
2. This site offers a potpourri of useful publications, forums, training information, and practical applications regarding resilience: **http://www.resiliency.com.**
3. ResilienceNet provides worldwide sources of current, reviewed information about human resilience. It provides information for helping children and families overcome adversities. Current resilience projects around the world are described and the site can be accessed at: **http://resilnet.uiuc.edu/.**
4. American Psychological Association Help Center site on resilience: Look for resilience under the Featured Topics tab accessed at: **http://www.apahelpcenter.org/.**
5. Resilience archives on ERIC: Type in resilience for the subject on the Education Resource Information Center (ERIC) database home page. Several articles will be retrieved: **http://www.eric.ed.gov/.**
6. This is the National Resilience Resource Center web site at the University of Minnesota: **http://www.cce.umn.edu/nrrc/index.html.**
7. Center for Effective Collaboration and Practice web site: Search site for resilience, which provides links to community or family approach to resilience: **http://cecp.air.org/site_search.asp.**
8. Resilience/Practice, Vol. 5, #1: This is a publication of the Center for Applied Research and Educational Improvement at the University of Minnesota. The entire volume focuses on resilience and includes cultural perspectives on resilience: **http://education.umn.edu/CAREI/Reports/Rpractice/Spring97/default.html.**
9. This site provides information on community resilience programs: **http://www.cedworks.com/communityresilience01.html.**
10. The Discovery Health Channel resource on resilience offers Ten Ways to Build Resilience with link to APA brochure "The Road to Resilience": **http://health.discovery.com/centers/mental/articles/resiliencetips.html.**
11. This site provides a gateway to links on the concepts of learned resourcefulness, resiliency, psychological hardiness, and related concepts as they apply to families and children, workplace stress, and personal development: **http://faculty.css.edu/dswenson/web/resilience.html.**
12. Resiliency in health promotion programs are discussed on this site: **http://www.hc-sc.gc.ca/ahc-asc/pubs/drugs-drogues/resiliency-ressortpsycholoique/programs-programmes_e.html.**

REFERENCES

Ahern, N. R. (2006). Adolescent resilience: an evolutionary concept analysis. *Journal of Pediatric Nursing, 21*(3), 175–185.

Ahern, N. R., Kiehl, E. M., Sole, M. L., & Byers, J. (2006). A review of instruments measuring resilience. *Issues in Comprehensive Pediatric Nursing, 29*(2), 103–125.

Antonovsky, A. (1979). *Health, stress, and coping.* San Francisco: Jossey-Bass.

Armstrong, L. (2000). *It's not about the bike: My journey back to life.* New York: Putnam.

Aroian, K. J., Schappler-Morris, N., Neary, S., Spitzer, A., & Tran, T. V. (1997). Psychometric evaluation of the Russian Language version of the Resilience Scale. *Journal of Nursing Measurement, 5*(2), 151–164.

Aronowitz, T. (2005). The role of "envisioning the future" in the development of resilience among at-risk youth. *Public Health Nursing, 22*(3), 200–208.

Bandura, A. (1977). Self-efficacy: Toward a unifying theory of behavioral change. *Psychological Review, 84,* 191–215.

Bedford, O., & Hwang, K. K. (2003). Guilt and shame in Chinese culture: A cross-cultural framework from the perspective of morality and identity. *Journal for the Theory of Social Behavior, 33*(2), 127–144.

Beery, T. A., Sommers, M. S., & Hall, J. (2002). Focused life stories of women with cardiac pacemakers. *Western Journal of Nursing Research, 24*(1), 7–23; discussion 23–27.

Black, C., & Forol-Gilboe, M. (2004). Adolescent mothers: Resilience, family health work and health-promoting practices. *Journal of Advanced Nursing, 48*(4), 351–360.

Block, J. (1980). The role of ego control and ego resiliency in the origins of behavior. *Development of Cognition/Minnesota Symposia on Child Psychology, 13.*

Board, R., & Ryan-Wenger, N. (2000). State of the science on parental stress and family functioning in pediatric intensive care units. *American Journal of Critical Care, 9*(2), 106–122; quiz 123–124.

Bosworth, K., & Earthman, E. (2002). From theory to practice: School leaders' perspectives on resiliency. *Journal of Clinical Psychology, 58*(3), 299–306.

Charon, J. M. (1998). The nature of the self. In J. M. Charon (Ed.), *Symbolic interactionism: An introduction, an interpretation, an integration* (6th ed., pp. 72–97). Upper Saddle River, NJ: Prentice-Hall.

Connor, K. M., & Davidson, J. R. (2003). Development of a new resilience scale: the Connor-Davidson Resilience Scale (CD-RISC). *Depression and Anxiety, 18*(2), 76–82.

Coyne, J. C., & Downey, G. (1991). Social factors and psychopathology: Stress, social support, and coping processes. *Annual Review of Psychology, 42,* 401–425.

Curtis, W. J., & Cicchetti, D. (2003). Moving research on resilience into the 21st century: theoretical and methodological considerations in examining the biological contributors to resilience. *Development and Psychopathology, 15*(3), 773–810.

Drummond, J., Kysela, G. M., McDonald, L., & Query, B. (2002). The family adaptation model: Examination of dimensions and relations. *Canadian Journal of Nursing Research, 34*(1), 29–46.

Dyer, J. G., & McGuinness, T. M. (1996). Resilience: Analysis of the concept. *Archives of Psychiatric Nursing, 10*(5), 276–282.

Felten, B. S. (2000). Resilience in a multicultural sample of community-dwelling women older than age 85. *Clinical Nursing Research, 9*(2), 102–123.

Felten, B. S., & Hall, J. M. (2001). Conceptualizing resilience in women older than 85: Overcoming adversity from illness or loss. *Journal of Gerontological Nursing, 27*(11), 46–53.

Fine, S. B. (1991). Resilience and human adaptability: Who rises above adversity? 1990 Eleanor Clarke Slagle Lecture. *American Journal of Occupational Therapy, 45*(6), 493–503.

Forsyth, G. L., Delaney, K. D., & Gresham, M. L. (1984). Vying for a winning position: Management style of the chronically ill. *Research in Nursing & Health, 7*(3), 181–188.

Freitas, A. L., & Downey, G. (1998). Resilience: a dynamic perspective. *International Journal of Behavioral Development, 22*(2), 263–285.

Friborg, O., Barlaug, D., Martinussen, M., Rosenvinge, J. H., & Hjemdal, O. (2005). Resilience in relation to personality and intelligence. *International Journal of Methods in Psychiatric Research, 14*(1), 29–42.

Friborg, O., Hjemdal, O., Rosenvinge, J. H., & Martinussen, M. (2003). A new rating scale for adult resilience: what are the central protective resources behind healthy adjustment? *International Journal of Methods in Psychiatric Research, 12*(2), 65–76.

Garmezy, N. (1974). The study of competence in children at risk for severe psychopathology. In C. Koupernik (Ed.), *The child in his family: Children at psychiatric risk* (Vol. 3, pp. 77–97). New York: Wiley.

Garmezy, N. (1981). *Children under stress: Perspectives on antecedents and correlates of vulnerability and resistance to psychopathology.* New York: John Wiley & Sons.

Garmezy, N. (1991). Resilience in children's adaptation to negative life events and stressed environments. *Pediatric Annals, 20,* 459–466.

Garmezy, N., Masten, A. S., & Tellegen, A. (1984). The study of stress and competence in children: A building block for developmental psychopathology. *Child Development, 55*(1), 97–111.

Haase, J. (1987). The components of courage in chronically ill adolescents. *Advances in Nursing Science, 9*(2), 64–80.

Haase, J. (2004). The Adolescent Resilience Model as a Guide to Interventions. Special Section: Proceedings from the 5th Annual State of the Science Workshop on Resilience and Quality of Life in Adolescents. *Journal of Pediatric Oncology Nursing, 21*(5), 289–299.

Haase, J. E., Britt, T., Coward, D. D., Leidy, N. K., & Penn, P. E. (1992). Simultaneous concept analysis of spiritual perspective, hope, acceptance and self-transcendence. *Image: Journal of Nursing Scholarship, 24*(2), 141–147.

Haase, J. E., Heiney, S. P., Ruccione, K. S., & Stutzer, C. (1999). Research triangulation to derive meaning-based quality-of-life theory: Adolescent resilience model and instrument development. *International Journal of Cancer Supplement, 12,* 125–131.

Haase, J. E., & Rostad, M. (1994). Experiences of completing cancer therapy: Children's perspectives. *Oncology Nursing Forum, 21*(9), 1483–1492; discussion 1493–1494.

Hauser, S. T., Vieyra, M. A., Jacobson, A. M., & Wertlieb, D. (1985). Vulnerability and resilience in adolescence: Views from the family. *Journal of Early Adolescence, 5,* 81–100.

Hauser, S. T., Vieyra, M. A., Jacobson, A. M., & Wertlieb, D. (1989). Family aspects of vulnerability and resilience in adolescence: A theoretical perspective. In T. Dugan & R. Coles (Eds.), *The child in our times: Studies in the development of resiliency.* New York: Brunner-Routledge.

Hawley, D. R., & DeHaan, L. (1996). Toward a definition of family resilience: Integrating life-span and family perspectives. *Family Process, 35*(3), 283–298.

Haz, A. M., Castillo, R., & Aracena, M. (2003). [Adaptation of the Multidimensional Trauma Recovery and Resilience (MTRR) questionnaire in a sample of Chilean mothers with a history of child abuse]. *Child Abuse and Neglect, 27*(7), 807–820.

Heilemann, M. V., Lee, K., & Kury, F. S. (2003). Psychometric properties of the Spanish version of the Resilience Scale. *Journal of Nursing Measurement, 11*(1), 61–72.

Heinzer, M. M. (1995). Loss of a parent in childhood: Attachment and coping in a model of adolescent resilience. *Holistic Nursing Practice, 9*(3), 27–37.

Henry, D. L. (2001). Resilient children: What they tell us about coping with maltreatment. *Social Work Health Care, 34*(3–4), 283–298.

Ho, D. Y. F., Chen, S. G., & Chiu, C. Y. (1991). Relational orientation: To find an answer for the methodology of Chinese social psychology. In K. S. Yang & K. K. Hwang (Eds.), *The psychology and behavior of Chinese people* (in Chinese). Taipei: Gui-Guan.

Hockenberry-Eaton, M., Dilorio, C., & Kemp, V. (1995). The relationship of illness longevity and relapse with self-perception, cancer stressors, anxiety, and coping strategies in children with cancer. *Journal of Pediatric Oncology Nursing, 12*(2), 71–79.

Hockenberry-Eaton, M., Kemp, V., & Dilorio, C. (1994). Cancer stressors and protective factors: Predictors of stress experienced during treatment for childhood cancer. *Research in Nursing & Health, 17*(5), 351–361.

Hollen, P. J., Hobbie, W. L., Finley, S. M., & Hiebert, S. M. (2001). The relationship of resiliency to decision making and risk behaviors of cancer-surviving adolescents. *Journal of Pediatric Oncology Nursing, 18*(5), 188–204.

Humphreys, J. C. (2001). Turnings and adaptations in resilient daughters of battered women. *Image: Journal of Nursing Scholarship, 33*(3), 245–251.

Humphreys, J. (2003). Resilience in sheltered battered women. *Issues in Mental Health Nursing, 24*(2), 137–152.

Hunter, A. J. (2001). A cross-cultural comparison of resilience in adolescents. *Journal of Pediatric Nursing, 16*(3), 172–179.

Hunter, A. J., & Chandler, G. E. (1999). Adolescent resilience. *Image: Journal of Nursing Scholarship, 31*(3), 243–247.

Hwang, K. K. (1997). Guanxi and mientze: Conflict resolution in Chinese Society. *International Communication Studies, 7*(1), 17–42.

Hwang, K. K. (2006). Constructive realism and Confucian relationalism: An epistemological strategy for the development of indigenous psychology. In U. Kim, K. S. Yang, & K. K. Hwang (Eds.), *Indigenous and cultural psychology: Understanding people in context.* New York: Springer.

Hymovich, D. P., & Roehnert, J. E. (1989). Psychosocial consequences of childhood cancer. *Seminars in Oncology Nursing, 5*(1), 56–62.

Jacelon, C. S. (1997). The trait and process of resilience. *Journal of Advanced Nursing, 25*(1), 123–129.

Kadner, K. D. (1989). Resilience. Responding to adversity. *Journal of Psychosocial Nursing & Mental Health Services, 27*(7), 20–25.

Kobasa, S. C. (1982). The hardy personality: Toward a social psychology of stress and health. *Social Psychology, 37,* 1–11.

Lee, I., Lee, E. O., Kim, H. S., Park, Y. S., Song, M., & Park, Y. H. (2004). Concept development of family resilience: A study of Korean families with a chronically ill child. *Journal of Clinical Nursing, 13*(5), 636–645.

Lothe, E. A., & Heggen, K. (2003). A study of resilience in young Ethiopian famine survivors. *Journal of Transcultural Nursing, 14*(4), 313–320.

Luthar, S. S., & Cicchetti, D. (2000). The construct of resilience: Implications for interventions and social policies. *Development & Psychopathology, 12*(4), 857–885.

Luthar, S. S., Cicchetti, D., & Becker, B. (2000). The construct of resilience: A critical evaluation and guidelines for future work. *Child Development, 71*(3), 543–562.

Mandleco, B. L., & Peery, J. C. (2000). An organizational framework for conceptualizing resilience in children. *Journal of Child and Adolescent Psychiatric Nursing, 13*(3), 99–111.

Masten, A. S. (1994). Resilience in individual development: Successful adaptation despite risk and adversity. In E. W. Gordon (Ed.), *Educational resilience in inner-city America: Challenges and prospects* (pp. 3–35). Hillsdale, NJ: Erlbaum.

Masten, A. S. (2001). Ordinary magic. Resilience processes in development. *American Psychologist, 56*(3), 227–238.

Masten, A. S., Best, K. M., & Garmezy, N. (1990). Resilience and development: Contributions from the study of children who overcome adversity. *Development and Psychopathology, 2,* 425–444.

Masten, A. S., & Coatsworth, J. D. (1998). The development of competence in favorable and unfavorable environments. Lessons from research on successful children. *American Psychologist, 53*(2), 205–220.

McAllister, M., & Walsh, K. (2003). CARE: A framework for mental health practice. *Journal of Psychiatric Mental Health Nursing, 10*(1), 39–48.

McCubbin, H., & McCubbin, M. (1996). Resiliency in families: A conceptual model of family adjustment and adaptation in response to stress and crisis. In H. I. McCubbin, A I. Thompson, & M. A. McCubbin (Eds.), *Family assessment: Resiliency, coping and adaptation—inventories for research and practice* (pp. 1–64). Madison, WI: University of Wisconsin System.

McCubbin, M., Balling, K., Possin, P., Frierdich, S., & Bryne, B. (2002). Family resiliency in childhood cancer. *Family Relations, 51*(2), 103–111.

McCubbin, M., & McCubbin, H. (1993). Family coping with health crisis: The Resiliency Model of Family Stress, Adjustment and Adaptation. In P. Winstead-Fry (Ed.),

Families, health, and illness (pp. 3–63). St. Louis: Mosby.

Mead, G. H. (1952). Mind, self and society. In C. W. Morris (Ed.), *Mind, self and society.* Chicago, Illinois: University of Chicago Press.

Morse, J. M., & Carter, B. J. (1995). Strategies of enduring and the suffering of loss: Modes of comfort used by a resilient survivor. *Holistic Nursing Practice, 9*(3), 38–52.

Murphy, L., & Moriarty, A. (1976). *Vulnerability, coping and growth from infancy to adolescence.* New Haven, CT: Yale University Press.

Nygren, B., Randstrom, K. B., Lejonklou, A. K., & Lundman, B. (2004). Reliability and validity of a Swedish language version of the Resilience Scale. *Journal of Nursing Measurement, 12*(3), 169–178.

Oshio, A., Kaneko, H., Nagamine, S., & Nakaya, M. (2003). Construct validity of the Adolescent Resilience Scale. *Psychological Reports, 93*(3 Pt 2), 1217–1222.

Patterson, J. M. (1995). Promoting resilience in families experiencing stress. *Pediatric Clinics of North America, 42*(1), 47–63.

Patterson, J. M. (2002). Understanding family resilience. *Journal of Clinical Psychology, 58*(3), 233–246.

Perkins, D. E., Luster, T., Villarruel, F. A. (1998). An ecological, risk-factor examination of adolescents' sexual activity in three ethnic groups. *Journal of Marriage and the Family, 60*, 600–623.

Pettit, G. S. (2000). Mechanisms in the cycle of maladaptation: The life-course perspective. *Prevention and Treatment, 3*(35).

Polk, L. V. (1997). Toward a middle-range theory of resilience. *Advances in Nursing Science, 19*(3), 1–13.

Rew, L., & Horner, S. D. (2003). Youth Resilience Framework for reducing health-risk behaviors in adolescents. *Journal of Pediatric Nursing, 18*(6), 379–388.

Rew, L., Taylor-Seehafer, M., Thomas, N. Y., & Yockey, R. D. (2001). Correlates of resilience in homeless adolescents. *Image: Journal of Nursing Scholarship, 33*(1), 33–40.

Richardson, G. E. (2002). The metatheory of resilience and resiliency. *Journal of Clinical Psychology, 58*(3), 307–321.

Rosenbaum, M. (1983). Learned resourcefulness as a behavioral repertoire for the self-regulation of internal events. In M. Rosenbaum, C. M. Franks, & Y. Jaffe (Eds.), *Perspectives on behavior therapy in the eighties* (pp. 54–73). New York: Springer Publishing Co.

Rutter, M. (1979). Protective factors in children's responses to stress and disadvantage. *Annals of the Academy of Medicine, Singapore, 8*(3), 324–338.

Rutter, M. (1987). Psychosocial resilience and protective mechanisms. *American Journal of Orthopsychiatry, 57*(3), 316–331.

Singer, B. H., & Ryff, C. (2001). *New horizons in health: An integrative approach.* Washington, DC: National Academy Press.

Sinnema, G. (1991). Resilience among children with special health-care needs and among their families. *Pediatric Annals, 20*(9), 483–486.

Smith, S. D. (1997). The retirement transition and the later life family unit. *Public Health Nursing, 14*(4), 207–216.

Stewart, M., Reid, G., & Mangham, C. (1997). Fostering children's resilience. *Journal of Pediatric Nursing, 12*(1), 21–31.

Svavarsdottir, E. K., McCubbin, M. A., & Kane, J. H. (2000). Well-being of parents of young children with asthma. *Research in Nursing & Health, 23*(5), 346–358.

Triandis, H. C., Bontempo, R., Villareal, M. J., Asai, M., & Lucca, N. (1988). Individualism and collectivism: Cross-culture perspectives on self-in-group relationships. *Journal of Personality and Social Psychology, 54*(2), 323–338.

Tusaie, K. R., & Patterson, K. (2006). Relationships among trait, situational, and comparative optimism: Clarifying concepts for a theoretically consistent and evidence-based intervention to maximize resilience. *Archives of Psychiatric Nursing, 20*(3), 144–150.

Vinson, J. A. (2002). Children with asthma: Initial development of the child resilience model. *Pediatric Nurse, 28*(2), 149–158.

Wagnild, G., & Young, H. M. (1990). Resilience among older women. *Image: Journal of Nursing Scholarship, 22*(4), 252–255.

Wagnild, G. M., & Young, H. M. (1993). Development and psychometric evaluation of the Resilience Scale. *Journal of Nursing Measurement, 1*(2), 165–178.

Waller, M. A. (2001). Resilience in ecosystemic context: Evolution of the concept. *American Journal of Orthopsychiatry, 71*(3), 290–297.

Wells, R., & Schwebel, A. (1987). Chronically ill children and their mothers: Predictors of resilience and vulnerability to hospitalization and surgical stress. *Developmental & Behavioral Pediatrics, 2*(2), 83–89.

Werner, E., & Smith, R. (1982). *Vulnerable but invincible: A longitudinal study of resilient children and youth.* New York: McGraw-Hill.

White, K. R. (1995). The transition from victim to victor: Application of the theory of mastery. *Journal of Psychosocial Nursing and Mental Health Services, 33*(8), 41–44.

White, N., Bichter, J., Koeckeritz, J., Lee, Y. A., & Munch, K. L. (2002). A cross-cultural comparison of family resiliency in hemodialysis patients. *Journal of Transcultural Nursing, 13*(3), 218–227.

Woodgate, R. L. (1999). Conceptual understanding of resilience in the adolescent with cancer: Part I. *Journal of Pediatric Oncology Nursing, 16*(1), 35–43.

Woodgate, R., & McClement, S. (1997). Sense of self in children with cancer and in childhood cancer survivors: A critical review. *Journal of Pediatric Oncology Nursing, 14*(3), 137–155.

Critical Analysis Exercises

Chapter 3 Analysis of Theory: Pain: A Balance Between Analgesia and Side Effects

■ **SHIRLEY M. MOORE**

INTERNAL CRITICISM

1. *Clarity.* The terms used and ideas conveyed in this theory are easy to understand. All terms are defined using words common to practicing nurses. The most unique idea expressed in the theory is the major concept of "a balance between analgesia and side effects" as a way to think about pain management. A clear definition is given of this new conceptualization of pain management. Additionally, all the propositions are expressed clearly and provide a coherent and comprehensive conceptualization.
2. *Consistency.* The description of this prescriptive theory is consistent in the use of concepts and definitions. The use of the terms and propositions are consistent with those used in other prescriptive theories. For example, the proposition specifying that nurses use appropriate multimodal interventions for pain management is prescriptive because it suggests that specific decisions and actions on the part of the nurse are likely to produce a particular outcome. In addition, consistent with prescriptive level theory, the propositions can be easily tested, using randomized controlled trials.
3. *Adequacy.* This theory presents a comprehensive approach to acute pain management. The theory addresses the affective and sensory dimensions to be considered in the management of acute pain and, as such, represents a more comprehensive approach than other current theories of acute pain management. The theory can be considered in its entirety or regarded as discrete steps in the pain management process. Despite the comprehensive and prescriptive nature of the theory, the number of propositions is manageable for the reader.
4. *Logical development.* The description of the theory clearly chronicles the historical evolution of knowledge about pain management and explains this theory's unique contributions to the field. The theory deductively incorporates previous knowledge and theoretical perspectives of pain management and is consistent with them. For example, the gate control theory of pain can be used to explain the mechanics of effect. This theory is also an exemplar of the utility of developing middle range theory inductively from clinical practice guidelines. The arguments of the theory are well supported and the conclusions are logical.

5. *Level of theory development.* In this prescriptive theory, specific choices and actions of the nurse to promote a balance between analgesia and side effects are posed. The theory is supported by some research; it has been tested in randomized controlled trials. Dr. Good has conducted research on the effects of nonpharmacological adjuvants as part of pain management. Knowledge about the behavioral and social cognitive mechanisms in some of the propositions of the theory is less developed. For example, little is known about the best ways to engage in goal setting for pain management, or timing the amount of information to provide for a patient when soliciting patient participation in acute pain management. Additionally, more research is needed about how the propositions may be influenced by cultural orientation.

EXTERNAL CRITICISM

1. *Reality convergence.* This theory is clearly reality based. It addresses the two dimensions of pain management, affective and sensory, that nurses observe in their clients. The assumptions of the theory represent the real world, a clinical reality to which every nurse can relate.
2. *Utility.* Acute pain management is a common problem in nursing. This is a pragmatic theory that nurses in practice and clinical researchers can easily use. Nurses can use this theory to generate testable hypotheses, both at the bedside and in full-scale research studies. Some hypotheses have been generated from this study, and the author describes empirical findings generated from them. The author suggests examples of additional hypotheses that can be tested. The theory can be used by practicing nurses to guide assessment and interventions with individual patients, as well as to guide quality assurance for groups of patients.
3. *Significance.* This theory has high significance. Symptom management is a central function of nurses, and managing pain is particularly important. Findings from studies testing the relationships posed in the propositions of this theory will have an immediate impact on nursing care and patients.
4. *Discrimination.* This theory is unique in that it is the only theory of pain management that focuses on the balance between analgesia and side effects. The theory has precise and clear boundaries, and the author has defined boundaries, clearly describing the phenomena that are and are not addressed by the theory. For example, the theory does not address acute pain management in children or management of chronic pain.
5. *Scope of theory.* The scope of this theory clearly meets the criteria for a middle range theory. It is broad enough to be applicable across a number of situations requiring acute pain management, yet narrow enough to be prescriptive for use with individual patients. It is middle range in that the propositions are abstract enough to be testable using research, but concrete enough to be directly applied in practice.
6. *Complexity.* Pain management is a complex idea. Thus, any theory that comprehensively addresses the phenomenon of pain management has the potential to be very complex and not easily understood. Dr. Good, however, has done an outstanding job of developing a parsimonious, easily understood theory. The clear descriptions of the terms, the commonly used language employed in labeling and describing the concepts, and the logical presentation of the propositions make this an easily understood theory despite the complexity of the underlying phenomenon. The use of diagrams of the propositions further reduces the complexity of the theory description.

About the Author

Shirley M. Moore, RN, PhD, FAAN, is Edward J. & Louise Mellon Professor of Nursing and Associate Dean for Research at Frances Payne Bolton School of Nursing, Case Western University, Cleveland, Ohio. She has taught nursing theory and knowledge-development courses at all levels of the nursing curriculum. Dr. Moore is a nurse researcher who, as principal investigator, has had multiple projects funded by the National Institute of Nursing Research. She has authored several articles on middle range theory development, including Good, M., & Moore, S. (1996). Clinical practice guidelines as a source of middle range theory: Focus on acute pain. Nursing Outlook, 44(2), 74–79.

Chapter 4 Analysis of Theory: Unpleasant Symptoms

■ KATHERINE J. BREDOW

INTERNAL CRITICISM

1. *Clarity.* The descriptions of the five main components of the Theory of Unpleasant Symptoms (TOUS) are clearly stated. They are described in the text and defined in the definition of key terms. Focusing on unpleasant symptoms (UPSs) as part of the lived experience, the theorists set out to design a model to explain the experience of UPSs as they occur in a dynamic clinical situation. Management techniques also emerged as a common factor in the author's early discussions on the development of the TOUS. Consideration should be given to including management techniques as a component of the model.

2. *Consistency.* The components are consistently used throughout the explanation of the theory. Development of the components are detailed in the references to the theorists' own symptom models (dispense and fatigue) and others symptom models (SIM and the Model of Symptom Management), and have been refined, as hypothesis testing in clinical practice and research has yielded new information. In the description of the theory there are three influencing components: physiological factors, psychological factors, and environmental factors. In the Definition of Key Terms, situational factors are the third influencing factor, of which environmental factors are a subset. Throughout the rest of the chapter, the terms are used in a congruent manner.

3. *Adequacy.* The theory explanation is succinct. The historical development of the theory was insightful and led to an understanding of the author's intent to make the symptom experience dynamic and more reflective of the real world. The theorists' goal was to construct a model to help the nurse understand all symptoms and their management. The focus of this theory is to understand the experience of UPSs. This is done by identifying antecedent factors, UPSs, and their influence on performance. It is suggested that an understanding of these components and their interrelationships will help the nurse to identify possible UPS-management interventions. Though inferred, it is not clearly stated where the management factor fits into the model. The diagram of the model is helpful in understanding the interrelationship of the factors.

4. *Logical development.* The theorists systematically set out to construct a theory to help the nurse to understand all symptoms and how to manage them. TOUS origins are founded in clinical observations, review of symptom literature, and collaboration with experts in theory development. It logically follows a line of thought of previous symptom work, expanding on it to build a theory that accounts for the antecedent factors, the dynamic experience of one or multiple symptoms, the performance, and their interrelationships. The use of established reliable and valid tools to measure some UPSs supports the logical foundation of TOUS. The examples of TOUS theory-based research helps to establish the usefulness and applicability to the nursing practice and research.

5. *Level of theory development.* TOUS fits the criteria of a middle range theory because it limits its scope and does not attempt to address all of the factors of the nursing metaparadigm. It provides a framework from which nurse researchers can generate hypothesis and research questions to better understand the dynamic experience of unpleasant symptoms.

EXTERNAL CRITICISM

1. *Reality convergence.* TOUS presents a comprehensive, holistic, and dynamic view of the unpleasant symptom experience. The underlying assumptions of TOUS ring true. Managing the care of people experiencing UPSs is a part of the real world of nursing. Increasing insight into the reality of the unpleasant symptom experience provides direction for management of the unpleasant symptoms patients experience.

2. *Utility.* The theory supports the development of research questions and study of the five components of TOUS. It has been applied to various populations experiencing UPSs and to caregivers distressed by their experience of UPSs in those they care for. Examples are given for both acute and chronic experiences of UPSs. Consideration of the research results led to a refinement of the TOUS. The interaction among components and their interrelationships with the other components were incorporated into the TOUS to make its utility even stronger.

3. *Significance.* Research conducted from hypotheses generated from the TOUS had a significant impact on the care that the nurses provided to patients. Since most clinical nurses deal in their practice with populations that experience UPSs, this theory offers a means of investigating the whole experience of health-threatening changes to patients perceived as normal functioning. It can be useful in gaining an understanding of the UPSs and management strategies.

4. *Discrimination.* The author tells the story of the development of the theory. The theorists constructed a unique theory that combined the essential components identified in earlier single-symptom models, to build a more inclusive, interactive dynamic theory for understanding the whole of UPSs. No other middle range theory addresses the multiple concepts of UPSs at the same time in one encompassing model. Because of the inclusion of situational factors, which are broad and have no clear boundaries, the TOUS is not as discriminating as it could be if it had not included this influencing factor. Moreover, the inclusion of culture and language, which have few definitive parameters, into the quality of symptoms makes the TOUS a less discriminating theory.

5. *Scope of theory.* The theory is useful for investigating one UPS or many UPSs. The scope of the TOUS can range from simple to complex, depending on the number of UPSs and variables the investigator chooses to study. Antecedents or influencing factors have the capability of being broad and all-encompassing, and a thorough assessment of all of these factors may be difficult.

6. *Complexity.* Initially, the TOUS seems succinct, logical, and practical. However, if it is applied to a complex, chronically ill patient with multiple problems, the task of considering all of the possible influencing factors, their interrelationships, and their congruent relationship to the various UPSs quickly becomes very complex. This is not to downplay the importance of a thorough assessment, but the more unpleasant symptoms that are entered into the model, the more complex it becomes.

About the Author
Kate Bredow, MA, RN, is a practicing school nurse, where she sees a variety of unpleasant symptoms in her patients every day. Her research experience dealt with the unpleasant symptom of sleep deprivation in the postpartum period.

Chapter 5 Analysis of Theory: The AACN Synergy Model

■ AMY REX SMITH

INTERNAL CRITICISM

1. *Clarity.* The contents of the AACN Synergy Model are understood with ease because the terminology is commonly used by nurses. The language accurately reflects acute care and critical care specialty practice. For example, patients are called patients, a word that both recognizes nurses' caring role and holds an appreciation of patients' vulnerability when critically ill. Further review of the descriptions of the eight patient characteristics demonstrates respect for patient individuality and empowerment of patients (to the extent that they are able) and of their families.
2. *Consistency.* Each component of the model is used in a consistent manner throughout the model, with no evidence of any inconsistencies. The relationships within the model are direct, such as the nurse–patient relationship, and as such are uncluttered, which supports consistency.
3. *Adequacy.* This model was developed to describe nursing practice in the hospital setting: 24-hour-a-day nursing care provided in a high-technology, complex, and often chaotic environment. It adequately captures the salient factors present in the setting.
4. *Logical development.* The process of the development of this model is described in this chapter in great detail. The model is unusual because it was developed by and for a specialty discipline, critical care nursing, rather than for all nursing situations. Despite the long history of prestigious certification in critical care nursing—the CCRN—leaders in the specialty recognized the need to move beyond using a task checklist and the medical perspective of physiological systems for the certification examinations. The process of model development was serial groups of carefully selected nurse leaders using a reflective and iterative process. This provided many checks and balances.
5. *Level of theory development.* The AACN Synergy Model was designed as a broad conceptual model of nursing. As such, it provides a starting point for middle range theory development (Fawcett, 2005). In general, its strength is in how it describes the real practice world of critical care nursing. In addition to the excellent description, the model provides a framework for patient

assessment and a structure to guide development of nurse expertise. It also attempts to prescribe good matches between nurses and patients, and because it posits that "synergy" occurs when these good matches happen, it could be seen as prescriptive. However, synergy, defined in the model as it is commonly understood as "something more than the sum of the parts," is not a measurable outcome and there is no way to tell if it has occurred or not. In this way, the model does not try to prescribe or predict any specific outcomes, only general measures not linked to any specific set of interventions. It only tells the "what is" and describes the ideal "what is."

As middle range theories are derived from the model, specific interventions and outcomes will be identified.

EXTERNAL CRITICISM

1. *Reality convergence.* The AACN Synergy Model is well matched to the real world of clinical nursing practice. It is meant to be used in the real world of the hospital environment and focuses attention exclusively on nurses and their patients.
2. *Utility.* The model is inherently useful. The model can be used every time a charge nurse makes a patient care assignment. It can also be used to design a curriculum to help nurses move from novice to expert and it can help to focus preceptors as they mentor new nurses on inpatient units. The model can be used to organize initial and ongoing patient assessments. Its use as a conceptual framework for research and theory development is only in the beginning stages, but the potential for its use in research is impressive. One of the reasons it has not been well used in research is that it still new, and it is difficult to study nurse–patient pairing. Thus far, most synergy-based studies focus on patients or nurses, not both. The challenges of developing research designs that are congruent with basic ideas of the model are a crucial next step for AACN members.
3. *Significance.* It is significant that the model is used for the certification examination of both patient care nurses (CCRNs) and advanced-practice nurses (CCNSs). As such, the model reflects certified practice. The model can be used to address a clinical issue, such as providing a structure for providing spiritual care in the intensive care unit (ICU) (Rex Smith, 2006).
4. *Discrimination.* The boundaries of this model appear to be well delineated, because they are clearly contained within the hospital setting. Consistent with all conceptual frameworks, however, the broad utility of the model is evident. The model has begun to be extended to the outpatient setting. Specifically, Hardin and Hussey (2003) presented a synergy model–based case study of advanced-practice nurse intervention with a congestive heart failure (CHF) patient in an outpatient clinic. So the boundaries as originally described in the model may be more fluid than the originators perceived.
5. *Scope of theory.* All four concepts of the nursing metaparadigm are addressed by this conceptual model: It includes the patient, the nurse, the environment, and health outcomes. This gives it a broad scope, broader than the middle range theories included in this book. Its scope is limited only by being designed for hospital-based nursing practice in acute care and critical care settings. Because of the focus on the nurse–patient relationship, the scope of the model is actually broader than it was originally conceived. In addition to the outpatient case study described previously, many of the nurse practitioner master's degree students at the University of Massachusetts Boston have selected this model for their final comprehensive paper.
6. *Complexity.* The model is less complex than many of the other nursing conceptual models. It is elegant in its simplicity, with a clear focus on the nurse–patient relationship. The synergy model

guides users to identify when optimal nurse–patient matches occur and what needs to be done to create matches when they have not yet occurred.

REFERENCES

Fawcett, J. (2005). *Contemporary nursing knowledge: Analysis and evaluation of nursing models and theories* (2nd ed.). Philadelphia: F.A. Davis.

Hardin, S., & Hussey, L. (2003). AACN synergy model for patient care case study of a CHF patient. *Critical Care Nurse, 23*(1), 73–76.

Rex Smith, A. (2006). Using the synergy model to provide spiritual care in critical care settings. *Critical Care Nurse, 26*(4), 41–47.

About the Author
Amy Rex Smith, DNSc, APRN, BC, is an Associate Professor at the University of Massachusetts Boston, where she coordinates the acute care/critical care clinical nurse specialist track. She is a board-certified advanced-practice nurse (clinical nurse specialist in adult health nursing). She maintains a clinical practice on a medical intermediate care unit at Brigham and Women's Hospital in Boston. She has a special interest in spiritual care of hospitalized patients. She has published using the AACN Synergy Model and is doing research using it as a conceptual framework.

Chapter 6 Analysis of Theory: Self-Efficacy

■ MARJORIE SIMPSON

INTERNAL CRITICISM

1. *Clarity.* Self-efficacy is a clearly defined theoretical framework, with main concepts that include efficacy expectations and outcome expectations as the sources of self-efficacy. Theoretical clarity is supported by the well-defined constructs within the framework and their relationship to each other, with self-efficacy preceding and impacting human behavior. The constructs and concepts incorporated into the self-efficacy theoretical framework are unique to the theory, and, therefore, their meanings are less likely to be misinterpreted.

2. *Consistency.* The relationships between the constructs included in self-efficacy remain consistently defined throughout the theoretical framework. In addition, the theme of causative capabilities as a belief that generates courses of action consistently serves as the foundation for the theory. Based on this premise, the theory of self-efficacy builds on the understanding that each individual's beliefs and past experiences influence his or her behavior.

3. *Adequacy.* The self-efficacy framework adequately explains and predicts behavior. Individuals with higher levels of self-efficacy for a specific behavior are more likely to attempt that behavior. The concept of outcome expectations offers an explanation for failure of an individual to attempt or adopt a behavior. According to the theory, the belief that a behavior will produce a worthwhile outcome is necessary for an individual to execute the behavior, regardless of the level of self-efficacy.

The completeness of the theory to predict behavior and explain situations when behaviors are not adopted supports the adequacy of the framework.

4. *Logical development.* The theory of self-efficacy was derived deductively from social cognitive theory, a model proposing that personal and environmental factors influence behavior. A basic assumption of this model is that individuals are human agents and have the ability to exercise control over their lives. This is congruent with other behavior change theories, and supports the logical development of the self-efficacy framework. In addition, the self-efficacy framework proceeds in a logical fashion. Efficacy expectations and outcome expectations are always antecedents to behavior and are reinforced when a behavior is successfully executed. In addition, the theory supports that enactive attainment is a strong influence over behavior and explains why self-efficacy for one behavior can be carried over to a different but similar behavior. These conclusions are logical and have been supported by previous nursing research.

5. *Level of theory development.* The self-efficacy theoretical model has been adapted and used in nursing research for many nursing interventions. Because the theory of self-efficacy accounts for new behaviors as well as lack of behavior change, it is predictive and can be used to explain an individual's responses to an intervention in both research and clinical settings. Therefore, self-efficacy as a middle range theory has been developed to a level that allows for purposeful nursing actions.

EXTERNAL CRITICISM

1. *Reality convergence.* An underlying assumption of the theory of self-efficacy is that most human behavior is determined by both intrinsic and extrinsic factors. Intrinsic factors include an individual's beliefs, and extrinsic factors include environmental influences that can be affected by an individual's actions. The influence of intrinsic and extrinsic factors on how people behave is reflected throughout nursing practice, and nurses frequently implement formal and informal interventions to alter these factors. For example, a rehabilitation nurse may demonstrate and instruct a patient in the use of adaptive equipment, and offer counseling or verbal persuasion to impact the patient's behavior. The actions of the nurse are altering the patient's self-efficacy for the use of adaptive equipment. In addition, addressing other physiological responses to illness, such as the unpleasant symptoms of pain and fatigue, is central to nursing and alters self-efficacy. Therefore, the theory of self-efficacy is grounded in reality and reflects the real world of nursing practice.

2. *Utility.* Core concepts that are central to the nursing profession include the interaction between the nurse, the patient, health, and the environment. This interaction often involves the nurse intervening to alter the intrinsic factors of the patient and the extrinsic environmental factors to facilitate behavior change and improve the patient's health. The self-efficacy theoretical framework is one that can generate researchable hypotheses on the interaction between these core nursing concepts, and can predict the outcomes of interventions, particularly those addressing the management of chronic illnesses and health promotion. Thus, it is useful both in research and practice.

3. *Significance.* Behavior change is an element that is essential to nurses in all specialties. The theory of self-efficacy is significant to the nursing profession because it offers a framework to generate hypotheses and conduct research to test behavioral change interventions. The research results derived from the self-efficacy framework can directly impact the way nurses practice. Self-efficacy measures can be used in clinical settings to identify individuals with low self-efficacy, and nurses can then develop approaches to increase self-efficacy to promote certain behaviors.

4. *Discrimination.* The self-efficacy theory can be used to generate and to test hypotheses that are unique to the diverse nursing profession. Because the framework is flexible, it can be adapted by all nursing specialties to the specific behaviors and conditions that are central in research and practice. Self-efficacy is operationalized using scales that measure strength and magnitude of self-efficacy for a specific behavior, as defined by the nurse researcher. The self-efficacy theory, therefore, is not only able to differentiate nursing from other disciplines, but is also able to distinguish and define the parameters of nursing specialties.

5. *Scope of theory.* The scope of the theory of self-efficacy is narrowly focused on the elements that influence behavior. Although the concept of behavior is comprehensive, the four sources of efficacy expectations and outcome expectations account for all of the factors that influence behavior. Therefore, self-efficacy is a middle range theory with a framework that is practical and applicable to all behavior-focused nursing research and practice.

6. *Complexity.* The theory of self-efficacy is complex enough to account for all intrinsic and extrinsic factors that influence human behavior. However, it is parsimonious enough that the relationships between the constructs within the theory are easily understood. The theoretical framework clearly defines and explains the concepts self-efficacy and behavior, as well as the constructs that include outcome expectations and the four sources of efficacy expectations. These variables that are incorporated into the theory are precise enough that they are easily understood and extensive enough to account for all human behavior.

About the Author

Marjorie Simpson, MS, CRNP, is a doctoral student and Clinical Instructor, School of Nursing, at the University of Maryland, Baltimore. Her research for her dissertation is on self-efficacy expectations in performance of restorative-care activities for nursing assistants. She has recently co-authored an article on measurement related to her research topic: Resnick, B., & Simpson, M. (2003). Reliability and validity testing self-efficacy outcome expectations scales for performing restorative care activities. Geriatric Nursing, 24(2), 2–7.

Chapter 7 Analysis of Theory: Chronic Sorrow

■ ANN M. SCHREIER

INTERNAL CRITICISM

1. *Clarity.* The description of the key concepts of the theory are clearly described and easily understood by the reviewer. The definition of chronic sorrow identifies it as a pervasive, permanent, periodic, and potentially progressive experience. The key concepts of loss, disparity, trigger events, and management methods are clearly defined, as well as the proposed relationship between these concepts. The theory is useful in understanding and anticipating various individuals' reactions to trigger events, such as the anniversary of a cancer diagnosis.

2. *Consistency.* The author consistently maintains the definitions of the key terms of loss experience, disparity, trigger events, and management methods. These key terms are congruent with the described research studies.

3. *Adequacy.* This theory explains what chronic sorrow is, as well as some of the common loss experiences that lead to chronic sorrow. However, it does not address why some individuals who have a loss experience do not experience chronic sorrow. In the example of bereaved individuals, 97% of the bereaved had symptoms of chronic sorrow (Eakes, Burke, & Hainsworth, 1999). Given that few of the subjects did not experience the symptoms labeled as chronic sorrow, the theory does address the experience of loss adequately. Future studies could examine whether there are predictors of those who will not experience chronic sorrow. Do individuals who do not experience chronic sorrow have different personality characteristics, or receive different health care interventions at the time of the loss? Another area that is open to future research is the identification of other conditions that commonly lead to chronic sorrow.

4. *Logical development.* The theoretical model of chronic sorrow is logically developed from the 10 qualitative studies conducted by the Consortium for Research on Chronic Sorrow. Because of the excellent base of qualitative studies, the theory aids in the understanding of the loss experience. With this research, the authors are able to draw conclusions and make arguments that are well supported by clinical and research data.

5. *Level of theory development.* The theory is appropriate to a middle range theory because it has a scope that is limited to the explanation of a single phenomena, that of response to loss.

EXTERNAL CRITICISM

1. *Reality convergence.* In clinical work with oncology patients, the theory makes sense of the reactions that nurses see, for example, in patients with a recurrence of the diagnosis of cancer, or to the stress patients experience when awaiting results from routine diagnostic tests during the remission period.

2. *Utility and discrimination.* Researchers could generate hypotheses based on the theoretical model. For instance, an appropriate hypothesis might be that parents of diabetic children, who participate in a 6-week support group, will demonstrate less discomfort from chronic sorrow than parents who do not participate in a support group. In addition, the author's work on an assessment instrument and its inclusion in this book clearly enhance the utility of the theory both for research and clinical practice. The theory of chronic sorrow is unique and specifically addresses grieving needs and the experience of loss.

3. *Significance.* This theoretical model lends itself to research on effectiveness of interventions for both caregivers and patients. In addition, the model can be used to determine what conditions are more likely to trigger an exacerbation of chronic sorrow and begin a chronic sorrow experience. With this knowledge, nurses will be able to anticipate needs and respond to these needs in an effective manner.

4. *Scope of theory.* The concepts and hypothesized relationships can easily be applied in clinical settings, and the score is narrow enough to fit the expectations of a middle range theory.

5. *Complexity.* The major concepts include loss experience, disparity, trigger events, chronic sorrow, and management methods. The conceptualization of the model is easily displayed in Figure 7-1 (theoretical model of chronic sorrow). Because the model is logical and cyclical, this figure

enhances the reader's understanding of the relationship between the variables. The model clearly delineates the subconcepts of internal versus external management, ineffective versus effective management, and discomfort versus increased comfort, as well as where appropriate intervention by nurses and other health care providers can occur. There are a limited number of variables, and the number appears to be sufficient to explain the phenomena. The description accompanying the theory is succinct and readily understood.

REFERENCE

Eakes, G. G., Burke, M. L., & Hainsworth, M. A. (1999). Chronic sorrow: The lived experience of bereaved individuals. *Illness, Crisis, and Loss, 7*(1), 172–182.

About the Author
Ann M. Schreier, RN, PhD, is Assistant Professor of Nursing, Department of Adult Health, East Carolina University, Greenville, North Carolina. She has served as a consultant and clinical director at the Hospice Society in Bethesda, Maryland. She has received external funding to conduct nursing research in the area of self-care and chronicity. She also has several research-related publications in the area of self-care, pain control, and patient education.

Chapter 8 Analysis of Theory: Social Support

■ JOANN P. WESSMAN

Dr. Schaffer presents several social support theories in her chapter. The present critique is focused on the body of middle range social support theories that she presents. Therefore, some criteria for the critique have been modified.

INTERNAL CRITICISM

The present critique will focus on clarity, consistency, adequacy, and level of theory development. The issue of logical development will not be considered inasmuch as this criterion is specific to one particular theory.

1. *Clarity.* The lack of a clear definition of social support is cited and evident throughout the chapter. Specifically, definitions lack the clarity to differentiate if social support encompasses interactions where (a) negative consequences occur for the provider or recipient, or (b) support providers are in "formal" categories such as professionals. It is unclear from the chapter discussion if social support can be considered to have occurred when it is not the intention of the provider to be helpful, but, indeed, support inadvertently is given. The author gives clear examples that differentiate meaning among emotional, information, instrumental, and appraisal kinds of support. Not as clear are the uses of the subconcepts structure and function.

2. *Consistency.* The lack of consistent use of the construct social support is identified in the chapter. When definitions vary widely, as they do, interpretations, principles, and methods will likewise lack consistency. The chapter section on clinical applications, particularly the use of social support as nursing intervention, highlights the diversity in conceptualizations of social support.

3. *Adequacy.* How adequate is the body of theories reviewed? Certainly the lack of definitional clarity and inconsistent use of definitional qualities diminishes adequacy. Yet, given these limitations, the robust nature of the concept, social support, is evident throughout the discussion. Yes, some definitional areas are ambiguous and inconsistent. However, the collection of theories reviewed does permit the nursing community to enter into meaningful dialog about the nature of social support. In this sense, the body of current theories possesses at least a degree of adequacy—meaningful conversations are evoked.

4. *Level of theory development.* It is interesting to note that among the theories of social support are elements of factor-isolating, explanatory, predictive, and prescriptive levels. Each theory cited attempts definition of the concept. Identification of variables related to social support, such as perceptions, timing, motivation, duration, direction, life stage, and source, offer a sense of factor-relating level of theory (explanation). The variability among instances of social support can be explained, at least to some degree, by these variables. We get a sense of explanation as to why not all instances of social support look identical, and relationships within the construct social support begin to emerge. Some social support theorists such as Norbeck clearly are mapping out relationships that can predict outcomes of nursing interventions aimed at enhancing social support. Clinical situations where social support interventions should be prescribed in a defined manner (predictive and prescriptive theory) are being identified.

EXTERNAL CRITICISM

Each of the six specific criteria of external criticism will be approached from the view of the body of several social support theories available to the nurse in practice and research applications. At times, specific social support theories will be isolated.

1. *Reality convergence.* Several of the social support theories converge well with "real world" nursing experiences. Chronically ill clients thrive when surrounded by supportive families and communities. Nursing's systems succeed when embedded in nurturing broader societal structures.

    The idea inherent in the buffer theory that social support modulates life stressors is one threaded throughout nursing literature. Design of care structures and referrals to type of caregiving facilities is shaped, in part, by the social supports available to the client to modulate stressors.

    Norbeck's model for using social support as intervention to improve health outcomes "rings true" with common nursing practices. Nurses routinely include family in client education programs because they expect family members to reinforce learning. Nurses often suggest support groups for clients experiencing complex, intense, and/or prolonged health challenges, believing that the group will be a source of healing and growth.

    Many more examples could be given. Social support theories have a high degree of reality convergence with lived nursing experiences.

2. *Utility.* How useful are present social support theories when applied in practice and research? Dr. Schaffer offers several specific examples to support the utility of social support theories for nursing. Her Table 8-2 offers specific clinical applications of social support theories that, in shaping meaningful interventions, reduce client stress and promote effective client coping. Examples are

offered on individual, dyadic, group, community, and systems levels. Clearly, social support theories are useful in a variety of clinical situations.

The examples of social support instruments described in Table 8-3 demonstrate the ability to operationalize social support theories in a way useful for research. The availability of specific instruments to measure social support in a valid and reliable manner is both useful and crucial to the researcher conducting quantitative studies. Schaffer and Lia-Hoagberg's study of the effects of social support on prenatal care and health behaviors of low-income women demonstrates the usefulness of present social support theories in guiding research. Present social support theories clearly are "birthing" useful instruments and studies.

3. *Significance.* Dr. Schaffer supports well her strong assertion that middle range social support theories are of significance to nursing. Social support influences health status, health behavior, use of health services, and health outcomes. Current social support theories help to explain this influence in a manner that permits meaningful intervention. The theories offer a way to apply the nursing process in the arena of interpersonal relationships of the client with supportive "others." Theories place the client within a relevant social context. Social support theories reflect the tradition within nursing to view the individual or family as an integral part of a rich fabric of relationships that define and reflect health.

4. *Discrimination.* The lack of definitional clarity and inconsistent use of the term *social support* among various theories adversely reflects on these theories' ability to discriminate social support from other related concepts. Perhaps this is the greatest limitation of the body of theories taken as a whole. (Individually, each social support theory may discriminate at a commendable level.)

   Norbeck's work reflects a strong attempt to develop social support theory in a manner that is unique to nursing. But many of the theorists are not nurses, and do not aim to develop the construct in a manner that discriminates nursing applications from those of other disciplines. This lack of discrimination is also a limitation of many social support theories.

5. *Scope of theory.* The social support theories discussed by Dr. Schaffer clearly are of appropriately circumscribed scope to be considered middle range theories. Their application to practice situations is direct because of this limited scope. Yet the theories are broad enough to encompass a specific type of interpersonal relationships at several levels from the individual to a given society.

6. *Complexity.* The complexity varies among the present social support theories. Some develop a limited number of variables; some, an extensive array. Dr. Schaffer notes that Brown's theory of social support develops one broad factor; in contrast, the model of Barerra is multidimensional. The lack of definitional consensus among social support theories creates an artificial complexity that functions in a negative manner.

SUMMARY

The present body of social support theories lacks a clear definition of the phenomenon. Like clarity, the criterion of consistency is not met. Even with these limitations, there is a sense in which the theories are adequately serving nursing to influence practice and research. Among the theories are elements of factor-isolating, explanatory, predictive, and prescriptive levels of theory development.

Looking at the criteria for external criticism, a positive picture is seen. There is strong reality convergence with the "real world" of nursing. The theories are proving to be useful both to practice and to research. Significance seems evident when looking at social support theories from the perspective of health status, health behaviors, use of health services, and health outcomes. Scope of theories seems clearly to be midrange. Only discrimination is a criterion unmet, and complexity, a criterion difficult to assess.

REFERENCES

Norbeck, J. S. (1981). Social Support: A model for clinical research and application. *Advances in Nursing Science, 3* (4), 43–59.

Schaffer, M. A. & Lia-Hoagberg, B. (1997). Effects of social support on prenatal care and health behaviours of low-income women. *Journal of Obstetric, Gynecologic, and Neonatal Nursing, 26* (4), 433–440.

About the Author

Joann P. Wessman, RN, PhD, is a Professor at Bethel University, St. Paul, Minnesota. She teaches nursing theory development and analysis at the graduate level. She has served as dissertation or thesis advisor to doctoral and master's students using middle range theory. Her recent research is in faith/health integration in church-affiliated frail elderly.

Chapter 9 Analysis of Theory: Caring

■ CECELIA I. ROSCIGNO

INTERNAL CRITICISM

1. *Clarity.* In Swanson's Theory of Caring, the structural components of the theory and the descriptions of their relations are made straightforward and easy to comprehend. In her theory, Swanson clarifies that the environment resembles an ecological model with nested levels both within the individual and outside the individual and explains how these environments interact with each other in both directions. This conceptualization clarifies that the client and the environment may be one in the same in some nursing practice settings.

2. *Consistency.* The structural components described, the definitions of those components, and the descriptions of their relations are clearly and consistently used throughout Swanson's publications on her theoretical work.

3. *Adequacy.* This theory presents a comprehensive and yet prescriptive approach to the nursing process that is consistent with nursing's values and mission. The theory addresses the parts of the process in relation to seeing the whole person in the context of his or her environments. The theory provides the discrete steps that lead to the whole process. Despite the comprehensive nature of the theory, the clear description of the necessary structural components makes it understandable and applicable.

4. *Logical development.* The Theory of Caring clearly describes the historical evolution of caring as a human attribute and describes how a caring interactional process between the nurse and his or her client(s) are particularly relevant to the nursing discipline or any discipline within health care. This is because all health care fields have at their core the altruistic values of service to society and promotion of health, which makes it necessary to take client's existential and sociocultural contexts into consideration. The theoretical model incorporated previous knowledge and yet, was also contrasted to extant descriptions of nursing's helping and caring role. The final conceptualization was later empirically tested by the theorist in her own research and further explicated in

her publications. For example, in a more recent publication, Swanson explains how her process of caring can be used to create healing environments that consider the whole person. The theorist's theoretical model is well supported by literature and the conclusions remain logical, consistent, and supported by some empirical evidence.

5. *Level of theory development.* The theory as currently conceptualized would be a middle range nursing theory that could be considered prescriptive. The theory has been used by the theorist and others to develop and test intervention programs. Further investigation is required to determine if the interventions provide more than increased client satisfaction but actually influence overall health and well-being.

EXTERNAL CRITICISM

1. *Reality convergence.* The Theory of Caring is clearly reality based beyond the discipline of nursing. It addresses the dimensions of human interaction that demonstrate a caring attitude. In fact, when developing and refining the theory, Swanson went beyond nursing—or any professional-based literature—using a literary meta-analysis to refine and explain the structural components of the theory and how they related. This gave the theory both clinical and social authenticity and makes it applicable to broader human interactions of any kind meant to be caring. In dissertation research, both children and parents describe the interactions they encountered following the child's traumatic brain injury, and across subjects, their descriptions of caring converge with the structures and meanings that Swanson described in her theory.

2. *Utility.* Because the structural components and their relationships are clearly explained, this theory can be used by nurses to generate testable questions or hypotheses, both at the bedside and for research generation. The theorist, herself, created a randomized controlled intervention program for couples following miscarriage. Other junior investigators have recently used it to guide their early programs of research inquiry and to develop preliminary intervention programs. The theory is also being instituted clinically in several health care settings, to guide health care interactions and intervention programs. More research is needed to validate whether guidance by this theory improves health care practitioner interactions or whether intervention programs guided by this theory improve clients' health-related outcomes or a more holistic sense of their own well-being. This latter outcome can be more difficult to capture in research. In practice, the theorist, herself, noted some limitations of capturing this caring process, especially with practitioners of various levels of expertise. She noted that novice nurses might be so focused on new tasks that they might miss the wholeness of the caring process described in Swanson's theory. She also noted that more experienced nurses may embed their caring processes in such an elaborate set of advanced skills that acknowledgment of the process could potentially be overlooked in an investigation.

3. *Significance.* Swanson's theory both is relevant and has tremendous significance to both the science and practice of nursing. This theory ties the key disciplinary values into the principles for framing what are ideal nursing research phenomena and what may guide improved professional interactions with clients. From a research perspective, this theory recognizes and incorporates that nursing is a human science that sees humans as wholes and advocates for understanding each person's health in terms of this whole. This theory also recognizes that both nursing practice and nursing research strive to understand the unique life existence of each person in order to appreciate the unique meanings the person may attach to his or her nurse–client interactions, social–environmental interactions,

and ultimately definitions of health and well-being. From a practice perspective, this theory points out that nurses need to clearly recognize how their interactions can influence the ecological environments, health, and overall well-being of the clients they serve in their practice and vice versa.

4. *Discrimination.* This theory is not the only theory of caring in nursing. Because caring is a universal concept to humans, the theory does not have precise and clear boundaries. Additionally, caring is a concept that is not unique to the profession of nursing alone. Other health care professions also have an altruistic and caring charge to their values. Thus, this theory has begun to be adopted in a variety of health care settings and across health care disciplines. Its appeal to the caring nature of all human interactions makes this theory have even broader societal implications, but does not limit its significance to the nursing profession.

5. *Scope.* The scope of this theory clearly meets the criteria for a middle range theory. It is broad enough to be applicable across a number of situations requiring caring interactions both professionally and nonprofessionally. However, the detail with which Swanson describes the processes of informed caring makes it prescriptive enough for application to individual situations, even to laypersons. The structural components of this theory are abstract enough to be testable, but are also concrete enough to be applicable to the clinical practice setting.

6. *Complexity.* Caring in the context of human interactions can be a complex and abstract idea, which could easily be difficult to understand. However, Dr. Swanson has presented comprehensible descriptions of the structural components and a logical presentation of how these components interrelate to each other. She makes it clear that with each client, the nurse must learn his or her uniqueness and use that to apply the nursing process. Swanson also uses a diagram to aid in illuminating this model.

About the Author
Cecelia I. Roscigno, MN, PhC, RN, CNRN, is a predoctoral research fellow and doctoral student at University of Washington. She is currently conducting a research study to learn children's perspectives of their life following a traumatic brain injury.

Chapter 10 Analysis of Theory: Interpersonal Relations

■ **SONJA J. MEIERS**
■ **KATHLEEN SHERAN**

INTERNAL CRITICISM

1. *Clarity.* This theory is rather complex when all aspects are considered. The major concepts are clearly defined and readily understandable, but numerous. The major concepts are nurse–patient relationship, phases of the nurse–patient relationship, roles of the nurse, psychobiological experiences, and psychological tasks. All concepts are generally at a high level of abstraction. The role of and importance of the nurse's self-understanding in the therapeutic relationship is clearly outlined.

2. *Consistency.* The theory is consistent and congruent in defining concepts throughout the original work. The focus on the nurse–patient relationship as central to practice and the concept of how the nurse intervenes are consistent with a theory based on interpersonal relations. Phases of the nurse–patient relationship, as originally defined, have been subsequently altered. This alteration has been from the defined phases of orientation, identification, exploitation, and termination, to the orientation, working, and resolution phases, with identification and exploitation now considered as subphases of the working phase. Concepts of anxiety, tension, unmet needs, frustration, and conflict are consistently presented as targets for the counseling role of the nurse. The worldview is phenomenological in nature and reinforced throughout the theory.

3. *Adequacy.* The theory is adequate in its ability to transfer to settings that allow the nurse time and opportunity to interact with the patient. Since the major foundations of the theory are deducted from disciplines other than nursing, the uniqueness is not found in the body of knowledge but, rather, in the therapeutic role of the nurse in interaction with the patient. Current weaknesses are its emphasis on the individual patient to the exclusion of family and community, the absence of pathophysiology, and a narrow set of cultural assumptions surrounding interpersonal interaction.

4. *Logical development.* Both inductive and deductive methods are used in development of the theory. The works of Freud, Havighurst, Sullivan, Maslow, and Rogers formed the deductive integration base for the hypothesis statements. Additionally, and most beneficial to nursing, Peplau's inductive approach is a well-formulated theory development process where observation of nursing practice with patients has resulted in identification of concepts of interest. Theoretical relationships between concepts are clearly presented in the statements of assumptions throughout the historical development of the theory. Within the theory, the role of the nurse is to facilitate the individual in his or her movement through the steps of the nursing process.

5. *Level of theory development.* This middle range theory is at the descriptive level. Classification of the phases of interpersonal relations between the nurse and patient is its focus. Specifically, interactional phenomena and intrapersonal and interpersonal phenomena of nursing situations and psychosocial phenomena are described.

EXTERNAL CRITICISM

1. *Reality convergence.* The basic underlying assumptions ring true and represent the real world of nursing, particularly in the specialty of psychiatric nursing. Definitions of major tradition domains of nurse, patient, health, and environment are similar to those used in practice. Elements of developmental psychology, humanistic psychology, and learning theory used in the theory are widely accepted premises within the discipline of nursing. The influence of Freud regarding the unconscious motivation of the patient as important to the nurse's role of assisting patients with management of anxiety is evident. These deductions from Freud, Sullivan, and others as they pertain to the nurse–patient interpersonal process are generally accepted, but may not be commonly understood or applied by the nurse generalist. The behaviorist perspective does provide an alternative and popular view of therapist–patient relationships.

2. *Pragmatic.* The theory can be operationalized in nursing practice settings that value the primacy of the interpersonal process intended to be therapeutic. It is most helpful for viewing and understanding the patient's psychobiological needs, and provides a method for assessing and intervening with these issues. The theory is applicable as a framework to teach the essential elements of therapeutic communication in nursing education.

3. *Utility.* This theory has not yet generated large numbers of research studies, though it meets the criteria of empirical adequacy for a middle range theory. Research that has been completed focuses on factors that influence the development of the nurse–patient relationship. Because many of the practice aspects of the theory have been inductively derived, instrument development has been limited. Therefore, measurement of variables within the theory has not been broadly achieved. Further demonstration of the link between the nurse–patient relationship, symptom relief, and the ultimate well-being of patients is needed.

4. *Significance.* The theory meets the criterion of significance for the discipline. The theory has been published, unchanged, since 1952 and continues to be useful, specifically in contemporary mental health nursing. Other nurse scientists have expanded use in areas such as therapeutic milieu, crisis, and family theory. The frequency of reference to the importance of and phases of the nurse–patient relationship in nursing textbooks and empirical studies attests to its continued utility.

5. *Discrimination.* Though the theorist is clear in distinctions between professional nursing practice and medicine in original works, there is not clear distinction between the important content of the nurse–patient relationship and the physician–patient relationship. The basic theory is easily applicable to a variety of helping professions and, though contributing its focus on the interaction to disciplinary development in nursing, is not limited uniquely to nursing.

6. *Scope of theory.* The theory is broad and can be applied in many practice domains, especially those nursing roles that assist the patient with interpersonal or intrapersonal difficulty. It does not provide concepts about pathophysiological or biological phenomena.

7. *Complexity.* The theory has breadth, life, and fluidity. The core of the theory is parsimonious (the relationship between the nurse and the patient). However, the theory describes several important related concepts that explain how to understand the nurse–patient interaction, creating complexity. If these concepts are considered part of the Theory of Interpersonal Relations, it meets the criterion for complexity. Application of the theory requires that the nurse be able to be both inductive and deductive when reasoning.

About the Authors

Sonja J. Meiers, PhD, MS, RN, is Associate Professor and Director of the Graduate Program at Minnesota State University, Mankato. Theory development is one of her areas of research interest. Kathleen Sheran, MS, RN, CNS, is Assistant Professor at Minnesota State University, Mankato. Her education, practice, and teaching background is in psychiatric–mental health nursing, all of which have made use of Peplau's Theory of Interpersonal Relations.

Chapter 11 Analysis of Theory: Modeling and Role-Modeling

■ MARTHA SOFIO

INTERNAL CRITICISM

1. *Clarity.* The theory is easy to understand. The language is simple and the concepts are clearly defined and used with consistency throughout the theory. The coined concept of affiliated individuation is one that does not immediately generate semantic clarity for the reader; however, it is clearly defined in this framework. It calls for further validation and concept analysis. The concept of self-care has a meaning in this framework that varies greatly from its general use, or use in other nursing theories. The concept of self-care knowledge as a subconscious component of person requires validation.

2. *Consistency.* Concepts remain consistently defined throughout the theoretical content. The concept of adaptation as an equilibrium level on a continuum of health and illness is consistent with the interpretation of person as a system adjusting in response to environmental stimuli. Stress is consistently presented as response to a stressor, and adaptation as a holistic response to experienced stressors. Other conceptual definitions of nurturance, object attachment, unconditional acceptance, self-care, holism, and health remain constant throughout the theory. The worldview is that of holistic human experience as related to mind–body interaction; however, it is not proposed to the extent of person/environment unity. The conceptualization of holism is addressed with consistency in reference to both client and nurse.

3. *Adequacy.* This theory is adequate in that its concepts and principles transfer readily into a variety of practice settings. The authors do not specify clinical situations for the use of this theory, and it is readily applicable to the care of individuals in almost all clinical settings. It is challenging, however, to extrapolate it to situations of family assessment and intervention. Because of the major use of theories from other disciplines, its exclusive differentiation for nursing is questionable.

4. *Logical development.* The theory evidences logical development. Deductively using differing external theoretical bases in the description of person, the author systematically presents theoretical relationships. Initially, theories are presented supporting how people are alike, followed by theoretical support for how people are different. These theoretical bases are then described in relationships called "linkages," which offer rich ground for hypothetical deductive research and development of nursing interventions. The theoretical bases and linkages are synthesized to aid in developing a conceptualization of the client's world, the process of which is called modeling. The nursing process is explicated through the use of role-modeling the developed model of the client's world. Specific interventions are subsumed under five generalized aims, all oriented to fulfilling the purpose of the model. All logical steps of the nursing process are intact.

5. *Level of theory development.* This theory is at the explanatory level. It provides clarity as to how to develop a model of the client's world, and proposes that use of that unique model in the role-modeling process will facilitate the client's adaptation. It is in this sense that

role-modeling or nurturance provides the basis for predictive and prescriptive nursing theory development.

EXTERNAL CRITICISM

1. *Reality convergence.* The basic premises of the theory easily converge with reality. The principles of growth and development, basic human needs, and adaptation to change and loss are commonly understood and generally accepted. The theory purports to be holistic, and the understanding of mind–body–spirit interaction is widely accepted within the discipline. The conceptualization of mutual goal planning is congruent with the values system of today's practitioners. The conceptualization of self-care knowledge, however, where the client knows what made him ill and what will make him better, might offer some difficulty in this regard.

2. *Utility.* The theory fulfills the criterion of utility. It readily gives the practicing nurse a framework with which to view the client, and from which to facilitate the client's plans for care. Detailed processes for collecting, aggregating, analyzing, and synthesizing data are provided. The theory easily lends itself to curricular development and student education. Adaptive potential, self-care, affiliated individuation, role-modeling, and multiple other conceptualizations offer important subject matter for the execution of nursing research.

3. *Significance.* The theory addresses essential issues in nursing, namely those of client assessment and intervention. Its most significant foci are those of mind–body interaction and mutual goal planning, which compel the nurse to respectively envision the client holistically and to empower him or her. The theory proposes multiple content areas supportive of research in the development of the discipline's body of knowledge.

4. *Discrimination.* A major limitation of the theory is its lack of capacity to discriminate nursing from other health professions and its interventions from other care-tending acts. It would be possible for a physician, psychologist, or social worker to implement this theory. The boundaries are open, and the extant acts and practices can flow inside or outside the discipline.

5. *Scope.* The theory is broad in scope and can be used in diverse practice domains.

6. *Complexity.* The theory is not parsimonious. It is complex and composed of multiple descriptive and explanatory components. The subject matter is rich and presented in great depth. The concept of person is dominant and the inter-relationship of theoretical variables is numerous.

About the Author
Martha Sofio, MS, RN, Assistant Professor at Metropolitan State University, St. Paul, Minnesota, is a certified nurse practitioner and certified hypnotherapist who studied with Helen Erickson. She teaches in both the graduate and undergraduate nursing programs at Metropolitan State University. Modeling and Role-Modeling is the theoretical foundation of its undergraduate curriculum.

Chapter 12 Analysis of Theory: Comfort

■ LINDA WILSON

INTERNAL CRITICISM

1. *Clarity.* The criterion of clarity is evaluated by how clearly the theory is presented and how easily it is understood by the reader (Barnum, 1990). Comfort Theory is clearly presented in the literature and can be easily read and understood by any reader. Through her program of research and numerous publications, Dr. Kolcaba clearly presents the development and evolution of the Comfort Theory.
2. *Consistency.* The criterion of consistency is evaluated by examining the definitions and repeated use of the terms of a theory (Barnum, 1990). Comfort Theory has several key concepts that are defined throughout the literature. In every publication, these key concepts are clearly and uniformly defined.
3. *Adequacy.* The criterion of adequacy is evaluated by how the theory accounts for the specialty to which it applies (Barnum, 1990). Comfort Theory can be applied to all populations. The three senses of comfort (ease, relief, and transcendence) and the contexts in which they occur (physical, social, psychospiritual, and environmental) account for comfort care with any patient.
4. *Logical development.* The criterion of logical development prescribes that the reasoning and conclusions of a theory be clearly presented (Barnum, 1990). Throughout the literature, the ongoing development of Comfort Theory is clearly presented in a reasonable and valid manner. In each of her publications, Dr. Kolcaba presents the theory and the logical reasoning that supports its evolution.
5. *Level of theory development.* To assess the level of theory development, the researcher needs to evaluate the research that has been completed using the theory (Barnum, 1990). At the time of this author's dissertation research (1998–2000), comfort and Comfort Theory had been clearly defined in the literature; therefore, studies testing explanatory theory using a correlational design were in order. Since that time, Dr. Kolcaba has published the development of the middle range Theory of Comfort. Comfort Theory meets the description of a middle range theory because it consists of several well-defined concepts and can be viewed as both general and complex (Fawcett & Downs, 1992).

EXTERNAL CRITICISM

1. *Reality convergence.* The criterion of reality convergence can be evaluated by examining the principles, interpretations, and method of a theory (Barnum, 1990). Both the concept of comfort and Comfort Theory have practical application to many populations. The essential principles and assumptions of Comfort Theory are clearly defined in the literature by Dr. Kolcaba and can easily be applied to any patient population. The logical development and presentation of the theory allows for easy interpretation and application of the theory in nursing research. Dr. Kolcaba's perception of the nursing world presents the patient and family who are cared for holistically.

2. *Utility.* The criterion of utility refers to the usefulness of the theory by nursing in any practice setting (Barnum, 1990). Comfort Theory can be applied to patients of all ages and in any practice setting. During dissertation research, this author was able to easily apply Comfort Theory to the population of hospitalized medical patients.

3. *Significance.* The criterion of significance is met if the theory contributes to the further development of nursing knowledge, and if it addresses essential nursing issues (Barnum, 1990). Comforting patients is a fundamental part of nursing care because comfort is a desired and expected patient outcome. Comfort Theory provides the basis for comfort care by presenting the three senses (ease, relief, and transcendence) and contexts (physical, social, psychospiritual, and environmental) in which the outcome of comfort occurs.

4. *Discrimination.* The criterion of discrimination is evaluated by the ability of the theory to differentiate nursing from other health professions and other caring acts (Barnum, 1990). Nurses care for patients holistically and in four contexts of human experience (physical, social, psychospiritual, and environmental) from which the outcome of comfort occurs.

5. *Scope of theory.* The criterion of scope of theory evaluates if the theory is broad or limited in scope (Barnum, 1990). The Theory of Comfort is broad in scope because it can be applied to patients of all ages and in various practice settings.

6. *Complexity.* The criterion of complexity allows the researcher the opportunity for explanation and interrelationship of multiple variables (Barnum, 1990). Comfort Theory allows the researcher the opportunity to examine comfort through the three senses of comfort (ease, relief, and transcendence) and the four contexts (physical, social, psychospiritual, and environmental) in which the outcome of comfort occurs. Any or all of these variables can be measured at one time. In addition, Comfort Theory posits relationships between nursing interventions, patient comfort, health-seeking behaviors, and institutional integrity. Any or all of these relationships can be tested through nursing research.

REFERENCES

Barnum, B. J. (1990). *Nursing theory: Analysis, application, evaluation.* Glenview, IL: Scott, Foresman, Little, Brown.

Fawcett, J., & Downs, F. S. (1992). *The relationship of theory and research* (2nd ed.). Philadelphia: F. A. Davis.

About the Author

Linda Wilson, RN, PhD, CPAN, CAPA, BC, is an Education Specialist for Nursing Continuing Education and Perianesthesia at Thomas Jefferson University Hospital in Philadelphia. Dr. Wilson used the Comfort Theory during her dissertation research, while studying adult hospitalized medical patients.

Chapter 13 Analysis of Theory: Health-Related Quality of Life

■ **LYNNE PLOETZ**

INTERNAL CRITICISM

1. *Clarity.* The detailed description of Wilson and Cleary's model of health-related quality of life (HRQOL) allows the reader to develop a clear understanding of the components and concepts involved in the theory. With a focus on patient outcomes, the authors (both physicians) indicate that health measures exist on a continuum of increasing complexity. They spell out five domains: biophysiological factors, symptoms, functioning, general health perceptions, and overall quality of life. They explain the health concepts involved in each level and relate these to general health perceptions and overall quality of life. In addition, they discuss the role of patient preferences and the emotional or psychological factors involved in HRQOL (Wilson & Cleary, 1995).
2. *Consistency.* The terminology used by Wilson and Cleary (1995) in explaining and discussing HRQOL is consistent throughout their paper. Because they are medical doctors, their terminology is congruent with nursing terminology and can readily be understood by nurses.
3. *Adequacy.* The questions asked by HRQOL are highly relevant to nursing research and practice, and exist on both individual and global scales. Using Wilson and Cleary's model, HRQOL thoroughly addresses the issues relevant to one's health perceptions and quality of life.
4. *Logical development.* Wilson and Cleary (1995) provide a well-researched argument that proceeds logically from their initial discussion on the role of HRQOL in research outcomes and how this can be used to improve patient outcomes. They identify the lack of a conceptual model of how different types or levels of patient outcomes relate to each other and to overall HRQOL, and propose a model that considers five main factors and their relationship to each other in determining overall HRQOL. The systems-type model flows logically from the description of these factors to define causal relationships between the factors.
5. *Level of theory development.* HRQOL is sufficiently defined and narrow to be considered an explanatory middle range theory. The practical nature of the theory allows the researcher to develop testable hypotheses regarding HRQOL in different patient populations.

EXTERNAL CRITICISM

1. *Reality convergence.* The HRQOL theory immediately "makes sense" to the nurse. This theory provides a framework for better understanding the relationship of illness and nursing interventions to patients' quality of life.
2. *Utility.* The HRQOL model is useful for nurses in both research and practice. Nurses in any discipline can identify hypotheses that can be tested by using the HRQOL model.
3. *Significance.* HRQOL is highly significant to nursing research and practice. As patients live longer with chronic illness because of improved diagnostics and therapeutics, research into nursing interventions that improve HRQOL becomes even more significant.

4. *Discrimination.* Because HRQOL is a multidisciplinary concept, boundaries could extend beyond nursing practice. When HRQOL is used as a framework for nursing research, care must be taken to provide clear boundaries regarding nursing interventions.

5. *Scope.* This model is sufficiently narrow in scope that research can focus on individuals as well as groups. However, studies could be designed that allow a broader scope, if desired.

6. *Complexity.* The HRQOL model by Wilson and Cleary is quite complex, with five determinants, each having multiple variables. However, the model allows the researcher to identify specific variables for study. Control of extraneous variables is necessary in any research study, and the thorough explanation of variables in the model would facilitate identification and control of those considered extraneous.

REFERENCE

Wilson, I. B., & Cleary, P. D. (1995). Linking clinical variables with health-related quality of life: A conceptual model of patient outcomes. *Journal of the American Medical Association, 273*(1), 59–65.

About the Author
Lynne Ploetz, RN, BS, is President and CEO of Matrix Advocare Network, Minneapolis. She is a nurse entrepreneur who works to improve her patients' health-related quality of life through innovative nursing practice. Ms. Ploetz is certified in gerontological nursing by the American Nurses Credentialing Center and is a certified case manager through the Commission for Case Management Certification. Several years ago, she started a geriatric case management company, Matrix AdvoCare Network. Today she employs 20 registered nurses, care consultants throughout Minnesota, who provide health advocacy and care consulting services to frail elderly and people with mental and physical disabilities.

Chapter 14 Analysis of Theory: Health Promotion

■ **MADELEINE J. KERR**

INTERNAL CRITICISM

1. *Adequacy.* The model broadly describes several factors that have relationships to health-promoting behavior. In comparison to some other models, the Pender Health Promotion Model is broader, in that the model includes a number of intrapersonal factors (such as perceived barriers to the behavior), interpersonal factors (such as social norms), and situational influences (such as availability of healthful options). A possible gap is the model's focus on individual health promotion. The model has implications for the health promotion of families and communities; however, use of multiple models would be ideal to address these populations. Tests of the initial Health Promotion Model in 38 studies have accounted for considerable variance in health-promoting lifestyle and several specific behaviors, such as exercise. The revised Health Promotion Model needs to be tested empirically.

2. *Clarity.* The phenomenon that the model seeks to explain is health-promoting behavior. This phenomenon has multiple definitions, but Pender's definition carefully circumscribes the limits of this phenomenon. Some readers may struggle with the concept, particularly in light of the traditional medical model with which so many nurses are familiar. While Pender offers that one major distinguishing feature between health promotion and health protection is motivation for the behavior, these may not be easily distinguished in practice. For instance, a client may engage in exercise for the dual benefits of increasing energy and avoiding cardiovascular disease and obesity. It is not clear how these dual motivations may affect the model.

Pender's model is presented in a language and style that is easily understood by nurses and other health professionals. A schematic illustrates relationships between concepts. She provides clear definitions of terms. Relationship statements are established in Pender, Murdaugh, and Parson's (2002) *Health Promotion in Nursing Practice* (4th ed.).

3. *Consistency.* Model terminology in definitions corresponds with use in relationship statements and throughout the description of the theory.

4. *Logical development.* The revised model includes clearly established assumptions, concepts, and relationships. Each of these is clearly labeled and presented to the reader.

The theoretical foundations of the model are attributed to several well-established theories of behavior. These theories include Feather's Expectancy Value Theory and Bandura's Social Cognitive Theory. Concepts that did not receive empirical support in the initial Health Promotion Model were dropped in the revised model. The rationale for each of the model revisions is explained, and detailed results of previous model-testing empirical studies are clearly presented in *Health Promotion in Nursing Practice* (4th ed.).

5. *Level of theory development.* The model represents a middle range theory in that it addresses a specific phenomenon. It is intended for use in providing health promotion services to clients.

EXTERNAL CRITICISM

1. *Reality convergence.* Pender's model describes phenomena of interest to nurses, and includes a variety of factors that are well known to experienced health professionals, such as client perceptions of barriers and benefits. The theory has been supported in a number of model-testing studies.

2. *Utility.* The theory can be operationalized to provide interventions in real-life settings. For example, Lusk, Kerr, Ronis, and Eakin (1999) used the Pender Health Promotion Model to identify factors influencing workers' use of hearing protection. This information was subsequently used to develop an educational intervention that increased this health behavior 20% from baseline. The model also is potentially useful for individually tailoring behavior change interventions to individuals with interactive computer communications.

Research shows the model to be useful for explaining and predicting client behavior in several important areas, including exercise and nutrition. The model has only recently begun to be used in the design of interventions, but may prove useful in guiding nurses to design cost-effective strategies to improve client health. The model provides a "framework for understanding the dimensions on which health promotion interventions can be based" (Pender et al., 2002, p. 75). However, the model does not guide the nurse using the framework in methods to develop interventions.

3. *Significance.* Health promotion as a phenomenon has enormous potential for the discipline of nursing. A change in focus from disease prevention to health promotion expands the role of

nursing in society, and has potential for greatly enhancing the well-being of society. Investment in diagnosis and treatment of disease has been the dominant model of health care until recently. However, the limitations of this model are now recognized more than ever, while the role of health behavior as a determinant of health is growing in recognition. The economic and nontangible advantages of investing in health promotion are gaining popularity in business and government. Because health behavior is a large and growing concern, having far-reaching consequences for the health and prosperity of society, the Health Promotion Model has great potential significance.

4. *Discrimination.* The Pender Health Promotion Model is unique within nursing, although it does bear some resemblance to theories of health behavior in the social and psychological sciences. However, its unique approach-oriented nature distinguishes it from other theories of health behavior that have an avoidance orientation. The model provides a framework for discriminating which concepts are relevant to specific health behaviors. Much work remains to be done to determine how the model can be applied to different behaviors, and in various cultural, developmental, and gender-based populations. The model focuses more on health promotion for individuals than on families, communities, and society.

5. *Scope.* The espoused scope of the theory is health-promoting behavior. Health-promoting behavior is directed toward increasing the level of well-being and self-actualization of a given individual or group (Pender et al., 2002, p. 34). Examples of health-promoting behavior provided by the authors include physical activity, nutrition, stress management, and social support. This range of behaviors is appropriate to middle range theory. However, the authors also describe the application of the model to health behavior beyond the scope of health promotion (e.g., use of hearing protection and environmental tobacco-smoke exposure). The success of the model in describing and explaining these client behaviors suggests that the model may have a scope of application beyond its original intent.

6. *Complexity.* The Pender Health Promotion Model uses relatively few (11, to be exact) concepts to address the complex phenomenon of health-promoting behavior. Relationships between even this small number of concepts are potentially large, however, because a single factor may have multiple relationships to other factors within the model. The authors seem to have achieved a balance between thoroughness and parsimony.

REFERENCES

Lusk, S., Kerr, M., Ronis, D., & Eakin, B. (1999). Applying the health promotion model to development of a worksite intervention. *American Journal of Health Promotion, 13*(4), 219–226.

Pender, N., Murdaugh, C., & Parsons, M. (2002). *Health promotion in nursing practice* (4th ed.). Upper Saddle River, NJ: Prentice Hall.

About the Author

Madeleine J. Kerr, PhD, RN, is Associate Professor in Public Health Nursing at the University of Minnesota School of Nursing, Minneapolis. She applied Pender's Health Promotion Model to the study of construction workers' hearing health behavior, and to the design of computer-based tailored educational interventions to promote use of hearing protection devices. She has also conducted one of the first cross-cultural tests of the Health Promotion Model with Mexican-American workers.

Chapter 15 Analysis of Theory: Deliberative Nursing Process

■ **MIMI DYE**

INTERNAL CRITICISM

1. *Clarity.* The theory demonstrates clarity in its specific definition of easily understood terms, and in its specific use of those terms as they are involved in the flow of communication and activities inherent in the Deliberative Nursing Process.
2. *Consistency.* The theory demonstrates consistency because the definition, use of terms, and formulation remain the same throughout.
3. *Adequacy.* The theory demonstrates adequacy because its scope includes any professional communication relevant to meeting patient needs at any level within and throughout the health care system. Implicit in the theory is that the nurse will validate the needs of a patient who is mute, cognitively impaired, or cognitively compromised, by means other than direct verbal communication, such as observations by the nurse or information provided by significant others.
4. *Logical development.* The theory demonstrates logical development from its premises to its product or outcome because the flow of ingredients explicitly used in the Deliberative Nursing Process reasonably leads one to the product or outcome, that is, improvement in the patient's immediate behavior.
5. *Level of theory development.* Because this theory is a situation-producing or prescriptive theory, it is Level IV theory. For instance, the nurse's greater understanding of the patient's need for help results in alleviating the patient's distress more effectively.

EXTERNAL CRITICISM

1. *Reality convergence.* The theory begins with the premise that the patients may have needs that they may not be able to express or meet without professional nursing assistance. Therefore, it is the responsibility of nurses to explore with patients whether or not they have such needs, and whether or not their nursing activities meet those needs. This theory includes using the Deliberative Nursing Process in any communication relevant to patient needs anywhere in the health care system. Essentially, it involves the patient as a crucial member of this communication system. Meeting patient needs with patients is widely accepted in nursing.
2. *Utility.* Since the theory offers the Deliberative Nursing Process as an explicit way to keep communication clear and has as its purpose ascertaining and meeting patient needs, it is useful to the administrator as well as to the practitioner. It is useful to the educator because it can be taught and practiced within the educational system. It is useful to the researcher because its variables lend themselves to research. The theory, therefore, has a high degree of utility for the nursing profession.
3. *Significance.* Since the theory focuses on nurse–patient communications and communications within the health care system relevant to meeting patients' health care needs, specifically, responding to

and relieving patients' immediate distress, the theory addresses the essential core issue in nursing—responding to and meeting patients' needs that cannot be met without professional nursing assistance. The theory contributes to nursing knowledge by offering the Deliberative Nursing Process, designed to ascertain and meet patients' needs and relieve patients' immediate distress. The theory can be taught. Its variables lend themselves to research. Therefore, the theory has immense significance for the nursing profession.

4. *Discrimination.* The theory constructs a system of nursing practice for nurses to fulfill a distinct professional function wherever they practice. The theory is inclusive for nurses in administration, education, and clinical practice in all specialties. The unique professional nursing function is to ascertain and meet patients' immediate needs for help when patients are unable to do so without professional nursing assistance. The product or outcome of this function is to relieve patients' distress. Therefore, this theory differentiates nursing from health professions.

5. *Scope of theory.* The scope of the theory is broadly applicable because it includes nursing communications relevant to meeting patients' health care needs in all specialties, wherever and however nurses are practicing, whether in administration, education, practice, or research.

6. *Complexity.* The theory offers a balance between parsimony and complexity. It is parsimonious in that its elements are few and include only those needed to describe and explain the theory. It is complex because communication between and among people can be complex and the dynamics of relationships including nurse–patient relationships can be complex.

About the Author
Mimi Dye, MSN, ARNP, is a former student and longtime friend of Ms. Orlando. She has recently served as a consultant to the New Hampshire Hospital Orlando Project.

Chapter 16 Analysis of Theory: Resilience

■ MARSHA L. ELLETT

INTERNAL CRITICISM

1. *Clarity.* According to the Adolescent Resilience Model (ARM), resilience may occur as a result of a process that includes deriving meaning from an adverse experience through interaction with others. The ARM is parsimonious, given the widespread agreement among researchers that resilience is a complex, multidimensional construct. The concepts of the model are named but are not explicitly defined. They are operationalized clearly by instruments derived from decision trees for the qualitative work. Three classes of protective factors—individual, family, and social—are hypothesized to positively affect resilience outcomes. The individual protective factors include courageous or positive coping and derived meaning. The familial protective factors include family atmosphere and support/resources available to the family. The social protective resources include health care resources and social integration. Two classes of factors are hypothesized to negatively

affect resilience: individual risk factor and illness-related stress factors. The individual risk factor is sustained defensive coping, and the illness-related stress factors include illness perspective and illness distress. The outcome factors of resilience include self-esteem, mastery/confidence, and self-transcendence, as well as quality of life, defined as a sense of well-being.

2. *Consistency.* There is consistency between the text and the model (Figure 16.2) in the social and family protective factors. However, the illness-related stress factors, including illness perspective and illness distress, in the text are referred to as symptom-related risk in the model and include illness perception, symptom distress, and severity of illness. This inconsistency in wording between the text and the model is somewhat confusing. Also, the only outcome variable depicted in the model is quality of life, so the relationships of self-esteem, mastery/confidence, and self-transcendence to quality of life are unclear.

3. *Adequacy.* A strength of the ARM is that it is an emerging model grounded in contextual experiences. It appears that defensive coping is an individual risk factor only if it is sustained. Progression to courageous coping can occur, which is positively related to resilience. Further refinement of the concepts will occur with continued use of the model.

4. *Logical development.* The ARM was developed first through qualitative studies that allowed the identification and clarification of concepts to be included in the model. Next, quantitative structural equation modeling was used to identify relationships among concepts. Then, qualitative methods were again used to evaluate these identified relationships.

5. *Level of theory development.* The ARM is only beginning to be used to guide nursing interventions; therefore, it is an emerging middle range theory.

EXTERNAL CRITICISM

1. *Reality convergence.* The assumptions underlying the ARM were not specifically stated as such; however, one assumption may be that persons with resilience require time to reflect on the meaning of their actions. Thus, Haase and colleagues state that resilience may occur through a process that includes deriving meaning from the experience through interaction with others. The ARM appears to reflect the real world of nursing and makes inherent sense to this reader. This model's ability to guide interventions is just beginning to be tested. The one described study testing the ARM aims to test the efficacy of a therapeutic music video intervention for adolescents and young adults during the acute phase of stem cell transplant. This indicates that the model has the potential to be useful in real-life settings.

2. *Utility.* The researchers state that several studies are currently being developed using the ARM, but only the study mentioned was described. In this study, the ARM was being used to generate hypotheses.

3. *Significance.* Any model that can guide nursing interventions to enhance resilience outcomes in adolescents and young adults faced with cancer would be highly significant.

4. *Discrimination.* Whether the ARM will guide hypothesis generation that could not be generated by other models of resilience is not known presently. At this time, the boundaries of resilience are inconsistent.

5. *Scope.* The scope of the ARM currently is narrow in that it is being studied in chronically ill adolescents, mostly those with cancer, and is being tested in practice. If the initial intervention research is successful, this reader can see expanding the scope of this model slightly to include

adolescents with other serious chronic illnesses and then, later, to chronically ill participants in different age groups facing different developmental tasks. The ARM has the potential to become more global in time with continued refinement.

6. *Complexity*. Given that resilience is a complex, multidimensional construct, the ARM is parsimonious, with few concepts that can be fairly easily understood without lengthy descriptions or explanations.

REFERENCE

Haase, J. E., Heiney, S. P., Ruccione, K. S., & Stutzer, C. (1999). Research triangulation to derive meaning/based quality of life theory: Adolescent resilience model and instrument development. *International Journal of Cancer Supplement, 12*, 125–131.

About the Author
Marsha Ellett, DNS, RN, is an Associate Professor at Indiana University School of Nursing, Indianapolis, and a pediatric clinical nurse specialist. She teaches pediatrics in both the baccalaureate and master's programs (Pediatric Clinical Nurse Specialist Program). Her research has focused on enteral tube placement in children and colic in infants. It is through her association with her colleague, Joan Haase, that she became familiar with the Adolescence Resilience Model. She identifies the model's utility to the practice of her specialty, in work with young people with chronic illnesses, such as Crohn's disease, ulcerative colitis, and chronic aggressive hepatitis.

Instruments

Burke/Eakes Chronic Sorrow Assessment Tool[©]

The questions below are asked about the effects that certain life events or situations may have on people over a period of time so that helping professionals can better meet their needs. In answering these questions, please focus on the impact that these life events or situations continue to have on your life. There are no right or wrong answers. You do not have to answer any or all of the questions and can stop without penalty of any kind. Thank you for taking the time to answer these questions.

DEMOGRAPHICS/BACKGROUND

1. Which of the following best describes your situation? (Please check only one)

   a) _____ Parent of disabled child (please specify the disability) _____

   b) _____ Person with a chronic condition (please specify the condition) _____

   c) _____ Caregiver of someone with a chronic or life-threatening illness (please specify the condition) _____

   d) _____ Bereaved person (please specify the relationship of deceased to you) _____

2. I have been dealing with this situation/loss for _____ years. (Please write in number of years)

3. Please provide the following information about yourself:

   a) Sex: _____ male _____ female

   b) Age: _____ years

   c) Marital status: _____ single _____ married _____ widowed _____ divorced
      _____ separated

© 2003 Eakes, G. G. & Burke, M. L.

3. (continued)

d) Religion: _____ Protestant _____ Catholic _____ Jewish

Other (please write in): _____

e) Ethnic origin: _____ Caucasian _____ Hispanic _____ African American

_____ American Indian _____ Asian

Other (please write in): _____

f) Please indicate your highest completed level of education:

a. Less than high school

b. High school graduate

c. Associate/technical degree

d. Bachelor's degree

e. Master's degree

f. PhD/MD or equivalent

g) Total family income per year from all sources before taxes:

a. Below $5,000

b. $5,001–10,000

c. $10,001–15,000

d. $15,001–20,000

e. $20,001–25,000

f. $25,001–30,000

g. $30,001–40,000

h. Over $40,000

DISPARITY

4. Even though some time may have passed since you began dealing with your situation/loss, you may still be coping with some ongoing issues and reactions. Please read the following statements and indicate if this is true for you. Remember, there are no right or wrong answers.

   a) I recognize the hole this situation/loss has created in my life.   ❏ True   ❏ False

   b) I think about the difference this situation/loss has made in my life.   ❏ True   ❏ False

   c) I experience changes in my life as a result of the situation/loss.   ❏ True   ❏ False

   d) I feel its effects in bits and pieces.   ❏ True   ❏ False

GRIEF-RELATED FEELINGS

The following are feelings you may have experienced as a result of your situation/loss.

5. At those times when you experience these feelings associated with your situation/loss, please indicate how upsetting they are for you. Remember, there are no right or wrong answers.

	Have Not Experienced	Have Experienced But Not Upsetting	Have Experienced, Somewhat Upsetting	Have Experienced, Very Upsetting
a) sad				
b) anxious				
c) angry				
d) overwhelmed				
e) heartbroken				
f) other (please specify):				

CHARACTERISTICS OF CHRONIC SORROW (PERVASIVE, PERMANENT, PERIODIC, POTENTIALLY PROGRESSIVE)

The questions below ask more about the feelings you may experience related to your situation/loss. Please mark the extent to which each statement below is true for you.

6. In describing my feelings about my situation/loss, I:

   a) have ups and downs. ❏ True ❏ False

   b) feel their effects on other parts of my life. ❏ True ❏ False

   c) feel them more strongly now than at first. ❏ True ❏ False

   d) believe they will impact me the rest of my life. ❏ True ❏ False

TRIGGERS

There may be certain times when you tend to experience the feelings associated with your situation/loss. Please read the following statements and indicate which are true for you.

7. These feelings about my situation/loss come up when I:

   a) have to seek medical care. ❏ True ❏ False

   b) realize all the responsibilities I have. ❏ True ❏ False

   c) compare where I am now with where others are in their lives. ❏ True ❏ False

   d) think of all I now have to do. ❏ True ❏ False

   e) meet someone else in the same situation. ❏ True ❏ False

   f) experience the anniversary of when this began. ❏ True ❏ False

   g) have a "special day" such as a birthday or holiday. ❏ True ❏ False

   h) other (please specify): _____

INTERNAL COPING MECHANISMS

The statements below are things you may have found helpful to you in managing the feelings associated with your situation/loss. Please indicate which is true for you.

8. It helps me deal with my feelings when I:

	Never Tried	Have Tried, But Not Helpful	Have Tried, Somewhat Helpful	Have Tried, Very Helpful
a) keep busy				
b) take one day at a time				
c) talk to someone close to me				
d) pray				
e) exercise				
f) count my blessings				
g) work on my hobbies				
h) express my feelings				
i) go to church, synagogue, or other place of worship				
j) talk with others in similar situations				
k) take a "can do" attitude				
l) talk with a minister, rabbi, or priest				
m) talk with a health professional				
n) focus on the positive				

o) other (please specify): _____

EXTERNAL COPING MECHANISMS

The following questions are to find out how helping professionals can assist people who are dealing with situations/losses such as yours. Please indicate which is true for you. Remember, there are no right or wrong answers.

9. It helps me deal with my feelings when helping professionals:

	Never Tried	Have Tried, But Not Helpful	Have Tried, Somewhat Helpful	Have Tried, Very Helpful
a) listen to me				
b) recognize my feelings				
c) answer me honestly				
d) allow me to ask questions				
e) take their time with me				
f) provide good care				

g) other (please specify): _____

Friends and family may also be helpful to you as you deal with the feelings associated with your situation/loss. Please read the following and indicate which is true for you.

10. It helps me deal with my feelings when family and friends:

	Never Tried	Have Tried, But Not Helpful	Have Tried, Somewhat Helpful	Have Tried, Very Helpful
a) listen to me				
b) have a positive outlook				
c) accept my feelings				
d) provide emotional support				
e) offer a helping hand				
f) acknowledge my situation/loss				

g) other (please specify): _____

Thank you for answering these questions. Please return the questionnaire at this time.

General Comfort Questionnaire

Thank you VERY MUCH for helping me in my study of the concept COMFORT. Below are statements that may describe your comfort right now. Four numbers are provided for each question; please circle the number you think most closely matches what you are feeling. Relate these questions to your comfort *at the moment you are answering the questions.*

	Strongly Agree			Strongly Disagree
1. My body is relaxed right now	4	3	2	1
2. I feel useful because I'm working hard	4	3	2	1
3. I have enough privacy	4	3	2	1
4. There are those I can depend on when I need help	4	3	2	1
5. I don't want to exercise	4	3	2	1
6. My condition gets me down	4	3	2	1
7. I feel confident	4	3	2	1
8. I feel dependent on others	4	3	2	1
9. I feel my life is worthwhile right now	4	3	2	1
10. I am inspired by knowing that I am loved	4	3	2	1
11. These surroundings are pleasant	4	3	2	1
12. The sounds keep me from resting	4	3	2	1
13. No one understands me	4	3	2	1
14. My pain is difficult to endure	4	3	2	1
15. I am inspired to do my best	4	3	2	1
16. I am unhappy when I am alone	4	3	2	1
17. My faith helps me to not be afraid	4	3	2	1
18. I do not like it here	4	3	2	1
19. I am constipated right now	4	3	2	1
20. I do not feel healthy right now	4	3	2	1
21. This room makes me feel scared	4	3	2	1
22. I am afraid of what is next	4	3	2	1

	Strongly Agree			Strongly Disagree
23. I have a favorite person(s) who makes me feel cared for	4	3	2	1
24. I have experienced changes that make me feel uneasy	4	3	2	1
25. I am hungry	4	3	2	1
26. I would like to see my doctor more often	4	3	2	1
27. The temperature in this room is fine	4	3	2	1
28. I am very tired	4	3	2	1
29. I can rise above my pain	4	3	2	1
30. The mood around here uplifts me	4	3	2	1
31. I am content	4	3	2	1
32. This chair (bed) makes me hurt	4	3	2	1
33. This view inspires me	4	3	2	1
34. My personal belongings are not here	4	3	2	1
35. I feel out of place here	4	3	2	1
36. I feel good enough to walk	4	3	2	1
37. My friends remember me with their cards and phone calls	4	3	2	1
38. My beliefs give me peace of mind	4	3	2	1
39. I need to be better informed about my health	4	3	2	1
40. I feel out of control	4	3	2	1
41. I feel crummy because I am not dressed	4	3	2	1
42. This room smells terrible	4	3	2	1
43. I am alone but not lonely	4	3	2	1
44. I feel peaceful	4	3	2	1
45. I am depressed	4	3	2	1
46. I have found meaning in my life	4	3	2	1
47. It is easy to get around here	4	3	2	1
48. I need to feel good again	4	3	2	1

Available at www.uakron.edu/comfort. No permission needed.

Code # _____   Date _____   Time _____

Comfort Behaviors Checklist: How is patient acting right now?
Please circle best response. *NA* = not applicable

	NA	No	Somewhat	Moderate	Strong
Vocalizations					
1. complaining	0	1	2	3	4
2. awake	0	1	2	3	4
3. moaning	0	1	2	3	4
4. content sounds/talk	0	1	2	3	4
5. crying/shouting	0	1	2	3	4
Motor Signs					
6. peaceful	0	1	2	3	4
7. agitated	0	1	2	3	4
8. rapid pacing	0	1	2	3	4
9. fidgety	0	1	2	3	4
10. muscles relaxed	0	1	2	3	4
11. rubbing an area	0	1	2	3	4
12. guarding	0	1	2	3	4
Behaviors					
13. anxious	0	1	2	3	4
14. accepts kindness	0	1	2	3	4
15. likes touch/ hand holding	0	1	2	3	4
16. appears depressed	0	1	2	3	4
17. able to rest	0	1	2	3	4
18. able to eat	0	1	2	3	4
19. calm, at ease	0	1	2	3	4
20. purposeless movements	0	1	2	3	4

	NA	No	Somewhat	Moderate	Strong
Facial					
21. grimaces/winces	0	1	2	3	4
22. relaxed expression	0	1	2	3	4
23. wrinkled brow	0	1	2	3	4
24. appears frightened or worried	0	1	2	3	4
25. smiles	0	1	2	3	4
Miscellaneous					
26. unusual breathing	0	1	2	3	4
27. focuses mentally	0	1	2	3	4
28. converses	0	1	2	3	4
29. awakens smoothly	0	1	2	3	4

If this is the *only* comfort/pain instrument being used, ask the patient:

30. Do you have any pain? No_____Yes _____ [Please rate your pain from 1 to 10, with 10 being the highest possible pain]. _____ (rating)

31. Taking everything into consideration, how comfortable are you right now? [Please rate your total comfort from 1 to 10, with 10 being the highest possible comfort.] _____ (rating)

Other open-ended comments

(change in medication use, recent injury, recent decline in functional status, staff reports of comfort/discomfort, changes in appetite, ambulation, etc.)

Adapted by K. Kolcaba from: Volicer, L. (1988). Management of advanced Alzheimer's dementia/The comfort checklist. In L. Volicer (Ed.), *Clinical management of Alzheimer's disease*. Rockville, MD: Aspen Publications.

Scoring of the Behaviors Checklist

1. *Subtract* number of "not applicable" (NA) from 29, to obtain **total answered.**

2. *Multiply* total answered (step 1) by 4, to obtain **total possible score.**

3. *Reverse code* numbers 1, 3, 5, 7, 8, 9, 11, 12, 13, 16, 20, 22, 23, and 25 to obtain **raw comfort responses.**

4. *Add* **raw comfort responses** (step 3) for all questions not marked NA, to obtain **actual comfort score.**

5. *Divide actual comfort score* (step 4) by *total possible score* (step 2) and round to two decimal places. (If the third decimal place is a 5 or greater, round the second decimal place up to the next number.)

6. Report score as a **2-digit number** (rounded percent without the % sign or decimal). *Higher scores* indicate *higher comfort.*

Comfort Behaviors Checklist © K. Kolcaba (2002).
Available at www.uakron.edu/comfort. No permission needed.

PAEDIATRIC ASTHMA QUALITY OF LIFE QUESTIONNAIRE WITH STANDARDISED ACTIVITIES (PAQLQ(S))

SELF-ADMINISTERED

© 1999

QOL TECHNOLOGIES LTD.

TM

For further information:

Elizabeth Juniper, MCSP, MSc
Professor
20 Marcuse Fields,
Bosham,
West Sussex,
PO18 8NA. UK
Tel: + 44 (0) 1243 572124
Fax: + 44 (0) 1243 573680
E-mail: juniper@qoltech.co.uk
Web: www.qoltech.co.uk

©   The PAQLQ(S) is copyrighted. It may not be altered, sold (paper or electronic), translated or adapted for another medium without the permission of Elizabeth Juniper.

PAEDIATRIC ASTHMA
QUALITY OF LIFE QUESTIONNAIRE (S)
SELF-ADMINISTERED

PATIENT ID _____

DATE _____

Page 1 of 5

Please complete **all** questions by circling the number that best describes how you have been during the **past week as a result of your asthma.**

HOW **BOTHERED** HAVE YOU BEEN DURING THE LAST WEEK DOING:

	Extremely Bothered	Very Bothered	Quite Bothered	Somewhat Bothered	Bothered a Bit	Hardly Bothered at All	Not Bothered
1. PHYSICAL ACTIVITIES (such as running, swimming, sports, walking uphill/ upstairs, and bicycling)?	1	2	3	4	5	6	7
2. BEING WITH ANIMALS (such as playing with pets and looking after animals)?	1	2	3	4	5	6	7
3. ACTIVITIES WITH FRIENDS AND FAMILY (such as playing at recess and doing things with your friends and family)?	1	2	3	4	5	6	7
4. COUGHING?	1	2	3	4	5	6	7

IN GENERAL, **HOW OFTEN** DURING THE LAST WEEK DID YOU:

	All of the Time	Most of the Time	Quite Often	Some of the Time	Once in a While	Hardly Any of the Time	None of the Time
5. Feel FRUSTRATED because of your asthma?	1	2	3	4	5	6	7

PAEDIATRIC ASTHMA
QUALITY OF LIFE QUESTIONNAIRE (S)
SELF-ADMINISTERED

PATIENT ID _____

DATE _____

	All of the Time	Most of the Time	Quite Often	Some of the Time	Once in a While	Hardly Any of the Time	None of the Time
6. Feel TIRED because of your asthma?	1	2	3	4	5	6	7
7. Feel WORRIED, CONCERNED, OR TROUBLED because of your asthma?	1	2	3	4	5	6	7

HOW **BOTHERED** HAVE YOU BEEN DURING THE LAST WEEK BY:

	Extremely Bothered	Very Bothered	Quite Bothered	Somewhat Bothered	Bothered a Bit	Hardly Bothered at All	Not Bothered
8. ASTHMA ATTACKS?	1	2	3	4	5	6	7

IN GENERAL, **HOW OFTEN** DURING THE LAST WEEK DID YOU:

	All of the Time	Most of the Time	Quite Often	Some of the Time	Once in a While	Hardly Any of the Time	None of the Time
9. Feel ANGRY because of your asthma?	1	2	3	4	5	6	7

HOW **BOTHERED** HAVE YOU BEEN DURING THE LAST WEEK BY:

	Extremely Bothered	Very Bothered	Quite Bothered	Somewhat Bothered	Bothered a Bit	Hardly Bothered at All	Not Bothered
10. WHEEZING?	1	2	3	4	5	6	7

IN GENERAL, HOW **OFTEN** DURING THE LAST WEEK DID YOU:

	All of the Time	Most of the Time	Quite Often	Some of the Time	Once in a While	Hardly Any of the Time	None of the Time
11. Feel IRRITABLE (cranky/grouchy) because of your asthma?	1	2	3	4	5	6	7

PAEDIATRIC ASTHMA
QUALITY OF LIFE QUESTIONNAIRE (S)
SELF-ADMINISTERED

PATIENT ID _____

DATE _____

HOW **BOTHERED** HAVE YOU BEEN DURING THE LAST WEEK BY:

	Extremely Bothered	Very Bothered	Quite Bothered	Somewhat Bothered	Bothered a Bit	Hardly Bothered at All	Not Bothered
12. TIGHTNESS IN YOUR CHEST?	1	2	3	4	5	6	7

IN GENERAL, **HOW OFTEN** DURING THE LAST WEEK DID YOU:

	All of the Time	Most of the Time	Quite Often	Some of the Time	Once in a While	Hardly Any of the Time	None of the Time
13. Feel DIFFERENT OR LEFT OUT because of your asthma?	1	2	3	4	5	6	7

HOW **BOTHERED** HAVE YOU BEEN DURING THE LAST WEEK BY:

	Extremely Bothered	Very Bothered	Quite Bothered	Somewhat Bothered	Bothered a Bit	Hardly Bothered at All	Not Bothered
14. SHORTNESS OF BREATH?	1	2	3	4	5	6	7

IN GENERAL, **HOW OFTEN** DURING THE LAST WEEK DID YOU:

	All of the Time	Most of the Time	Quite Often	Some of the Time	Once in a While	Hardly Any of the Time	None of the Time
15. Feel FRUSTRATED BECAUSE YOU COULDN'T KEEP UP WITH OTHERS?	1	2	3	4	5	6	7
16. WAKE UP DURING THE NIGHT because of your asthma?	1	2	3	4	5	6	7
17. Feel UNCOMFORTABLE because of your asthma?	1	2	3	4	5	6	7

PAEDIATRIC ASTHMA
QUALITY OF LIFE QUESTIONNAIRE (S)
SELF-ADMINISTERED

PATIENT ID _____

DATE _____

	All of the Time	Most of the Time	Quite Often	Some of the Time	Once in a While	Hardly Any of the Time	None of the Time
18. Feel OUT OF BREATH because of your asthma?	1	2	3	4	5	6	7
19. Feel you COULDN'T KEEP UP WITH OTHERS because of your asthma?	1	2	3	4	5	6	7

IN GENERAL, **HOW OFTEN** DURING THE LAST WEEK DID YOU:

	All of the Time	Most of the Time	Quite Often	Some of the Time	Once in a While	Hardly Any of the Time	None of the Time
20. Have trouble SLEEPING AT NIGHT because of your asthma?	1	2	3	4	5	6	7
21. Feel FRIGHTENED BY AN ASTHMA ATTACK?	1	2	3	4	5	6	7

THINK ABOUT ALL THE ACTIVITIES THAT YOU DID IN THE PAST WEEK:

	Extremely Bothered	Very Bothered	Quite Bothered	Somewhat Bothered	Bothered a Bit	Hardly Bothered at All	Not Bothered
22. How much were you bothered by your asthma during these activities?	1	2	3	4	5	6	7

PAEDIATRIC ASTHMA
QUALITY OF LIFE QUESTIONNAIRE (S)
SELF-ADMINISTERED

PATIENT ID _____

DATE _____

Page 5 of 5

IN GENERAL, **HOW OFTEN** DURING THE LAST WEEK DID YOU:

	All of the Time	Most of the Time	Quite Often	Some of the Time	Once in a While	Hardly Any of the Time	None of the Time
23. Have difficulty taking a DEEP BREATH?	1	2	3	4	5	6	7

DOMAIN CODE:

Symptoms: 4, 6, 8, 10, 12, 14, 16, 18, 20, 23
Activity Limitation: 1, 2, 3, 19, 22
Emotional Function: 5, 7, 9, 11, 13, 15, 17, 21

Index

Page numbers followed by "t" denote tables; those followed by "f" denote figures; and those followed by "b" denote boxes.

DRC0910